T-Cell Immunology

T-Cell Immunology

Edited by Josiah Robinson

STATES
ACADEMIC PRESS
www.statesacademicpress.com

States Academic Press,
109 South 5th Street,
Brooklyn, NY 11249, USA

Visit us on the World Wide Web at:
www.statesacademicpress.com

ISBN: 978-1-63989-508-3

Cataloging-in-Publication Data

T-cell immunology / edited by Josiah Robinson.
p. cm.
Includes bibliographical references and index.
ISBN 978-1-63989-508-3
1. T cells--Immunology. 2. T cells. 3. Immunology. I. Robinson, Josiah.
QR185.8.T2 T34 2022
616.079 7--dc23

Table of Contents

Preface

It is often said that books are a boon to mankind. They document every progress and pass on the knowledge from one generation to the other. They play a crucial role in our lives. Thus I was both excited and nervous while editing this book. I was pleased by the thought of being able to make a mark but I was also nervous to do it right because the future of students depends upon it. Hence, I took a few months to research further into the discipline, revise my knowledge and also explore some more aspects. Post this process, I begun with the editing of this book.

T-cells are a type of white blood cells that play an important role in the adaptive immune response. T-cell receptors are present on the surface of T-cells which distinguish them from the other cells. The T-cells are formed in the bone marrow from the hematopoietic stem cells. These are the stem cells that give rise to different types of blood cells. T-cells do not mature in the bone marrow. The developing cells migrate to thymus where they mature into several different types of T-cells. The differentiated subtypes of T-cells have a major role in controlling and shaping the immune response. This book is compiled in such a manner, that it will provide in-depth knowledge about the T-cells. It includes some of the vital pieces of work being conducted across the world, on various topics related to T-cells. This book serves as a valuable source of reference for graduate and post graduate students.

I thank my publisher with all my heart for considering me worthy of this unparalleled opportunity and for showing unwavering faith in my skills. I would also like to thank the editorial team who worked closely with me at every step and contributed immensely towards the successful completion of this book. Last but not the least, I wish to thank my friends and colleagues for their support.

Editor

1

Cellular-level versus receptor-level response threshold hierarchies in T-cell activation

Hugo A. van den Berg[1]*, Kristin Ladell[2], Kelly Miners[2], Bruno Laugel[2], Sian Llewellyn-Lacey[2], Mathew Clement[2], David K. Cole[2], Emma Gostick[2], Linda Wooldridge[2], Andrew K. Sewell[2], John S. Bridgeman[2] and David A. Price[2,3]

[1] *University of Warwick, Coventry, UK*
[2] *Institute of Infection and Immunity, Cardiff University, Cardiff, UK*
[3] *Vaccine Research Center, National Institute of Allergy and Infectious Diseases, National Institutes of Health, Bethesda, MD, USA*

Edited by:
Nick Gascoigne, Scripps Research Institute, USA

Reviewed by:
Nick Gascoigne, Scripps Research Institute, USA
Edward John Collins, The University of North Carolina at Chapel Hill, USA

***Correspondence:**
Hugo A. van den Berg, University of Warwick, Coventry CV4 7AL, UK
e-mail: hugo@maths.warwick.ac.uk

Peptide-MHC (pMHC) ligand engagement by T-cell receptors (TCRs) elicits a variety of cellular responses, some of which require substantially more TCR-mediated stimulation than others. This threshold hierarchy could reside at the receptor level, where different response pathways branch off at different stages of the TCR/CD3 triggering cascade, or at the cellular level, where the cumulative TCR signal registered by the T-cell is compared to different threshold values. Alternatively, dual-level thresholds could exist. In this study, we show that the cellular hypothesis provides the most parsimonious explanation consistent with data obtained from an in-depth analysis of distinct functional responses elicited in a clonal T-cell system by a spectrum of biophysically defined altered peptide ligands across a range of concentrations. Further, we derive a mathematical model that describes how ligand density, affinity, and off-rate all affect signaling in distinct ways. However, under the kinetic regime prevailing in the experiments reported here, the TCR/pMHC class I (pMHCI) dissociation rate was found to be the main governing factor. The CD8 coreceptor modulated the TCR/pMHCI interaction and altered peptide ligand potency. Collectively, these findings elucidate the relationship between TCR/pMHCI kinetics and cellular function, thereby providing an integrated mechanistic understanding of T-cell response profiles.

Keywords: T-cell activation, T-cell cross-reactivity, T-cell receptor

INTRODUCTION

T lymphocyte antigen receptors mediate adaptive immune responses via interactions with disease-associated peptide ligands presented on the surface of target cells by major histocompatibility complex (MHC) molecules. In the case of $CD8^+$ T-lymphocytes (CTLs), which constitute the classical T-cell effector subset, the clonotypically expressed T-cell receptors (TCRs) engage specific peptide-MHC class I (pMHCI) molecules to elicit several functions that are instrumental in eliminating the pathogenic threat (1).

The six hyper-variable complementarity-determining regions (CDRs) of the TCR govern molecular interactions with pMHCI (2). These CDRs confer the specificity of molecular recognition, allowing CTLs to attack diseased cells without causing undue harm to healthy cells (1). Nonetheless, a certain degree of degeneracy within the antigen recognition system is unavoidable (3). Indeed, ample experimental evidence supports the notion that a single TCR clonotype can interact productively with numerous peptide ligands, which typically vary in their ability to elicit different types of cellular response (4–14). Furthermore, some cellular responses are more readily evoked than others (15–18). It seems reasonable to explain this phenomenon by postulating a hierarchy of thresholds. Such a hierarchy may reside either at the level of individual TCR/CD3 complexes or at the cellular level. In the former scenario, the threshold parameters relate to distinct components of the TCR triggering process, with different responses being elicited at different stages in the development of a mature signalosome. Essentially, this is the kinetic discrimination model proposed by Rabinowitz et al. (19), whereby early responses require a shorter TCR/pMHCI dwell-time than late responses. This model is logically distinct from the kinetic proofreading model that accounts for the existence of dwell-time thresholds *per se* (20).

In the cellular-level scenario, TCR triggering delivers a stereotypical signal that elicits distinct responses across a single quantitative gradient (e.g., concentration of the relevant signaling factor). The contrast between these two scenarios is illustrated diagrammatically in **Figure 1**. A third possibility is that the hierarchy comprises a combination of both receptor-level and cellular-level modes. It has hitherto been unclear which of these three alternatives prevails in T-cell signaling.

In this study, we used a mathematical model to investigate the extent to which each of the three possibilities (receptor-level hierarchy, cellular-level hierarchy, or a combination of both) agree with experimental data. Our model accounts for the functional sensitivity of TCR-mediated responses to a given pMHCI ligand on the basis of TCR/pMHCI interaction kinetics. The concept that TCR/pMHCI kinetics governs functional sensitivity was pioneered by Lanzavecchia et al. (21) and subsequently formulated as a mathematical model (22, 23). Bridgeman et al. (24) recently summarized the available evidence across reported systems.

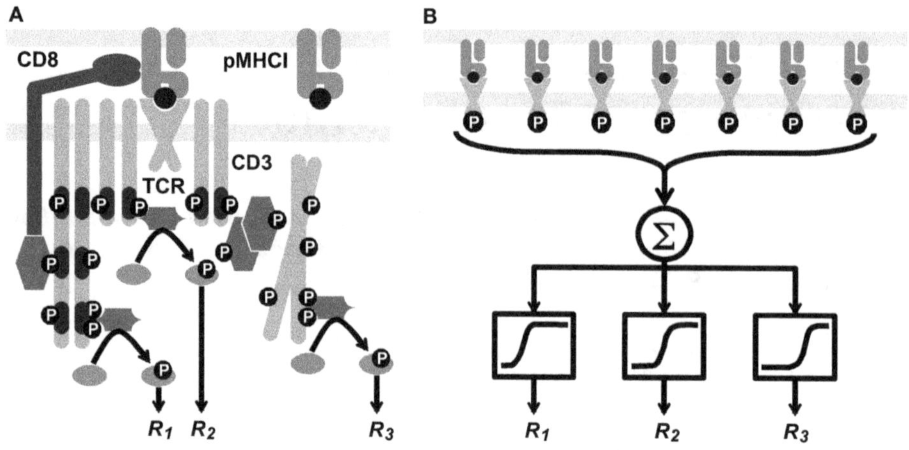

FIGURE 1 | Two hypotheses on the level of the response hierarchy. (A) Signaling cascades are initiated at different points along the TCR/CD3 reaction pathway, which includes phosphorylation events and the docking of kinases and linker proteins. Thus, responses R_1, R_2, and R_3 would correspond to distinct values of the TCR triggering threshold, i.e., $T_R^{[1]} < T_R^{[2]} < T_R^{[3]}$. **(B)** Cellular integration of signals from the triggered TCRs is shown as a summation (Σ) box. This signal passes through a non-linear threshold that determines whether the cell will respond. Here, R_1, R_2, and R_3 represent various cellular responses, such as the expression of different cytokine species. Each receives the same integrated signal W as an input, but different values of W are required to initiate a response. This is depicted schematically by sigmoid curves whose midpoint lies to the left, in the middle, or to the right. These differences correspond to distinct values of the cellular activation threshold, i.e., $W_{act}^{[1]} < W_{act}^{[2]} < W_{act}^{[3]}$. These two hypotheses are not mutually exclusive.

Analysis of TCR/pMHCI interaction kinetics demonstrates that functional sensitivity is not dependent on a single biophysical parameter, but rather on the interplay between association rate, dissociation rate, and ligand densities (23, 25, 26). Under the experimental conditions prevailing in the present study, however, the dissociation rate (the reciprocal of the mean dwell-time of the TCR/pMHCI interaction) emerged as the dominant biophysical parameter. Moreover, we estimated the extent to which the CD8 coreceptor modulates this parameter using data from parallel experiments conducted in the absence of an extracellular MHCI/CD8 interaction.

Five distinct cellular responses were investigated: (i) mobilization of the degranulation marker CD107a; (ii) secretion of macrophage inflammatory protein 1-β (MIP-1β); (iii) secretion of tumor necrosis factor-α (TNF-α); (iv) secretion of interleukin-2 (IL-2); and (v) secretion of interferon-γ (IFN-γ). Measured simultaneously and independently by flow cytometry, the magnitude of each response was quantified as a function of fluorescence and plotted against peptide concentration. The resulting dose-response curves indicated that the five cellular responses were elicited by pMHCI stimulation according to a pronounced hierarchy. Analysis of these curves by means of the mathematical model, in conjunction with biophysical data, indicated that the cellular-level response threshold hierarchy hypothesis provides the most parsimonious explanation.

MATERIALS AND METHODS

EXPERIMENTAL PROCEDURES

Cells and peptide ligands

The CTL clone ILA1 recognizes residues 540–548 (ILAKFLHWL in single-letter amino acid code, abbreviated as ILA) of the human telomerase reverse transcriptase protein presented in the context of the human MHCI allotype HLA-A*0201 (HLA-A2). Cell culture was performed as described previously (27). The altered peptide ligands used in this study are referred to here as 3G, 5Y, 8T, 8E, and 3G8T; these ligands were largely characterized previously (27, 28), and display equivalent binding to HLA-A2 (29).

Bioassay

Stable C1R transfectants expressing wild-type HLA-A2 (C1R-A2) or CD8-null HLA-A2 (C1R-A2null), the α3 domain of which contains the double mutation D227K/T228A that abrogates CD8 binding (30), were pulsed with peptide as indicated for 1 h at 37°C. For each condition, assays were set up simultaneously in 96-well plates using 4.5×10^5 C1R cells per well, thereby ensuring that all cellular parameters were consistent across ligand stimulations. Subsequently, brefeldin A (10 μg/ml; BD Biosciences) and monensin (0.7 μl/ml; BD Biosciences) were added together with a pre-titred concentration of the directly conjugated monoclonal antibody (mAb) αCD107a-FITC [BD Pharmingen; Ref. (31)]. Serum-starved CTLs, incubated in Roswell Park Memorial Institute (RPMI) medium (Life Technologies) containing 2% fetal calf serum (FCS) for 16 h prior to assay, were subsequently added at 9×10^5 cells per well. After incubation for 6 h, which generally allows sufficient time for even the most sluggish response to appear, cells were washed in phosphate-buffered saline (PBS) containing 1% FCS and incubated for 10 min at room temperature with Aqua fixable live/dead cell stain (Life Technologies) to enable the exclusion of dead cells from the analysis. Pre-titred concentrations of αCD3-H7allophycocyanin (BD Biosciences), αCD8-QD705 (Life Technologies), and αCD19-V500 (BD Horizon) were then added for 20 min at 4°C. After two further washes in PBS/1% FCS, cells were fixed/permeabilized using a Cytofix/Cytoperm™ kit (BD Biosciences) according to the manufacturer's instructions, then stained intracellularly with pre-titred concentrations of

αMIP-1β-PE (BD Pharmingen), αIFNγ-V450 (BD Horizon), αIL-2-allophycocyanin (BD Pharmingen), and αTNFα-PECy7 (BD Pharmingen) for 20 min at 4°C.

Flow cytometry

Stained cell samples were acquired and recorded using a customized FACS Aria II flow cytometer (BD Biosciences) equipped for the simultaneous detection of 18 fluorescent parameters. Polychromatic analyses were conducted using FlowJo software version 9.5.2 (TreeStar Inc.). The following gating tree was applied: (i) single cells were identified based on their light scatter properties; (ii) Boolean gating was carried out to exclude artifacts and fluorochrome aggregates; (iii) viable $CD3^{+}CD19^{-}$ events were selected; (iv) outliers were eliminated in a side-scatter versus CD3 display; and (v) gates were set on cells positive for individual functional read-outs. The frequencies and median fluorescence intensity (MFI) values of each functional response were exported for data analysis to *Excel* and onward for simultaneous curve fitting in *Mathematica.*

Surface plasmon resonance

Soluble TCR, derived from the ILA1 CTL clone, was manufactured as described previously (32, 33). Binding analysis by surface plasmon resonance (SPR) was performed using a BIAcore T100™ equipped with a CM5 sensor chip (34). Biotinylated pMHCI (200–400 response units) was immobilized to streptavidin, which was chemically linked to the chip surface. The pMHCI was injected at a slow flow rate (10 μl/min) to ensure uniform distribution on the chip surface. Combined with the small amount of pMHCI bound to the chip surface, this reduced the likelihood of dissociation rate limiting mass transfer effects. The ILA1 TCR was purified and concentrated to $\sim$100 μM on the day of SPR analysis to reduce the likelihood of TCR aggregation affecting the results. At least 5 serial dilutions were prepared in duplicate and injected over the relevant sensor chips at a flow rate of 45 μl/min. All experiments were conducted at 25°C. Results were analyzed using *BIAevaluation, Excel,* and *Origin.*

THEORY AND DATA ANALYSIS

Assumptions

The assumptions of the TCR triggering model are as follows: (i) TCRs on the T-cell surface become "triggered" (i.e., are induced to become signalosomes) during an interaction with a pMHCI ligand; and (ii) the T-cell accumulates the signals emanating from triggered TCRs over space (cell:cell interface) and time (duration of cell:cell interaction), proceeding with a response when this signal exceeds a cellular activation threshold. The mathematical formulation of these assumptions is based on the kinetics of the TCR/pMHCI interaction.

The TCR triggering rate equation

The model describes the kinetics of interactions between TCR and pMHCI molecules in the interface area between a T-cell and an antigen-presenting cell (APC). This area is occupied by TCRs on the T-cell side of the interaction and by pMHCI complexes on the APC side. Let R_T be the total number of TCRs and Z_T be the total number of pMHCI molecules. Both are subject to a conservation law:

$$R_T = C + R \tag{1}$$

$$Z_T = C + Z \tag{2}$$

where C is the number of TCR/pMHCI complexes, R is the number of TCRs not engaged in a complex (i.e., "free" TCR molecules) and Z is the number of free pMHCI molecules. Kinetic equilibrium is expressed by the law of mass action equation:

$$k_{\text{on}} RZ = k_{\text{off}} C. \tag{3}$$

This equation, together with equations (1) and (2), leads to a quadratic in C with solution

$$C = \frac{R_T + Z_T + k_{\text{off}}/k_{\text{on}}}{2}\left(1 - \sqrt{1 - \frac{4R_T Z_T}{R_T + Z_T + k_{\text{off}}/k_{\text{on}}}}\right) \tag{4}$$

(the other root is irrelevant since it exceeds both R_T and Z_T). The rate at which TCRs are being triggered can be expressed as the rate at which TCR/pMHCI complexes dissociate times the probability that any given TCR/pMHCI association event results in a triggering of the associated TCR/CD3 complex:

$$W = k_{\text{off}}\; C\; P_{\text{trig}} \tag{5}$$

where W denotes the TCR triggering rate and P_{trig} the triggering probability for an individual interaction event. Since triggering of a TCR/CD3 complex requires completion of a series of phosphorylation and docking events, it is reasonable to assume that triggering can only happen if the peptide ligand remains engaged for at least a certain amount of time. This minimum duration is the *TCR triggering threshold* T_R. If the lifetime of the TCR/pMHCI complex is exponentially distributed, the triggering probability is given by:

$$P_{\text{trig}} = \exp\{-k_{\text{off}} T_R\}. \tag{6}$$

Combined, equations (4–6) yield the general triggering rate equation:

$$W = \frac{k_{\text{off}} \exp\{-k_{\text{off}} T_R\}}{2}\,(R_T + Z_T + k_{\text{off}}/k_{\text{on}}) \times \left(1 - \sqrt{1 - \frac{4R_T Z_T}{R_T + Z_T + k_{\text{off}}/k_{\text{on}}}}\right). \tag{7}$$

Simple forms in special cases [equations (13–15)] are obtained by using the first-order approximation to the square root in equation (7).

Connecting the theoretical model to experimental observations

The available data comprise cellular response measurements (read-outs) of T-cell activation following exposure to APCs incubated with various peptide ligands across a range of concentrations, as well as TCR/pMHCI association and dissociation rates for each peptide ligand, measured via SPR. To relate these measurements to the TCR triggering theory, a number of auxiliary assumptions are required. In particular, if Y is the peptide incubation concentration, the following proportionality is assumed:

$$Z_T = \alpha Y. \quad (8)$$

If K_D is the dissociation constant determined via SPR, the following proportionality is assumed:

$$\frac{k_{\text{off}}}{k_{\text{on}}} = \kappa K_D. \quad (9)$$

The proportionality constant κ is required to convert rates as measured via SPR to the 2-dimensional environment of the cell:cell interaction area. To connect the model to data, two compound parameters are introduced: $\zeta = \alpha/\kappa$ (dimensionless), and $\rho = R_T/\kappa$ (M). With these parameters, the TCR triggering rate $w = W/\kappa$ (in M·s^{-1}) assumes a simpler form:

$$w = \frac{k_{\text{off}} \exp\{-k_{\text{off}} T_R\}}{2} (\rho + \zeta Y + K_D) \times \left(1 - \sqrt{1 - \frac{4\rho\zeta Y}{\rho + \zeta Y + K_D}}\right). \quad (10)$$

The read-out in the present study is median fluorescence intensity (MFI), which is a valid measure of activation in view of its good correlation with the fraction of responding cells. Accordingly, the read-out U is assumed to be proportional to the fraction of responding cells. This assumption is validated by response data at the level of individual cells (see Results below). The equation for the read-out is as follows:

$$U = U_{\min} + (U_{\max} - U_{\min})\,\mathbb{P}(\text{respond}) \quad (11)$$

where $U_{\min}$ and $U_{\max}$ are nuisance parameters associated with the read-out procedure; these parameters take specific values for each type of cellular response and are assumed not to vary across peptide ligands. The probability that a T-cell responds is modeled as follows:

$$\mathbb{P}(\text{respond}) = \mathbb{P}(w_{\text{act}} \le w) \quad (12)$$

where w is the scaled TCR triggering rate given by equation (10) and w_{act} is the *cellular activation threshold.* This latter quantity is assumed to have a log-normal distribution over the population of T-cells in the experiment. Stochastic variation between the T-cells within the responding population is thus taken into account. The parameters are estimated by simultaneous least-squares fitting over the set of available ligands and read-outs. The median of the log-normal distribution provides the estimate of w_{act}.

Implementation of response hierarchy hypotheses

We examined five different cellular responses and compared three hypotheses: (i) for each type of cellular response, both T_R and w_{act} have distinct values; (ii) there is a common value of T_R across responses, whereas w_{act} has a different value for each response; and (iii) there is a common value of w_{act} across responses, whereas T_R has a different value for each response. As the least-squares fit is carried out simultaneously, these hypotheses can be implemented by specifying either common or particular values for these parameters.

RESULTS

KINETIC PARAMETERS AND LIGAND NUMBERS INTERACT TO DETERMINE THE RATE OF TCR TRIGGERING

The triggering equation (7) reduces to various simplified forms, depending on which receptors are kinetically limiting. These forms are of immunological interest since they illuminate the controversy over which kinetic parameter primarily governs T-cell activation. First, if the term $k_{\text{off}}/k_{\text{on}}$ is much larger than both R_T and Z_T, which applies when both cells have introduced comparatively low numbers of ligands into the interaction area, the following approximation is accurate:

$$W = R_T Z_T k_{\text{on}} \exp\{-k_{\text{off}} T_R\} \quad (k_{\text{off}}/k_{\text{on}} \gg \max\{R_T, Z_T\}), \quad (13)$$

that is, the triggering rate will be proportional to both TCR and pMHCI numbers: signaling is *affinity-limited.*

On the other hand, if the cells express numbers of ligands in the interaction area that are much larger than the 2-dimensional dissociation constant $k_{\text{off}}/k_{\text{on}}$, there are two further good approximations:

$$W = R_T k_{\text{off}} \exp\{-k_{\text{off}} T_R\} \quad (k_{\text{off}}/k_{\text{on}} \ll Z_T) \quad (14)$$
$$W = Z_T k_{\text{off}} \exp\{-k_{\text{off}} T_R\} \quad (k_{\text{off}}/k_{\text{on}} \ll R_T); \quad (15)$$

in the first case, signaling is *TCR-limited* and in the second, it is *MHC-limited.* These equations imply that under the receptor-limited regimes, the TCR triggering rate displays an optimum relative to k_{off} at the point $k_{\text{off}} = T_R^{-1}$, whereas under the affinity-limited regime, W increases monotonically in k_{on} and decreases monotonically in k_{off}.

When both R_T and Z_T are much larger than $k_{\text{off}}/k_{\text{on}}$, the TCR triggering rate is proportional to $\min\{R_T, Z_T\}$ as shown in **Figure 2A**, whereas at lower receptor densities, $W \propto R_T Z_T$ as per equation (13). The transition between the two regimes happens where the receptor densities traverse the 2-dimensional dissociation constant $k_{\text{off}}/k_{\text{on}}$. Thus, depending on receptor densities, the triggering rate may be affected solely by changes in R_T (TCR copy numbers), Z_T (pMHCI copy numbers), or both. The MHC-limited case corresponds to the serial triggering (serial engagement) hypothesis proposed by Valitutti et al. (35–37); however, the present theory is more general in the sense that the serial triggering mechanism arises as a special case.

Figure 2B shows that the TCR triggering rate increases with both k_{on} and mean dwell-time k_{off}^{-1} when k_{on} is low (relative to receptor densities; scaling is explained in the legend to **Figure 2**). However, when k_{on} increases, the triggering rate exhibits a weak dependence on k_{on} and a non-monotone dependence on k_{off}, attaining a maximum at $k_{\text{off}} = 1/T_R$.

The *avidity effect* is routinely exploited to determine the functional sensitivity of the TCR to a given ligand. This effect hinges on mutual compensation by pMHC ligand numbers and the TCR

A

B

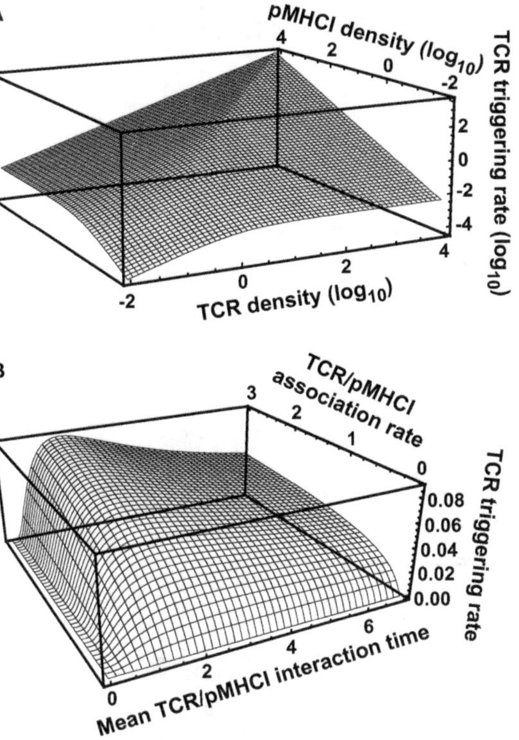

FIGURE 2 | TCR triggering rate depends on TCR/pMHCI association and dissociation rates as well as the densities of TCR and pMHCI molecules. **(A)** Dependence of the rate of TCR triggering on receptor densities. Quantities are dimensionless: TCR triggering rate is scaled as $WT_R^2 k_{on}$, TCR density is scaled as $R_T k_{on}/k_{off}$, pMHCI density is scaled as $Z_T k_{on}/k_{off}$, and $k_{off} = 1/T_R$ is assumed (this means that the ligand is optimal under MHC-limited conditions). **(B)** Dependence of the rate of TCR triggering on kinetic parameters. The dependence on the mean TCR/pMHCI interaction time ($1/k_{off}$) is non-monotone, indicating that a maximally strong agonist must satisfy $k_{off} = 1/T_R$. In contrast, the dependence on k_{on} is monotone. Affinity is customarily expressed by the dissociation constant $K_D = k_{off}/k_{on}$. Accordingly, whether or not an improvement of affinity correlates with an enhanced TCR triggering rate depends on where the system is initially located on the surface of the graph, as well as on the relative contributions that changes in association and dissociation rates make to the overall change in affinity. Quantities are dimensionless: TCR triggering rate is scaled as $WT_R/(R_T + Z_T)$, association rate is scaled as $k_{on}T_R(R_T + Z_T)$, and the mean lifetime of the interaction is scaled as $1/(k_{off}T_R)$. Here, $R_T = Z_T$. Similar qualitative behavior results when the two ligand densities are unequal.

triggering rate per ligand; i.e., a T-cell can be activated by a strong agonist even at low copy numbers whereas a poor agonist may be effective but only at sufficiently high copy numbers. In equation (15), copy numbers are expressed by Z_T and the intrinsic quality of the ligand is expressed by the quantity $k_{off}\exp\{-k_{off}T_R\}$. The latter attains a maximum at $k_{off} = 1/T_R$. If the triggering rate W needs to exceed a certain threshold value to activate the T-cell, sufficient pMHCI copy numbers can compensate for a suboptimal intrinsic triggering rate. However, increasing Z_T may transfer the system into the TCR-limited regime (**Figure 2B**), under which conditions pMHCI density-based compensation cannot be achieved, *cf.* equation (14). Moreover, physiological bounds must exist on how many copies can be present in the interaction area and poor agonists will be unable to activate the T-cell unless unusually high numbers of the ligand are presented (e.g., the cell transcribes very large quantities of the protein).

INTERCELLULAR VARIATION IN RESPONSE HIERARCHY THRESHOLDS

An overview of the experimental data is provided in **Figure 3**. In keeping with the avidity effect, the fraction of cells that exhibited at least n distinct responses (where $1 \leq n \leq 5$) increased with peptide concentration; individual ligands differed with respect to the minimal concentration required to elicit n cellular responses. There was appreciable variability with regard to which functions were elicited, as depicted in **Figure 3B**, which displays the data obtained at peptide concentrations of 10^{-6} M. The responses generally conformed to the following series:

$$\text{MIP-1}\beta < \text{CD107a} < \text{TNF}\alpha < \text{IL-2} < \text{IFN-}\gamma$$

(with the lowest threshold on the left). However, a small proportion of cells exhibited a slightly different ordering of threshold values, as would be expected given the natural variability between cells with respect to the threshold value of any one given response.

These results indicate that, for each response, there is variation between cells with respect to the cellular threshold value. This supports the assumption made in the section *Connecting the theoretical model to experimental observations* above, namely that the sigmoid dose-response shape of the population-level read-out can be accounted for by postulating a statistical distribution at the cell population level with respect to the cellular threshold for any given response.

THE RESPONSE HIERARCHY RESIDES AT THE LEVEL OF CELLULAR SIGNAL INTEGRATION

The parameters of the mathematical model were estimated by means of least-squares fitting of model predictions to the data; the biophysical data are summarized in **Table 1** and **Figure A1** in the Appendix. **Figure 4** shows the results of least-squares curve fitting for the dual-hierarchy hypothesis, the receptor-level response hierarchy hypothesis, and the cellular-level response hierarchy hypothesis. The goodness-of-fit should be assessed in the light of the parsimoniousness of the model. There is less than one parameter per curve. This compares favorably to the standard practice of fitting a separate sigmoid model to each curve, which requires three or more parameters per curve. The fit is very good for such extreme parameter-count efficiency.

There is no substantial difference in the quality of fit between the dual-threshold model and the cellular-threshold model, whereas the fit to the receptor-threshold model is consistently less good. Thus, the data are best explained by postulating a hierarchy only at the level of the cellular activation threshold.

The MIP-1β response was found to have the lowest activation threshold. Relative to this value, the ratios of median threshold values were found to be as follows: CD107a/MIP-1$\beta = 1.44$; TNFα/MIP-1$\beta = 11.7$; IL-2/MIP-1$\beta = 225$; and IFN-γ/MIP-1$\beta = 231$. These findings broadly agree with the consensus series derived from the data reported in **Figure 3**. The estimated median activation threshold values are markedly higher for IL-2 and IFN-γ, which required a stimulus over two orders of magnitude larger compared to the more readily elicited responses.

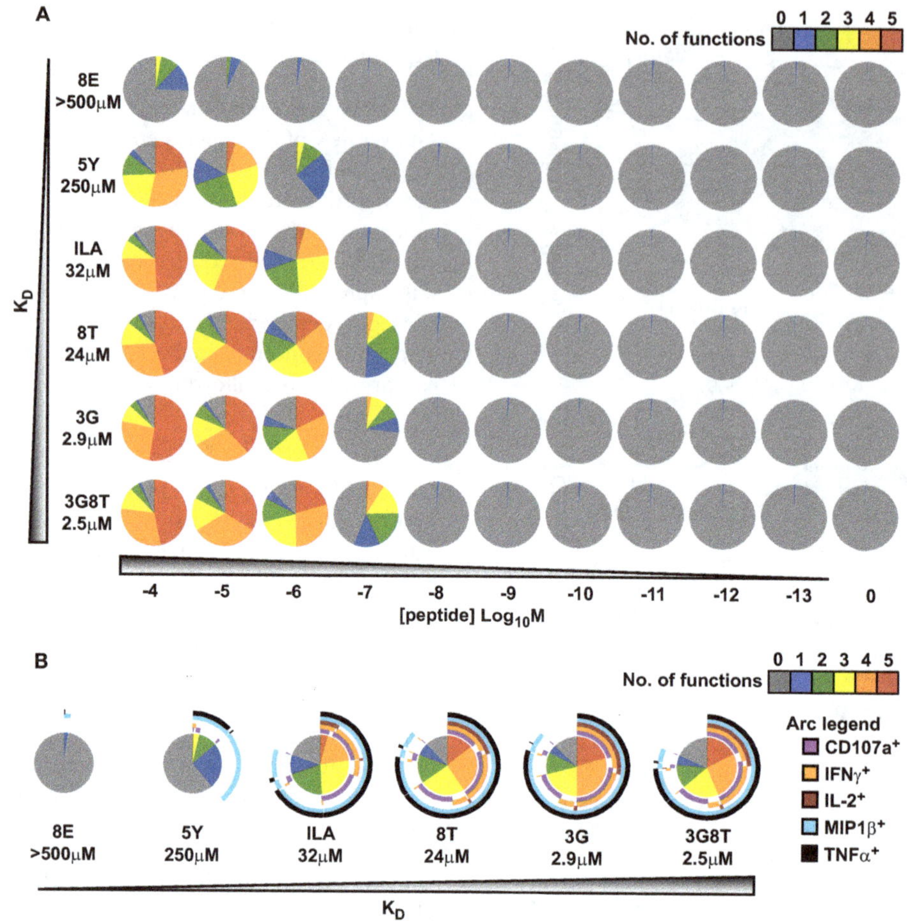

FIGURE 3 | Functional variation at the cell population level in response to six different peptide ligands. The CTL clone ILA1 was stimulated for 6 h with peptide-pulsed C1R-A2 targets as indicated. Five functional read-outs (CD107a, MIP-1β, TNF-α, IL-2, and IFN-γ) were measured via flow cytometry. The 8E peptide was included as an extremely weak ligand. **(A)** Overview of functional profiles. Pie chart segments represent the fraction of cells expressing the number of functions indicated in the key. **(B)** Detailed analysis of functional profiles at [peptide] = 10^{-6} M. Pie charts are extended with arcs defining expressed functions as indicated in the key.

Table 1 | Biophysical parameters.

Ligand	On-rate ($M^{-1}s^{-1}$)	Off-rate (s^{-1})	K_D (M)
3G8T	19,500	0.049	2.5×10^{-6}
3G	16,000	0.047	2.9×10^{-6}
8T	4,000	0.095	2.4×10^{-5}
ILA	4,100	0.13	3.2×10^{-5}
5Y	1,300	0.32	2.5×10^{-4}

The kinetics of the TCR/pMHCI interaction for the 5Y and 3G8T ligands are reported here for the first time; it should be noted that the 5Y data are subject to a comparatively greater potential measurement error due to their rapidity.

MHCI/CD8 BINDING MODULATES FUNCTIONAL SENSITIVITY

The experiments described above were repeated using C1R-A2null cells as APCs, which cannot productively engage the CD8 coreceptor (38). It is well-attested that the MHCI/CD8 interaction modulates the TCR/pMHCI association rate (k_{on}), the TCR/pMHCI dissociation rate (k_{off}), and the receptor-level triggering threshold (T_R) (27, 38, 39). Multipliers can be used to model these effects. For example, k_{off} is replaced throughout by $\gamma_{off}k_{off}$ where γ_{off} represents the effect of abrogating the MHCI/CD8 interaction and $\gamma_{off} > 1$ since CD8 stabilizes the TCR/pMHCI interaction (38–40). The parameter γ_{off} was set to 2.16, the value reported by Wooldridge et al. (38).

Since the prevailing kinetic regime in the experiments described here is MHC limitation, the parameter γ_{on} for the association rate could not be estimated and was set to 1. This leaves a single free parameter, γ_R, for the data obtained with C1R-A2null APCs. Data fits are shown in **Figure 5**, with $\gamma_R = 1.14$ (the least-squares estimate) for the receptor threshold T_R. This value indicates that the MHCI/CD8 interaction decreases the TCR triggering threshold by 13%.

DISCUSSION

T-cells can exhibit a variety of cellular responses to TCR-mediated stimulation, some of which are elicited far more readily than

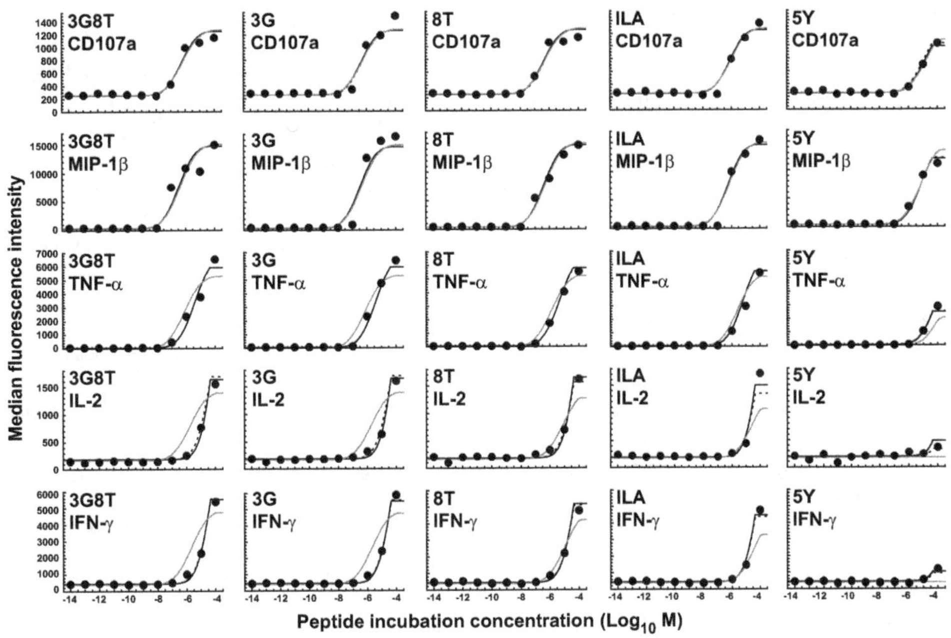

FIGURE 4 | Dose-response curves for five peptide ligands and five cellular responses. Solid black curves correspond to the dual-threshold model in which both the receptor-level and the cellular-level thresholds have different values for different cellular responses. Solid gray curves correspond to the receptor-level threshold model in which the receptor-level thresholds have different values for different cellular responses, but the cellular activation threshold is constant. Dashed curves correspond to the cellular-level threshold model in which the cellular activation thresholds have different values for different cellular responses, but the receptor-level threshold is constant.

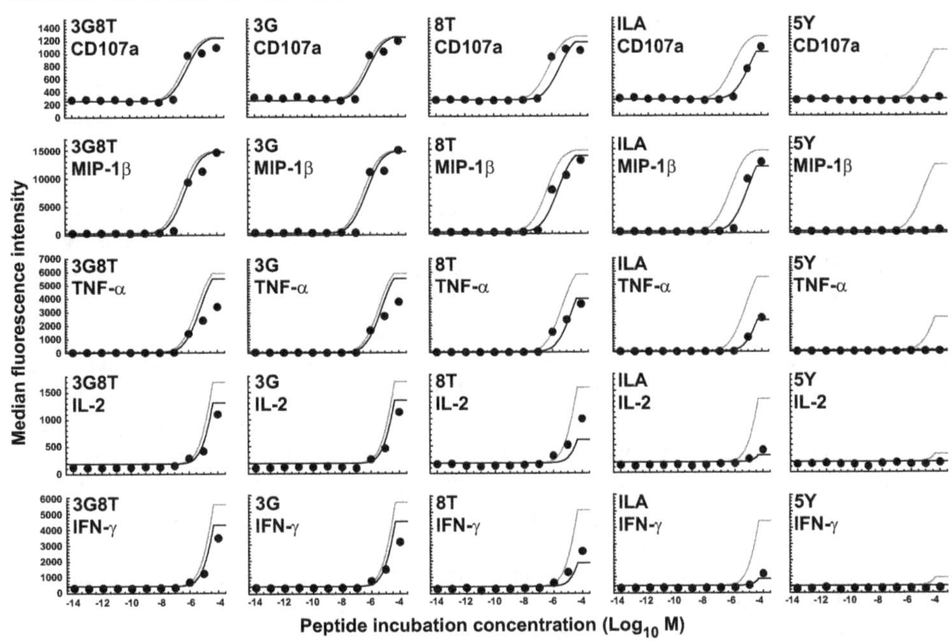

FIGURE 5 | Dose-response curves for five peptide ligands and five cellular responses in the absence of the MHCI/CD8 interaction. All curves correspond to the cellular-level threshold model in which the cellular activation thresholds have different values for different cellular responses, but the receptor-level threshold is constant. Black curves are the fits to the data shown. Gray curves correspond to the situation in which the MHCI/CD8 interaction is present. Parameter values are as in the previous figure. Two new parameters (γ_{off} and γ_R) have been introduced and estimated to account for the absence of the CD8 effect; γ_{off} was set to 2.16 and γ_R was estimated as the sole remaining free parameter.

others. In particular, different responses require different levels of stimulation in terms of ligand densities present on the APC surface. Such threshold differences might be postulated at the receptor level (different response pathways branch off at different stages in the sequence of signaling events), and/or at the cellular level (the TCR signal received by the T-cell needs to exceed different threshold values for different responses). The present study suggests that the cellular-level hypothesis is the most parsimonious explanation consistent with the data. Furthermore, the role of the CD8 coreceptor as a modulator of T-cell functional sensitivity is confirmed by the present findings, which indicate that the MHCI/CD8 interaction decreases the TCR/pMHCI dissociation rate as well as the duration of TCR/pMHCI contact required to activate the T-cell.

A key consideration for the interpretation of our results is the standardized nature of the system. Determinative cellular factors, such as TCR density, membrane constituency, and the expression of costimulatory/inhibitory molecules, were fixed across all conditions, which means that these extraneous factors can be discounted as discriminative because only ligand nature and concentration varied between stimulations. These built-in controls justify the simplifying assumptions from which the mathematical model was derived.

The present findings certainly do not exclude the existence of a receptor-level hierarchy. Indeed, the co-existence of hierarchies at both the receptor and cellular levels may explain the data equally well. However, the hypothesis that the response hierarchy resides solely at the receptor level is contradicted by the present findings. A threshold hierarchy at the level of cellular activation would imply that the functional responses are located downstream from signaling pathways that share a common starting point (the triggered TCR or signalosome). Further detailed molecular studies of the CD3-complex phosphorylation cascade would be required to rule out a receptor-level hierarchy definitively.

Our mathematical model elucidates the contrasting roles played by the dissociation rate and the affinity constant as determinants of T-cell functional sensitivity, with TCR and pMHCI molecular densities governing the limitation regime under which the kinetics operate. The disappearance of the optimum behavior as the system moves from the receptor-limited to the affinity-limited regime can be studied experimentally by increasing TCR density. This shift was first predicted by Van den Berg et al. (23) and confirmed experimentally by Gonzales et al. (41). Furthermore, the pattern of dependence on k_{on} and k_{off} shown in **Figure 2B** may account for the discrepancies between the findings of Kalergis et al. (42), who reported such an optimal dwell-time ($= k_{off}^{-1}$), and the findings of Holler et al. (43), who reported monotone dependence. The shift along the k_{on} axis may also explain the observations of Irving et al. (26), who observed that affinity modulates the dependence on k_{off}. In the experimental system studied here, the TCR is stimulated under MHC-limited conditions. This means that the optimum-type dependence on k_{off} prevails. This is shown in **Figure 6**, where the calculated TCR triggering rate (at 10^{-5} M) is plotted against k_{off}. The effect of k_{on} is so slight that the curves overlap almost perfectly for the five ligands. Even under MHC-limited conditions, however, k_{on} remains a crucial determinant of functional sensitivity, in view of the fact that the ratio of k_{off} and k_{on} determines the transition between affinity-limited and

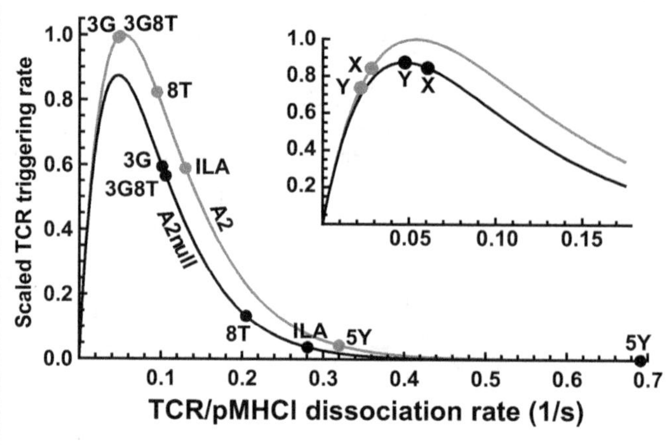

FIGURE 6 | Differential effects of CD8 modulation on functional sensitivity. TCR triggering rate, scaled with respect to the optimal ligand under MHC-limited conditions, as a function of k_{off}, comparing the wild-type MHCI/CD8 interaction ("A2") to the abrogated MHCI/CD8 interaction ("A2null"). The positions for the five ligands are indicated. The inset shows two hypothetical ligands: "X," which is unaffected by the absence of the CD8 interaction, and "Y," which is optimal under the MHC-null condition.

ligand-limited signaling, as illustrated schematically in **Figure 7**. Thus, the association rate and the dissociation rate play distinct roles in T-cell activation, consistent with reports of dominant effects associated with each of these biophysical parameters under different conditions (24, 44); these differences also explain earlier observations on the interplay of kinetic parameters and receptor numbers (41, 45, 46).

In the presence of the wild-type MHCI/CD8 interaction, the ligands 3G and 3G8T are virtually optimal, whereas abrogation of MHCI/CD8 binding leads to a reduction in functional sensitivity. In virtue of the non-linear character of the curve, the magnitude of the reduction varies considerably across ligands. Two parameters (γ_{on} and γ_R) suffice to capture these effects. The ILA ligand evokes a triggering rate approximately one order of magnitude less than optimal under C1R-A2null conditions. Nonetheless, the data show that strongly attenuated but discernible responses can be elicited at sufficiently high presentation levels, in keeping with Wooldridge et al. (14), who reported that a ligand could be physiologically significant even at an estimated ~2.1 orders of magnitude below the optimal ligand for a responding T-cell clone.

Although all ligands studied here become less potent when presented by C1R-A2null cells, the model predicts that this is not necessarily the case. Indeed, the functional sensitivity to a ligand marked "X" in the inset of **Figure 6** is unaffected when the MHCI/CD8 interaction is abrogated. Moreover, ligand "Y" becomes optimal in the absence of the CD8 effect (so that the T-cell has a higher functional sensitivity to this ligand under CD8-null conditions). The existence of such ligands would imply that T-cells can "tune" to distinct cognate ligands by up- or down-regulating their CD8 coreceptors. This effect would greatly amplify the ability of T-cells to reconcile extensive cross-reactivity with the avoidance of self-recognition.

The hypothetical ligands "X" and "Y" are strongly heteroclitic. Peptides of this nature occur markedly less frequently than

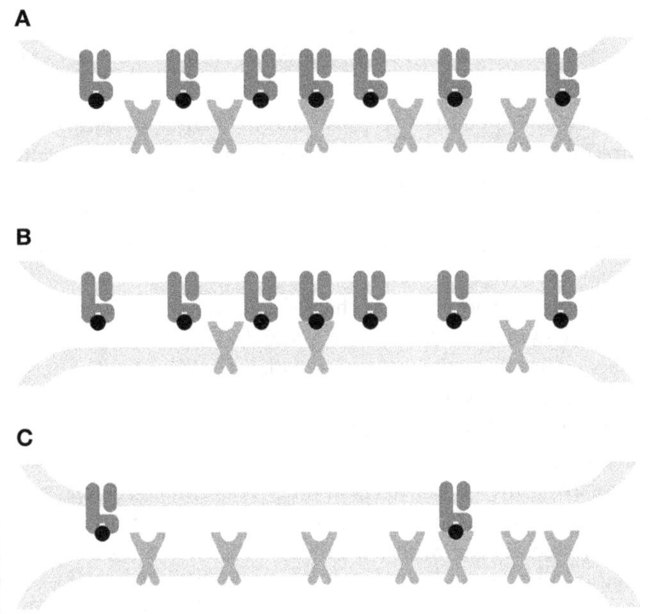

FIGURE 7 | Interplay between kinetic parameters and receptor densities. (A) Affinity-limited: the TCR triggering rate is proportional to the densities of both receptors. **(B)** TCR-limited: the TCR triggering rate is proportional to the TCR density and is monotone decreasing in k_{off}. **(C)** MHC-limited: the TCR triggering rate is proportional to the MHC density and has an optimum k_{off}. The affinity $K_D = k_{off}/k_{on}$ governs the transitions between these kinetic regimes.

homoclitic ligands, which makes them more challenging to detect and characterize. Nonetheless, work is ongoing to demonstrate the existence of such anomalous ligands, using combinatorial peptide library screening combined with importance sampling (14) in the presence of different extracellular contributions from the CD8 coreceptor (29).

The effect of CD8 on the value of the TCR triggering threshold is consistent with the conclusions of Van den Berg et al. (39) and may be due to the association of TCR/CD3 with protein tyrosine kinases such as p56lck, which expedites the immunoglobulin family tyrosine-based activation motif phosphorylation sequence (47). This agrees with the observation that the CD8 $\alpha\beta$ hetero-dimer is more potent as a coreceptor than the $\alpha\alpha$ homo-dimer (48, 49), perhaps due to interactions with other signalosome components mediated by the palmitoylated CD8 β chain (50), which interacts with myristoylated p56lck. Docking of CD8 to the TCR/CD3 complex may also be driven by initial activation (51). The kinetics of CD8 binding after TCR/pMHC contact was analyzed previously by Van den Berg and Sewell (52). More recently, Mukhopadhyay et al. (53) developed a model that explicitly accounts for the interplay between the CD3 phosphorylation cascade and p56lck, ZAP-70, and CD45.

The dissociation rates determined by SPR were assumed to be indicative of the normal interaction in this study. In reality, these values might be more true to the case where the MHCI/CD8 interaction is absent. Assuming the latter would not dramatically alter the qualitative conclusions of this study, but would lead to a slight adjustment in the interpretation of the parameter estimates. Most importantly, the value found for the TCR triggering threshold T_R would be adjusted down from 17.46 to 15.26 s.

Values based on SPR experiments are best regarded as 3-dimensional, representative of ligands in solution. However, the TCR/pMHCI interaction takes place in a 2-dimensional environment, which essentially reduces spatial degrees of freedom of molecular motion and introduces dynamics related to the forces that constrain the molecules to this environment (54). Consequently, rate constants may be different in two dimensions as opposed to three dimensions. In particular, 2-dimensional dissociation rates can be substantially faster (55). The ratio between the 3-dimensional and 2-dimensional affinities is a length measure, denoted h and called the confinement length (56, 57). Wu et al. demonstrated that h is proportional to the range of motion available to the free forms of the interacting ligands along the spatial axis perpendicular to the two parallel membranes. Thus, the intermembrane separation provides an upper bound, and if the ranges of motion do not differ too much, it is reasonable to assume that the confinement length is roughly the same for all mutants involved.

The use of a fixed receptor duration might appear simplistic given the complexity of the events that are required to trigger a TCR/CD3 complex, but the law of large numbers provides indirect support for a simple assumption: the true waiting-time-till-triggering is a composite of a large number of stochastic durations which tends to regress it on the mean value. In fact, the number of terms is itself a random variate due to the possibility of alternative routes in the activation pathway of the complex (such processes are termed "compound stochastic"). The complexity illustrated in **Figure 1** effectively underpins a simple assumption, viz. that there is a fixed, stereotypical receptor threshold T_R.

The parameters T_R and w_{act} are both subject to further modulation. By varying the levels of the CD8 coreceptor, surface molecules such as CD45, and cytosolic concentrations of kinases, phosphorylases, and linker proteins in the immediate vicinity of the CD3 complex, the T-cell can adjust the effective value of the receptor triggering threshold T_R (29, 30, 38, 39, 58–61). The value of the cellular activation threshold w_{act} is modulated by costimulation ("signal 2"). Moreover, the T-cell can actively modulate its receptiveness to this signal by adjusting the relative levels of CD28 and CD152 (52, 62). Furthermore, the maintenance of tolerance requires continual dynamic tuning of the cellular activation threshold (63, 64). Conceivably, these mechanisms provide an additional "multiplier" that modulates w_{act} over and above the factors that set w_{act} to different values for different responses.

The data on intercellular response variability (**Figure 3**) support the assumption that the distribution of responsiveness in terms of MFI can be attributed to intercellular variation in the triggering threshold. However, the observed variability may also arise from differences in the numbers of TCR and pMHCI molecules present in the T-cell/APC interaction area. Mathematically, this model is slightly more involved because interactions can now be distributed over different kinetic regimes. Nonetheless, apart from this technical difficulty, the resulting model is mathematically equivalent; this follows from the properties of the log-normal distribution. Thus, the analysis is not substantially affected by this alternative explanation of the intercellular variability. Experimentally, the two hypotheses could be distinguished by following an individual T-cell over a series of interactions and responses. If cellular thresholds for the various responses remain largely constant, there would be little event-to-event variation according to the former hypothesis; in contrast, the receptor copy number hypothesis would predict considerable event-to-event variation.

In addition, there may be variability with respect to antigen presentation levels across the experimental APC population, due to differential antigen exposure and stochastic effects in antigen acceptance from the incubation medium. However, it can be shown that the resulting variance is not such as to make a substantial contribution to overall variability, for instance by following the argument presented in Appendix C of Van den Berg et al. (22).

When the TCR/pMHCI ternary complex dissociates, the covalent modifications and multimeric aggregations that the CD3 complex undergoes during the gradual transition to signalosome status are reversed, both by thermal agitation and the action of phosphorylases. In the present model, it has been assumed that this "reset" occurs much more rapidly than the typical time required for the TCR/CD3 complex to encounter the next non-null pMHCI ligand. However, given that the molecules have to drift away from each other through diffusion in the 2-dimensional arena of the T-cell/APC interface, there is a possibility of rapid rebinding to the *same* pMHCI molecule before the CD3 complex has had sufficient time to "reset." This rapid rebinding is equivalent to a diminishment of the effective off-rate; a basic model capturing this effect has been proposed by Aleksic et al. (65). Extending the present model with this effect is straightforward in principle, albeit at the cost of an additional parameter. Furthermore, the number of complexes with other pMHCI species is ignored in equation (1). This is valid if the vast majority of all other ligands consists of null agonists. An analysis that takes the entire presentation profile (all pMHCI species present) into account can be found in Van den Berg et al. (22, 23).

A further aspect of the cellular activation threshold that has been left implicit in the present treatment is the duration of the T-cell/APC interaction. If this contact is initiated at t_0 and is terminated at t_1, the cumulative signal transmitted to the cytosolic signaling machinery is given by an integral:

$$Q = \int_{t_0}^{t_1} W(\tau)d\tau. \tag{16}$$

In fact, this quantity Q is presumed to be directly compared to a threshold. However, $Q/(t_1 - t_0)$ is proportional to the activation threshold as defined in the present study. Indeed, variability in the duration of the contact is one of the sources of stochasticity underlying the log-normal response curve used to fit the dose-response curves.

A related phenomenon is that of TCR down-regulation (66–68), whereby triggered TCRs are gradually removed from the cell surface. This affects the integral in equation (16); Van den Berg et al. (23) discuss how the model can be extended to take this effect into account. TCR down-regulation can in fact be exploited by the T-cell to gauge both k_{on} and k_{off} independently. As indicated in **Figure 2A**, if the system starts in the MHC-limited regime, gradual removal of TCR molecules will result in a transition to the TCR-limited regime, where a sudden drop of the instantaneous signal results. At the point of change-over, $R_T \approx Z_T$. This means that the T-cell can, in principle, glean a rough estimate of the biophysical rate parameters k_{off} and k_{on} by combining information from the gross signal and the number of down-regulated TCRs at the transition point. This mechanism can only function in the ligand-limited regime, not in the affinity-limited regime.

In conclusion, the present study confirms that a response hierarchy exists with respect to the strength of TCR stimulation required to elicit various cellular responses. Moreover, a combination of experimentation and mathematical modeling indicates that this hierarchy resides at the cellular level rather than at the level of the individual receptor molecules. Functional sensitivity is generally enhanced by the CD8 coreceptor, although the theory indicates that the MHCI/CD8 interaction can depress TCR signaling for certain heteroclitic ligands.

ACKNOWLEDGMENTS

This work was supported by the Biotechnology and Biological Sciences Research Council (grant BB/H001085/1). The authors are grateful to Brenda Hartman (NIH/VRC) for expert assistance with graphics.

REFERENCES

1. Parham P. *The Immune System.* New York: Garland Publishing (2000).
2. Rudolph MG, Stanfield RL, Wilson IA. How TCRs bind MHCs, peptides, and coreceptors. *Annu Rev Immunol* (2006) **24**:419–66. doi:10.1146/annurev.immunol.23.021704.115658
3. Mason D. A very high level of crossreactivity is an essential feature of the T-cell receptor. *Immunol Today* (1998) **19**: 395–404. doi:10.1016/S0167-5699(98)01299-7
4. Wraith DC, Bruun B, Fairchild PJ. Cross-reactive antigen recognition by an encephalitogenetic T cell receptor. *J Immunol* (1992) **149**:3765–70.
5. Bhardwaj V, Kumar V, Geysen HM, Sercarz EE. Degenerate recognition of a dissimilar antigenic peptide by myelin basic protein. Implications for thymic education and autoimmunity. *J Immunol* (1993) **151**:5000–10.
6. Reay PA, Kantor RM, Davis MM. Use of global amino acid replacements to define the requirements for MHC binding and T cell recognition of moth cytochrome c (93–103). *J Immunol* (1994) **152**:3946–3957.
7. Evavold BD, Sloan-Lancaster J, Wilson KJ, Rothbard JB, Allen PM. Specific T cell recognition of minimally homologous peptides: evidence for multiple endogenous ligands. *Immunity* (1995) **2**: 655–63. doi:10.1016/1074-7613(95)90010-1
8. Wucherpfennig KW, Strominger JL. Molecular mimicry in T cell-mediated autoimmunity: viral peptides activate human T cell clones specific for myelin basic protein. *Cell* (1995) **80**: 695–705. doi:10.1016/0092-8674(95)90348-8
9. Ignatowicz L, Rees W, Pacholczyk R, Ignatowicz H, Kushnir E, Kappler J, et al. T cells can be activated by peptides that are unrelated in sequence to their selecting peptide. *Immunity* (1997) **7**: 179–186. doi:10.1016/S1074-7613(00)80521-X
10. Hemmer B, Fleckenstein BT, Vergelli M, Jung G, McFarland H, Martin R, et al. Identification of high potency microbial and self ligands for a human autoreactive class II-restricted T cell clone. *J Exp Med* (1997) **185**:1651–1659. doi:10.1084/jem.185.9.1651
11. Bachmann MF, Speiser DE, Zakarian A, Ohashi PS. Inhibition of TCR triggering by a spectrum of altered peptide ligands suggests the mechanism for TCR antagonism. *Eur J Immunol* (1998) **28**:3110–9. doi:10.1002/(SICI)1521-4141(199810)28:10<3110::AID-IMMU3110>3.0.CO;2-5

12. Wilson DB, Wilson DH, Schroder K, Pinilla C, Blondelle S, Houghten RA, et al. Specificity and degeneracy of T cells. *Mol Immunol* (2004) **40**:1047–1055. doi:10.1016/j.molimm.2003.11.022
13. Ishizuka J, Grebe K, Shenderov E, Peters B, Chen Q, Peng Y, et al. Quantitating T cell cross-reactivity for unrelated peptide antigens. *J Immunol* (2009) **183**:4337–45. doi:10.4049/jimmunol.0901607
14. Wooldridge L, Ekeruche-Makinde J, van den Berg HA, Skowera A, Miles JJ, Tan MP, et al. A single autoimmune T cell receptor recognizes more than a million different peptides. *J Biol Chem* (2012) **287**:1168–77. doi:10.1074/jbc.M111.289488
15. Valitutti S, Müller S, Dessing M, Lanzavecchia A. Different responses are elicited in cytotoxic T lymphocytes by different levels of T cell receptor occupancy. *J Exp Med* (1996) **183**:1917–1921. doi:10.1084/jem.183.4.1917
16. Itoh Y, Germain RN. Single cell analysis reveals regulated hierarchical T cell antigen receptor signaling thresholds and intraclonal heterogeneity for individual cytokine responses of CD4+ cells. *J Exp Med* (1997) **186**:757–766. doi:10.1084/jem.186.5.757
17. Hemmer B, Stefanova I, Vergelli M, Germain RN, Martin R. Relationships among TCR ligand potency, thresholds for effector function elicitation, and the quality of early signaling events in human T cells. *J Immunol* (1998) **160**:5807–5814.
18. Price DA, Sewell AK, Dong T, Tan R, Goulder PJR, Rowland-Jones SL, et al. Antigen-specific release of β-chemokines by anti-HIV-1 cytotoxic T lymphocytes. *Curr Biol* (1998) **8**:355–8. doi:10.1016/S0960-9822(98)70138-1
19. Rabinowitz JD, Beeson C, Lyons DS, Davis MM, McConnell HM. Kinetic discrimination in T-cell activation. *Proc Natl Acad Sci U S A* (1996) **93**:1401–1405. doi:10.1073/pnas.93.4.1401
20. McKeithan TW. Kinetic proofreading in T-cell receptor signal transduction. *Proc Natl Acad Sci U S A* (1995) **92**:5042–5046. doi:10.1073/pnas.92.11.5042
21. Lanzavecchia A, Iezzi G, Viola A. From TCR engagement to T cell activation: a kinetic view of T cell behavior. *Cell* (1999) **96**:1–4. doi:10.1016/S0092-8674(00)80952-6
22. van den Berg HA, Rand DA, Burroughs NJ. A reliable and safe T cell repertoire based on low-affinity T cell receptors. *J Theor Biol* (2001) **209**:465–486. doi:10.1006/jtbi.2001.2281
23. van den Berg HA, Burroughs NJ, Rand DA. Quantifying the strength of ligand antagonism in TCR triggering. *Bull Math Biol* (2002) **64**:781–808. doi:10.1006/bulm.2002.0302
24. Bridgeman JS, Sewell AK, Miles JJ, Price DA, Cole DK. Structural and biophysical determinants of $\alpha\beta$ T-cell antigen recognition. *Immunology* (2012) **135**:9–18. doi:10.1111/j.1365-2567.2011.03515.x
25. van den Berg HA, Rand DA. Quantitative theories of T-cell responsiveness. *Immunol Rev* (2007) **216**:81–92. doi:10.1111/j.1600-065X.2006.00491.x
26. Irving M, Zoete V, Hebeisen M, Schmid D, Baumgartner P, Guillaume P, et al. Interplay between T cell receptor binding kinetics and the level of cognate peptide presented by major histocompatibility complexes governs CD8+ T cell responsiveness. *J Biol Chem* (2012) **287**:23068–78. doi:10.1074/jbc.M112.357673
27. Laugel B, van den Berg HA, Gostick E, Cole DK, Wooldridge L, Boulter J, et al. Different T cell receptor affinity thresholds and CD8 coreceptor dependency govern cytotoxic T lymphocyte activation and tetramer binding properties. *J Biol Chem* (2007) **282**:23799–810. doi:10.1074/jbc.M700976200
28. Melenhorst JJ, Scheinberg P, Chattopadhyay PK, Lissina A, Gostick E, Cole DK, et al. Detection of low avidity $CD8^+$ T cell populations with coreceptor-enhanced peptide-major histocompatibility complex class I tetramers. *J Immunol Methods* (2008) **338**:31–9. doi:10.1016/j.jim.2008.07.008
29. Wooldridge L, Laugel B, Ekeruche J, Clement M, van den Berg HA, Price DA, et al. CD8 controls T cell cross-reactivity. *J Immunol* (2010) **185**:4625–32. doi:10.4049/jimmunol.1001480
30. Purbhoo MA, Boulter JM, Price DA, Vuidepot A-L, Hourigan CS, Dunbar PR, et al. The human CD8 coreceptor effects cytotoxic T cell activation and antigen sensitivity primarily by mediating complete phosphorylation of the T cell receptor ζ chain. *J Biol Chem* (2001) **276**:32786–32792. doi:10.1074/jbc.M102498200
31. Betts MR, Brenchley JM, Price DA, De Rosa SC, Douek DC, Roederer M, et al. Sensitive and viable identification of antigen-specific $CD8^+$ T cells by a flow cytometric assay for degranulation. *J Immunol Methods* (2003) **281**:65–78. doi:10.1016/S0022-1759(03)00265-5
32. Cole DK, Pumphrey NJ, Boulter JM, Sami M, Bell JI, Gostick E, et al. Human TCR-binding affinity is governed by MHC class restriction. *J Immunol* (2007) **178**:5727–34.
33. Cole DK, Yuan F, Rizkallah PJ, Miles JJ, Gostick E, Price DA, et al. Germ line-governed recognition of a cancer epitope by an immunodominant human T-cell receptor. *J Biol Chem* (2009) **284**:27281–9. doi:10.1074/jbc.M109.022509
34. Cole DK, Rizkallah PJ, Boulter JM, Sami M, Vuidepot A, Glick M, et al. Computational design and crystal structure of an enhanced-affinity mutant human CD8 $\alpha\alpha$ coreceptor. *Proteins* (2007) **67**:65–74. doi:10.1002/prot.21176
35. Valitutti S, Müller S, Cella M, Padovan E, Lanzavecchia A. Serial triggering of many T-cell receptors by a few peptide-MHC complexes. *Nature* (1995) **375**:148–151. doi:10.1038/375148a0
36. Valitutti S, Lanzavecchia A. Serial triggering of TCRs: a basis for the sensitivity and specificity of antigen recognition. *Immunol Today* (1997) **18**:299–304. doi:10.1016/S0167-5699(97)80027-8
37. Valitutti S. The serial engagement model 17 years after: from TCR triggering to immunotherapy. *Front Immunol* (2012) **3**:272. doi:10.3389/fimmu.2012.00272
38. Wooldridge L, van den Berg HA, Glick M, Gostick E, Brenchley JM, Douek DC, et al. Interaction between the CD8 coreceptor and MHC class I stabilizes TCR-antigen complexes at the cell surface. *J Biol Chem* (2005) **280**:27491–27501. doi:10.1074/jbc.M500555200
39. van den Berg HA, Wooldridge L, Laugel B, Sewell AK. Coreceptor CD8-driven modulation of T cell antigen receptor specificity. *J Theor Biol* (2007) **249**:395–408. doi:10.1016/j.jtbi.2007.08.002
40. Luescher IF, Vivier E, Layer A, Mahiou J, Godeau F, Malissen B, et al. CD8 modulation of T-cell antigen receptor-ligand interactions on living cytotoxic T lymphocytes. *Nature* (1995) **373**:353–356. doi:10.1038/373353a0
41. Gonzales PA, Carreño LJ, Coombs D, Mora JE, Palmeiri E, Goldstein B, et al. T cell receptor binding kinetics required for T cell activation depend on the density of the cognate ligand of the antigen-presenting cell. *Proc Natl Acad Sci U S A* (2005) **102**:4824–4829. doi:10.1073/pnas.0500922102
42. Kalergis AM, Boucheron N, Doucey M-A, Palmieri E, Goyarts EC, Vegh Z, et al. Efficient T cell activation requires an optimal dwell-time of interaction between the TCR and the pMHC complex. *Nat Immunol* (2001) **2**:229–34. doi:10.1038/85286
43. Holler PD, Lim AR, Cho BK, Rund LA, Kranz DM. $CD8^-$ T cell transfectants that express a high affinity T cell receptor exhibit enhanced peptide-dependent activation. *J Exp Med* (2001) **194**:1043–1052. doi:10.1084/jem.194.8.1043
44. Carreño LJ, González PA, Kalergis AM. Modulation of T cell function by TCR/pMHC binding kinetics. *Immunobiology* (2006) **211**:47–64. doi:10.1016/j.imbio.2005.09.003
45. Govern CC, Paczosa MK, Chakraborty AK, Huseby ES. Fast on-rates allow short dwell time ligands to activate T cells. *Proc Natl Acad Sci U S A* (2010) **107**:8724–9. doi:10.1073/pnas.1000966107
46. Dushek O, Aleksic M, Wheeler RJ, Zhang H, Cordoba S-P, Peng Y-C, et al. Antigen potency and maximal efficacy reveal a mechanism of efficient T cell activation. *Sci Signal* (2011) **4**:ra39. doi:10.1126/scisignal.2001430
47. Arcaro A, Grégoire C, Bakker TR, Baldi L, Jordan M, Goffin L, et al. CD8β endows CD8 with efficient coreceptor function by coupling T cell receptor/CD3 to raft-associated CD8/p56^{lck} complexes. *J Exp Med* (2001) **194**:1485–95. doi:10.1084/jem.194.10.1485
48. Bosselut R, Kubo S, Guinter T, Kopacz JL, Altman JD, Feigenbaum L, et al. Role of CD8β domains in CD8 coreceptor function: importance for MHC I binding, signaling, and positive selection of $CD8^+$ T cells in the thymus. *Immunity* (2000) **12**:409–418. doi:10.1016/S1074-7613(00)80193-4
49. Gangadharan D, Cheroute H. The CD8 isoform CD8$\alpha\alpha$ is not a functional homologue of the TCR co-receptor CD8$\alpha\beta$. *Curr Opin Immunol* (2004) **16**:264–270. doi:10.1016/j.coi.2004.03.015
50. Arcaro A, Grégoire C, Boucheron N, Stolz S, Palmer E, Malissen B, et al. Essential role of CD8 palmitoylation in CD8 coreceptor function. *J Immunol* (2000) **165**:2068–2076.
51. Laugel B, Cole DK, Clement M, Wooldridge L, Price DA, Sewell AK. The multiple roles of the CD8 coreceptor in T cell biology: opportunities for the selective modulation of self-reactive cytotoxic T cells. *J*

Leukoc Biol (2011) **90**:1089–99. doi:10.1189/jlb.0611316
52. van den Berg HA, Sewell AK. Dynamic tuning of T cell receptor specificity by co-receptors and costimulation. In: Molina-París C, Lythe G, editors. *Mathematical Models and Immune Cell Biology*. Berlin: Springer-Verlag (2011) pp. 47–73.
53. Mukhopadhyay H, Cordoba S-P, Maini PK, van der Merwe PA, Dushek O. Systems model of T cell receptor proximal signaling reveals emergent ultrasensitivity. *PLoS Comput Biol* (2013) **9**:e1003004. doi:10.1371/journal.pcbi.1003004
54. Wu Y, Vendome J, Shapiro L, Ben-Shaul A, Honig B. Transforming binding affinities from three dimensions to two with application to cadherin clustering. *Nature* (2011) **475**:510–4. doi:10.1038/nature10183
55. Zarnitsyna V, Zhu C. T cell triggering: insights from 2D kinetics analysis of molecular interactions. *Phys Biol* (2012) **9**:045005. doi:10.1088/1478-3975/9/4/045005
56. Bell GI. Models for the specific adhesion of cells to cells. *Science* (1978) **200**:618–27. doi:10.1126/science.347575
57. Bell GI, Dembo M, Bongrand P. Cell adhesion. Competition between nonspecific repulsion and specific bonding. *Biophys J* (1984) **45**:1051–64. doi:10.1016/S0006-3495(84)84252-6
58. Werlen G, Palmer E. The TCR signalosome: a dynamic structure with expanding complexity. *Curr Opin Immunol* (2002) **14**:299–305. doi:10.1016/S0952-7915(02)00339-4
59. Filipp D, Zhang J, Leung BL, Shaw A, Levin SD, Veillette A, et al. Regulation of Fyn through translocation of activated Lck into lipid rafts. *J Exp Med* (2003) **197**:1221–1227. doi:10.1084/jem.20022112
60. Maile R, Siler CA, Kerry SE, Midkiff KE, Collins EJ, Frelinger JA. Peripheral "CD8 tuning" dynamically modulates the size and responsiveness of an antigen-specific T cell pool in vivo. *J Immunol* (2005) **174**:619–627.
61. Park J-H, Adoro S, Lucas PJ, Sarafova SD, Alag AS, Doan LL, et al. 'Coreceptor tuning': cytokine signals transcriptionally tailor CD8 coreceptor expression to the self-specificity of the TCR. *Nat Immunol* (2007) **8**:1049–58. doi:10.1038/ni1512
62. Collins AV, Brodie DW, Gilbert RJC, Iaboni A, Manso-Sancho R, Stuart DI, et al. The interaction properties of costimulatory molecules revisited. *Immunity* (2002) **17**:201–10. doi:10.1016/S1074-7613(02)00362-X
63. Grossman Z, Paul WE. Adaptive cellular interactions in the immune system: the tunable activation threshold and the significance of subthreshold responses. *Proc Natl Acad Sci U S A* (1992) **89**:10365–10369. doi:10.1073/pnas.89.21.10365
64. van den Berg HA, Rand DA. Dynamics of T cell activation threshold tuning. *J Theor Biol* (2004) **228**:397–416. doi:10.1016/j.jtbi.2004.02.002
65. Aleksic M, Dushek O, Zhang H, Shenderov E, Chen J-L, Cerundolo V, et al. Dependence of the T cell antigen receptor on the T cell receptor-peptide MHC confinement time. *Immunity* (2010) **32**:1–12. doi:10.1016/j.immuni.2009.11.013
66. Lauritsen JPH, Christensen MD, Dietrich J, Kastrup J, Ødum N, Geisler C. Two distinct pathways exist for down-regulation of the TCR. *J Immunol* (1998) **161**:260–267.
67. Liu H, Rhodes M, Wiest DL, Vignali DAA. On the dynamics of TCR:CD3 complex cell surface expression and downmodulation. *Immunity* (2000) **13**:665–675. doi:10.1016/S1074-7613(00)00066-2
68. Sousa J, Carneiro J. A mathematical analysis of TCR serial triggering and down-regulation. *Eur J Immunol* (2000) **30**:3219–3227. doi:10.1002/1521-4141(200011)30:11<3219::AID-IMMU3219>3.0.CO;2-7

2

Co-receptor CD8-mediated modulation of T-cell receptor functional sensitivity and epitope recognition degeneracy

Barbara Szomolay[1], Tamsin Williams[2], Linda Wooldridge[3] and Hugo Antonius van den Berg[1]*

[1] University of Warwick, Coventry, UK
[2] Institute of Infection and Immunity, Cardiff University School of Medicine, Cardiff, UK
[3] Faculty of Medical and Veterinary Sciences, University of Bristol, Bristol, UK

Edited by:
Bruno Laugel, Cardiff University School of Medicine, UK

Reviewed by:
Brian M. Baker, University of Notre Dame, USA
Yoram Louzoun, Bar-Ilan University, Israel

***Correspondence:**
Hugo Antonius van den Berg, University of Warwick, Systems Biology, Coventry, CV4 7AL, UK
e-mail: hugo@maths.warwick.ac.uk

The interaction between T-cell receptors (TCRs) and peptide epitopes is highly degenerate: a TCR is capable of interacting productively with a wide range of different peptide ligands, involving not only cross-reactivity proper (similar epitopes elicit strong responses), but also polyspecificity (ligands with distinct physicochemical properties are capable of interacting with the TCR). Degeneracy does not gainsay the fact that TCR recognition is fundamentally specific: for the vast majority of ligands, the functional sensitivity of a given TCR is virtually null whereas this TCR has an appreciable functional sensitivity only for a minute fraction of all possible ligands. Degeneracy can be described mathematically as the probability that the functional sensitivity, of a given TCR to a randomly selected ligand, exceeds a set value. Variation of this value generates a statistical distribution that characterizes TCR degeneracy. This distribution can be modeled on the basis of a Gaussian distribution for the TCR/ligand dissociation energy. The kinetics of the TCR and the MHCI molecule can be used to transform this underlying Gaussian distribution into the observed distribution of functional sensitivity values. In the present paper, the model is extended by accounting explicitly for the kinetics of the interaction between the co-receptor and the MHCI molecule. We show that T-cells can modulate the level of degeneracy by varying the density of co-receptors on the cell surface. This could allow for an analog of avidity maturation during incipient T-cell responses.

Keywords: T-cell receptor, co-receptor CD8, degeneracy, functional sensitivity, ligand focusing, mathematical model

INTRODUCTION

Thymus-derived lymphocytes (T-cells) recognize peptide antigens via antigen-specific receptors (TCRs); in particular, $CD8^+$ cytotoxic T lymphocytes (CTLs) recognize short peptides presented by major histocompatibility complex (MHC) class I molecules (1). Estimates of the human TCR diversity suggest that there are $\sim 10^8$ different antigen receptors in the naïve T-cell pool (2), which raises the question how such a limited TCR repertoire can provide effective immunity to perhaps over 10^{15} distinct pMHCs (2). The discrepancy suggests that even while TCRs are highly specific, a considerable degree of degeneracy remains (we use *degeneracy* as a term of art to cover both polyspecificity and cross-reactivity). The central importance of degeneracy was first pointed out by Mason (3) and later confirmed by others such as (4). Experimental and mathematical studies confirm that TCR recognition is highly degenerate: a single TCR may be able to recognize, at physiologically relevant degrees of functional sensitivity, over one million different peptides in the context of a single MHCI molecule (2, 5), an estimate that takes into account the binding specificity of the MHC molecule, but not the additional selection imposed by the stringency requirements of peptide cleavage and processing in the presentation pathway. The latter constitutes an epitope diversity filter that is instrumental in regulating the immunovisibility of salient epitopes (6). The issue of whether there exists an optimal level of TCR repertoire diversity was reviewed by Nikolich-Žuglich et al. (7), and various authors have reviewed the functional repercussions at the systems level (8–10).

The interaction between TCR and pMHCI ligand can be modulated by the co-receptor CD8 in several ways: (i) promoting the association of TCR and pMHCI; (ii) stabilizing the TCR/pMHCI interaction; and (iii) enhancing the rate at which the TCR/CD3 complex attains signaling status by association of TCR/CD3 with protein tyrosine kinases such as $p56^{lck}$ and adaptor molecules such as LAT and LIME (5, 11–16). The first of these three mechanisms modifies the affinity of the TCR/pMHCI interaction, whereas the third alters the time it takes for an engaged TCR/CD3 complex to attain full signalosome status. In particular, CD8 can enhance the TCR/pMHCI association rate by 50%, and reduce the TCR/pMHCI dissociation rate by at least 50% (16, 17), and CD8 modulates the rate of immune receptor tyrosine-based activation motif (ITAM) phosphorylation, by recruiting TCR/pMHCI complexes to membrane micro-domains at a rate which depends on the affinity of pMHCI/CD8 binding (16).

These findings suggest that CD8 not only controls degeneracy, but also differentially regulates functional sensitivity, that is, the T-cell can increase its sensitivity for one ligand, while reducing it for others. By varying the level of CD8 expression, the T-cell can increase its sensitivity to the disease-associated antigen, while at the same time decreasing its sensitivity to antigens associated with healthy conditions. This novel mode of co-receptor action could be critical in ensuring that the TCR repertoire retains the ability to respond to antigenic challenges, while avoiding autoimmunity.

T-cell antigen recognition can be expressed in terms of its *functional sensitivity* (18). One of the main determinants of functional sensitivity is the rate at which a single agonist copy elicits TCR triggering. Functional sensitivity depends on bio-molecular parameters such as the TCR/pMHCI on-rate and off-rate. The molecular kinetics at the T-cell:antigen-presenting cell (APC) interface determine this relationship. This kinetic theory resolves the long-standing controversy over whether T-cell activation is governed by affinity or off-rate (cf. (19, 20)); the theory shows that *both* parameters play a role, but in the so-called MHC-limited regime, the off-rate is the main governing factor. However, the on-rate and the off-rate together determine whether or not the kinetics is MHC-limited (21–23).

The aim of the present study is to explore the kinetic basis of the role of CD8 in regulating degeneracy and functional sensitivity. Our model generalizes the classical kinetic proofreading model, as proposed by McKeithan (24), and later modified by others (21, 22, 25–27). The kinetic proofreading model assumes that the TCR needs to remain bound to a pMHC in order for the TCR/CD3 complex to become fully activated, via several modification steps such as phosphorylation of several tyrosine residues on the TCR complex, and recruitment and subsequent activation of ZAP-70 (28).

The statistics of TCR degeneracy is modeled by relating the TCR/pMHCI mean interaction time with the dissociation energy according to Arrhenius theory. We show that by varying the total co-receptor density and key kinetic parameters, the T-cell can modulate the level of degeneracy. Furthermore, we compare our results with experimental data for HLA A*0201 mutants with altered binding affinity for CD8.

THEORY: TCR/pMHCI/CD8 KINETICS AND TCR DEGENERACY

We assume (i) that the TCR/CD3 complex on the T-cell surface becomes triggered (achieves signalosome status) during an interaction with a pMHCI ligand if it undergoes n ITAM phosphorylations, where n is a positive integer; and (ii) that the presence of a CD8 molecule bound to the pMHCI ligand affects the TCR/pMHCI association and dissociation rates, as well as the rate at which the TCR/CD3 complex progresses through the phosphorylation sequence. The co-receptor CD8 is associated with TCR/CD3 with tyrosine kinases such as $p56^{lck}$, which phosphorylates tyrosine residues within the ITAMs.

To determine the kinetics of the TCR/pMHCI/CD8 interactions, consider the four binding states of a pMHCI molecule, labeled (I–IV) in **Figure 1A**. The states in which the TCR and the pMHCI ligand are bound can be further subdivided into different states according to the number of phosphorylated ITAMs, as shown in **Figure 1B**. The transition rate between these states is n/T_R, where T_R is the average time required to go through the entire sequence. The notation T_R emphasizes that this quantity is the average time for the TCR/CD3 complex to become triggered. We call this the *TCR triggering threshold*. Typical values of TCR triggering threshold T_R are in the range of 5–15 s (29).

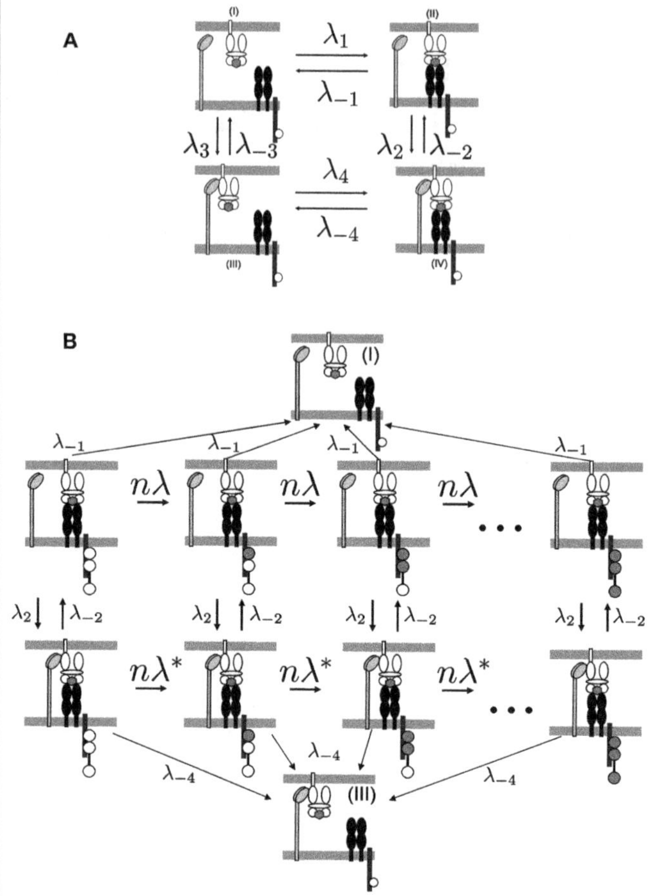

FIGURE 1 | TCR/pMHCI/CD8 interactions represented in the model. (A) Kinetics of TCR/pMHCI/CD8 complex formation. TCRs and CD8s are located on the T-cell side and pMHCIs on the APC side. Four possible states are shown: in (I) and (II), pMHCI is not bound to CD8 whereas in (III) and (IV), pMHCI is bound to CD8; in (I) and (III), pMHCI is not bound to TCR/CD3 whereas in (II) and (IV), pMHCI is bound to TCR/CD3. Transition rates between these four states are indicated with forward rates labeled as λ_i and backward rates labeled as λ_{-i} (where $i = 1, 2, 3, 4$). The white circles in the tails of the TCR/CD3 complex represent the ITAMs, which are present on the cytoplasmic tails of the γ, δ, the two ε, and the two ζ polypeptide chains of the CD3 complex; only one such tail is indicated here, for clarity. There are n such ITAMs, with only three shown here for the sake of clarity. This part of the kinetic scheme is assumed to be in equilibrium. **(B)** The TCR/pMHCI bound states (II) and (IV) are further subdivided into n states each depending on the number of phosphorylated ITAMs, resulting in a Markov chain. The triggered states are the right-most ones where all n ITAMs have been phosphorylated (indicated as filled-in circles). At each state a reversal (at rate λ_{-1} or λ_{-4}) to the unbound states (I) or (III), respectively, can occur. Transitions between the sequences occur at rates λ_2 and λ_{-2}. Left-to-right transitions within the sequences correspond to ITAM phosphorylation by kinases such as $p56^{lck}$ and ZAP-70, at rate $n\lambda = n/T_R$ in the sequence with CD8 unbound and at rate $n\lambda^* = n/T_R^*$ in the chain with CD8 bound. The Markov chain serves to calculate the TCR triggering probability and is not assumed to be in equilibrium.

KINETIC EQUATIONS

The model describes the kinetics of the interactions between the TCR, pMHCI molecules, and co-receptor CD8 in the contact area between a T-cell and an APC. This area is occupied by TCRs and

CD8s on the T-cell side and by pMHCIs on the APC side, whereby CD8 binds pMHCI at a distinct site of the TCR/pMHCI complex. ITAMs are located on the ζ-chains of the CD3 complex associated with the TCR and are represented schematically in **Figure 1B**.

Interactions between TCR, pMHCI, and CD8

Key quantities in the model (summarized in **Table 1**) are the densities of free receptors on the T-cell and free ligands on the APC, which can also form complexes with the receptors. The surface densities of the TCR, CD8, and pMHCI molecules are subject to the following conservation laws:

$$M_T = M + M_R + M_X + M_{XR}\,, \tag{1}$$
$$X_T = X + M_X + M_{XR}\,, \tag{2}$$
$$R_T = R + M_R + M_{XR}\,, \tag{3}$$

which state that for each species, the total density must equal the sum of all bound forms plus the free density. We define pseudo-unimolecular association rates $\lambda_i (i=1, \ldots, 4)$ as follows (see **Figure 1A**):

$$\lambda_1 = \Lambda_1 R,\ \lambda_2 = \Lambda_2 X, \tag{4}$$
$$\lambda_3 = \Lambda_3 X,\ \lambda_4 = \Lambda_4 R, \tag{5}$$

where $\Lambda_1 - \Lambda_4$ are the two-dimensional association rates ($\mathrm{cm}^2\mathrm{s}^{-1}$) for TCR/pMHCI or CD8/pMHCI binding. Two-dimensional dissociation constants (cm^{-2}) are defined as follows:

$$K_1 = \frac{\lambda_{-1}}{\lambda_1} R, \tag{6}$$
$$K_2 = \frac{\lambda_{-2}}{\lambda_2} X, \tag{7}$$
$$K_3 = \frac{\lambda_{-3}}{\lambda_3} X, \tag{8}$$
$$K_4 = \frac{\lambda_{-4}}{\lambda_4} R, \tag{9}$$

In order for a system of reactions to be in thermal equilibrium, each individual reaction must be at equilibrium (the principle of detailed balance):

$$\begin{aligned} &\lambda_1 M = \lambda_{-1} M_R,\ \lambda_2 M_R = \lambda_{-2} M_{XR}, \\ &\lambda_3 M = \lambda_{-3} M_X,\ \lambda_4 M_X = \lambda_{-4} M_{XR}, \end{aligned} \tag{10}$$

from which it follows that $K_1K_2 = K_3K_4$. Combining this with the conservation laws with we obtain:

$$\begin{aligned} M &= \frac{M_T}{C},\ M_R = \frac{M_T\lambda_1}{C\lambda_{-1}}, \\ M_X &= \frac{M_T\lambda_3}{C\lambda_{-3}},\ M_{XR} = \frac{M_T\lambda_1\lambda_2}{C\lambda_{-1}\lambda_{-2}}, \end{aligned} \tag{11}$$

where

$$C = 1 + \frac{\lambda_1}{\lambda_{-1}} + \frac{\lambda_3}{\lambda_{-3}} + \frac{\lambda_1\lambda_2}{\lambda_{-1}\lambda_{-2}}. \tag{12}$$

Table 1 | Model parameters and variables.

M	Free pMHCI density
M_R	TCR/pMHCI density without CD8 bound
M_X	pMHCI/CD8 density without TCR bound
M_{XR}	TCR/pMHCI/CD8 density
X	Free CD8 density
R	Free TCR density
M_T	Total pMHCI density
X_T	Total CD8 density
R_T	Total TCR density

These results can also be expressed in terms of standard affinity constants:

$$\begin{aligned} M_R &= \frac{M_T R}{K_1 + R + XK_1/K_3 + RX/K_2}, \\ M_X &= \frac{M_T X}{K_3 + X + RK_3/K_1 + RX/K_4}, \\ M_{XR} &= \frac{M_T XR}{K_1K_2 + RK_2 + XK_4 + RX}. \end{aligned} \tag{13}$$

The co-receptor CD8 modulates the rate of TCR triggering. Three major modulatory functions of the co-receptor have been documented: modulation of TCR/pMHCI on-rate, TCR/pMHCI off-rate, and of the ITAM phosphorylation rate. These effects can be represented by dimensionless multipliers.

(i) enhanced TCR/pMHCI on-rate:

$$\Lambda_4 = \gamma_{\mathrm{on}}\Lambda_1 \text{ where } \gamma_{\mathrm{on}} \geq 1;$$

(ii) reduced TCR/pMHCI off-rate:

$$\lambda_{-4} = \gamma_{\mathrm{off}}\lambda_{-1} \text{ where } 0 < \gamma_{\mathrm{off}} \leq 1;$$

(iii) increased phosphorylation rate, which is equivalent to a reduced TCR triggering threshold T_R^*

$$\lambda = \gamma_R \lambda^*, \text{ where } \gamma_R \leq 1 \text{ and } \lambda = \tfrac{1}{T_R} \text{ and } \lambda^* = \tfrac{1}{T_R^*}. \tag{14}$$

It is sometimes convenient to combine the on-rate and off-rate effects into a single coefficient, as follows:

$$\gamma_{\mathrm{kin}} = \frac{\gamma_{\mathrm{off}}}{\gamma_{\mathrm{on}}} = \frac{K_4}{K_1} = \frac{K_2}{K_3}, \text{ where } 0 < \gamma_{\mathrm{kin}} \leq 1. \tag{15}$$

From equation (15), we have $\gamma_{\mathrm{kin}} \leq \gamma_{\mathrm{off}}$. We rewrite M_R, M_X, and M_{XR}, as given by equation (13), in terms of γ_{kin}:

$$\begin{aligned} M_R &= M_T \frac{R/K_1}{1 + R/K_1 + X/K_3 + RX/(K_1K_3\gamma_{\mathrm{kin}})}, \\ M_X &= M_T \frac{X/K_3}{1 + R/K_1 + X/K_3 + RX/(K_1K_3\gamma_{\mathrm{kin}})}, \\ M_{XR} &= M_T \frac{RX/(K_1K_3)}{\gamma_{\mathrm{kin}}(1 + X/K_3 + R/K_1) + XK_3/(RK_1)}. \end{aligned} \tag{16}$$

To non-dimensionalize this system, we introduce the following dimensionless quantities:

$$x = \frac{X}{K_3}, \quad r = \frac{R}{K_1}, \quad x_T = \frac{X_T}{K_3}, \quad r_T = \frac{R_T}{K_1},$$
$$\kappa = \frac{K_1}{K_3}, \quad m_T = \frac{M_T}{K_1}. \tag{17}$$

It follows from equation (17) that $M_T/K_3 = \kappa m_T$. By equations (16) and (17), we have the following non-linear system of equations that determines the surface densities of free and bound receptors of all species:

$$x_T = x + \kappa m_T \frac{x}{1 + x + r + xr/\gamma_{\text{kin}}} + \kappa m_T \frac{xr}{\gamma_{\text{kin}}(1 + x + r) + xr},$$
$$r_T = r + m_T \frac{r}{1 + x + r + xr/\gamma_{\text{kin}}} + m_T \frac{xr}{\gamma_{\text{kin}}(1 + x + r) + xr}. \tag{18}$$

This system is readily solved numerically for x and r, given the parameters γ_{kin}, κ, r_T, and m_T.

The TCR triggering rate

The functional sensitivity of the TCR is represented in the present model as the rate at which TCR/CD3 complexes attain signalosome status. To calculate this TCR triggering rate, which we shall denote by W, consider the Markov chain as depicted in **Figure 1B**, which is best thought of as a system of two coupled linear Markov chains. The TCR/CD3 complex has to undergo n phosphorylations for the TCR to be triggered. When the co-receptor is not bound to the TCR/pMHCI complex, individual phosphorylation steps proceed at rate $n/T_R \equiv n\lambda$ whereas when the co-receptor is engaged, this rate is $n/T_R^* \equiv n\lambda^* \geq n\lambda$. The factor n arises simply as a matter of scaling, so that the average time to progress through the chain of phosphorylations equals T_R.

In reality, signalosome formation involves several other types of event besides ITAM phosphorylation, such as binding of ZAP-70, engagement of LAT, and so on. To avoid cumbersome notation we shall formulate the model as if ITAM phosphorylation were the only type of event; the essential theory is not materially affected by this simplification. We do not assume an equilibrium state for the Markov chain: the complex starts at zero phosphorylations at the beginning of every encounter with a pMHCI ligand and proceeds forward stochastically.

The pMHCI/TCR/CD3 complex may not attain the nth state (triggered state), but instead the pMHCI/TCR engagement may terminate, which happens at rate λ_{-1} when the co-receptor is not bound and at rate $\lambda_{-4} \leq \lambda_{-1}$ when the co-receptor is engaged. We assume that upon TCR/pMHCI dissociation the CD3 complex reverts to the basal state of zero ITAM phosphorylations sufficiently rapidly that the TCR/CD3 complex will be in this completely unphosphorylated state when the next encounter with a pMHCI molecule occurs. Essentially, this means that the CD3 complex is more susceptible to the action of phosphorylases and/or less susceptible to the action of kinases when the TCR is not engaged. A mechanistic explanation underpinning this assumption lies outside the scope of the present model.

The probability that the TCR/CD3 complex will undergo another ITAM phosphorylation is given by

$$\mathbb{P}_a^0 = \frac{n\lambda}{\lambda_{-1} + n\lambda + \lambda_2} \tag{19}$$

in the case where the co-receptor CD8 is not engaged and by

$$\mathbb{P}_a^* = \frac{n\lambda^*}{\lambda_{-4} + n\lambda^* + \lambda_{-2}} \tag{20}$$

when CD8 is engaged. The following expression gives the probability that the system switches from the chain with CD8 unbound to the chain with CD8 bound:

$$\mathbb{P}_b^0 = \frac{\lambda_2}{\lambda_{-1} + n\lambda + \lambda_2} \tag{21}$$

whereas the system will switch from CD8-unbound to CD8-bound with probability

$$\mathbb{P}_b^* = \frac{\lambda_{-2}}{\lambda_{-4} + n\lambda^* + \lambda_{-2}}. \tag{22}$$

TCR triggering requires completion of all steps before the TCR/pMHCI complex comes apart. We shall find an expression for the probability that the CD3 complex will ultimately attain completion when starting from i completed steps. Let $\mathbb{P}_i^0$ denote this probability for the case with CD8 unbound and $\mathbb{P}_i^*$ for the case with CD8 bound. The TCR triggering probability is then found as $\mathbb{P}_0^0$ if CD8 is unbound when pMHCI docks the TCR, and $\mathbb{P}_0^*$ if CD8 is bound. These triggering probabilities allow us to calculate the TCR triggering rate W. In particular, W can be expressed as the rate at which TCR/pMHCI complexes dissociate, times the probability that whenever a given TCR/pMHCI docking commences, the CD3 complex is ultimately triggered (the probabilities P_0^0 and P_0^*). In formula, this statement is represented as follows:

$$W = M\lambda_1 \mathbb{P}_0^0 + M_X \lambda_4 \mathbb{P}_0^* \tag{23}$$

which, by the principle of detailed balance, can be rewritten in terms of *dissociation rates*, as follows:

$$W = R\lambda_{-1}\mathbb{P}_0^0 + M_{XR}\lambda_{-4}\mathbb{P}_0^*. \tag{24}$$

The law of total probability yields the following system of coupled difference equations:

$$\begin{bmatrix} \mathbb{P}_{i-1}^0 \\ \mathbb{P}_{i-1}^* \end{bmatrix} = \frac{1}{1 - \mathbb{P}_b^0\mathbb{P}_b^*} \begin{bmatrix} \mathbb{P}_a^0 & \mathbb{P}_b^0\mathbb{P}_a^* \\ \mathbb{P}_b^*\mathbb{P}_a^0 & \mathbb{P}_a^* \end{bmatrix} \begin{bmatrix} \mathbb{P}_i^0 \\ \mathbb{P}_i^* \end{bmatrix} \tag{25}$$

which can be solved to give

$$\begin{bmatrix} \mathbb{P}_0^0 \\ \mathbb{P}_0^* \end{bmatrix} = \frac{1}{(1 - \mathbb{P}_b^0\mathbb{P}_b^*)^n} \begin{bmatrix} \mathbb{P}_a^0 & \mathbb{P}_b^0\mathbb{P}_a^* \\ \mathbb{P}_b^*\mathbb{P}_a^0 & \mathbb{P}_a^* \end{bmatrix}^n \begin{bmatrix} 1 \\ 1 \end{bmatrix} \tag{26}$$

where we have used the boundary condition

$$P_n^0 = P_n^* = 1. \tag{27}$$

This boundary condition expresses the basic assumption that triggering is attained when the sequence has been completed. To render the equations dimensionless, we introduce the following parameters:

$$\nu = \frac{\Lambda_2 K_3}{\lambda}, \alpha = \frac{\lambda_{-1}}{\lambda}, \delta = \frac{\lambda_{-2}}{\lambda}. \quad (28)$$

The scaled (dimensionless) TCR triggering rate is then given by the following expression:

$$w = \alpha(\epsilon \mathbb{P}_0^0 + \zeta\gamma_{\text{off}}\mathbb{P}_0^*) \quad (29)$$

where

$$w = \frac{W}{K_1 m_T \lambda}; \quad (30)$$

$$\varepsilon = \frac{r}{1 + x + r + xr/\gamma_{\text{kin}}}; \quad (31)$$

$$\zeta = \frac{xr}{\gamma_{\text{kin}}(1 + x + r) + xr}. \quad (32)$$

The scaled TCR triggering rate w depends on ten dimensionless parameters (**Table 2**).

STATISTICAL FORMULATION OF TCR DEGENERACY

To express TCR degeneracy mathematically, we consider the distribution of the triggering rate over the set of peptide ligands. This is just the set of w_{ij}-values for a given TCR clonotype i over pMHCI ligands j. The distribution can be represented by plotting the probability $\mathbb{P}(w_{ij} > \omega)$ as a function of ω. Such a graph shows how many randomly selected peptides would have triggering rate w larger than a set value ω. Let T_{ij} denote the mean dwell time of the TCR/pMHCI interaction for TCR clonotype i and pMHCI species j so that T_{ij}^{-1} is the TCR/pMHCI off-rate λ_{-1} (we have thus far suppressed subscripts for clone i and ligand j to keep notation uncluttered). Arrhenius theory furnishes the following relationship with the dissociation energy barrier ΔU_{ij}:

$$T_{ij} = T_0 \exp(\Delta U_{ij}), \quad (33)$$

where T_0 is the frequency factor and ΔU_{ij} is expressed in Boltzmann units. We assume that the dissociation energy barrier arises as a result of a large number of individual reaction steps at the TCR/pMHCI interface. If these combine additively, then the Central Limit Theorem implies that ΔU_{ij} has a Gaussian distribution. Letting $u_{ij} = \Delta U_{ij} - \ln\{T_R/T_0\}$ we have $u_{ij} \sim N(-\mu, \sigma^2)$, where $\mu > 0$ and σ are the underlying parameters of the normal distribution N. The assumption that the mean is negative is a consequence of the fact that for the vast majority of TCR/pMHCI complexes the mean dwell time is less than the typical time required to complete the chain of ITAM phosphorylations. It now follows that the dimensionless parameter α, associated with the TCR/pMHCI off-rate, is log-normally distributed.

RESULTS

We investigated the effect of variations of the total CD8 density on the functional sensitivity of hypothetical ligands with various TCR/pMHCI off-rates. All variables and parameters are dimensionless (scaled) in the model simulations. The scaled parameters are summarized in **Table 2** and their scaling is defined in equations (14), (15), (17), and (28).

Table 2 | Dimensionless (scaled) parameters that govern functional sensitivity.

m_T	Scaled total pMHCI density
x_T	Scaled total CD8 density
r_T	Scaled total TCR density
α	Scaled TCR/pMHCI off-rate without CD8 bound
δ	Scaled pMHCI/CD8 off-rate with TCR bound
ν	Scaled kinetic effect of pMHCI/CD8 interactions with and without TCR
κ	Ratio of dissociation constants K_1 and K_3
γ_{off}	Factor by which CD8 modulates TCR/pMHCI off-rate
γ_{kin}	Factor by which CD8 modulates the TCR/pMHCI affinity
γ_R	Factor by which CD8 modulates the TCR triggering threshold

LIGAND FOCUSING AND CD8-MEDIATED CONTROL OF DEGENERACY

Figure 2A shows the scaled functional sensitivity w as a function of scaled total CD8 density x_T with different scaled TCR/pMHCI off-rates α. A striking feature is the dip at $x_T \approx 50$, suggesting that at this CD8 density the T-cell is minimally responsive. As the scaled total CD8 density increases above $x_T \approx 50$, the scaled functional sensitivity increases for all hypothetical ligands.

It can be observed that a ligand with $\alpha = 2.5$ (solid line) and a ligand with $\alpha = 0.5$ (dotted line) show opposing changes in the scaled functional sensitivity: a ligand that is less potent at low CD8 becomes more potent at high CD8 and *vice versa.* Hence, changes in CD8 expression levels can differentially affect the potency of ligands, each of which is potentially a strong agonist. In effect, the T-cell can tune in on a specific ligand and thus control ligand promiscuity. We call this the principle of *ligand focusing.*

The corresponding degeneracy curves $\mathbb{P}(w > \omega)$ for different scaled total CD8 densities are shown in **Figure 2B**. The effect of the increase in co-receptor density on the sensitivity and degeneracy is indicated: sensitivity is a change in the horizontal direction (modulating the triggering threshold) and degeneracy is a change in the vertical direction (controlling cross-reactivity). As the scaled total CD8 density increases up to $x_T \approx 50$, the degeneracy curves $P(w > \omega)$ move to the left from the curve without CD8 ($x_T = 0$): degeneracy and sensitivity decrease. By contrast, as the scaled total CD8 density increases above $x_T \approx 50$, the degeneracy curves move to the right, which means that degeneracy and sensitivity both increase. The overall effect is that the T-cell becomes more degenerate as CD8 levels increase. Thus, in addition to the focusing effect, the co-receptor also governs the overall degeneracy of the T-cell.

A high degree of degeneracy can increase the risk autoimmune disease. On the other hand, too low a degree of degeneracy could compromise the immune system's ability to mount a timely and efficient response. To analyze these risks, suppose that the T-cell is activated if its integrated TCR triggering rate exceeds a certain value, termed *cellular activation threshold.* A simple model is to

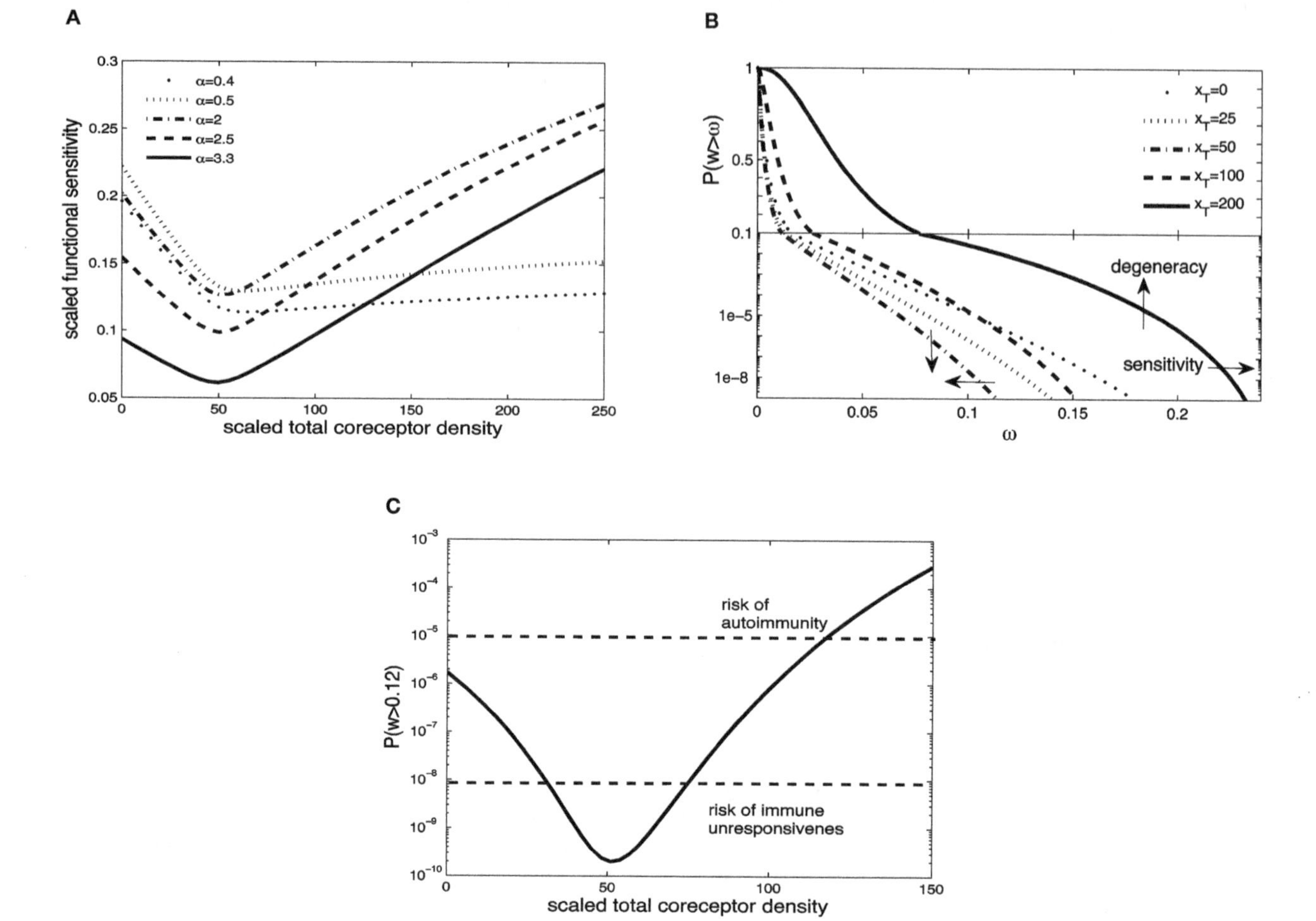

FIGURE 2 | (A) Scaled functional sensitivity w as a function of scaled total CD8 density x_T for various scaled TCR/pMHCI off-rates α. **(B)** Degeneracy curves $\mathbb{P}(w > \omega)$ for various scaled total CD8 density x_T. **(C)** The probability $\mathbb{P}(w > \omega)$ as a function of CD8 density x_T, at a set value of functional sensitivity $\omega = 0.12$. The operating range of the probability $\mathbb{P}$ is shown as a function of x_T with dashed lines at $\mathbb{P}(w > 0.12) = 10^{-8}$ and $\mathbb{P}(w > 0.12) = 10^{-5}$. Parameter values: $\delta = 300$, $\nu = 0.5$, $n = 100$, $\gamma_{kin} = 0.5$, $\gamma_{off} = 0.5$, $\gamma_R = 0.3$, $\kappa = 5$, $m_T = 10$, $r_T = 10$. The log-normal distribution has mean 2 and SD 0.2.

assume that the T-cell is activated if

$$Z_j T_I w_{ij} > W_{act} \tag{34}$$

where Z_j is the presentation level of ligand j, T_I is the duration of the T-cell:APC interaction, and W_{act} is the activation threshold. For a given Z_j and T_I, there is a critical w_{ij} which is the minimum value required to satisfy equation (34). Suppose for instance that this corresponds to $w_{ij} = 0.12$. The corresponding probabilities $\mathbb{P}(w > 0.12)$ are plotted in **Figure 2C**. Given the estimates of the TCR repertoire size, normal immune function is probably confined to an operating range of probabilities 10^{-8} to 10^{-5}. **Figure 2C** shows how the level of CD8 can regulate the responsiveness to remain within this band; if the activation probability drops below this range, the risk of not responding to a pathogen looms, whereas at much elevated activation probabilities, the risk of autoimmunity is heightened.

MODES OF CD8-MEDIATED MODULATION OF FUNCTIONAL SENSITIVITY

Figures 3 and **4** exhibit the co-receptor effect on functional sensitivity in two parameter scenarios, where we assume a weak ($\nu = 0.05$) or a strong ($\nu = 300$) kinetic effect of pMHCI/CD8 interactions, respectively. When the kinetic parameter ν is small, increasing the levels of CD8 on the T-cell surface leads to enhanced functional sensitivity of ligands with $\alpha > 1$, as shown in **Figure 3A**. By contrast, ligands with low off-rates ($\alpha < 1$) become less potent when CD8 levels are increased. These opposite effects demonstrate CD8-mediated focusing on particular ligands.

Figure 3B shows the effect of increasing CD8 levels on a ligand that is optimal in the absence of CD8. When the modulatory effect of CD8 on the TCR triggering threshold is modest (γ_R is near 1), the ligand becomes less potent as levels of CD8 are increased. On the other hand, when CD8 has a strong effect on the TCR triggering threshold (low γ_R, since the time required to trigger the TCR/CD3 complex is shortened), increasing the levels of CD8 on the cell surface enhances the functional sensitivity to the ligand.

The effect of CD8 levels on functional sensitivity is shown in **Figure 4A**. For each ligand, there is an optimal CD8 level which depends on that ligand's TCR/pMHCI off-rate α. This shows that the T-cell can favor the signaling strength of a given ligand by

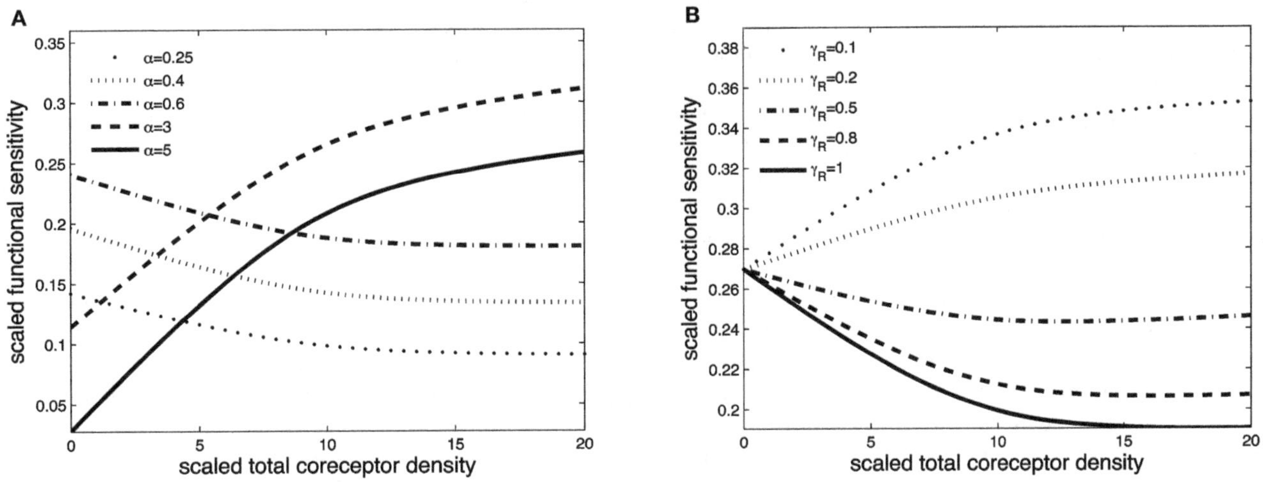

FIGURE 3 | Scaled functional sensitivity w as a function of scaled total CD8 density x_T. **(A)** Curves for various values of the scaled TCR/pMHCI off-rate α. **(B)** Curves for various values of the factor γ_R by which CD8 modulates the TCR triggering threshold. Parameter values in **(A,B)**: $\delta = 2.5$, $\nu = 0.05$, $n = 100$, $\gamma_{kin} = 0.5$, $\gamma_{off} = 0.5$, $\gamma_R = 0.5$, $\kappa = 1$, $m_T = 10$, $r_T = 10$, $\alpha = 1$.

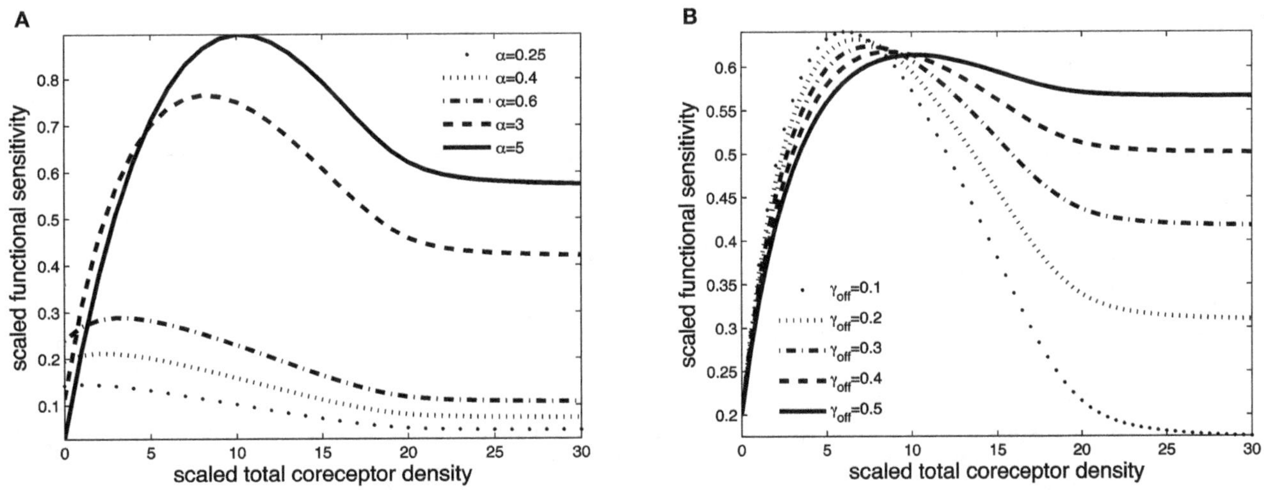

FIGURE 4 | Scaled functional sensitivity w as a function of scaled total CD8 density x_T. **(A)** Curves for various values of the scaled TCR/pMHCI off-rate α. **(B)** Curves for various values of the dimensionless factor γ_{off} expressing the modulatory effect of CD8 on the TCR/pMHCI off-rate. Parameter values in **(A,B)** $\delta = 3$, $\nu = 300$, $n = 100$, $\gamma_{kin} = 0.05$, $\gamma_{off} = 0.2$, $\gamma_R = 0.5$, $\kappa = 2$, $m_T = 10$, $r_T = 10$, $\alpha = 2$.

adjusting the density of CD8 molecules on its surface. As one would expect, the modulatory effect is most profound when the relative effect that the co-receptor exerts on the TCR/pMHCI off-rate is greatest; this is shown in **Figure 4B**. When CD8 alters the off-rate strongly, the functional sensitivity is strongly depressed when CD8 levels are increased beyond the optimal level, whereas for a moderate value of the modulatory multiplier γ_{off}, the functional sensitivity remains at near-optimal levels when CD8 levels are increased. The value of γ_{off} may be expected to be different for different TCR/ligand combinations. In particular, when CD8 makes a substantial contribution to the binding energy, the multiplier γ_{off} will be low, and the co-receptor role in governing ligand optimality will be more pronounced.

CO-RECEPTOR MODULATION OF DEGENERACY VIA ALTERED pMHCI/CD8 BINDING AFFINITY

Wooldridge et al. (5, 30, 31) have shown that (i) increased pMHCI/CD8 interaction results in enhanced recognition of pMHCI by cytotoxic T-cells and (ii) increased pMHCI/CD8 interaction impairs pMHCI recognition specificity, suggesting that the pMHCI-CD8 interaction is essential in regulating the balance between optimal T-cell cross-reactivity and T-cell antigen specificity (32). These findings suggest that an optimal pMHCI/CD8 strength exists that yields maximum pMHCI sensitivity without loss of specificity. Motivated by these results, we consider a hypothetical scenario in which pMHCI mutant molecules with altered binding affinity for CD8 modulate TCR degeneracy.

In keeping with (17), the following pMHCI mutants are considered: A245V representing weak pMHCI/CD8 affinity ($K_D = 498\,\mu M$), wild-type ($K_D = 137.1\,\mu M$), Q115E representing slightly enhanced affinity ($K_D = 97.94\,\mu M$), and A2/α3k^b with enhanced affinity ($K_D = 10.87\,\mu M$). These values are based on Surface Plasmon Resonance experiments and should be regarded as "three-dimensional," relating to the ligands in solution. However, the TCR/pMHCI interaction takes place in the "two-dimensional" environment of the T-cell:contact area, which essentially reduces spatial degrees of freedom of molecular motion and, moreover, introduces dynamics related to the forces that constrain the molecules to this environment, such as rotations with respect to the membrane plane, membrane fluctuations, and the translational motion of the membranes themselves (33). Furthermore, cooperativity interactions, such as the involvement of the co-receptor, may be profoundly altered. As a result, the rate constants can be markedly different in the "two-dimensional" environment; in particular, two-dimensional dissociation rates can be substantially faster (28). The ratio between the three- and two-dimensional affinities is a length measure, denoted h and called the confinement length (34, 35). Wu et al. (33) demonstrated that h is proportional to the range of motion available to the free forms of the interacting ligands along the spatial axis perpendicular to the two parallel membranes. Thus the inter-membrane separation distance provides an upper bound, and if the ranges of motion are broadly comparable, we may assume that the confinement length is roughly the same for all mutants involved.

The two-dimensional dissociation constant for pMHCI/CD8 interaction without TCR bound, K_3, appears in the scaled parameters κ, x_T, and ν. Hence, by taking K_3 to be proportional to K_D for a given pMHCI mutant, we can simulate the impact of the altered pMHC/CD8 binding affinity on TCR degeneracy and sensitivity. **Figure 5A** shows the scaled functional sensitivity w as a function of scaled TCR/pMHCI off-rate α for the four hypothetical pMHCI mutants.

The co-receptor CD8 can modulate the specificity of antigen recognition, as shown in **Figure 5B**. Each TCR degeneracy curve corresponds to a given pMHCI mutant, where the one with the strongest pMHCI/CD8 binding affinity (A2/α3k^b) is the most degenerate, with the largest antigen sensitivity. The three regions are a schematic representation of the overall pattern of CD8$^+$ T-cell antigen specificity, as defined by Cole et al. (32). With increasing strength of pMHCI/CD8 affinity, as indicated by the arrow, the recognition efficiency of partially CD8-dependent ligands is enhanced and the spectrum of CD8$^+$ T-cell antigen degeneracy becomes wider. Enhancing the kinetic effect of pMHCI/CD8 interactions (setting $\nu \gg 1$) results in the reversed pattern, as shown in **Figure 5C**.

Whereas in the MHC-limited kinetic regime, the behavior is as shown in **Figure 5B**, the degeneracy curves for the various mutants overlap in the TCR-limited regime. This suggests that excess levels of ligand, relative to the available levels of TCR molecules, can diminish the importance of the interaction between pMHCI and CD8. In principle, this endows the APC with a means to "override" the ligand focusing exerted by the T-cell, allowing a professional APC, such as a dendritic cell, to force a naïve T-cell, with which it has conjugated, to be maximally degenerate.

DISCUSSION

The co-receptors CD4 and CD8 are glycoproteins that modulate the interactions of the TCR with pMHCI and pMHCII molecules, by binding to invariant sites on these molecules (10). It is well-established that the co-receptors differentially regulate the responsiveness of the TCR to the ligand and thereby modulate TCR specificity (1). In particular, CD8 is known to affect both the on-rate and the off-rate of the TCR/pMHCI interaction (17, 36). This allows the co-receptor to differentially regulate the strengths of the various *potentially* strong agonists of the TCR. This accords with the finding that the strength of pMHCI/CD8 interaction is a determinant of T-cell degeneracy (5). This ligand focusing effect remains to be observed experimentally, to the best of our knowledge. Perhaps this is only to be expected inasmuch as the experimenter has to search for ligands that are sub-optimal under standard conditions but become better or worse agonists when CD8 levels are manipulated. Research is presently underway to identify such ligands and we anticipate that the phenomenon will be confirmed and eventually emerge as a pervasive "design principle" of cellular adaptive immunity.

Co-receptor-directed ligand focusing may allow the T-cell response to an antigen challenge to undergo an adaptive evolution that would be functionally analogous to affinity maturation in B-cell immunity. Moreover, CD8 modulation could allow for an elevated degeneracy among the earliest responding clones. This would ensure that at least one or more responding clones are activated sufficiently early in the course of the infection. Moreover, a gradual restriction of the degeneracy, coupled with an increase in functional sensitivity to the salient epitope, would then reduce the degeneracy of the response, which would gradually evolve from oligoclonal to one that is dominated by an optimally tuned single clone.

Disrupting the pMHCI/CD8 interaction impairs the ability of T-cells to recognize antigens. In particular, T-cell activation can be abrogated if the pMHCI/CD8 interaction is blocked (32), whereas increases in pMHCI/CD8 affinity have the opposite effect (37, 38). The contribution of CD8 to increase functional sensitivity appears to be crucial for weaker agonists (36). A comprehensive evaluation of clonal CD8$^+$ T-cell degeneracy using combinatorial peptide libraries and APCs expressing mutant HLA A*0201 molecules with altered pMHCI/CD8 affinity has shown that the co-receptor enhances T-cell degeneracy by increasing the range of agonist ligands that can elicit T-cell activation (5). Furthermore, increasing the affinity of CD8 for HLA A*0201 by at least an order of magnitude resulted in the loss of cognate antigen specificity (5, 31). The affinity of the pMHCI/CD8 interaction may be directly linked to TCR degeneracy: increased pMHCI/CD8 interaction enhances CD8$^+$ T-cell antigen sensitivity, but reduces CD8$^+$ T-cell antigen specificity (32). This agrees with our main finding that variation of the co-receptor effect regulates the degree of T-cell degeneracy and antigen specificity.

A cornerstone of the present theory is that a certain amount of degeneracy is unavoidable, in view of the vast universe of possible peptides and the relatively modest number of TCR clonotypes that even a large mammal might be able to maintain in its standing repertoire. Moreover, salient epitopes, those associated with a disease state, and non-salient ones, such as self-peptides

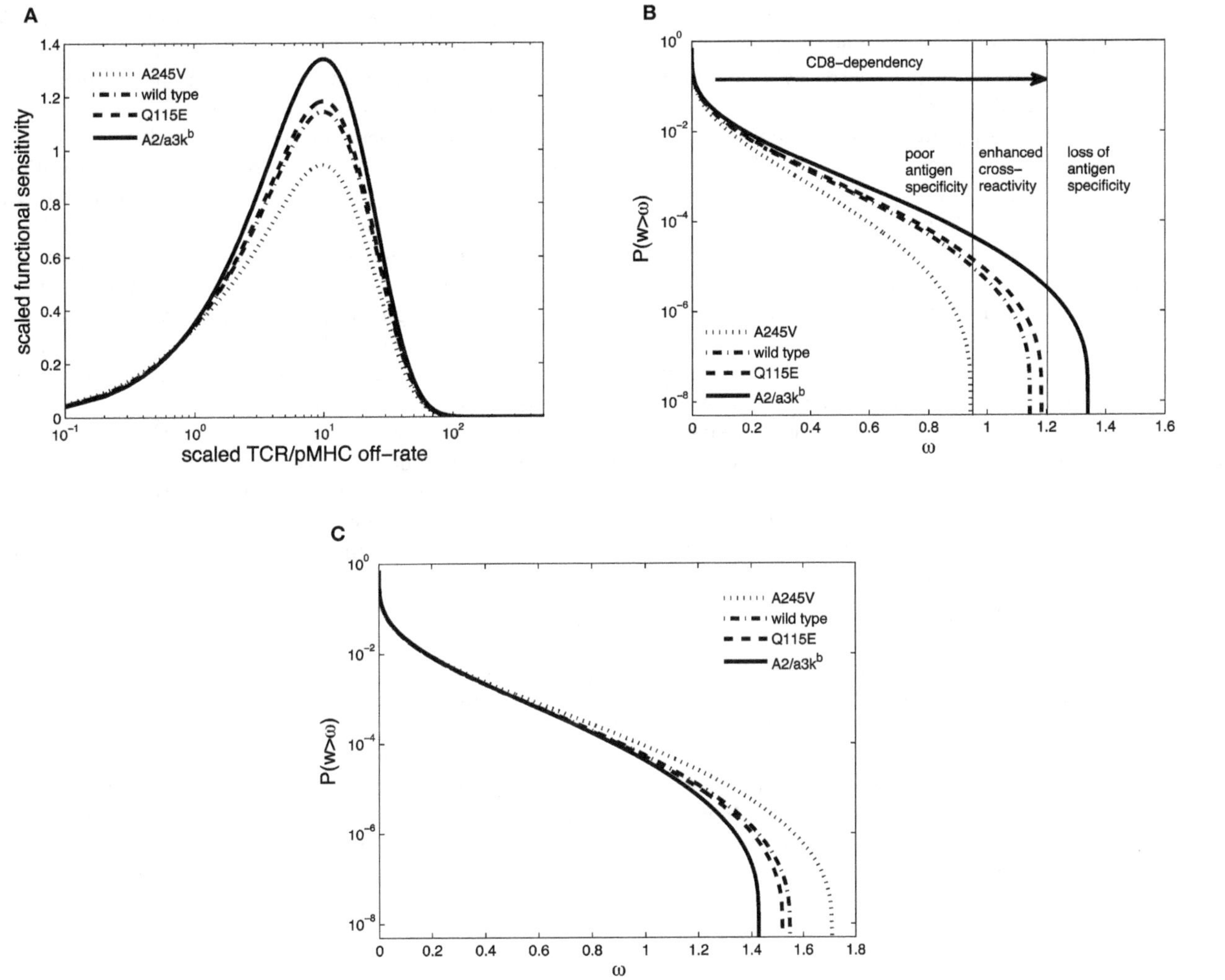

FIGURE 5 | (A) Scaled functional sensitivity w as a function of scaled TCR/pMHCI off-rate α. **(B)** Degeneracy curves $\mathbb{P}(w > \omega)$ for HLA A*0201 mutants with altered binding affinity for CD8: A245V (dotted line), wild-type (semi-dashed line), Q115E (dashed line), and A2/α3k^b (solid line). The three regions represent the overall pattern of CD8$^+$ T-cell antigen specificity and the arrow indicates the strength of pMHCI/CD8 interaction. **(C)** Degeneracy curves $\mathbb{P}(w > \omega)$ for HLA A*0201 mutants with altered binding affinity for CD8. The parameter values are the same as in A except for $\nu = 10$. Parameter values in **(A,B)**: $\delta = 0.2$, $\nu = 0.05$, $n = 100$, $\gamma_{kin} = 0.5$, $\gamma_{off} = 0.5$, $\gamma_R = 0.2$, $\kappa = 1$, $m_T = 10$, $r_T = 10$, $x_T = 10$. The log-normal distribution has mean 5 and SD 0.5.

for which immune tolerance is required, will of necessity be "finely interleaved" subsets of the peptide universe (a mathematician would say that one subset is "dense" in the other), lest the tolerant subset forms a target for the rapidly evolving pathogens: the system cannot work if molecular mimicry is readily attained. From these two premises, it follows that a TCR must be degenerate, and also that this degeneracy must be susceptible to exquisite modulation. Against this line of reasoning a case could be made that the size of the ligand universe is effectively much smaller. For instance, if one considers n-mer peptides that are anchored to the MHC binding groove at a positions, and the region of the TCR that interacts with the peptide (roughly speaking, the CDR3 loop) makes contacts with c of the amino acid residues in the m-mer (so that $0 < m \leq n - a$), then there are $20^m(n-a)!/(m!(n-a-m)!)$ effectively distinct pMHCI ligands as seen by the TCR. To give an extreme example, with $n = 9$, $a = 2$, and $m = 1$, this works out as just $20 \times 7 = 140$ distinct ligands. Perhaps the estimate $m = 4$ is more realistic: this gives only $20^4 \times 35 = 5.6 \times 10^6$ functionally distinct ligands, which is of the same order as the TCR repertoire size. Whereas there may be some merit to this argument, its underlying image, essentially of CDR3 as a tape recorder head that interacts with only m amino acid residues and is indifferent to the $n - m$ other ones, is a gross oversimplification. The physical behavior of the m amino acid residues at the contact sites cannot fail to be influenced by the $n - m$ remaining ones (including the a anchor residues). This is overwhelmingly apparent not just from the basic principles of molecular dynamics, but also from the typical results obtained with combinatorial peptide library scans. A case in point is the finding that changes at the anchor position result in changes in the center of the peptide and therefore influence TCR binding (39, 40).

The present model indicates that intermediate levels of CD8 are associated with the lowest functional sensitivity. This suggests the following mechanism to maintain quiescent (naïve) T-cells in a relatively unresponsive state. When the T-cell receives the appropriate stimuli, it either up-regulates or down-regulates the co-receptor and a specific subset of its potential agonists "comes into focus." Such signals are known to be transmitted via cytokine profiles in the T-cell's surroundings (15) as well as costimulatory receptor-mediated signals transmitted by professional APCs (41). When no harm is detected, the default response of the naïve T-cells would be to "de-tune" whenever a strong signal is registered. Detuning of T-cells via alterations of CD8 expression levels, under control of cytokine stimuli, has been reported (42) and the connection between functional sensitivity, tolerance, and CD8 expression levels is well-established (14, 43, 44). On the other hand, when harm is detected and transmitted via a pro-inflammatory cytokine profile, the T-cell's response would invert and the tendency would become to "tune in" to any supra-threshold stimulation. On a molecular-cellular level, this would involve a scanning mechanism whereby the stimulus would make the cell enter a mode in which it gradually alters the CD8 expression level whilst the received TCR signal (which will shift in magnitude as the CD8 level changes) feeds back onto this pathway. To the best of our knowledge, the molecular details of such a regulatory pathway have not been elucidated to date. However, we believe that it is well within the regulatory capabilities of cellular signaling networks; we have previously discussed similar mechanisms in more depth (45, 46).

Whilst the model includes the key components of TCR triggering, many important aspects have been omitted. In particular, we have neglected the spatial dynamics of TCR, CD8, and pMHCI within the immunological synapse, where the relative concentrations of $p56^{lck}$ and CD45 will determine how quickly partially phosphorylated TCR/CD3 will reset to the basic state (47). A functional consequence of the exclusion of phosphorylases, for instance, could be the ability of the TCR/CD3 complex to be triggered over subsequent interactions with ligands that would in a normal context only have weak functional sensitivity.

In addition to kinetics of the interaction between TCR, MHCI, and CD8, we have only considered ITAM phosphorylation steps. It is well known that phosphorylated ITAMs orchestrate the activation of the Src-related protein tyrosine kinases which initiate TCR signaling. These kinases induce tyrosine phosphorylation of several polypeptides, including the transmembrane adaptors. Protein tyrosine phosphorylation subsequently leads to the activation of multiple pathways such as ERK, NF-κB, and NFAT (48, 49). Moreover, negative regulation of TCR signaling is key to avoiding hyper-activation. Notwithstanding the additional layers of complexity which our simple model ignores, we believe that the system of two linked proofreading chains as presented here does capture, in a qualitative sense, the essence of TCR triggering.

In summary, the present findings suggest that the co-receptor CD8 can differentially modulate functional sensitivity to its potential agonists, thereby modulating TCR degeneracy in a tunable fashion. The ligand focusing mechanism would allow each T-cell to have a wide range of potential agonists, even while only one of these would be a ligand of high functional sensitivity at any particular moment in time.

ACKNOWLEDGMENTS

This work was supported by the Biotechnology and Biological Sciences Research Council (grant BB/H001085/1) and the Wellcome Trust (Grants WT079848MA, WT096454AIA, and WT099067AIA). The authors are indebted to the reviewers for their constructive comments.

REFERENCES

1. Parham P. *The Immune System*. New York: Garland Publishing (2000).
2. Wooldridge L, Ekeruch-Makinde J, van den Berg HA, Skowera A, Miles JJ, Tan MP, et al. A single autoimmune T cell receptor recognizes more than a million different peptides. *J Biol Chem* (2012) **287**:1168–77. doi:10.1074/jbc.M111.289488
3. Mason D. A very high level of crossreactivity is an essential feature of the T-cell receptor. *Immunol Today* (1998) **19**:395–404. doi:10.1016/S0167-5699(98)01299-7
4. Wilson DB, Wilson DH, Schroder K, Pinilla C, Blondelle S, Houghten RA, et al. Specificity and degeneracy of T cells. *Mol Immunol* (2004) **40**:1047–55. doi:10.1016/j.molimm.2003.11.022
5. Wooldridge L, Laugel B, Ekeruche J, Clement M, van den Berg HA, Price DA, et al. CD8 controls T cell cross-reactivity. *J Immunol* (2010) **185**:4625–32. doi:10.4049/jimmunol.1001480
6. van den Berg HA, Rand DA. Antigen presentation on MHC molecules as a diversity filter that enhances immune efficacy. *J Theor Biol* (2003) **224**:249–67. doi:10.1016/S0022-5193(03)00162-0
7. Nikolich-Žuglich J, Slifka MK, Messaoudi I. The many important facets of T-cell repertoire diversity. *Nat Rev Immunol* (2004) **4**:123–32. doi:10.1038/nri1292
8. Regner M. Cross-reactivity in T-cell recognition. *Immunol Cell Biol* (2001) **79**:91–100. doi:10.1046/j.1440-1711.2001.00994.x
9. van den Berg HA, Molina-París C, Sewell AK. Specific T-cell activation in an unspecific T-cell repertoire. *Sci Prog* (2011) **94**:245–64. doi:10.3184/003685011X13139280383942
10. Sewell AK. Why must T cells be cross-reactive? *Nat Rev Immunol* (2012) **12**:669–77. doi:10.1038/nri3279
11. Purbhoo MA, Boulter JM, Price DA, Vuidepot A-L, Hourigan CS, Dunbar PR, et al. The human CD8 coreceptor effects cytotoxic T cell activation and antigen sensitivity primarily by mediating complete phosphorylation of the T cell receptor ζ chain. *J Biol Chem* (2001) **276**:32786–32792. doi:10.1074/jbc.M102498200
12. Werlen G, Palmer E. The TCR signalosome: a dynamic structure with expanding complexity. *Curr Opin Immunol* (2002) **14**:299–305. doi:10.1016/S0952-7915(02)00339-4
13. Filipp D, Zhang J, Leung BL, Shaw A, Levin SD, Veillette A, et al. Regulation of Fyn through translocation of activated Lck into lipid rafts. *J Exp Med* (2003) **197**:1221–1227. doi:10.1084/jem.20022112
14. Maile R, Siler CA, Kerry SE, Midkiff KE, Collins EJ, Frelinger JA. Peripheral "CD8 tuning" dynamically modulates the size and responsiveness of an antigen-specific T cell pool in vivo. *J Immunol* (2005) **174**:619–627.
15. Park J-H, Adoro S, Lucas PJ, Sarafova SD, Alag AS, Doan LL, et al. 'Coreceptor tuning': cytokine signals transcriptionally tailor CD8 coreceptor expression to the self-specificity of the TCR. *Nat Immunol* (2007) **8**:1049–58. doi:10.1038/ni1512
16. van den Berg HA, Wooldridge L, Laugel B, Sewell AK. Coreceptor CD8-driven modulation of T cell antigen receptor specificity. *J Theor Biol* (2007) **249**:395–408. doi:10.1016/j.jtbi.2007.08.002
17. Wooldridge L, van den Berg HA, Glick M, Gostick E, Laugel SLHB, Milicic A, et al. Interaction between the CD8 coreceptor and major histocompatibility complex class I stabilizes T cell receptor-antigen complexes at the cell surface. *J Biol Chem* (2005) **280**:27491–501. doi:10.1074/jbc.M500555200
18. Wooldridge L, Lissina A, van den Berg HA, Price DA, Sewell AK. Tricks with tetramers: how to get the most from multimeric peptide-MHC. *Immunology* (2009) **126**:147–64. doi:10.1111/j.1365-2567.2008.02848.x

19. Kalergis AM, Boucheron N, Doucey M, Palmieri E, Goyarts EC, Vegh Z, et al. Efficient T cell activation requires an optimal dwell-time of interaction between the TCR and the pMHC complex. *Nat Immunol* (2001) **2**:229–34. doi:10.1038/85286
20. Tian S, Maile R, Collins EJ, Frelinger JA. $CD8^+$ T cell activation is governed by TCR-peptide/MHC affinity, not dissociation rate. *J Immunol* (2007) **179**:2952–60.
21. van den Berg HA, Rand DA, Burroughs NJ. A reliable and safe T cell repertoire based on low-affinity T cell receptors. *J Theor Biol* (2001) **209**:465–486. doi:10.1006/jtbi.2001.2281
22. van den Berg HA, Burroughs NJ, Rand DA. Quantifying the strength of ligand antagonism in TCR triggering. *Bull Math Biol* (2002) **64**:781–808. doi:10.1006/bulm.2002.0302
23. van den Berg HA, Ladell K, Miners K, Laugel B, Llewellyn-Lacey S, Clement M, et al. Cellular-level versus receptor-level response threshold hierarchies in T-cell activation. *Front Immunol* (2013) **4**:250. doi:10.3389/fimmu.2013.00250
24. McKeithan TW. Kinetic proofreading in T-cell receptor signal transduction. *Proc Natl Acad Sci U S A* (1995) **92**:5042–6. doi:10.1073/pnas.92.11.5042
25. Rabinowitz JD, Beeson C, Lyons DS, Davis MM, McConnell HM. Kinetic discrimination in T-cell activation. *Immunology* (1996) **93**:1401–5.
26. Dushek O, Das R, Coombs D. A role for rebinding in rapid and reliable T cell responses to antigen. *PLoS Comput Biol* (2009) **50**:e1000578. doi:10.1371/journal.pcbi.1000578
27. Jansson AA. A mathematical framework for analyzing T cell receptor scanning of peptides. *Biophys J* (2010) **99**:2717–25. doi:10.1016/j.bpj.2010.08.024
28. Zarnitsyna V, Zhu C. T cell triggering: insights from 2D kinetics analysis of molecular interactions. *Phys Biol* (2012) **9**(4):045005. doi:10.1088/1478-3975/9/4/045005
29. Valitutti S, Lanzavecchia A. Serial triggering of TCRs: a basis for the sensitivity and specificity of antigen recognition. *Immunol Today* (1997) **18**:299–304. doi:10.1016/S0167-5699(97)80027-8
30. Wooldridge L, Lissina A, Vernazza J, Gostick E, Laugel B, Hutchinson SL, et al. Enhanced immunogenicity of CTL antigens through mutation of the CD8 binding MHC class I invariant region. *Eur J Immunol* (2007) **37**:1323–33. doi:10.1002/eji.200636765
31. Wooldridge L, Clement M, Lissina A, Edwards ES, Ladell K, Ekeruche J, et al. MHC class I molecules with superenhanced CD8 binding properties bypass the requirement for cognate TCR recognition and nonspecifically activate CTLs. *Immunol* (2010) **184**:3357–66. doi:10.4049/jimmunol.0902398
32. Cole DK, Laugel B, Clement M, Price DA, Wooldridge L, Sewell AK. The molecular determinants of CD8 co-receptor function. *Immunology* (2012) **137**:139–48. doi:10.1111/j.1365-2567.2012.03625.x
33. Wu Y, Vendome J, Shapiro L, Ben-Shaul A, Honig B. Transforming binding affinities from three dimensions to two with application to cadherin clustering. *Nature* (2011) **475**:510–4. doi:10.1038/nature10183
34. Bell GI, Dembo M, Bongrand P. Cell adhesion. Competition between nonspecific repulsion and specific bonding. *Biophys J* (1984) **45**:1051–64. doi:10.1016/S0006-3495(84)84252-6
35. Bell GI. Models for the specific adhesion of cells to cells. *Science* (1978) **200**:618–27. doi:10.1126/science.347575
36. Laugel B, van den Berg HA, Gostick E, Cole DK, Wooldridge L, Boulter J, et al. Different T cell receptor affinity thresholds and CD8 coreceptor dependence govern cytotoxic T lymphocyte activation and tetramer binding properties. *J Biol Chem* (2007) **282**:23799–810. doi:10.1074/jbc.M700976200
37. Holler PD, Lim AR, Cho BK, Rund LA, Kranz DM. $CD8^-$ T cell transfectants that express a high affinity T cell receptor exhibit enhanced peptide-dependent activation. *J Exp Med* (2001) **194**:1043–52. doi:10.1084/jem.194.8.1043
38. Holler PD, Kranz DM. Quantitative analysis of the contribution of TCR/pepMHC affinity and CD8 to T cell activation. *Immunity* (2003) **18**:255–264. doi:10.1016/S1074-7613(03)00019-0
39. Chen J-L, Stewart-Jones G, Bossi G, Lissin NM, Wooldridge L, Man Lik Choi E. Structural and kinetic basis for heightened immunogenicity of T cell vaccines. *J Exp Med* (2005) **8**:1243–55. doi:10.1084/jem.20042323
40. Cole DK, Edwards ESJ, Wynn KK, Clement M, Miles JJ, Ladell K. Modification of MHC anchor residues generates heteroclitic peptides that alter TCR binding and T cell recognition. *J Immunol* (2010) **185**:2600–10. doi:10.4049/jimmunol.1000629
41. Salomon B, Bluestone JA. Complexities of CD28/B7: CTLA-4 costimulatory pathways in autoimmunity and transplantation. *Annu Rev Immunol* (2001) **19**:225–252. doi:10.1146/annurev.immunol.19.1.225
42. Xiao Z, Mescher MF, Jameson SC. Detuning CD8 T cells: down-regulation of CD8 expression, tetramer binding, and response during CTL activation. *J Exp Med* (2007) **204**:2667–77. doi:10.1084/jem.20062376
43. Zhang L, Fung-Leung W, Miller RG. Down-regulation of CD8 on mature antigen-reactive T cells as a mechanism of peripheral tolerance. *J Immunol* (1995) **155**:3464–71.
44. Demotte N, Colau D, Ottaviani S, Godelaine D, Van Pel A, Boon T. A reversible functional defect of CD8+ T lymphocytes involving loss of tetramer labeling. *Eur J Immunol* (2002) **32**:1688–97. doi:10.1002/1521-4141(200206)32:6<1688::AID-IMMU1688>3.0.CO;2-9
45. van den Berg HA, Rand DA. Dynamics of T cell activation threshold tuning. *J Theor Biol* (2004) **228**:397–416. doi:10.1016/j.jtbi.2004.02.002
46. van den Berg HA, Sewell AK. Dynamic tuning of T cell receptor specificity by co-receptors and costimulation. In: Molina-París C, Lythe G editors. *Mathematical Models and Immune Cell Biology*. Berlin: Springer-Verlag (2011). p. 47–73.
47. Dushek O. Elementary steps in T cell receptor triggering. *Front Immunol* (2012) **2** 91. doi:10.3389/fimmu.2011.00091
48. Davis MM. A new trigger for T cells. *Cell* (2002) **110**:285–7. doi:10.1016/S0092-8674(02)00865-6
49. Okkenhaug K, Vanhaesebroeck B. PI3K in lymphocyte development, differentiation and activation. *Nat Rev Immunol* (2003) **4**:317–30. doi:10.1038/nri1056

3

Structural and biophysical insights into the role of CD4 and CD8 in T cell activation

Yili Li[1,2], Yiyuan Yin[3] and Roy A. Mariuzza[1,2]*

[1] W. M. Keck Laboratory for Structural Biology, Institute for Bioscience and Biotechnology Research, University of Maryland, Rockville, MD, USA
[2] Department of Cell Biology and Molecular Genetics, University of Maryland, College Park, MD, USA
[3] Department of Antibody Engineering, Genentech, South San Francisco, CA, USA

Edited by:
Bruno Laugel, Cardiff University, UK

Reviewed by:
Paula Kavathas, Yale University, USA
Cheng Zhu, Georgia Institute of Technology, USA
Simon John Davis, University of Oxford, UK
Rose Zamoyska, University of Edinburgh, UK

***Correspondence:**
Roy A. Mariuzza, Institute for Bioscience and Biotechnology Research, University of Maryland, 9600 Gudelsky Drive, Rockville, MD 20850, USA
e-mail: rmariuzz@umd.edu

T cell receptors (TCRs) recognize peptides presented by MHC molecules (pMHC) on an antigen-presenting cell (APC) to discriminate foreign from self-antigens and initiate adaptive immune responses. In addition, T cell activation generally requires binding of this same pMHC to a CD4 or CD8 co-receptor, resulting in assembly of a TCR–pMHC–CD4 or TCR–pMHC–CD8 complex and recruitment of Lck via its association with the co-receptor. Here we review structural and biophysical studies of CD4 and CD8 interactions with MHC molecules and TCR–pMHC complexes. Crystal structures have been determined of CD8αα and CD8αβ in complex with MHC class I, of CD4 bound to MHC class II, and of a complete TCR–pMHC–CD4 ternary complex. Additionally, the binding of these co-receptors to pMHC and TCR–pMHC ligands has been investigated both in solution and *in situ* at the T cell–APC interface. Together, these studies have provided key insights into the role of CD4 and CD8 in T cell activation, and into how these co-receptors focus TCR on MHC to guide TCR docking on pMHC during thymic T cell selection.

Keywords: CD4, CD8, MHC, T cell receptor, structure, T cell activation

INTRODUCTION

Adaptive immunity depends on specific recognition by an αβ T cell receptor (TCR) of an antigenic peptide bound to a major histocompatibility complex (pMHC) molecule on an antigen-presenting cell (APC). However, TCR–pMHC interactions alone do not efficiently trigger T cells, requiring the participation of the co-receptors CD4 and CD8 (1–4). These transmembrane glycoproteins mark different T cell subsets. CD4 is expressed on Th1, Th2, and Th17 helper cells, as well as on CD4 regulatory T cells (Tregs); CD8 is expressed on cytotoxic T lymphocytes (CTLs) and CD8 Tregs. CD4 and CD8 enhance T cell signaling by binding MHC class II (CD4) or MHC class I (CD8) molecules on APCs. The interaction of CD4 with MHC class II greatly reduces the number of antigenic peptides required for T cell activation (5) and substantially increases cytokine production by helper T cells (1). Likewise, the CD8–MHC class I interaction enhances the antigen sensitivity and response of cytotoxic T cells to pMHC ligands (6).

The principal role of the CD4 and CD8 co-receptors is to recruit the Src tyrosine kinase p65lck (Lck) to the TCR–pMHC complex following co-receptor binding to MHC, resulting in assembly of a TCR–pMHC–CD4 or TCR–pMHC–CD8 ternary complex (7–10). Recruitment of Lck occurs via its association with the cytoplasmic tail of CD4 or CD8. The accompanying increase in the local concentration of Lck promotes phosphorylation of immunoreceptor tyrosine activation motifs (ITAMs) in the cytoplasmic tails of CD3 subunits associated with the TCR in the TCR–CD3 complex, leading to the recruitment and activation of Zap-70. Activated Zap-70 phosphorylates LAT and SLP-76, which function as scaffolds to recruit other signaling molecules to the downstream T cell signaling apparatus that regulates T cell activation, proliferation, and differentiation. The targeted delivery of Lck to TCR by CD4 or CD8 during thymic selection is believed to impose MHC restriction on the developing αβ TCR repertoire (11). In support of this idea, αβ TCRs in mice lacking co-receptors and MHC are not biased toward pMHC ligands, but instead display antibody-like recognition specificities (12, 13).

This review focuses on structural and biophysical studies of CD4 and CD8 interactions with MHC molecules. Crystal structures have been determined of CD8αα and CD8αβ in complex with MHC class I, of CD4 bound to MHC class II, and, most recently, of a complete TCR–pMHC–CD4 ternary complex. In addition, the binding of these co-receptors to pMHC and TCR–pMHC ligands has been investigated both in solution and *in situ*. Collectively, these studies have provided critical insights into the role of CD4 and CD8 in T cell activation and in guiding TCR docking on pMHC during T cell development.

INTERACTION OF CD8 WITH MHC CLASS I

CD8 exists as two isoforms, CD8αα and CD8αβ, which are expressed on different cell types and appear to have different functions. CD8ββ homodimers have also been reported, but these lack MHC-binding activity and their significance is unknown (14). Whereas CD8αα is found on γδ T cells, intestinal intraepithelial T lymphocytes, and natural killer (NK) cells, CD8αβ is expressed on αβ TCR thymocytes and CTLs. The function of CD8αα remains obscure, but it has been implicated in the negative regulation of intestinal intraepithelial T lymphocytes (15). By contrast, CD8αβ is clearly required for positive selection of $CD8^+$ T cells in the thymus (16–18) and for activation of $CD8^+$ T cells in the periphery (19). In both CD8αα and CD8αβ, Lck associates with the CD8α chain. In addition, ligation of CD8αβ by MHC, in the absence of TCR engagement, results in apoptosis of a proportion of double-positive thymocytes, which may be a mechanism for removing thymocytes that have failed positive selection (20).

Fluorescence resonance energy transfer experiments have shown that, during T cell activation, the TCR binds initially to pMHC, and that CD8 then binds to the same pMHC as the TCR, leading to formation of a TCR–pMHC–CD8 complex (21). This order of engagement ensures that the specific TCR–pMHC interaction dominates T cell recognition. As measured by surface plasmon resonance (SPR), CD8 binds very weakly to MHC class I in both mouse and human, with little influence of the MHC-bound peptide (21–23). In the mouse, the average binding affinity for CD8αβ (K_D~50 μM) is similar to that for CD8αα (~70 μM), with some variation depending on the particular MHC class I allele. The human CD8–MHC class I interaction is weaker still, averaging ~150 μM (24–26). In both cases, these affinities are 10- to 100-fold lower than for most TCR–pMHC interactions.

In overall agreement with these SPR results, *in situ* measurements of the mouse CD8–MHC class I interaction gave an affinity several orders of magnitude lower than that of TCR for pMHC (27). These experiments used a micropipette adhesion frequency assay to measure the adhesion kinetics of live T cells interacting with pMHC ligands presented on surrogate APCs. The two-dimensional (2D) binding parameters derived from this technique are thought to more accurately reflect biological interactions in membranes than the three-dimensional (3D) parameters derived from SPR, in which fluid-phase receptors and ligands are removed from their cellular environment (28).

Although the affinity of CD8 for MHC class I is weak, recent 2D affinity measurements support the idea that CD8 contributes significantly to stabilizing the TCR–pMHC interaction at the T cell–APC interface (9). These experiments revealed that the TCR–pMHC–CD8 trimolecular interaction generates synergy over the simple sum of the individual TCR–pMHC and pMHC–CD8 interactions, and that this cooperativity amplifies peptide discrimination. Thus, in addition to its primary role of recruiting Lck to the TCR–pMHC complex, a secondary function of CD8 is to reinforce TCR binding to the pMHC ligand. Whether the CD4 co-receptor also promotes cooperative binding remains to be determined.

The micropipette adhesion frequency assay also revealed that the kinetics of the TCR–pMHC–CD8 trimolecular interaction at the T cell membrane proceeds in two stages (9). The first consists of TCR-dominant binding to agonist pMHC. This triggers a second stage involving an upregulation of CD8-dependent adhesion after a 1 s delay. The second stage requires Lck kinase activity to initiate CD8 binding to the same pMHC ligand engaged by the TCR, generating synergy. It remains to be established whether the TCR–pMHC–CD4 trimolecular interaction involves a similar sequence of events.

STRUCTURES OF CD8 BOUND TO MHC CLASS I

CD8αβ is a heterodimeric type I transmembrane glycoprotein, whose α and β chains are each composed of an immunoglobulin (Ig)-like domain connected by a long stalk to a transmembrane domain and a cytoplasmic tail, with Lck bound to the CD8α tail. By contrast, the CD8αα homodimer comprises only the α chain. Four structures of CD8αα or CD8αβ bound to MHC class I molecules have been reported: (1) the complex between human CDαα and HLA-A*0201 (29); (2) the complex between human CD8αα and HLA-A*2402 (30); (3) the complex between mouse CD8αα and H-2K^b (31); and (4) the complex between mouse CD8αβ and H-2D^d (23).

In the CD8αβ–H-2D^d complex (23), the CD8αβ heterodimer contacts only the α3 domain of the MHC class I heavy chain (**Figure 1A**). By contrast, CD8αα also contacts the α2 domain and β_2-microglobulin (β_2m) in the CDαα–HLA-A*0201 (29), CD8αα–HLA-A*2402 (30), and CD8αα–H-2K^b complexes (31) (**Figure 1C**). The CD8β subunit occupies a position equivalent to that of the CD8α1 subunit in the three CD8αα–MHC class I structures, which places CD8β proximal to the T cell membrane. The CD8α subunit of CD8αβ is located in the same position as the CD8α2 subunit, distal from the T cell and near the C-terminus of the MHC class I α3 domain (**Figures 1A,C**). Nearly all MHC class I residues that mediate key interactions with CD8αα or CD8αβ are non-polymorphic, which explains the largely allele-independent nature of CD8 binding.

For both CD8αα and CD8αβ, the main binding interaction is with a protruding loop in the α3 domain of the MHC class I molecule (CD loop), corresponding to residues 220–228 (**Figures 1B,D**). This loop is flexible in the absence of CD8, but is stabilized by CD8 binding. In the CD8αα–MHC class I structures, the two CDR3-like loops of the CD8α subunits clamp onto the central β-turn portion of the CD loop in an antibody-like manner, as do the two CDR3-like loops of CD8αβ (23, 29–31). In addition, CD8αα contacts the α2 domain and β_2m through its CD8α1 subunit, whereas the corresponding CD8β subunit of CD8αβ contacts only α3. Of particular note in the CD8αβ–H-2D^d complex is Gln226 of H-2D^d, a highly conserved residue among MHC class I alleles and the only one that interacts with both CD8α and CD8β (**Figure 1B**).

ROLE OF THE CD8 STALK REGION IN CO-RECEPTOR FUNCTION

The Ig-like domains of CD8α and CD8β are tethered to the T cell membrane by long stalk regions comprising ~45 residues for CD8α and ~35 residues CD8β (32). These stalk regions, which are rich in threonine, serine, and proline residues, are heavily *O*-glycosylated at multiple sites in all species studied (33). The stalk of CD8αβ undergoes developmentally programed *O*-glycan modification controlled by the sialyltransferase ST3 Gal-I, which catalyzes addition of sialic acid to core 1 *O*-linked glycans (34). In particular, immature CD4$^+$CD8$^+$ thymocytes exhibit lower levels of CD8 sialylation than mature thymocytes (32, 34, 35). Decreased sialylation of the CD8αβ stalk was found to markedly increase the affinity of CD8 for MHC class I, as measured by MHC tetramer binding, thereby affecting T cell selection (34, 35). Enhanced CD8αβ binding at the CD4$^+$CD8$^+$ stage facilitates elimination of autoreactive T cells in the thymus. However, once a double-positive thymocyte has differentiated to the CD8$^+$ stage, *O*-glycan sialylation of the CD8αβ stalk reduces co-receptor affinity for pMHC, requiring a stronger TCR–pMHC interaction for T cell activation in the periphery (34, 35).

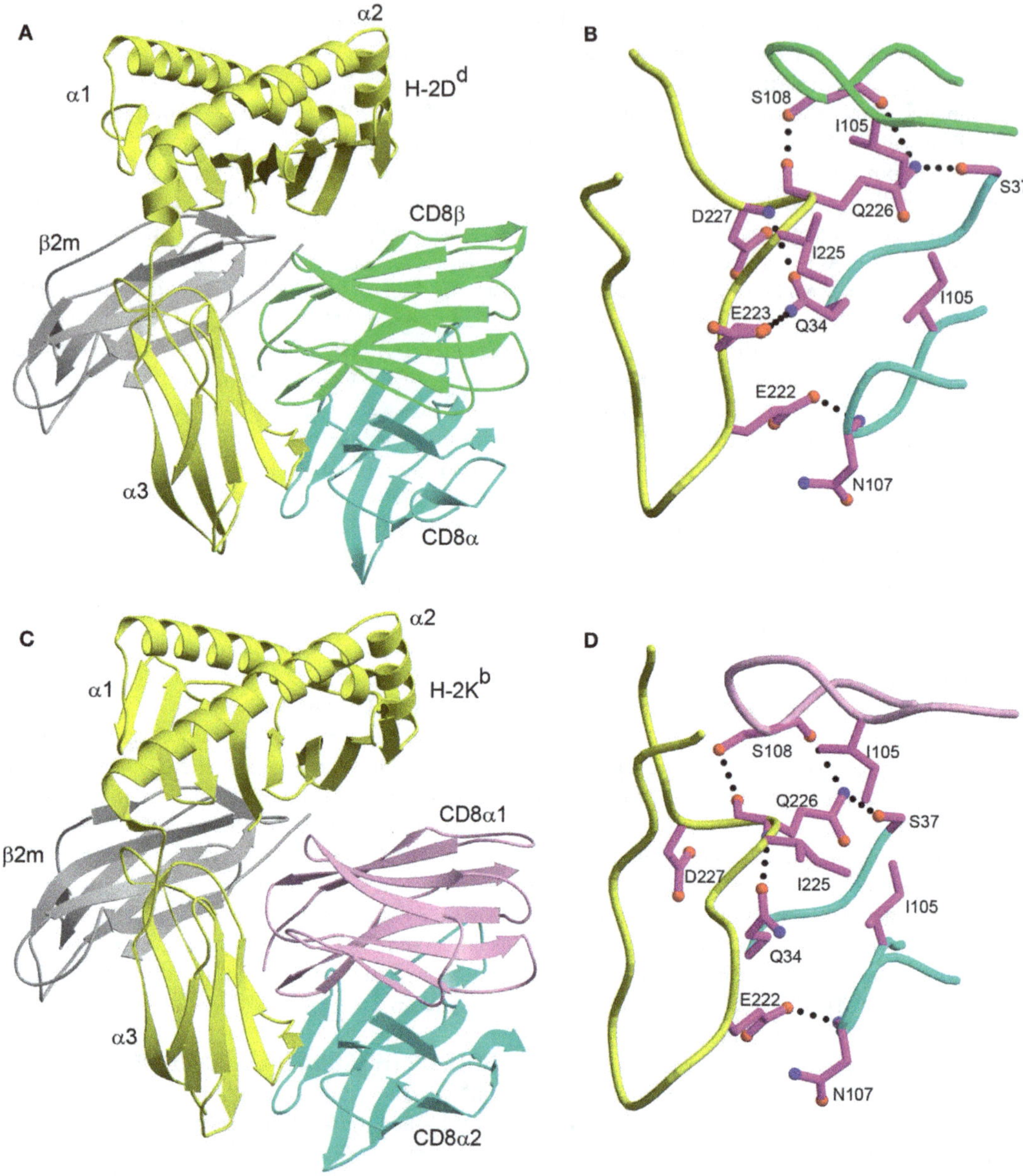

FIGURE 1 | Comparison of CD8αβ–H-2D^d and CD8αα–H-2K^b complexes. **(A)** Ribbon diagram of the CD8αβ–H-2D^d complex (Protein Data Bank accession code 3DMM) (23). MHC α chain, yellow; β_2m, gray; CD8α, cyan; CD8β, green. **(B)** Interaction between the CDR-like loops of CD8αβ and the H-2D^d α3 CD loop. The side chains of contacting residues are shown in ball-and-stick representation with carbon atoms in magenta, nitrogen atoms in blue, and oxygen atoms in red. Hydrogen bonds are drawn as dotted black lines. **(C)** Ribbon diagram of the CD8αα–H-2K^b complex (1BQH) (31). MHC α chain, yellow; β_2m, gray; CD8α1, pink; CD8α2, cyan. **(D)** Interaction between the CDR-like loops of CD8αα and the H-2K^b α3 CD loop.

The structural basis for reduced CD8αβ affinity for MHC class I upon sialylation of the stalk region is unknown. One possibility is that sialylation alters the association or orientation of the Ig-like domains of the CD8αβ heterodimer, reducing its capacity to bind MHC class I (34). However, Merry et al. (36) found that sialylation had little or no effect on the overall structure of CD8, insofar as sialylated and non-sialylated forms of soluble CD8αα exhibited indistinguishable hydrodynamic properties. This suggests that the results of Moody et al. (34) and Daniels et al. (35) might be explained by avidity effects arising from aggregation of unsialylated CD8 on the T cell surface that increase MHC tetramer binding (36).

Irrespective of the underlying mechanism, the finding that developmentally regulated glycosylation of the CD8αβ stalk can modulate MHC binding at the cell surface demonstrates that the stalk has a specialized role in co-receptor function, beyond simply attaching the MHC-binding domains to the T cell membrane. The long CD8αβ stalk may also allow a possible *cis* interaction between CD8 and MHC class I expressed on the same T cell (37), in addition to the established *trans* interaction between CD8 and MHC class I expressed on different cells. Interestingly, the stalk regions of other immune system receptors have also been recently found to play prominent roles in receptor function. For example, the long stalk regions of Ly49 NK cell receptors enable binding to MHC class I in *cis* or *trans* configurations (38). Additionally, the stalk domain of the activating NK receptor NKp30 is critical for NK cell killing and may contribute directly to binding its tumor cell ligand B7-H6 (39).

No 3D structural information is available for the stalk regions of CD8αβ or CD8αα, since the stalks, when included in the constructs used for protein expression, were mostly or entirely disordered in the CD8–MHC class I crystal structures (23, 29–31). Although this has been interpreted to mean that that the CD8 stalk is highly flexible, it should be emphasized that the stalks completely lacked glycosylation because the CD8 proteins were produced in bacteria. However, there is biophysical evidence that *O*-glycosylation may significantly restrict the flexibility of the stalks. Studies of mucins have demonstrated that *O*-glycans stiffen polypeptides through steric interactions between peptide-linked *N*-acetylgalactosamine residues and adjacent peptide residues (40, 41). Moreover, *O*-glycans in the CD8 stalk polypeptides were found to reduce the overall extension of the stalk from a theoretical maximum of 3.4 Å per residue to 2.6 Å per residue, indicating rigidification (36, 42). Therefore, *O*-glycosylation may limit the mobility of the CD8 head group relative to the T cell membrane, an important consideration in evaluating co-receptor interactions with TCR–pMHC during thymic selection and peripheral antigen recognition, as discussed below.

STRUCTURES OF CD4 BOUND TO MHC CLASS II

CD4 is a monomeric type I transmembrane glycoprotein consisting of four Ig-like extracellular domains connected by a short stalk to a transmembrane domain and a cytoplasmic tail that interacts with Lck. CD4 binds MHC class II with exceptionally low affinity compared to all other leukocyte cell–cell recognition molecules characterized to date, whose K_Ds typically fall in the 1–100 μM range, as measured by SPR (43, 44). For the CD4–MHC class II interaction, K_Ds have been estimated to range from ~200 μM (for human CD4 binding to mouse MHC class II) (45) to >2 mM (for human CD4 binding to human MHC class II) (43). These affinities are substantially weaker than those for CD8–MHC class I interactions, which range from ~10 μM (for mouse CD8αβ binding to H-2D^d) (23) to ~150 μM (for human CD8αα binding to HLA-A*0201) (26). Presumably, evolution has calibrated the affinity of CD4 for MHC class II to enable peripheral T cells to respond efficiently to the very low abundance of foreign pMHC molecules on APCs (sensitivity), yet avoid activation by the far greater number of self-pMHC molecules (discrimination), which could cause autoimmunity.

The ability of CD4 to recognize highly polymorphic MHC class II molecules is central to its function as a co-receptor (1). In humans, MHC class II molecules are encoded by three separate loci (HLA-DR, -DQ, and -DP), while in mice they are encoded by two loci (I-A and I-E). For HLA-DR, most variability derives from the β-chain, with >700 known alleles at the population level, whereas there are only three α-chain variants. In contrast, both α- and β-chains of HLA-DQ and -DP are polymorphic (46). Two structures of CD4 bound to MHC class II molecules have been reported: (1) the complex between human CD4 (domains D1 and D2) and mouse I-A^k to 4.3 Å resolution (47); and (2) the complex between human CD4 (domains D1 and D2) and human HLA-DR1 to 2.4 Å resolution (48). These structures readily explain the ability of CD4 to recognize multiple MHC class II alleles.

The CD4–I-A^k and CD4–HLA-DR1 complexes display similar overall topologies, although only the higher-resolution CD4–HLA-DR1 structure permitted an atomic-level description of the CD4–MHC class II interface. In both complexes, CD4 binds MHC class II through its membrane-distal D1 domain, which contacts the membrane-proximal α2 and β2 domains of the MHC class II molecule (**Figure 2A**). CD4 uses two discontinuous regions to engage MHC class II in a concavity formed by the α2 and β2 domains (**Figure 2B**). The first region, composed of β-strands C′ and C″, exclusively contacts the β2 domain. The second region, comprising a short 3_{10} helix within the loop connecting β-strands D and E, binds solely to the α2 domain.

Figure 2C shows sequence alignments of the α- and β-chains of selected HLA-DR, -DP, and -DQ alleles in the regions where HLA-DR1 contacts CD4. For the β-chains, 11 of 12 CD4-contacting residues are absolutely conserved in these human MHC class II molecules, and 1 is conservatively substituted (Val116Ile in HLA-DQ). For the α-chains, all three CD4-contacting residues (Glu88, Thr90, Leu176) are invariant across human MHC class II alleles. Hence, the remarkable cross-reactivity of CD4 is attributable to the targeting of non-polymorphic residues in the concavity formed by the α2 and β2 domains of HLA-DR, -DP, and -DQ. For I-A^k, 11 of 14 CD4-contacting residues are identical to those of HLA-DR1, while for I-E^k 12 of 14 are identical (**Figure 2C**). All non-identical residues are conservatively substituted in both molecules. Therefore, CD4 almost certainly engages all human and mouse MHC class II molecules in the same manner as it does HLA-DR (48).

STRUCTURE OF A TCR–pMHC–CD4 TERNARY COMPLEX

The low affinity of CD4 for MHC class II presented a major technical obstacle to crystallizing a TCR–pMHC–CD4 ternary complex. To overcome this obstacle, *in vitro* directed evolution by yeast surface display was used to increase the affinity of CD4 for MHC class II (49). Affinity maturation by yeast display relies on expression of a library of mutants on the surface of yeast, followed by selection of variants with improved affinity (50). The D1 domain of human CD4 was subjected to *in vitro* random mutagenesis, and the resulting mutant library was displayed on yeast by fusion to agglutinin protein Aga2p (48). Because CD4 binds MHC class II very weakly (43, 45), the CD4 library was sorted by flow cytometry using HLA-DR1 tetramers, rather than monomers, to increase the avidity of the selecting ligand. In this way, a CD4 mutant that bound HLA-DR1 with $K_D = 9$ μM was isolated, compared with no detectable binding for wild-type CD4, even at high concentrations (400 μM). The CD4 mutant exhibited similar affinity for HLA-DR4 ($K_D = 10$ μM), in agreement with the ability of CD4 to recognize all HLA-DR alleles, as discussed above.

The affinity-matured CD4 mutant contained two substitutions in the D1 domain: Gln40Tyr and Thr45Trp. In the mutant

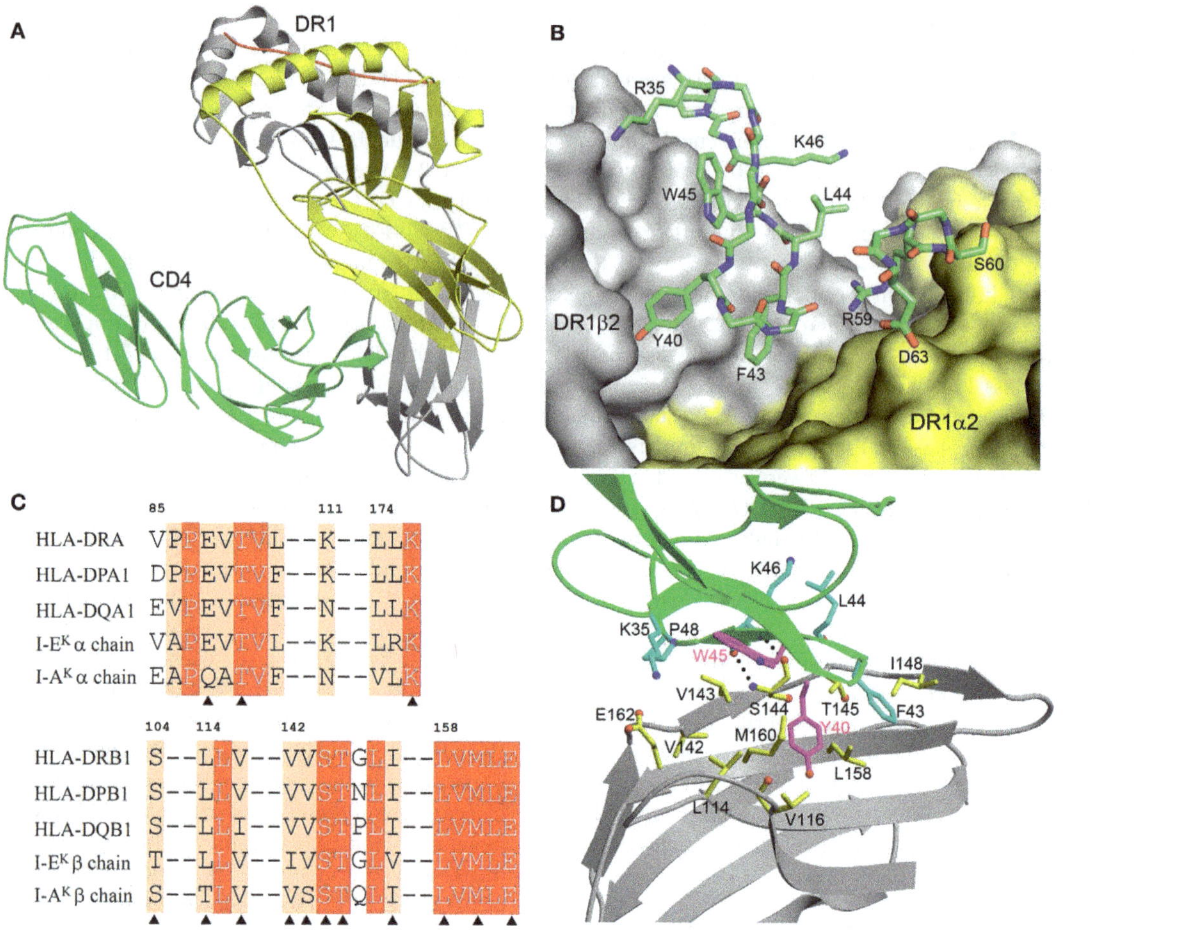

FIGURE 2 | Structure of a human CD4–MHC class II complex. (A) CD4 (green) contacts the α2 (yellow) and β2 (gray) domains of HLA-DR1 through its D4 domain (3S4S) (48). The MHC-bound peptide is red. **(B)** The CD4–HLA-DR1 binding interface. The two regions of CD4 (residues 35–48 and 59–63) that contact HLA-DR1 are shown in stick representation with carbon atoms in green, oxygen atoms in red, and nitrogen atoms in blue. The molecular surface of HLA-DR1 that interacts with CD4 is depicted with the α2 domain in yellow and the β2 domain in gray. **(C)** Sequence alignment of the CD4-contacting regions of the α- and β-chains of different human and mouse MHC class II alleles. Residues that contact CD4 in the CD4–HLA-DR1 structure are marked with triangles. White characters on a red background show residues that are strictly conserved across human or mouse MHC class II molecules. Black characters on a tan background are conservatively substituted residues. **(D)** Close-up view of the interactions between an affinity-matured CD4 mutant (green) and the HLA-DR1 β2 domain (gray). The side chains of interacting residues are shown in ball-and-stick representation with carbon atoms in cyan (CD4) or yellow (HLA-DR1), oxygen atoms in red, and nitrogen atoms in blue. The mutated Tyr40 and Trp45 residues of CD4 are in magenta. Hydrogen bonds are drawn as dotted black lines.

CD4–HLA-DR1 structure (48), CD4 Trp45 is located at the center of the interface with HLA-DR1, where its bulky side chain makes multiple hydrophobic contacts with DR1 β2 Val143 (**Figure 2D**). Similarly, CD4 Tyr40 is surrounded by apolar DR1 β2 residues Leu114, Val116, Leu158, and Met160, resulting in increased hydrophobic interactions at the mutation site. Together, the Gln40Tyr and Thr45Trp mutations improved shape and chemical complementarity with HLA-DR1, thereby stabilizing the CD4–HLA-DR1 complex.

The enhanced affinity of this CD4 mutant made possible the crystallization and structure determination of a complete TCR–pMHC–CD4 ternary complex involving a human autoimmune TCR (MS2-3C8), a self-peptide from myelin basic protein (MBP) bound to HLA-DR4, and CD4 (49) (**Figure 3A**). The TCR–pMHC–CD4 complex resembles a pointed arch in which both TCR and CD4 are tilted rather than oriented vertically. The TCR and CD4 molecules each make an angle of ~65° with the T cell surface. The apex of the arch is formed by the α2 and β2 domains of HLA-DR4 and the D1 domain of CD4. MS2-3C8 engages MBP via the canonical docking mode of αβ TCRs (51), in which the TCR adopts a central diagonal orientation over pMHC (52, 53). There are no direct contacts between TCR and CD4 (**Figure 3A**), in agreement with an earlier prediction (47).

The CD4 molecule bound to TCR–pMHC retains the overall extended conformation observed in different crystal forms of unbound CD4 (54), with some hinge-like variability at the D2–D3 junction. The limited segmental flexibility of CD4 implies that any

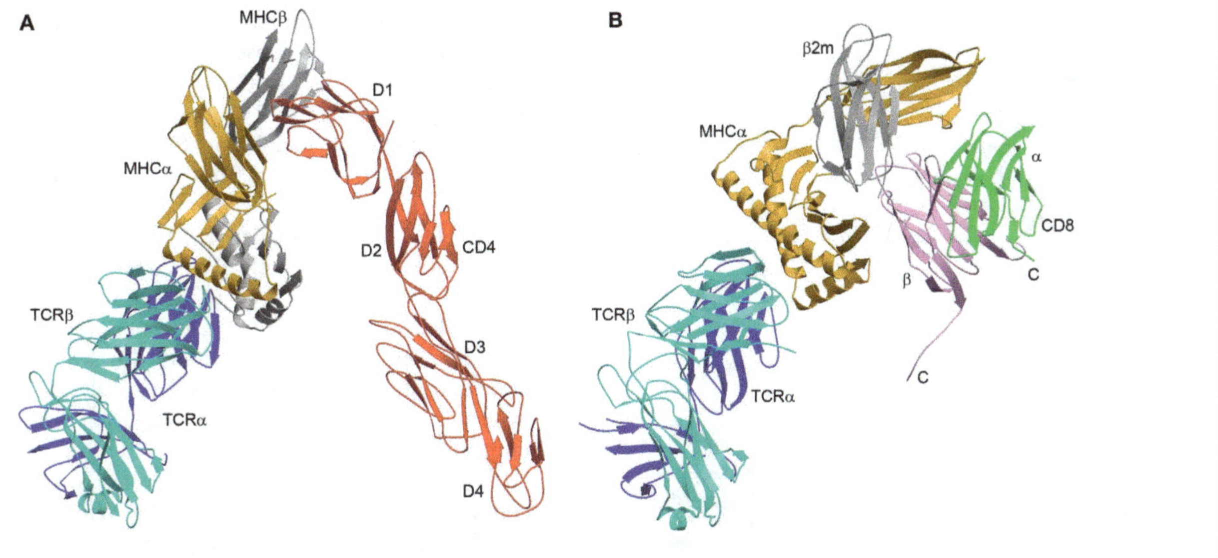

FIGURE 3 | Comparison of TCR–pMHC–CD4 and TCR–pMHC–CD8 ternary complexes. (A) Crystal structure of a TCR–pMHC–CD4 complex (MS2-3C8–MBP–DR4–CD4) oriented as if the TCR and CD4 molecules are attached to the T cell at the bottom and the MHC class II molecules is attached to an opposing APC at the top (3T0E) (49). TCR α chain, blue; TCR β chain, cyan; MHC α chain, yellow; MHC β chain, gray; CD4, red. **(B)** Hypothetical model of the TCR–pMHC–CD8 complex. The model was constructed by superposing the CD8αβ–H-2D^d complex (3DMM) (23) onto a TCR–H-2D^b complex (3PQY) through the MHC class I molecule. A portion of the CD8β stalk region was visible in the crystal structure and points toward the T cell membrane. The C-termini of the CD8α and CD8β chains are labeled. The orientation of the TCR–pMHC complex is the same as in **(A)**. TCR α chain, blue; TCR β chain, cyan; MHC α chain, yellow; $β_2$m, gray; CD8α, green; CD8β, violet.

significant variations in overall complex architecture must arise from differences in TCR docking on pMHC.

The absence of direct contacts between TCR and CD4 explains how these molecules can simultaneously, yet independently, bind to pMHC. Importantly, the wide separation (~70 Å) between the membrane-proximal TCR Cα/Cβ module and CD4 D4 domain provides ample room for the placement of TCR-associated CD3εγ, εδ, and ζζ subunits (**Figure 4A**), which transmit activation signals to the T cell (55). Although no crystal structure is available for the TCR–CD3 complex, mutational studies have identified docking sites for the ectodomains of CD3εδ and CD3εγ, which interact with the TCR through adjacent Cα DE and Cβ CC′ loops, respectively (56–58). Based on this information, CD3εγ and CD3εδ would be situated inside the TCR–pMHC–CD4 arch, wedged between the TCR and T cell membrane (**Figure 4A**). In the organization of the TCR–CD3 complex proposed by Fernandes et al. (58), only CD3γ and CD3δ contact the TCR, whereas CD3ε projects away from the receptor. The relative proximity of CD3ε to CD4 in the TCR–pMHC–CD4 complex, compared to CD3γ or CD3δ, may confer preference to CD3ε in the ITAM phosphorylation cascade upon Lck recruitment by CD4 (**Figure 4A**).

The ectodomain of CD3ζ, which is only nine amino acids in length, has not been implicated in interactions with the TCR ectodomain, and so is not shown in **Figure 4A**. However, mutational analysis of the transmembrane regions of TCR and CD3 subunits has established that CD3ζζ is associated with TCRα in the T cell membrane (59).

It has been proposed that, in resting T cells, CD3ε ITAMs are sequestered in the membrane, and that activation results in ITAM exposure to Src kinases (60). If so, the TCR–pMHC–CD4 structure suggests a possible mechanism by which this may occur. If the TCR shifts from an upright to a tilted orientation upon formation of the TCR–pMHC–CD4 complex (**Figure 3A**), this movement could potentially drive the CD3 ectodomains, situated inside the TCR–pMHC–CD4 arch, into the T cell membrane. This in turn could cause displacement of CD3ε ITAMs from the membrane and their phosphorylation by Lck.

THE TCR–pMHC–CD4 COMPLEX AND MODELS FOR TCR TRIGGERING

There is considerable controversy over the mechanism of TCR triggering, and a variety of models have been proposed to explain how pMHC binding to TCR initiates signaling across the T cell membrane (55). Some of these models invoke dimerization (or oligomerization) of CD4 (54), MHC (61), or TCR (57) as a means of enhancing phosphorylation of CD3 ITAMs by increasing the proximity of associated tyrosine kinases. The plausibility of these models can be assessed in terms of the geometrical constraints imposed by the TCR–pMHC–CD4 structure.

The structure of human CD4 D1–D4 in unbound form showed that CD4 molecules form dimers through the D4 domain, at least in the crystal (54). This observation suggested that D4–D4-associated CD4 dimers might contribute to T cell activation by cross-linking TCR–pMHC complexes (54, 62). However, the TCR–pMHC–CD4 structure is incompatible with this idea. In a hypothetical model constructed by superposing the TCR–pMHC–CD4 structure onto the D4–D4-associated CD4 dimer, the distance between the C-termini of the D4 domains and the T cell surface is too far (~40 Å) to be spanned by the eight-residue stalk region of CD4 (49). Similarly, the finding that some HLA-DR

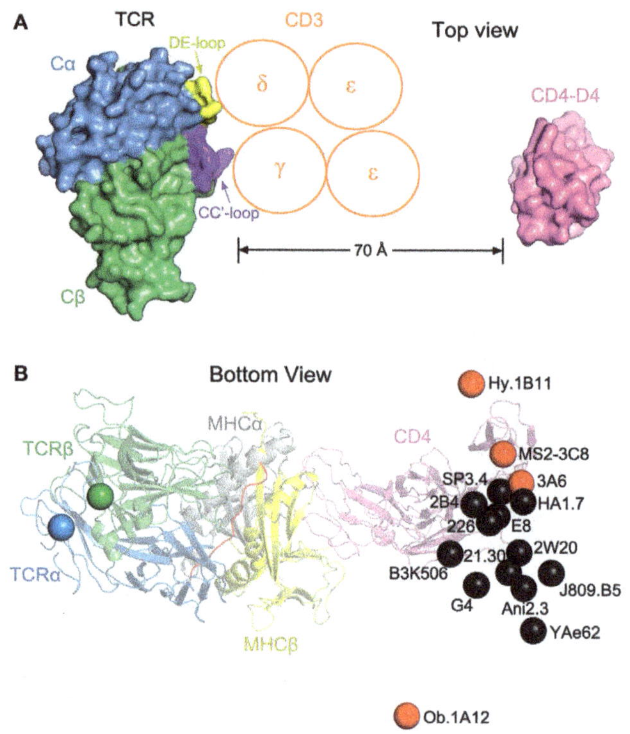

FIGURE 4 | Orientation of TCR and CD4 in TCR–pMHC–CD4 complexes. **(A)** Top view of the MS2-3C8–MBP–DR4–CD4 complex (**Figure 3A**), as if looking down on the T cell. The membrane-proximal TCR $C\alpha/C\beta$ domains and the CD4 D4 domain are depicted in surface representation. Other domains and pMHC are omitted for clarity. TCR $C\alpha$, blue; TCR $C\beta$, green; CD4 D4, pink. The proposed arrangement of the ectodomains of $CD3\varepsilon\gamma$ and $CD3\varepsilon\delta$ (58) is shown in relation to docking sites identified by mutational analyses (56, 58): $C\alpha$ DE loop (yellow) and $C\beta$ CC′ loop (dark blue). The Ig-like ectodomains of $CD3\varepsilon\gamma$ and $CD3\varepsilon\delta$ are drawn as orange circles. In this arrangement, only $CD3\gamma$ and $CD3\delta$ contact the TCR. $CD3\varepsilon$ projects away from the TCR, toward CD4. **(B)** Bottom view of the MS2-3C8–MBP–DR4–CD4 complex, as if looking up from inside the T cell. On the left side, the C-termini of the extracellular portions of the α and β chains of TCR MS2-3C8, as defined in the crystal structure (49), are indicated by blue and green spheres, respectively. On the right side, the C-terminus of the extracellular portion of CD4 in the complex with MS2-3C8 and HLA-DR4 is marked by a red sphere labeled MS2-3C8. The right side also shows the predicted position of the C-terminus of CD4 in 15 hypothetical ternary complexes constructed using other TCR–pMHC class II structures [human: HA1.7 (1JH8), Ob.1A12 (1YMM), 3A6 (1ZGL), E8 (2IAM), Hy.1B11 (3PL6), G4 (4E41); SP3.4 (4GG6); Ani2.3 (4H1L); mouse: B3K506 (3C5Z), 2W20 (3C6L), YAe62 (3C60), 21.30 (3MBE); J806.B5 (3RDT); 2B4 (3QIB); 226 (3QIU)]. In each case, the C-terminus of CD4 is marked by a colored sphere labeled with the name of the corresponding TCR. Autoimmune TCRs (MS2-3C8, Ob.1A12, 3A6, Hy.1B11) are red; anti-foreign (HA1.7, B3K506, 2W20, 21.30, YAe62, SP3.4, Ani2.3, J805.B5, 2B4, 226) and anti-tumor TCRs (E8, G4) are black. The TCR–pMHC–CD4 complexes were modeled by superposing each TCR–pMHC class II structure onto the MS2-3C8–MBP–DR4–CD4 complex through the $C\alpha/C\beta$ domains of the TCRs. The anti-foreign and anti-tumor TCRs (black spheres) form a cluster that mostly excludes the autoimmune TCRs (red spheres), with Hy.1B11, MS2-3C8, and 3A6 on one side of the cluster and Ob.1A12 on the other.

molecules crystallize as dimers (61, 63) suggested a mechanism for T cell triggering in which an MHC class II dimer cross-links two TCRs. However, the CD4-binding site on HLA-DR4 almost completely overlaps the putative HLA-DR dimerization site, which would preclude formation of such MHC class II dimers (49).

Recently, it was proposed that TCRs can dimerize in the T cell membrane via $C\alpha$–$C\alpha$ interactions, and that the resulting juxtaposition of two TCR–pMHC complexes facilitates signaling through the membrane (57, 64). Consistent with this model, the putative site of $C\alpha$–$C\alpha$ dimerization is on the outside of the TCR–pMHC–CD4 arch, opposite the sites mediating TCR–CD3 interactions (**Figure 4A**) (49). As such, CD4 would not interfere sterically with TCR dimerization through the $C\alpha$ domain. However, a survey of 22 TCR–pMHC crystal structures failed to reveal any $C\alpha$–$C\alpha$ contacts consistent with biologically relevant TCR dimerization (65). More tellingly, the $C\alpha$ domain contains two conserved *N*-linked glycans at positions that would preclude the hypothesized TCR dimerization via $C\alpha$–$C\alpha$ interactions.

Several recent studies have demonstrated that physical force applied to the TCR–CD3 complex can activate T cells (66–68). This finding has led to the concept of the TCR as an anisotropic mechanosensor that converts mechanical energy into a biochemical signal upon specific pMHC ligation as a T cell moves over APCs during immune surveillance (66). While it is unknown how pulling on the TCR–CD3 complex can be transduced to the T cell interior, one possibility is that pMHC binding leads to a conformational change in the CD3 cytoplasmic tails, allowing ITAM phosphorylation by Src kinases. This process may be facilitated by the CD4 (or CD8) co-receptor, whose binding to the TCR–pMHC complex could promote dissociation of CD3 ITAMs from the cytoplasmic side of the T cell membrane and their exposure to Lck, as discussed above.

CO-RECEPTORS AND TCR–pMHC DOCKING ORIENTATION

The TCR–pMHC–CD4 complex provides a basis for understanding how the CD4 and CD8 co-receptors focus TCR on MHC to guide TCR docking on pMHC during thymic T cell selection. Structural studies of numerous (>25) TCR–pMHC complexes have demonstrated remarkable similarities in the overall topology of TCR binding to pMHC, regardless of MHC class I or class II restriction (52, 53). Typically, the TCR is positioned diagonally over the center of the composite surface created by the peptide and the MHC α-helices that flank the peptide-binding groove, with $V\alpha$ situated over the N-terminal half of the peptide, and $V\beta$ over the C-terminal half, although the exact angle and pitch of TCR engagement vary.

Two competing (though not mutually exclusive) hypotheses have been proposed to explain this roughly conserved diagonal binding mode. The first maintains that co-evolution of TCR and MHC genes has led to specific interaction motifs between the germline-encoded CDR1 and CDR2 loops of TCRs and the α-helices of MHC proteins (53, 69–73). According to the second hypothesis, TCR docking topology is guided by the CD4 and CD8 co-receptors during T cell development in order to achieve intracellular juxtaposition of co-receptor-bound Lck with CD3 ITAMs (11–13, 49, 71, 72, 74, 75). According this view, it is the need for co-receptor function during thymic T cell selection that restricts the geometry of TCR–pMHC recognition and eliminates from positive selection $CD4^+CD8^+$ double-positive thymocytes expressing

TCRs unable to engage pMHC in a manner that generates a signal to induce maturation.

The arch-shaped TCR–pMHC–CD4 complex establishes anchor points for TCR and CD4 on the T cell membrane, thereby imposing constraints on the orientation of CD3 relative to Lck associated with CD4 on the cytoplasmic side of the membrane. **Figure 4B** shows the position of the C-terminus of CD4 observed in the complex with TCR MS2-3C8 and HLA-DR4, as well as the predicted position of the C-terminus of CD4 in hypothetical ternary complexes constructed using 15 other TCR–pMHC class II structures, both human and mouse. Except for the human autoimmune TCR Ob.1A12 (76), the C-termini of CD4 in these modeled complexes are grouped in a loose cluster that includes the C-terminus of CD4 in the MS2-3C8–MBP–DR4–CD4 complex. Differences in the position of the CD4 membrane anchor point are attributable to variations in the diagonal docking topology of the TCR–pMHC complexes, which places CD3εγ and CD3εδ inside the TCR–pMHC–CD4 arch, opposite CD4 (**Figure 4A**). If the TCR–pMHC docking polarity were reversed (i.e., Vα over the C-terminus of the peptide and Vβ over the N-terminus), CD3εγ and CD3εδ would be positioned outside, rather than inside, the TCR–pMHC–CD4 arch. The much greater distance between CD4-bound Lck and CD3 ITAMs would likely hinder ITAM phosphorylation by Lck, thereby preventing positive selection of T cells bearing TCRs with the reversed polarity, or their activation in the periphery. We therefore propose that the diagonal docking topology of TCR–pMHC complexes reflects not only genetically encoded interactions with MHC (53, 69), but also the requirement to form a ternary complex with the CD4 or CD8 co-receptor that is geometrically competent to deliver a maturation signal to $CD4^+CD8^+$ thymocytes during T cell selection.

Nonetheless, some flexibility must exist within the overall signaling complex to accommodate variations in TCR–pMHC docking geometry that affect the location of anchor points for TCR and CD4 on the T cell membrane (**Figure 4B**). Given the rigidity of the CD4 ectodomain (49), this flexibility most likely resides in interactions involving the flexible cytoplasmic tails of CD3 and CD4 with Lck, which itself can adopt multiple conformations (77). The flexibility of the cytoplasmic domains of CD3 is supported by circular dichroism analysis and disorder prediction algorithms (78). By both methods, the cytoplasmic domains of CD3ζ, CD3ε, CD3γ, and CD3δ were found to be intrinsically unstructured, random-coil proteins in both monomeric and oligomeric states, and in the presence or absence of lipids.

Of the 16 TCRs in **Figure 4B**, 4 are autoimmune (Hy.1B11, MS2-3C8, 3A6, Ob.1A12). These TCRs, which were isolated from different multiple sclerosis patients, recognize MBP self-peptides bound to HLA-DQ1 (Hy.1B11), HLA-DR4 (MS2-3C8), HLA-DR2a (3A6), or HLA-DR2b (Ob.1A12). T cells expressing these four autoimmune TCRs escaped negative selection in the thymus yet still retained the ability to productively engage self-antigens in the periphery. The remaining 12 TCRs recognize foreign antigens, such as influenza virus hemagglutinin (HA1.7) and moth cytochrome c (2B4, 226), or tumor antigens (G4, E8). In **Figure 4B**, the C-termini of CD4 in the 16 TCR–pMHC–CD4 complexes sweep out an arc of ~70°, with autoimmune TCRs Ob.1A12 and Hy.1B11 at the two extremities. Strikingly, the 12 anti-foreign or tumor-specific TCRs form a relatively tight cluster that effectively excludes the four autoimmune TCRs, with Ob.1A12 on one side of the cluster and Hy.1B11, MS2-3C8, and 3A6 on the other. Because CD4-bound Lck would be positioned differently with respect to CD3 ITAMs inside the T cell, phosphorylation of CD3 ITAMs by Lck may be differentially affected in TCR–pMHC–CD4 complexes involving anti-foreign versus autoimmune TCRs. In this way, the geometry of the TCR–pMHC–CD4 complex could modulate TCR signaling, and thereby directly impact T cell development and autoimmunity.

IMPLICATIONS FOR THE TCR–pMHC–CD8 TERNARY COMPLEX

Although no structure of a TCR–pMHC–CD8 ternary complex has been reported, a hypothetical model may be constructed by superposing the CD8αβ–H-$2D^d$ complex (23) onto a representative TCR–pMHC class I complex through the shared MHC class I molecule (**Figure 3B**). The model is consistent with the idea that the shorter CD8β stalk helps orient the cytoplasmic domains of CD8αβ for their role in signal transduction (23, 79). However, in the absence of structural information on the CD8 stalk, the model cannot establish anchor points for TCR and CD8 on the T cell membrane, as did the TCR–pMHC–CD4 structure (**Figure 3A**). While the TCR–pMHC–CD8 complex is probably not as conformationally constrained as the TCR–pMHC–CD4 complex, *O*-glycosylation of the CD8 stalk likely restricts its flexibility (36, 42), as discussed above. By limiting the mobility of the MHC-binding head group of CD8 in this way, *O*-glycosylation would impose constraints on the orientation of CD3 subunits relative to CD8-bound Lck, as does the rigid CD4 structure (**Figure 4A**).

Even with *O*-glycosylation, the proline-rich CD8 stalk is likely to be less stiff than the four tandem Ig-like domains of CD4. This flexibility may help compensate for variations in TCR–pMHC docking geometry to facilitate intracellular juxtaposition of CD8-bound Lck with CD3 ITAMs. The cytoplasmic tails of the CD3 subunits would provide additional flexibility within the overall TCR–pMHC–CD8 signaling complex, just as in the TCR–pMHC–CD4 complex.

FUTURE DIRECTIONS

Much more is known about the biophysics of CD8 interactions with TCR–pMHC at the T cell–APC interface than in the case of CD4. For example, whereas *in situ* studies have demonstrated that TCR and CD8 bind cooperatively to pMHC, and that this synergy amplifies peptide discrimination (9), there is no comparable information for CD4. Conversely, whereas the structure of a TCR–pMHC–CD4 complex has been reported (49), that of a TCR–pMHC–CD8 complex remains to be determined.

Until now, most studies of autoimmunity have emphasized reduced TCR affinity for self-pMHC as the main reason autoreactive T cells sometimes escape negative selection in the thymus (80). However, it is also possible that the altered docking topologies observed in autoimmune TCR–pMHC complexes (81) may modulate T cell signaling by altering interactions with CD4 or CD8. In fact, autoimmune TCRs appear to segregate from anti-foreign TCRs in terms of the geometry of the corresponding TCR–pMHC–CD4 ternary complexes (**Figure 4B**). This hypothesis clearly merits further investigation, particularly in view of an emerging appreciation for the role of TCR docking geometry on T cell signaling (49, 71).

The TCR–pMHC–CD4 structure, in conjunction with mutational data on TCR–CD3 ectodomain interactions, suggests that CD3εγ and CD3εδ are located under the TCR–pMHC–CD4 arch, facing CD4 (**Figure 4A**). However, the current reality is that we only have nebulous ideas about the molecular architecture of the TCR–CD3 complex. Direct structural analysis of the TCR–CD3 complex will be required to establish anchor points for CD3 and CD4 on the T cell membrane. This information, combined with the known pairings of the transmembrane helices of the TCR and CD3 chains from mutational analysis (TCRα–CD3εδ, TCRα–CD3ζζ, and TCRβ–CD3εγ) (59), will reveal the intracellular organization of CD3 ITAMs relative to each other, and relative to Lck bound to the CD4 or CD8 co-receptor.

ACKNOWLEDGMENTS

This work was supported by Grants from the National Institutes of Health (AI036900 and AI073654) to Roy A. Mariuzza.

REFERENCES

1. Janeway CA Jr. The T cell receptor as a multicomponent signalling machine: CD4/CD8 coreceptors and T cell activation. *Annu Rev Immunol* (1992) **10**:645–54. doi:10.1146/annurev.immunol.10.1.645
2. Zamoyska R. CD4 and CD8: modulators of T-cell receptor recognition of antigen and of immune responses? *Curr Opin Immunol* (1998) **10**:82–7. doi:10.1016/S0952-7915(98)80036-8
3. Singer A, Bosselut R. CD4/CD8 coreceptors in thymocyte development, selection, and lineage commitment: analysis of the CD4/CD8 lineage decision. *Adv Immunol* (2004) **83**:91–131. doi:10.1016/S0065-2776(04)83003-7
4. Laugel B, van den Berg HA, Gostick E, Cole DK, Wooldridge L, Boulter J, et al. Different T cell receptor affinity thresholds and CD8 coreceptor dependence govern cytotoxic T lymphocyte activation and tetramer binding properties. *J Biol Chem* (2007) **282**:23799–810. doi:10.1074/jbc.M700976200
5. Irvine DJ, Purbhoo MA, Krogsgaard M, Davis MM. Direct observation of ligand recognition by T cells. *Nature* (2002) **419**:845–9. doi:10.1038/nature01076
6. Holler PD, Kranz DM. Quantitative analysis of the contribution of TCR/pepMHC affinity and CD8 to T cell activation. *Immunity* (2003) **18**:255–64. doi:10.1016/S1074-7613(03)00019-0
7. Li QJ, Dinner AR, Qi S, Irvine DJ, Huppa JB, Davis MM, et al. CD4 enhances T cell sensitivity to antigen by coordinating Lck accumulation at the immunological synapse. *Nat Immunol* (2004) **5**:791–9. doi:10.1038/ni1095
8. Artyomov MN, Lis M, Devadas S, Davis MM, Chakraborty AK. CD4 and CD8 binding to MHC molecules primarily acts to enhance Lck delivery. *Proc Natl Acad Sci U S A* (2010) **107**:16916–21. doi:10.1073/pnas.1010568107
9. Jiang N, Huang J, Edwards LJ, Liu B, Zhang Y, Beal CD, et al. Two-stage cooperative T cell receptor-peptide major histocompatibility complex-CD8 trimolecular interactions amplify antigen discrimination. *Immunity* (2011) **34**:13–23. doi:10.1016/j.immuni.2010.12.017
10. van der Merwe PA, Cordoba SP. Late arrival: recruiting coreceptors to the T cell receptor complex. *Immunity* (2011) **34**:1–3. doi:10.1016/j.immuni.2011.01.001
11. Van Laethem F, Tikhonova AN, Singer A. MHC restriction is imposed on a diverse T cell repertoire by CD4 and CD8 co-receptors during thymic selection. *Trends Immunol* (2012) **33**:437–41. doi:10.1016/j.it.2012.05.006
12. Van Laethem F, Sarafova SD, Park JH, Tai X, Pobezinsky L, Guinter TI, et al. Deletion of CD4 and CD8 coreceptors permits generation of αβT cells that recognize antigens independently of the MHC. *Immunity* (2007) **27**:735–50. doi:10.1016/j.immuni.2007.10.007
13. Tikhonova AN, Van Laethem F, Hanada K, Lu J, Pobezinsky LA, Hong C, et al. αβ T cell receptors that do not undergo major histocompatibility complex-specific thymic selection possess antibody-like recognition specificities. *Immunity* (2012) **36**:79–81. doi:10.1016/j.immuni.2011.11.013
14. Devine L, Kieffer LJ, Aitken V, Kavathas PB. Human CD8β, but not mouse CD8β, can be expressed in the absence of CD8α as a ββ homodimer. *J Immunol* (2000) **164**:833–8.
15. Cheroutre H, Lambolez F. Doubting the TCR coreceptor function of CD8α/α. *Immunity* (2008) **28**:149–56. doi:10.1016/j.immuni.2008.01.005
16. Fung-Leung WP, Schilham MW, Rahemtulla A, Kündig TM, Vollenweider M, Potter J, et al. CD8 is needed for development of cytotoxic T cells but not helper T cells. *Cell* (1991) **65**:443–9. doi:10.1016/0092-8674(91)90462-8
17. Crooks ME, Littman DR. Disruption of T lymphocyte positive and negative selection in mice lacking the CD8 β chain. *Immunity* (1994) **1**:277–85. doi:10.1016/1074-7613(94)90079-5
18. Nakayama K, Negishi I, Kuida K, Louie MC, Kanagawa O, Nakauchi H, et al. Requirement for CD8 β chain in positive selection of CD8-lineage T cells. *Science* (1994) **263**:1131–3. doi:10.1126/science.8108731
19. Moebius U, Kober G, Griscelli AL, Hercend T, Meuer SC. Expression of different CD8 isoforms on distinct human lymphocyte subpopulations. *Eur J Immunol* (1991) **21**:1793–800. doi:10.1002/eji.1830210803
20. Grebe KM, Clarke RL, Potter TA. Ligation of CD8 leads to apoptosis of thymocytes that have not undergone positive selection. *Proc Natl Acad Sci U S A* (2004) **101**:10410–5. doi:10.1073/pnas.0402079101
21. Yachi PP, Ampudia J, Zal T, Gascoigne NR. Altered peptide ligands induce delayed CD8-T cell receptor interaction – a role for CD8 in distinguishing antigen quality. *Immunity* (2006) **25**:203–11. doi:10.1016/j.immuni.2006.05.015
22. Garcia KC, Scott CA, Brunmark A, Carbone FR, Peterson PA, Wilson IA, et al. CD8 enhances formation of stable T-cell receptor/MHC class I molecule complexes. *Nature* (1996) **384**:577–81. doi:10.1038/384577a0
23. Wang R, Natarajan K, Margulies DH. Structural basis of the CD8 αβ/MHC class I interaction: focused recognition orients CD8 β to a T cell proximal position. *J Immunol* (2009) **183**:2554–64. doi:10.4049/jimmunol.0901276
24. Wyer JR, Willcox BE, Gao GF, Gerth UC, Davis SJ, Bell JI, et al. T cell receptor and coreceptor CD8 αα bind peptide-MHC independently and with distinct kinetics. *Immunity* (1999) **10**:219–25. doi:10.1016/S1074-7613(00)80022-9
25. Gao GF, Willcox BE, Wyer JR, Boulter JM, O'Callaghan CA, Maenaka K, et al. Classical and nonclassical class I major histocompatibility complex molecules exhibit subtle conformational differences that affect binding to CD8αα. *J Biol Chem* (2000) **275**:15232–8. doi:10.1074/jbc.M909946199
26. Cole DK, Dunn SM, Sami M, Boulter JM, Jakobsen BK, Sewell AK. T cell receptor engagement of peptide-major histocompatibility complex class I does not modify CD8 binding. *Mol Immunol* (2008) **45**:2700–9. doi:10.1016/j.molimm.2007.12.009
27. Huang J, Edwards LJ, Evavold BD, Zhu C. Kinetics of MHC-CD8 interaction at the T cell membrane. *J Immunol* (2007) **179**:7653–62.
28. Zhu C, Jiang N, Huang J, Zarnitsyna VI, Evavold BD. Insights from *in situ* analysis of TCR-pMHC recognition: response of an interaction network. *Immunol Rev* (2013) **251**:49–64. doi:10.1111/imr.12016
29. Gao GF, Tormo J, Gerth UC, Wyer JR, McMichael AJ, Stuart DI, et al. Crystal structure of the complex between human CD8αα and HLA-A2. *Nature* (1997) **387**:630–4. doi:10.1038/42523
30. Shi Y, Qi J, Iwamoto A, Gao GF. Plasticity of human CD8αα binding to peptide-HLA-A*2402. *Mol Immunol* (2011) **48**:2198–202. doi:10.1016/j.molimm.2011.05.009

31. Kern PS, Teng MK, Smolyar A, Liu JH, Liu J, Hussey RE, et al. Structural basis of CD8 coreceptor function revealed by crystallographic analysis of a murine CD8αα ectodomain fragment in complex with H-2K^b. *Immunity* (1998) **9**:519–30. doi:10.1016/S1074-7613(00)80635-4
32. Casabó LG, Mamalaki C, Kioussis D, Zamoyska R. T cell activation results in physical modification of the mouse CD8β chain. *J Immunol* (1994) **152**:397–404.
33. Rudd PM, Elliott T, Cresswell P, Wilson IA, Dwek RA. Glycosylation and the immune system. *Science* (2001) **291**:2370–6. doi:10.1126/science.291.5512.2370
34. Moody AM, Chui D, Reche PA, Priatel JJ, Marth JD, Reinherz EL. Developmentally regulated glycosylation of the CD8αβ coreceptor stalk modulates ligand binding. *Cell* (2001) **107**:501–12. doi:10.1016/S0092-8674(01)00577-3
35. Daniels MA, Devine L, Miller JD, Moser JM, Lukacher AE, Altman JD, et al. CD8 binding to MHC class I molecules is influenced by T cell maturation and glycosylation. *Immunity* (2001) **15**:1051–61. doi:10.1016/S1074-7613(01)00252-7
36. Merry AH, Gilbert RJ, Shore DA, Royle L, Miroshnychenko O, Vuong M, et al. O-glycan sialylation and the structure of the stalk-like region of the T cell co-receptor CD8. *J Biol Chem* (2003) **278**:27119–28. doi:10.1074/jbc.M213056200
37. Santos SG, Powis SJ, Arosa FA. Misfolding of major histocompatibility complex class I molecules in activated T cells allows *cis*-interactions with receptors and signaling molecules and is associated with tyrosine phosphorylation. *J Biol Chem* (2004) **279**:53062–70. doi:10.1074/jbc.M408794200
38. Back J, Malchiodi EL, Cho S, Scarpellino L, Schneider P, Kerzic MC, et al. Distinct conformations of Ly49 natural killer cell receptors mediate MHC class I recognition in *trans* and *cis*. *Immunity* (2009) **31**:598–608. doi:10.1016/j.immuni.2009.07.007
39. Hartmann J, Tran TV, Kaudeer J, Oberle K, Herrmann J, Quagliano I, et al. The stalk domain and the glycosylation status of the activating natural killer cell receptor NKp30 are important for ligand binding. *J Biol Chem* (2012) **287**:31527–39. doi:10.1074/jbc.M111.304238
40. Shogren R, Gerken TA, Jentoft N. Role of glycosylation on the conformation and chain dimensions of *O*-linked glycoproteins: light scattering studies of ovine submaxillary mucin. *Biochemistry* (1989) **28**:5525–36. doi:10.1021/bi00439a029
41. Gerken TA, Butenhof JK, Shogren R. Effects of glycosylation on the conformation and dynamics of *O*-linked glycoproteins: carbon-13 NMR studies of ovine submaxillary mucin. *Biochemistry* (1989) **28**:5536–43. doi:10.1021/bi00439a030
42. Shore DA, Wilson IA, Dwek RA, Rudd PM. Glycosylation and the function of the T cell co-receptor CD8. *Adv Exp Med Biol* (2005) **564**:71–84. doi:10.1007/0-387-25515-X_12
43. Davis SJ, Ikemizu S, Evans EJ, Fugger L, Bakker TR, van der Merwe PA. The nature of molecular recognition by T cells. *Nat Immunol* (2003) **4**:217–24. doi:10.1038/ni0303-217
44. Cole DK, Pumphrey NJ, Boulter JM, Sami M, Bell JI, Gostick E, et al. Human TCR-binding affinity is governed by MHC class restriction. *J Immunol* (2007) **178**:5727–34.
45. Xiong Y, Kern P, Chang H, Reinherz E. T cell receptor binding to a pMHCII ligand is kinetically distinct from and independent of CD4. *J Biol Chem* (2001) **276**:5659–67. doi:10.1074/jbc.M009580200
46. Robinson J, Mistry K, McWilloam H, Lopez R, Parham P, Marsh SGE. The IMGT/HLA database. *Nucleic Acids Res* (2011) **39**:D1171–6. doi:10.1093/nar/gkq998
47. Wang JH, Meijers R, Xiong Y, Liu JH, Sakihama T, Zhang R, et al. Crystal structure of the human CD4 N-terminal two-domain fragment complexed to a class II MHC molecule. *Proc Natl Acad Sci U S A* (2001) **98**:10799–804. doi:10.1073/pnas.191124098
48. Wang XX, Li Y, Yin Y, Mo M, Wang Q, Gao W, et al. Affinity maturation of human CD4 by yeast surface display and crystal structure of a CD4–HLA-DR1 complex. *Proc Natl Acad Sci U S A* (2011) **108**:15960–5. doi:10.1073/pnas.1109438108
49. Yin Y, Wang XX, Mariuzza RA. Crystal structure of a complete ternary complex of T-cell receptor, peptide-MHC, and CD4. *Proc Natl Acad Sci U S A* (2012) **109**:5405–10. doi:10.1073/pnas.1118801109
50. Gai SA, Wittrup KD. Yeast surface display for protein engineering and characterization. *Curr Opin Struct Biol* (2007) **17**:467–73. doi:10.1016/j.sbi.2007.08.012
51. Yin Y, Li Y, Kerzic MC, Martin R, Mariuzza RA. Structure of a TCR with high affinity for self-antigen reveals basis for escape from negative selection. *EMBO J* (2011) **30**:1137–48. doi:10.1038/emboj.2011.21
52. Rudolph MG, Stanfield RL, Wilson IA. How TCRs bind MHCs, peptides, and coreceptors. *Annu Rev Immunol* (2006) **24**:419–66. doi:10.1146/annurev.immunol.23.021704.115658
53. Marrack P, Scott-Browne JP, Dai S, Gapin L, Kappler JW. Evolutionarily conserved amino acids that control TCR-MHC interaction. *Annu Rev Immunol* (2008) **26**:171–203. doi:10.1146/annurev.immunol.26.021607.090421
54. Wu H, Kwong PD, Hendrickson WA. Dimeric association and segmental variability in the structure of human CD4. *Nature* (1997) **387**:527–30. doi:10.1038/387527a0
55. van der Merwe PA, Dushek O. Mechanisms of T cell receptor triggering. *Nat Rev Immunol* (2010) **11**:47–55. doi:10.1038/nri2887
56. Kuhns MS, Davis MM. Disruption of extracellular interactions impairs T cell receptor-CD3 complex stability and signaling. *Immunity* (2007) **26**:357–69. doi:10.1016/j.immuni.2007.01.015
57. Kuhns MS, Girvin AT, Klein LO, Chen R, Jensen KD, Newell EW, et al. Evidence for a functional sidedness to the αβ TCR. *Proc Natl Acad Sci U S A* (2010) **107**:5094–9. doi:10.1073/pnas.1000925107
58. Fernandes RA, Shore DA, Vuong MT, Yu C, Zhu X, Pereira-Lopes S, et al. The T-cell receptor is a structure capable of initiating signaling in the absence of large conformational rearrangements. *J Biol Chem* (2012) **287**:13324–35. doi:10.1074/jbc.M111.332783
59. Call ME, Pyrdol J, Wiedmann M, Wucherpfennig KW. The organizing principle in the formation of the T cell receptor-CD3 complex. *Cell* (2002) **111**:967–79. doi:10.1016/S0092-8674(02)01194-7
60. Xu C, Gagnon E, Call ME, Schnell JR, Schwieters CD, Carman CV, et al. Regulation of T cell receptor activation by dynamic membrane binding of the CD3ε cytoplasmic tyrosine-based motif. *Cell* (2008) **135**:702–13. doi:10.1016/j.cell.2008.09.044
61. Brown JH, Jardetzky TS, Gorga JC, Stern LJ, Urban RG, Strominger JL, et al. Three-dimensional structure of the human class II histocompatibility antigen HLA-DR1. *Nature* (1993) **364**:33–9. doi:10.1038/364033a0
62. Moldovan MC, Sabbagh L, Breton G, Sékaly RP, Krummel MF. Triggering of T cell activation via CD4 dimers. *J Immunol* (2006) **176**:5438–45.
63. Ghosh P, Amaya M, Mellins E, Wiley DC. The structure of an intermediate in class II MHC maturation: CLIP bound to HLA-DR3. *Nature* (1995) **378**:457–62. doi:10.1038/378457a0
64. Kuhns MS, Badgandi HB. Piecing together the family portrait of TCR–CD3 complexes. *Immunol Rev* (2012) **250**:120–43. doi:10.1111/imr.12000
65. Wang JH, Reinherz EL. Revisiting the putative TCR Cα dimerization model through structural analysis. *Front Immunol* (2013) **4**:16. doi:10.3389/fimmu.2013.00016
66. Kim ST, Takeuchi K, Sun ZY, Touma M, Castro CE, Fahmy A, et al. The αβ T cell receptor is an anisotropic mechanosensor. *J Biol Chem* (2009) **284**:31028–37. doi:10.1074/jbc.M109.052712
67. Li YC, Chen BM, Wu PC, Cheng TL, Kao LS, Tao MH, et al. Cutting edge: mechanical forces acting on T cells immobilized via the TCR complex can trigger TCR signaling. *J Immunol* (2010) **184**:5959–63. doi:10.4049/jimmunol.0900775
68. Judokusumo E, Tabdanov E, Kumari S, Dustin ML, Kam LC. Mechanosensing in T lymphocyte activation. *Biophys J* (2012) **102**:L5–7. doi:10.1016/j.bpj.2011.12.011
69. Garcia KC, Adams JJ, Feng D, Ely LK. The molecular basis of TCR germline bias for MHC is surprisingly simple. *Nat Immunol* (2009) **10**:143–7. doi:10.1038/ni.f.219
70. Scott-Browne JP, White J, Kappler JW, Gapin L, Marrack P. Germline-encoded amino acids in the αβ T-cell receptor control thymic selection. *Nature* (2009) **458**:1043–6. doi:10.1038/nature07812
71. Adams JJ, Narayanan S, Liu B, Birnbaum ME, Kruse AC, Bowerman NA, et al. T cell receptor signaling is limited by docking geometry to peptide-major histocompatibility complex. *Immunity* (2011) **35**:681–93. doi:10.1016/j.immuni.2011.09.013
72. Garcia KC. Reconciling views on T cell receptor germline bias for MHC. *Trends Immunol* (2012) **33**:429–36. doi:10.1016/j.it.2012.05.005
73. Deng L, Langley RJ, Wang Q, Topalian SL, Mariuzza RA. Structural insights into the editing of germ-line-encoded interactions between T-cell receptor and MHC

class II by Vα CDR3. *Proc Natl Acad Sci U S A* (2012) **109**:14960–5. doi: 10.1073/pnas.1207186109

74. Buslepp J, Wang H, Biddison WE, Appella E, Collins EJ. A correlation between TCR Vα docking on MHC and CD8 dependence: implications for T cell selection. *Immunity* (2003) **19**:595–606. doi: 10.1016/S1074-7613(03)00269-3
75. Mazza C, Malissen B. What guides MHC-restricted TCR recognition? *Semin Immunol* (2007) **19**: 225–35. doi:10.1016/j.smim.2007.03.003
76. Hahn M, Nicholson MJ, Pyrdol J, Wucherpfennig KW. Unconventional topology of self peptide-major histocompatibility complex binding by a human autoimmune T cell receptor. *Nat Immunol* (2005) **6**:490–6. doi:10.1038/ni1187
77. Boggon TJ, Eck MJ. Structure and regulation of Src family kinases. *Oncogene* (2004) **23**:7918–27. doi: 10.1038/sj.onc.1208081
78. Sigalov AB, Aivazian DA, Uversky VN, Stern LJ. Lipid-binding activity of intrinsically unstructured cytoplasmic domains of multichain immune recognition receptor signaling subunits. *Biochemistry* (2006) **45**:15731–9. doi:10.1021/bi061108f
79. Rettig LL, McNeill L, Sarner N, Guillaume P, Luescher I, Tolaini M, et al. An essential role for the stalk region of CD8 β in the coreceptor function of CD8. *J Immunol* (2009) **182**:121–9.
80. Goodnow CC, Sprent J, Fazekas de St Groth B, Vinuesa CG. Cellular and genetic mechanisms of self tolerance and autoimmunity. *Nature* (2005) **435**:590–7. doi:10.1038/nature03724
81. Wucherpfennig KW, Call MJ, Deng L, Mariuzza RA. Structural alterations in peptide-MHC recognition by self-reactive T cell receptors. *Curr Opin Immunol* (2009) **21**:590–5. doi:10.1016/j.coi.2009.07.008

4

Immune parameters to consider when choosing T-cell receptors for therapy

Scott R. Burrows[1,2] and John J. Miles[1,2,3] *

[1] Human Immunity Laboratory and Cellular Immunology Laboratory, Queensland Institute of Medical Research, Brisbane, QLD, Australia
[2] School of Medicine, The University of Queensland, Brisbane, QLD, Australia
[3] Institute of Infection and Immunity, Cardiff University School of Medicine, Cardiff, Wales, UK

Edited by:
Bruno Laugel, Cardiff University School of Medicine, UK

Reviewed by:
Liisa Kaarina Selin, University of Massachusetts Medical School, USA
Mirjam Heemskerk, Leiden University Medical Center, Netherlands

Correspondence:
John J. Miles, Human Immunity Laboratory, Queensland Institute of Medical Research, 300 Herston Road, Herston, Brisbane, QLD 4006, Australia
e-mail: john.miles@qimr.edu.au

T-cell receptor (TCR) therapy has arrived as a realistic treatment option for many human diseases. TCR gene therapy allows for the mass redirection of T-cells against a defined antigen while high affinity TCR engineering allows for the creation of a new class of soluble drugs. However, deciding which TCR blueprint to take forward for gene therapy or engineering is difficult. More than one quintillion TCR combinations can be generated by somatic recombination and we are only now beginning to appreciate that not all are functionally equal. TCRs can exhibit high or low degrees of HLA-restricted cross-reactivity and alloreact against one or a combination of HLA alleles. Identifying TCR candidates with high specificity and minimal cross-reactivity/alloreactivity footprints before engineering is obviously highly desirable. Here we will summarize what we currently know about TCR biology with regard to immunoengineering.

Keywords: T-cell epitope, T-cell receptor, T-cell engineering

BACKGROUND

The αβ T-cell receptor (TCR) is one of the most variable proteins known to science (1) with the human V(D)J recombination system capable of generating hundreds of trillion of unique αβ TCR molecules (2). This incredibly vast receptor reserve is our immune systems' core defense against the torrent of hypervariable microorganisms and pathogenic challenges encountered over the course of life. During thymopoiesis, the TCR recombination machinery uses "cut-and-paste" transposition to incise and rearrange 174 variable (TRAV and TRBV), diversity (TRBD), joining (TRAJ and TRBJ), and constant (TRAC and TRBC) TCR gene segments on chromosomes 7 (TRB loci) and 14 (TRA loci) into around seven-and-a-half million distinctive gene combinations (2). This chromosomal recombination process generates only around 10% of total TCR diversity with the remaining 90% of diversity generated through further exonuclease activity and the addition of random, non-template-dependent nucleotides (N-nucleotides) across the V(D)J junction by the enzyme terminal deoxynucleotidyl transferase (TdT) (3). The collective sum of this recombination event is a theoretical 10^{15}–10^{20} structurally unique αβ TCR molecules (1, 4, 5). Due to size constraints (2), the human immune system only houses an infinitely small slice of the full repertoire. In an adult human, this equates to 10^{12} T-cells (6, 7) bearing around 2.5×10^6 unique αβ TCR structures (6), with the upper bounds comprising 10^8–10^{11} unique αβ TCR structures per individual (6, 7).

The αβ TCR is a glycosylated, membrane-integral surface protein comprising one α-chain and one β-chain (2). The two chains fold and fuse via cysteine–cysteine disulfide linkers to produce a single, functional heterodimeric receptor (8, 9). The outward facing and solvent-exposed edge of the heterodimer bears six highly flexible complementarity determining region (CDR) loops. The CDR1 and CDR2 loops are encoded by the germline TRAV and TRBV genes and generally function to fix the TCR to the major histocompatibility complex (MHC) platform. Conversely, the CDR3 loops are encoded by the somatically hypervariable V(D)J junction and classically function to engage the peptide (p) cradled in the MHC groove (8, 9), although variations on CDR binding geometry have been noted (9).

A TCR engages its cognate pMHC as a single, composite ligand, and docks in an approximately diagonal fashion that slightly varies in pivot and tilt from complex to complex (9, 10). One steady constant of TCR/pMHC engagement is that the CDR3α loop is positioned toward the direction of the peptide N-terminus and the CDR3β loop is positioned toward the direction of the peptide C-terminus and variation in this geometry has not been seen to date (9, 10), however extreme terminal focusing has been recently observed (11). The TCR/pMHC docking process can be very fluid and conformational changes to the TCR, peptide, and MHC have all been observed suggesting that both interfaces often adjust to each other to find a compatible binding solution (9). Biophysical data show that TCR binding is stratified based on function. TCRs that engage pMHC class-I (pMHC-I) targets bind strongly with a mean affinity three time stronger than TCRs that engage pMHC class-II (pMHC-II) targets (8). Likewise, TCRs are further stratified based on whether the antigen target is of self or foreign origin, with foreign-reactive TCRs binding cognate pMHC with a mean affinity 10 times stronger than TCRs that bind self pMHC (8).

In spite of the large number of TCR receptor "options" available in the naive repertoire, T-cell repertoires deployed against pMHC antigens often exhibit ordered and predictable TCR gene architecture [reviewed (2, 12)]. This phenomenon, termed TCR bias, can result in residue-identical memory clonotypes being found across multiple individuals sharing a common MHC allele. The mechanisms behind the appearance of these "public" T-cell responses are still being determined (2) but is thought to involve both biases in recombination during thymopoiesis (13) and some optimal, structural-based, filtering event during antigen-driven selection (14–20). For this filtering event, it appears the peptide is the determining factor during repertoire formation (21) with TCR repertoire assembly not dependent on antigen source, presenting MHC allele or immunodominance hierarchy. Once a memory T-cell repertoire is established, it appears to remain relatively consistent both in terms of clonotype stability and clonotype frequency over decades of life (22, 23).

Adoptive cell therapy (ACT) using antigen-specific T-cells has proven to be a remarkably effective experimental treatment option for Epstein–Barr virus malignancies (24), cytomegalovirus infection (25), and melanoma (26). Given these promising results, many groups have turned toward TCR gene transfer as a simpler, faster, and more homogeneous technique for generating ACTs. Here, antigen-specific αβ TCR genes are delivered into recipient T-cells using a γ-retroviral vector, lentiviral vector, or transposon [reviewed (26)]. Another parallel approach for TCR therapy is to engineer high affinity mutants from natural αβ TCR "blueprints" using yeast display (27) or phage display (28). These TCR mutants can have their binding affinities amplified logarithmically to the low pM K_D range (28) while still retaining high specificity for antigen (28, 29). Affinity enhanced TCR can be used in two ways. First the mutants can be gene transferred into T-cells to increase antigen sensitivity and polyfunctionality (30). Second, the mutants can be used in soluble form to deliver therapeutic payloads to cells bearing the appropriate pMHC targets (31). Importantly, before considering a receptor for therapeutic ends, a number of parameters should be considered regarding the genetics and biology of the human TCR.

CONSIDERATION ONE: CROSS-REACTIVITY

The first parameter to considering when applying TCR therapy is the cross-reactivity profile of the candidate receptor. A theoretical proposal (32) predicted that the αβ TCR must intrinsically encode a high degree of cross-reactivity in order to provide sufficient coverage against the huge constellation of pMHC complexes that could be encountered in nature. Through the use of combinatorial peptide libraries (CPLs), that comprise almost all possible peptides of a particular length, this theory was recently tested experimentally and proven (33, 34). In the context of a single MHC, a single αβ TCR can recognize over one million different peptides as well or better than its cognate ligand (34). Whether this is the case for *all* TCRs is under active investigation. Very recent CPL data suggests that TCRs have sliding cross-reactive intensities (35) and, at least for pMHC-I-specific TCRs, an explicit preference for peptides of defined length. Thus, cross-reactivity for peptides outside a TCRs "programmed length preference" is unlikely.

Given the intrinsic cross-reactivity of TCRs, it is tempting to select for TCR that engage multiple target pMHC. Indeed, this "multiple birds with one stone" approach could dramatically boost therapeutic efficacy of a candidate TCR *in vivo*. However, caution is advised in this pursuit as it has recently been shown that multi-pMHC specific TCR can result in serious side effects (36). Here, a therapeutic TCR that recognized multiple MAGE-derived peptides resulted in neurological toxicity when administered to melanoma patients as TCR gene therapy. Off-target toxicity was thought to be due to one of the MAGE peptides being expressed in the brain. This localized expression profile was not previously known.

Another parameter to consider (on top of the large numbers of proteogenic peptides T-cells can recognize) is the issue of "transformed self." It is known that αβ T-cells can engage proteogenic peptides containing post-translational modifications, such as phosphorylation (37), glycosylation (38), citrullination (39), and dimerization (40). Whether a given αβ TCR also cross-recognizes large numbers of modified peptides is yet to be determined. In addition to classical pMHC-I and pMHC-II targets, αβ TCR are also now known to bind a growing list of classical and non-classical MHC molecules which cradle an extraordinary diverse array of organic and inorganic compounds (41). TCR ligands can include proteogenic peptides in HLA-E (42), lipids in the cluster of differentiation 1 (CD1) molecule (41, 43), vitamin metabolites in MHC-I related (MR1) molecules (44), small molecule drugs in MHC-I (45), and the empty platform of human hemochromatosis protein (HFE) (46).

Precisely mapping the complete cross-reactive profile of a therapeutic TCR candidate across the thousands of classical and non-classical MHC alleles which present a combined universe of organic and inorganic compounds is currently possible but difficult. Basic approaches are available for assessment (**Table 1**). For instance, scanning a group of candidate TCRs across a CPL library can quickly rule out receptors with extensive pMHC cross-reactivity footprints. From these select receptors, blasting the raw CPL data across the human proteome may identify self peptides which could drive off-target activity *in vivo*. Candidate TCR with minimal cross-reactivity footprints as suggested by CPL scanning could then advance to *in vitro* testing on multi-cell subsets. Here, various cell types (monocytes, DCs, T-cells, B-cells, fibroblasts, epithelial cells, etc.) that express the HLA restriction allele of interest could be used as target cells to determine potential TCR cross-reactivity with self pMHC molecules. Target cells could be derived from primary sorted cells and/or cell lines.

CONSIDERATION TWO: ALLOREACTVITY

As mentioned above, a significant degree of degeneracy in peptide recognition likely evolved to ensure that the TCR repertoire has the capacity to recognize the enormous variety of foreign peptides that are encountered throughout life. Furthermore, broadly reactive T-cells may aid primary and memory responses where memory T-cells for one pathogen are reactivated by a different infectious agent (47). However, limited specificity of self-MHC-restricted T-cells is also the basis of the alloresponse and its associated clinical problems.

T-cell allorecognition occurs when the immune system is presented with MHC molecules of a different allotype to that of the host. Alloreactivity becomes clinically significant in the case of solid-organ grafts or bone marrow transplants in which mismatched MHC molecules can potentially result in organ graft rejection or graft versus-host disease (GVHD). This response can be either direct, in which the T-cells mount an immune response to the foreign-pMHC, or indirect, a chronic self-MHC restricted response resulting from polymorphism in the processed antigen that can include peptides from allogeneic MHC molecules (48). It is estimated that up to 0.1–1% of T-cells are alloreactive toward a given allogeneic MHC molecule (49). However, the probability of

Table 1 | Pre-clinical testing options for therapeutic TCR candidates.

Parameter to consider when choosing a candidate TCR for therapy	Testing option/s
Could the candidate TCR cross-react with a peptide presented by an autologous classical and non-classical MHC molecule?	Scan the candidate TCR across different primary cell subset targets (monocytes, DCs, B-cells, T-cells) sorted from prospective patients. Scan the candidate TCR across PBMC and cell lines (monocytes, DCs, B-cells, T-cells, fibroblast, epithelial) from a library of HLA allele matched healthy donors. Scan the candidate TCR across peptide length-matched CPL to establish a metric of cross-reactivity potential.
Could the candidate TCR alloreact with a peptide presented by a mismatched MHC molecule?	Scan the candidate TCR across an extensive, fully HLA haplotyped cell line library. The cell line library should contain HLA alleles found at high frequency in the target population.
Are the germline sequences for the candidate TCR donor/patient matched?	Compare the TRAV, TRAJ, TRBV, and TRBJ sequences of the candidate TCR with patient TR loci. Polymorphisms in these genes may alter the effectiveness of the therapeutic TCR *in vivo*. Additionally, if the donor/patient TR alleles do not match, or if the patient has a key TR allele deleted, there is a possibility that a patient-derived immune response could be mobilized against the "foreign" TCR.
Could the candidate TCR steer functional phenotype of recipient T-cells when used in gene therapy?	Transduce the candidate TCR in naive T-cells *in vitro* or into mice with human immune system components. Prime the cultures with differing concentrations of cognate Ag and monitor cell fate decisions. Note temporal and final ratios in effector, memory and Tfh differentiation. Transduce the candidate TCR in memory T-cells *in vitro*. Prime the cultures with differing concentrations of cognate Ag and monitor if cell fate is altered when compared to phenotype pre-transduction.

a TCR reacting with any allogeneic MHC molecules is obviously much higher due to MHC polymorphism, and this is a potential problem for TCR therapy.

There are numerous reports of T-cell clones with dual specificity for an allo-MHC molecule and a nominal antigen complexed with self-MHC (50). The best characterized example is the response to the Epstein–Barr virus epitope FLRGRAYGL, that binds to HLA-B8, in which CTL clones were isolated that cross-reacted with one of three common alloantigens (HLA-B44, B14, or B35) (51, 52). Interestingly, the HLA-B44 alloreactive TCR [which has also been shown to alloreact with HLA-B∗5501 (53)] is a public TCR that dominates the response to this viral epitope in most HLA-B8$^+$ people (54, 55). By examining the response to this viral epitope in individuals who co-expressed HLA-B8 and one of the alloantigen targets, subdominant TCRs were identified that were not alloreactive (55, 56). Such TCRs would be the obvious choice for use in TCR therapy, and this approach could be used in other systems to identify non-alloreactive TCRs for therapeutic use where the dominant receptors are alloreactive.

Many other T-cell clones have been shown to cross-react with alloantigens, and work from Frans Claas's group has shown that up to 45% of virus-reactive T-cell clones from humans are alloreactive (50). Allo-HLA cross-reactivity was shown from T-cell clones raised against a range of viruses including cytomegalovirus, varicella-zoster virus, and influenza (50). These included both CD8$^+$ and CD4$^+$ clones alloreacting with MHC-I and MHC-II molecules, respectively, and surprisingly, they also included two distinct cytomegalovirus-reactive, MHC-I-restricted T-cell clones that recognized allogeneic MHC-II molecules (57).

The obvious way to manage the problem of T-cell alloreactivity in the context of TCR therapy is to perform preliminary *in vitro* screens of the TCR for cross-recognition of cell lines expressing a wide range of allo-HLA alleles. The limitation here is that it will be near impossible to screen against the huge variety of HLA molecules, given there are over 6,000 known class-I alleles and over 1,000 class-II alleles. Furthermore, alloreactive T-cells are generally also specific for one or more "self"-peptides presented by the allo-HLA molecule, and these may not be presented by cells from all tissues, or they could be derived from polymorphic gene products and are therefore not presented by all individuals or cell lines. For example, the EBV-reactive TCR described above is specific for a "self"-peptide derived from an ATP binding cassette protein ABCD3 which is presented by allo-HLA-B44 and shares only one residue with the viral peptide (58). This peptide appears to be presented at different levels in distinct tissues based on the recent observation that these T-cells recognize HLA-B44$^+$ lymphoid cells but not epithelial and endothelial cells (59).

Although T-cell cross-reactivity with alloantigens has not proven to be a major problem in adoptive T-cell transfer clinical trials, it is an issue that should not be ignored in future trials of TCR therapy. Testing for cross-reactivity with one or more alloantigens is currently possible *in vitro* through target cell screening across large allo cell libraries (50, 53).

CONSIDERATION THREE: POLYMORPHISM

As with vaccines that elicit T-cell responses against a limited number of epitopes, TCR-based therapeutic approaches need to address the important issue of polymorphism in the genes involved in antigen presentation and those encoding for the target peptide antigens. Viral antigens are particularly prone to accumulating escape mutations, and so TCRs that recognize regions of viral proteins that are critical for viral fitness and are therefore highly conserved (60) should be favored for TCR therapy. Genetic instability is also a common feature of cancer cells, often resulting in the selection of antigenic variants by T-cells which allow cancer cells to escape destruction (61). The simultaneous administration of multiple TCRs that target different epitopes should circumvent these problems to some extent. Another potential mechanism through which human genetic polymorphism could create problems is if a TCR, transferred into an unrelated recipient, cross-reacts with a polymorphic self-peptide which it had not encountered during thymic negative selection, leading to damage of healthy tissue.

HLA polymorphism is also a major consideration that restricts the potential value of individual TCRs to a limited subset of any given population. As mentioned above, a huge number of HLA alleles have now been identified and therefore TCR therapy will need to be personalized to ensure recognition of epitopes presented by relevant HLA alleles. TCRs that recognize antigenic peptides that are presented by multiple HLA alleles are also valuable candidates for TCR therapy. A degree of degeneracy in HLA-peptide binding has been demonstrated whereby multiple class-I alleles can share common sequence motifs due to homology of amino acids within the major pockets of the peptide binding cleft, and these groups of alleles are referred to as HLA supertypes. Based on HLA structural similarities and overlapping peptide binding motifs, nine major HLA supertypes have been proposed (62). Examples of TCRs that have the capacity to recognize individual peptides bound to multiple members of an HLA supertype have been described (63–66). These TCRs with promiscuous HLA restriction can often accommodate differences in the exposed HLA α-helix residues between the restricting MHC and foreign MHC antigens that present the same peptide.

As with the MHC genes, allelic sequence variation is also a feature of the TCR and this issue needs to be addressed in the context of TCR therapy. Several sequencing studies have revealed considerable polymorphism within the TRAV and TRBV gene segments (67, 68). In one study, the TCR loci from 40 individuals across four ethnic groups were fully sequenced, and more than 550 SNPs were found, with many being situated in coding/regulatory regions of functional TCR genes and several causing null and non-functional mutations. On average, the coding region of each TCR variable gene contained two SNPs, with many more found in the 5′, 3′ and intronic sequences of these segments. A total of 51 SNPs in the TRA locus and 72 SNPs in the TRB locus were found to result in amino acid changes (67, 68).

The extensive variability within the TCR gene segments raises the interesting possibility that, unless the TCR genetics are matched between donor and recipient, some TCR gene products will be seen as foreign antigens and could elicit an immune response that limits the efficacy of transferred TCRs. Particularly strong immune responses could be expected in patients with deletions or inactivating polymorphisms that prevent expression of certain TRBV genes. There are seven frequently occurring inactivating polymorphisms in functional TRBV gene segments and a large (21.5 kb) insertion/deletion related polymorphism in the TRB locus encompassing two V gene segments (67–70). In the latter case, two functional variable β genes, *TRBV6-2/TRBV6-3* and *TRBV4-3*, are frequently deleted in all major ethnic groups (68, 70, 71). TCRs that are encoded by V genes that include common polymorphisms could perhaps be avoided for use in TCR therapy.

CONSIDERATION FOUR: FUNCTIONAL PHENOTYPE

Recent evidence suggests that different TCRs expressed by T-cell clones of the same pMHC specificity can have different effects on immune phenotype (72). When challenged with pathogen, clonotypically distinct naive T-cells were observed to give rise to differing ratios of Th1 and Tfh progeny. These alternate differentiation programs were dependent on pMHC dwell time and/or Ag density. Interestingly, this data suggests that different TCR clonotypes of the same pMHC specificity may impart differential effects on total immune function through varying effects on macrophage activity and antibody section by B-cells. An additional complexity in this area is the observation that after priming, a single naive T-cell can have multiple fates when proceeding down the cell differentiation pathway (73, 74). Thus, determining exactly which differentiation program a candidate TCR induces is an important parameter when considering a receptor for therapeutic use.

CONCLUDING REMARK

The TCR is an extremely effective tool for targeting biological and non-biological molecules and vast opportunity exists to exploit these receptors therapeutically. However, TCRs are highly polymorphic by nature and intrinsically encode a considerable degree of differential functionality and cross-reactivity across a number of MHC and MHC-like molecules. These factors require that therapeutic TCR candidates are donor/patient matched and undergo the most comprehensive *in vitro* cross-reactivity testing we can perform with present technology. The goal of this testing should be the identification of receptor candidates with predictable cell differentiation "programs" and minimal and traceable cross-reactivity/alloreactivity footprints.

REFERENCES

1. Shortman K, Egerton M, Spangrude GJ, Scollay R. The generation and fate of thymocytes. *Semin Immunol* (1990) **2**:3–12.
2. Miles JJ, Douek DC, Price DA. Bias in the alphabeta T-cell repertoire: implications for disease pathogenesis and vaccination. *Immunol Cell Biol* (2011) **89**:375–87. doi:10.1038/icb.2010.139
3. Cabaniols JP, Fazilleau N, Casrouge A, Kourilsky P, Kanellopoulos JM. Most alpha/beta T cell receptor diversity is due to terminal deoxynucleotidyl transferase. *J Exp Med* (2001) **194**:1385–90. doi:10.1084/jem.194.9.1385
4. Davis MM, Bjorkman PJ. T-cell antigen receptor genes and T-cell recognition. *Nature* (1988) **334**:395–402. doi:10.1038/334395a0
5. Lieber MR. Site-specific recombination in the immune system. *FASEB J* (1991) **5**:2934–44.
6. Arstila TP, Casrouge A, Baron V, Even J, Kanellopoulos J, Kourilsky P. A direct estimate of the human alphabeta T cell receptor diversity. *Science* (1999) **286**:958–61. doi:10.1126/science.286.5441.958
7. Arstila TP, Casrouge A, Baron V, Even J, Kanellopoulos J, Kourilsky P. Diversity of human alpha beta T cell receptors. *Science* (2000) **288**:1135. doi:10.1126/science.288.5469.1135a
8. Bridgeman JS, Sewell AK, Miles JJ, Price DA, Cole DK. Structural and biophysical determinants of alpha-beta T-cell antigen recognition. *Immunology* (2012) **135**:9–18. doi:10.1111/j.1365-2567.2011.03515.x

9. Gras S, Burrows SR, Turner SJ, Sewell AK, McCluskey J, Rossjohn J. A structural voyage toward an understanding of the MHC-I-restricted immune response: lessons learned and much to be learned. *Immunol Rev* (2012) **250**:61–81. doi:10.1111/j.1600-065X.2012.01159.x
10. Rudolph MG, Stanfield RL, Wilson IA. How TCRs bind MHCs, peptides, and coreceptors. *Annu Rev Immunol* (2006) **24**:419–66. doi:10.1146/annurev.immunol.23.021704.115658
11. Liu YC, Miles JJ, Neller MA, Gostick E, Price DA, Purcell AW, et al. Highly divergent T-cell receptor binding modes underlie specific recognition of a bulged viral peptide bound to a HLA class I molecule. *J Biol Chem* (2013) **288**:15442–54. doi:10.1074/jbc.M112.447185
12. Turner SJ, Doherty PC, McCluskey J, Rossjohn J. Structural determinants of T-cell receptor bias in immunity. *Nat Rev Immunol* (2006) **6**:883–94. doi:10.1038/nri1977
13. Venturi V, Price DA, Douek DC, Davenport MP. The molecular basis for public T-cell responses? *Nat Rev Immunol* (2008) **8**:231–8. doi:10.1038/nri2260
14. Gras S, Chen Z, Miles JJ, Liu YC, Bell MJ, Sullivan LC, et al. Allelic polymorphism in the T cell receptor and its impact on immune responses. *J Exp Med* (2010) **207**:1555–67. doi:10.1084/jem.20100603
15. Gras S, Saulquin X, Reiser JB, Debeaupuis E, Echasserieau K, Kissenpfennig A, et al. Structural bases for the affinity-driven selection of a public TCR against a dominant human cytomegalovirus epitope. *J Immunol* (2009) **183**:430–7. doi:10.4049/jimmunol.0900556
16. Ishizuka J, Stewart-Jones GB, van der Merwe A, Bell JI, McMichael AJ, Jones EY. The structural dynamics and energetics of an immunodominant T cell receptor are programmed by its Vbeta domain. *Immunity* (2008) **28**:171–82. doi:10.1016/j.immuni.2007.12.018
17. Kjer-Nielsen L, Clements CS, Purcell AW, Brooks AG, Whisstock JC, Burrows SR, et al. A structural basis for the selection of dominant alphabeta T cell receptors in antiviral immunity. *Immunity* (2003) **18**:53–64. doi:10.1016/S1074-7613(02)00513-7
18. Stewart-Jones GB, McMichael AJ, Bell JI, Stuart DI, Jones EY. A structural basis for immunodominant human T cell receptor recognition. *Nat Immunol* (2003) **4**:657–63. doi:10.1038/ni942
19. Tynan FE, Burrows SR, Buckle AM, Clements CS, Borg NA, Miles JJ, et al. T cell receptor recognition of a 'super-bulged' major histocompatibility complex class I-bound peptide. *Nat Immunol* (2005) **6**:1114–22. doi:10.1038/ni1257
20. Tynan FE, Reid HH, Kjer-Nielsen L, Miles JJ, Wilce MC, Kostenko L, et al. A T cell receptor flattens a bulged antigenic peptide presented by a major histocompatibility complex class I molecule. *Nat Immunol* (2007) **3**:268–76. doi:10.1038/ni1432
21. Koning D, Costa AI, Hoof I, Miles JJ, Nanlohy NM, Ladell K, et al. CD8+ TCR repertoire formation is guided primarily by the peptide component of the antigenic complex. *J Immunol* (2013) **190**:931–9. doi:10.4049/jimmunol.1202466
22. Miles JJ, Silins SL, Brooks AG, Davis JE, Misko I, Burrows SR. T-cell grit: large clonal expansions of virus-specific CD8+ T cells can dominate in the peripheral circulation for at least 18 years. *Blood* (2005) **106**:4412–3. doi:10.1182/blood-2005-06-2261
23. Neller MA, Burrows JM, Rist MJ, Miles JJ, Burrows SR. High frequency of herpesvirus-specific clonotypes in the human T cell repertoire can remain stable over decades with minimal turnover. *J Virol* (2013) **87**:697–700. doi:10.1128/JVI.02180-12
24. Bollard CM, Rooney CM, Heslop HE. T-cell therapy in the treatment of post-transplant lymphoproliferative disease. *Nat Rev Clin Oncol* (2012) **9**:510–9. doi:10.1038/nrclinonc.2012.111
25. Sellar RS, Peggs KS. Therapeutic strategies for the prevention and treatment of cytomegalovirus infection. *Expert Opin Biol Ther* (2012) **12**:1161–72. doi:10.1517/14712598.2012.693471
26. Park TS, Rosenberg SA, Morgan RA. Treating cancer with genetically engineered T cells. *Trends Biotechnol* (2011) **29**:550–7. doi:10.1016/j.tibtech.2011.04.009
27. Richman SA, Healan SJ, Weber KS, Donermeyer DL, Dossett ML, Greenberg PD, et al. Development of a novel strategy for engineering high-affinity proteins by yeast display. *Protein Eng Des Sel* (2006) **19**:255–64. doi:10.1093/protein/gzl008
28. Li Y, Moysey R, Molloy PE, Vuidepot AL, Mahon T, Baston E, et al. Directed evolution of human T-cell receptors with picomolar affinities by phage display. *Nat Biotechnol* (2005) **23**:349–54. doi:10.1038/nbt1070
29. Dunn SM, Rizkallah PJ, Baston E, Mahon T, Cameron B, Moysey R, et al. Directed evolution of human T cell receptor CDR2 residues by phage display dramatically enhances affinity for cognate peptide-MHC without increasing apparent cross-reactivity. *Protein Sci* (2006) **15**:710–21. doi:10.1110/ps.051936406
30. Varela-Rohena A, Molloy PE, Dunn SM, Li Y, Suhoski MM, Carroll RG, et al. Control of HIV-1 immune escape by CD8 T cells expressing enhanced T-cell receptor. *Nat Med* (2008) **14**:1390–5. doi:10.1038/nm.1779
31. Liddy N, Bossi G, Adams KJ, Lissina A, Mahon TM, Hassan NJ, et al. Monoclonal TCR-redirected tumor cell killing. *Nat Med* (2012) **18**:980–7. doi:10.1038/nm.2764
32. Mason D. A very high level of crossreactivity is an essential feature of the T-cell receptor. *Immunol Today* (1998) **19**:395–404. doi:10.1016/S0167-5699(98)01299-7
33. Sewell AK. Why must T cells be cross-reactive? *Nat Rev Immunol* (2012) **12**:669–77. doi:10.1038/nri3279
34. Wooldridge L, Ekeruche-Makinde J, van den Berg HA, Skowera A, Miles JJ, Tan MP, et al. A single autoimmune T cell receptor recognizes more than a million different peptides. *J Biol Chem* (2012) **287**:1168–77. doi:10.1074/jbc.M111.289488
35. Ekeruche-Makinde J, Miles JJ, van den Berg HA, Skowera A, Cole DK, Dolton G, et al. Peptide length determines the outcome of TCR/peptide-MHCI engagement. *Blood* (2013) **121**:1112–23. doi:10.1182/blood-2012-06-437202
36. Morgan RA, Chinnasamy N, Abate-Daga D, Gros A, Robbins PF, Zheng Z, et al. Cancer regression and neurological toxicity following anti-MAGE-A3 TCR gene therapy. *J Immunother* (2013) **36**:133–51. doi:10.1097/CJI.0b013e3182829903
37. Mohammed F, Cobbold M, Zarling AL, Salim M, Barrett-Wilt GA, Shabanowitz J, et al. Phosphorylation-dependent interaction between antigenic peptides and MHC class I: a molecular basis for the presentation of transformed self. *Nat Immunol* (2008) **9**:1236–43. doi:10.1038/ni.1660
38. Dowling W, Thompson E, Badger C, Mellquist JL, Garrison AR, Smith JM, et al. Influences of glycosylation on antigenicity, immunogenicity, and protective efficacy of ebola virus GP DNA vaccines. *J Virol* (2007) **81**:1821–37. doi:10.1128/JVI.02098-06
39. Hill JA, Bell DA, Brintnell W, Yue D, Wehrli B, Jevnikar AM, et al. Arthritis induced by posttranslationally modified (citrullinated) fibrinogen in DR4-IE transgenic mice. *J Exp Med* (2008) **205**:967–79. doi:10.1084/jem.20072051
40. Chen W, Yewdell JW, Levine RL, Bennink JR. Modification of cysteine residues in vitro and in vivo affects the immunogenicity and antigenicity of major histocompatibility complex class I-restricted viral determinants. *J Exp Med* (1999) **189**:1757–64. doi:10.1084/jem.189.11.1757
41. Adams EJ, Luoma AM. The adaptable major histocompatibility complex (MHC) fold: structure and function of nonclassical and MHC class I-like molecules. *Annu Rev Immunol* (2013) **31**:529–61. doi:10.1146/annurev-immunol-032712-095912
42. Sullivan LC, Hoare HL, McCluskey J, Rossjohn J, Brooks AG. A structural perspective on MHC class Ib molecules in adaptive immunity. *Trends Immunol* (2006) **27**:413–20. doi:10.1016/j.it.2006.07.006
43. Rossjohn J, Pellicci DG, Patel O, Gapin L, Godfrey DI. Recognition of CD1d-restricted antigens by natural killer T cells. *Nat Rev Immunol* (2012) **12**:845–57. doi:10.1038/nri3328
44. Kjer-Nielsen L, Patel O, Corbett AJ, Le Nours J, Meehan B, Liu L, et al. MR1 presents microbial vitamin B metabolites to MAIT cells. *Nature* (2012) **491**:717–23. doi:10.1038/nature11605
45. Illing PT, Vivian JP, Dudek NL, Kostenko L, Chen Z, Bharadwaj M, et al. Immune self-reactivity triggered by drug-modified HLA-peptide repertoire. *Nature* (2012) **486**:554–8. doi:10.1038/nature11147
46. Rohrlich PS, Fazilleau N, Ginhoux F, Firat H, Michel F, Cochet M, et al. Direct recognition by alphabeta cytolytic T cells of Hfe, a MHC class Ib molecule without antigen-presenting function. *Proc Natl Acad Sci U S A* (2005) **102**:12855–60. doi:10.1073/pnas.0502309102
47. Welsh RM, Che JW, Brehm MA, Selin LK. Heterologous immunity between viruses. *Immunol Rev* (2010) **235**:244–66.

48. Ely LK, Burrows SR, Purcell AW, Rossjohn J, McCluskey J. T-cells behaving badly: structural insights into alloreactivity and autoimmunity. *Curr Opin Immunol* (2008) **20**:575–80. doi:10.1016/j.coi.2008.07.006
49. Suchin EJ, Langmuir PB, Palmer E, Sayegh MH, Wells AD, Turka LA. Quantifying the frequency of alloreactive T cells in vivo: new answers to an old question. *J Immunol* (2001) **166**:973–81.
50. Amir AL, D'Orsogna LJ, Roelen DL, van Loenen MM, Hagedoorn RS, de Boer R, et al. Allo-HLA reactivity of virus-specific memory T cells is common. *Blood* (2010) **115**:3146–57. doi:10.1182/blood-2009-07-234906
51. Burrows SR, Khanna R, Burrows JM, Moss DJ. An alloresponse in humans is dominated by cytotoxic T lymphocytes (CTL) cross-reactive with a single Epstein-Barr virus CTL epitope: implications for graft-versus-host disease. *J Exp Med* (1994) **179**:1155–61. doi:10.1084/jem.179.4.1155
52. Burrows SR, Silins SL, Khanna R, Burrows JM, Rischmueller M, McCluskey J, et al. Cross-reactive memory T cells for Epstein-Barr virus augment the alloresponse to common human leukocyte antigens: degenerate recognition of major histocompatibility complex-bound peptide by T cells and its role in alloreactivity. *Eur J Immunol* (1997) **27**:1726–36. doi:10.1002/eji.1830270720
53. D'Orsogna LJ, Amir AL, Zoet YM, van der Meer-Prins PM, van der Slik AR, Kester MG, et al. New tools to monitor the impact of viral infection on the alloreactive T-cell repertoire. *Tissue Antigens* (2009) **74**:290–7. doi:10.1111/j.1399-0039.2009.01311.x
54. Argaet VP, Schmidt CW, Burrows SR, Silins SL, Kurilla MG, Doolan DL, et al. Dominant selection of an invariant T cell antigen receptor in response to persistent infection by Epstein-Barr virus. *J Exp Med* (1994) **180**:2335–40. doi:10.1084/jem.180.6.2335
55. Burrows SR, Silins SL, Moss DJ, Khanna R, Misko IS, Argaet VP. T cell receptor repertoire for a viral epitope in humans is diversified by tolerance to a background major histocompatibility complex antigen. *J Exp Med* (1995) **182**:1703–15. doi:10.1084/jem.182.6.1703
56. Gras S, Burrows SR, Kjer-Nielsen L, Clements CS, Liu YC, Sullivan LC, et al. The shaping of T cell receptor recognition by self-tolerance. *Immunity* (2009) **30**:193–203. doi:10.1016/j.immuni.2008.11.011
57. Rist M, Smith C, Bell MJ, Burrows SR, Khanna R. Cross-recognition of HLA DR4 alloantigen by virus-specific CD8+ T cells: a new paradigm for self-/nonself-recognition. *Blood* (2009) **114**:2244–53. doi:10.1182/blood-2009-05-222596
58. Macdonald WA, Chen Z, Gras S, Archbold JK, Tynan FE, Clements CS, et al. T cell allorecognition via molecular mimicry. *Immunity* (2009) **31**:897–908. doi:10.1016/j.immuni.2009.09.025
59. D'Orsogna LJ, Roelen DL, van der Meer-Prins EM, van der Pol P, Franke-van Dijk ME, Eikmans M, et al. Tissue specificity of cross-reactive allogeneic responses by EBV EBNA3A-specific memory T cells. *Transplantation* (2011) **91**:494–500. doi:10.1097/TP.0b013e318207944c
60. Peut V, Kent SJ. Fitness constraints on immune escape from HIV: implications of envelope as a target for both HIV-specific T cells and antibody. *Curr HIV Res* (2006) **4**:191–7. doi:10.2174/157016206776055110
61. Liu JQ, Bai XF. Overcoming immune evasion in T cell therapy of cancer: lessons from animal models. *Curr Mol Med* (2008) **8**:68–75. doi:10.2174/156652408783565531
62. Sette A, Sidney J. Nine major HLA class I supertypes account for the vast preponderance of HLA-A and -B polymorphism. *Immunogenetics* (1999) **50**:201–12. doi:10.1007/s002510050594
63. Burrows SR, Elkington RA, Miles JJ, Green KJ, Walker S, Haryana SM, et al. Promiscuous CTL recognition of viral epitopes on multiple human leukocyte antigens: biological validation of the proposed HLA A24 supertype. *J Immunol* (2003) **171**:1407–12.
64. Fleischhauer K, Tanzarella S, Wallny HJ, Bordignon C, Traversari C. Multiple HLA-A alleles can present an immunodominant peptide of the human melanoma antigen Melan-A/MART-1 to a peptide-specific HLA-A*0201+ cytotoxic T cell line. *J Immunol* (1996) **157**:787–97.
65. Khanna R, Burrows SR, Nicholls J, Poulsen LM. Identification of cytotoxic T cell epitopes within Epstein-Barr virus (EBV) oncogene latent membrane protein 1 (LMP1): evidence for HLA A2 supertype-restricted immune recognition of EBV-infected cells by LMP1-specific cytotoxic T lymphocytes. *Eur J Immunol* (1998) **28**:451–8. doi:10.1002/(SICI)1521-4141(199802)28:02<451::AID-IMMU451>3.3.CO;2-L
66. Threlkeld SC, Wentworth PA, Kalams SA, Wilkes BM, Ruhl DJ, Keogh E, et al. Degenerate and promiscuous recognition by CTL of peptides presented by the MHC class I A3-like superfamily: implications for vaccine development. *J Immunol* (1997) **159**:1648–57.
67. Mackelprang R, Livingston RJ, Eberle MA, Carlson CS, Yi Q, Akey JM, et al. Sequence diversity, natural selection and linkage disequilibrium in the human T cell receptor alpha/delta locus. *Hum Genet* (2006) **119**:255–66. doi:10.1007/s00439-005-0111-z
68. Subrahmanyan L, Eberle MA, Clark AG, Kruglyak L, Nickerson DA. Sequence variation and linkage disequilibrium in the human T-cell receptor beta (TCRB) locus. *Am J Hum Genet* (2001) **69**:381–95. doi:10.1086/321297
69. Mackelprang R, Carlson CS, Subrahmanyan L, Livingston RJ, Eberle MA, Nickerson DA. Sequence variation in the human T-cell receptor loci. *Immunol Rev* (2002) **190**:26–39. doi:10.1034/j.1600-065X.2002.19003.x
70. Seboun E, Robinson MA, Kindt TJ, Hauser SL. Insertion/deletion-related polymorphisms in the human T cell receptor beta gene complex. *J Exp Med* (1989) **170**:1263–70. doi:10.1084/jem.170.4.1263
71. Zhao TM, Whitaker SE, Robinson MA. A genetically determined insertion/deletion related polymorphism in human T cell receptor beta chain (TCRB) includes functional variable gene segments. *J Exp Med* (1994) **180**:1405–14. doi:10.1084/jem.180.4.1405
72. Tubo NJ, Pagan AJ, Taylor JJ, Nelson RW, Linehan JL, Ertelt JM, et al. Single naive CD4+ T cells from a diverse repertoire produce different effector cell types during infection. *Cell* (2013) **153**:785–96. doi:10.1016/j.cell.2013.04.007
73. Gerlach C, van Heijst JW, Swart E, Sie D, Armstrong N, Kerkhoven RM, et al. One naive T cell, multiple fates in CD8+ T cell differentiation. *J Exp Med* (2010) **207**:1235–46. doi:10.1084/jem.20091175
74. Stemberger C, Huster KM, Koffler M, Anderl F, Schiemann M, Wagner H, et al. A single naive CD8+ T cell precursor can develop into diverse effector and memory sub-

5

Individual MHCI-restricted T-cell receptors are characterized by a unique peptide recognition signature

Linda Wooldridge*

Institute of Infection and Immunity, Cardiff University School of Medicine, Heath Park, Cardiff, UK

Edited by:
Bruno Laugel, Cardiff University, UK

Reviewed by:
Eric Huseby, University of Massachusetts, USA
Klaus Dornmair, LMU Munich, Germany

Correspondence:
Linda Wooldridge, Institute of Infection and Immunity, Cardiff University School of Medicine, Heath Park, Cardiff CF14 4XN, UK
e-mail: wooldridgel@cardiff.ac.uk

Effective immunity requires that a limited TCR repertoire is able to recognize a vast number of foreign peptide-MHCI (peptide-major histocompatibility complex class I) molecules. This challenge is overcome by the ability of individual TCRs to recognize large numbers of peptides. Recently, it was demonstrated that MHCI-restricted TCRs can recognize up to 10^6 peptides of a defined length. Astonishingly, this remarkable level of promiscuity does not extend to peptides of different lengths, a fundamental observation that has broad implications for $CD8^+$ T-cell immunity. In particular, the findings suggest that effective immunity can only be achieved by mobilization of "length-matched" $CD8^+$ T-cell clonotypes. Overall, recent findings suggest that every TCR is specific for a unique set of peptides, which can be described as a unique "peptide recognition signature" (PRS) and consists of three components: (1) peptide length preference, (2) number of peptides recognized; and, (3) sequence identity (e.g., self versus pathogen derived). In future, the ability to de-convolute peptide recognition signatures across the normal and pathogenic repertoire will be essential for understanding the system requirements for effective $CD8^+$ T-cell immunity and elucidating mechanisms which underlie $CD8^+$ T-cell mediated disease.

Keywords: MHCI-peptide length, T-cell crossreactivity, vaccination, autoimmunity, alloreactivity

INTRODUCTION

$CD8^+$ T cells are important for the control of viral infection and the natural eradication of cancer. $CD8^+$ T cells recognize short peptides presented at the target cell surface bound to major histocompatibility complex class I (MHCI) molecules (1). Recognition of peptide-MHCI (pMHCI) is mediated by the alpha beta T-cell receptor (TCR). Initially, it was thought that MHCI molecules predominantly presented peptides of between 8 and 10 amino acids in length. However, subsequent studies demonstrated that peptides of between 11 and 14 amino acids in length are also presented and can be highly immunogenic (2). In fact, many longer peptides can be immunodominant over completely overlapping shorter peptides that also bind to the same MHCI allele (3–6). Thus, it is now well established that MHCI can present peptides of between 8 and 14 amino acids in length. A vast array of peptides within this length range can be generated from permutations of the twenty proteogenic L-amino acids (1.7×10^{18}). Of course, not all of these peptide sequences occur in the current database of natural proteins. However, it is vital that the TCR repertoire is poised to recognize vast numbers of peptide sequences, even if not identified to date, in order to adapt and deal with changes in pathogen diversity.

The MHCI-presented peptide repertoire is constrained by factors such as the specificity of antigen processing pathway components (proteasome, ERAAP/ERAP1, tapasin, and TAP) and the HLA type of the individual (7, 8). As a result, conservative estimates suggest that only ~1% of the peptide universe can be processed and presented at the cell surface in the context of MHCI (9). However, this still leaves a staggering 1.7×10^{16} peptides of different lengths to which a relatively small number of TCRs (~25 million) (10) must be able to respond appropriately. Therefore, in order to understand the requirements for effective $CD8^+$ T-cell immunity, it is important to understand how a limited TCR repertoire responds and adapts to the vast number of possible different epitopes across a length spectrum.

INDIVIDUAL TCRs CAN RECOGNIZE LARGE NUMBERS OF PEPTIDES OF A DEFINED LENGTH

It has been appreciated for many years that individual TCRs can recognize multiple ligands (11–18). Initial studies of TCR degeneracy were conducted using small numbers of peptide analogs (typically less than 200). The development of combinatorial peptide library (CPL) screening which was pioneered by Houghten et al. (19, 20) allowed for a more comprehensive analysis of TCR degeneracy and the ability to define much larger numbers of candidate peptide analogs (21). A more recent study examined ~4,000 peptides, although it must be appreciated that this number still only represents an extremely small portion of the entire peptide universe (18).

Estimates of TCR degeneracy were initially performed using data from peptide library screening. Elegant studies which were conducted by two independent groups estimated that individual MHCII-restricted TCRs can recognize ~10^6 peptides (22, 23). A similar analysis performed by Wilson and colleagues suggested that MHCI-restricted TCRs exhibit lower levels of degeneracy (24). However, approaches performed using small peptide sets or library screening alone preclude a comprehensive analysis of the entire peptide universe and as such, may result in an underestimate of TCR degeneracy. In order to address this possibility, a recent study developed an approach to quantify TCR degeneracy that can be used to probe the entire peptide universe of a defined length.

This approach involves a combination of sampling from motif-restricted peptide sets and sampling from the entire peptide universe with bias toward those peptides predicted to elicit a response (termed CPL-based importance sampling) (25). The approach was used to construct a degeneracy curve which revealed, in the initial application of this strategy, that an individual MHCI-restricted TCR (1E6) can recognize over one million different decamer peptides in the context of a single MHCI at physiologically relevant concentrations. Furthermore, it was possible to identify peptides that were up to 100-fold more potent than the cognate peptide for this particular TCR. To date, this study represents the most comprehensive quantification of MHCI-restricted TCR degeneracy (25). However, continued development of techniques that allow rapid and accurate quantification of TCR degeneracy are essential if we are to understand the role that this phenomenon plays in common T-cell mediated diseases.

The ability of individual TCRs to recognize large numbers of peptides provides an explanation for how a limited TCR repertoire can provide effective immune coverage against all possible foreign pMHCI that can be encountered. However this analysis was confined to a single autoimmune TCR which may represent the extreme end of the cross-reactivity spectrum. In order to understand the system requirements for effective CD8$^+$ T-cell immunity, it will be important to measure how this phenomenon varies across the normal TCR repertoire. It is tempting to speculate that variations in levels of TCR degeneracy may contribute to the pathogenesis of disease. In fact there is emerging evidence to suggest that this is indeed the case. For example, several studies suggest that levels of TCR degeneracy can influence disease outcome during infection with viruses such as HIV-1 that have a high mutation rate (26–29). Overall more information is required about how TCR degeneracy varies across the normal TCR repertoire and the role that variations play in the pathogenesis of disease.

TCRs EXHIBIT AN EXPLICIT PREFERENCE FOR MHCI-BOUND PEPTIDE LENGTH

It is clear that TCRs can recognize a large number of peptides of a defined length and it would seem logical that this flexibility could extend to the recognition of peptides of different lengths, as this would maximize the ability of the TCR repertoire to provide broad antigenic coverage. In order to examine this possibility, a recent study utilized a series of combinatorial peptide libraries, ranging from 8 to 13 amino acids in length, to perform a comprehensive analysis of peptide length preference across a panel of CD8$^+$ T-cell clones raised against a range of pMHCI antigens spanning different peptide lengths derived from both foreign and self antigens (30). An unexpected feature of the TCR/pMHCI interaction was discovered by showing that any given TCR exhibits an explicit preference for a single MHCI-bound peptide length (30). This MHCI-bound peptide length preference was identical to the length of the original peptide which had been used to derive each clone. Furthermore, this unexpected finding applied to all TCRs examined regardless of antigenic specificity and MHCI restriction. Importantly, peptide length preference was shown to be an intrinsic feature of the TCR and not determined by differential MHCI-peptide binding. A very small number of agonists of non-preferred length were identified, but the incidence of this phenomenon was extremely rare and recognition was generally sub-optimal when compared to peptides of the preferred length. Interestingly, however, agonists of non-preferred length identified were entirely distinct in sequence, with a different amino acid residue at every position. As described above, CPL-based importance sampling revealed that the 1E6 TCR can recognize over one million different 10mer peptides at a functional sensitivity equivalent to or greater than index (25). In contrast, the 1E6 TCR was not capable of recognizing any 8, 9, 11, 12, or 13mer peptides within this functional sensitivity range. Thus, individual MHCI-restricted TCRs exhibit an explicit preference for a single MHCI-peptide length (30). The next challenge will be to explain how a repertoire of TCRs that display a stringent preference for peptide length can provide effective immune coverage against all peptide lengths that can be presented by MHCI. To address this question, it will be important to examine how peptide length preference varies across the entire TCR repertoire.

IMPLICATIONS OF MHCI-BOUND PEPTIDE LENGTH PREFERENCE FOR CD8$^+$ T-CELL IMMUNITY

The TCR/pMHCI interaction is pivotal in all aspects of CD8$^+$ T-cell immunity including thymic development, naive T-cell survival, and recognition of foreign pMHCI in the periphery. Peptide length determines the outcome of TCR/pMHCI engagement and, as such, has far-reaching implications (**Box 1**). Firstly, the findings predict that the thymic epithelial cell (TEC) (31, 32) surface must display peptides of multiple different lengths to ensure that an appropriately diverse CD8$^+$ T-cell repertoire undergoes positive and negative selection before being released into the periphery. Once in the periphery, continual TCR engagement of low affinity self-derived pMHCI molecules is essential for naive T-cell survival (33, 34). Here, peptides of non-preferred length may actually play a very important role because signaling below the threshold for T-cell activation may be sufficient for the delivery of survival signals.

Box 1 | Implications of peptide length preference.

A: Implications for CD8$^+$ T-cell immunity

- Thymic development: TECs must display peptides of multiple lengths
- Naive T-cell survival: mediated by recognition of defined length peptides
- Effective CD8$^+$ T-cell immunity: requires "length-matched" clonotypes
- Protective vaccination: must elicit "length-matched" clonotypes

B: Implications for disease pathogenesis

- Identification of ligands that trigger CD8$^+$ T-cell expansions in autoimmunity and hematological disease: length preference must be established
- Rare peptides of non-preferred length peptides with entirely disparate sequence: may represent a novel mechanism underlying molecular mimicry
- Alloreactivity: an important consideration in the identification of alloreactive ligands

Importantly, the findings imply that the CD8$^+$ T-cell repertoire is compartmentalized with respect to peptide length preference, such that effective immunity can only be achieved by mobilization of the appropriate "length-matched" antigen-specific CD8$^+$ T-cell clonotypes (30). To understand the system requirements for effective CD8$^+$ T-cell immunity, it will therefore be necessary to examine how peptide length preference varies across the normal TCR repertoire and how different "peptide length footprints" overlap to provide effective coverage across all peptide lengths. The length preference phenomenon also informs our understanding of the requirements for effective peptide vaccination. For example, it was recently observed that the heteroclitic 10mer epitope ELAGIGILTV derived from MART-1/Melan-A, which is commonly used in melanoma clinical trials, primes a population of CD8$^+$ T cells that is very poor at cross-recognizing the dominant naturally presented 9mer epitope AAGIGILTV (35, 36). These findings may explain, at least in part, the poor objective response rates observed in these trials (37). Accordingly, such findings suggest that peptide length is likely to be an important consideration in the provision of effective CD8$^+$ T-cell immunity and the response to peptide vaccination.

IMPLICATIONS OF MHCI-BOUND PEPTIDE LENGTH PREFERENCE FOR DISEASE PATHOGENESIS

As well as playing a critical role in CD8$^+$ T-cell immunity, the TCR/pMHCI interaction can result in inappropriate CD8$^+$ T-cell activity in situations such as autoimmunity, hematological disorders, and transplant rejection (alloreactivity). Factors that influence the outcome of TCR/pMHCI engagement, such as peptide length, therefore impact on our understanding of disease pathogenesis. Transient, asymptomatic CD8$^+$ T-cell expansions are relatively common and often associated with viral infections. However, in certain disease states, monoclonal/oligoclonal CD8$^+$ T-cell expansions with a differentiated phenotype persist, suggesting an exaggerated response to an immunodominant antigen. Monoclonal CD8$^+$ T-cell expansions are a characteristic feature of T-LGL leukemia (38), but can also be triggered by drugs [e.g., protein tyrosine kinase inhibitors (39)]. Oligoclonal expansions have been observed in various autoimmune diseases [e.g., multiple sclerosis (40, 41), rheumatoid arthritis (42), and aplastic anemia (43)]. To date, there has been no attempt to identify the origin of the ligands that drive these potentially pathogenic CD8$^+$ T-cell populations. This is a priority for the future because it will yield information about the pathogenesis of these important diseases. In order to achieve this goal, the dominant pathogenic T-cell clone must be isolated and the peptide length preference defined. This will narrow the search and allow the selection of length-appropriate peptide libraries to enable ligand hunting.

Alloreactivity represents a major barrier to transplantation and, as such, there is a pressing need to understand the molecular and structural basis of this phenomenon (44, 45). This is especially important considering that substantial efforts are being made to increase the number of available donors despite the fact that, in the last decade, little progress has been made in understanding how to reduce the risks and severity of transplant rejection. It is well established that alloreactive T-cells are highly prevalent within the T-cell repertoire. However, the mechanisms that underlie this phenomenon remain unclear. Originally, it was thought that alloreactivity was mediated by TCR recognition of foreign MHC ("MHC-centric"). More recently, however, it has become increasingly apparent that the alloreactive TCR/pMHCI interaction can be highly peptide-dependent ("peptide-centric") (46–48). In fact, it appears that peptide specificity is profound when self-MHCI and foreign-MHCI are closely related (49). Further studies are required to determine whether alloreactive TCR/pMHCI interactions exhibit the levels of promiscuity that typify autologous TCR/pMHCI interactions. It will also be important to examine the possibility that alloreactive TCR/pMHCI interactions may exhibit a peptide length preference. This will facilitate the identification of alloreactive ligands and allow characterization of the peptide repertoire recognized in the context of non-self MHCI (30).

INDIVIDUAL MHCI-RESTRICTED TCRs ARE CHARACTERIZED BY A UNIQUE PEPTIDE RECOGNITION SIGNATURE

Taken together, recent observations suggest that every TCR is specific for a unique set of peptides, which can be described as a unique "peptide recognition signature" (PRS) (**Figure 1**). The PRS of individual TCRs comprises three different components: (i) an explicit preference for a single MHCI-peptide length; (ii) the number of peptide sequences recognized at the preferred length, which can be very large (up to $\sim 10^6$ different peptides); and, (iii) the sequence identity of the recognized peptides, many of which will be biologically relevant. The sequence identity of the peptides recognized by an individual TCR is the most important component of the PRS (**Figure 1**). Many of the peptide sequences recognized by individual TCRs can appear in a large number of self proteins or pathogen derived proteins. If these sequences can be naturally processed and presented at the cell surface then the TCR will have the opportunity to mount a response to them *in vivo*. If a TCR can respond to naturally processed sequences from more than one pathogen then this will allow a single TCR to provide immunity to more than one infection. This phenomenon [often referred to as "heterologous immunity" (50, 51)] is extremely important for the provision of effective immunity and an example of the immense benefits that can be gained from TCR degeneracy. However, the ability to be able to recognize both self and pathogen derived pMHCI has the potential to be highly pathogenic and provides a mechanistic basis for "molecular mimicry," which is the widely hypothesized cause of autoimmune disease (52). Although good examples of molecular mimicry exist in mouse models of disease there is still a lack of concrete evidence for this in human autoimmune disease (52). It is very important that this question is answered in the context of human disease. The ability to de-convolute the PRS of TCRs involved in autoimmune disease will be of immense interest in the future.

APPROACHES THAT CAN BE USED TO DE-CONVOLUTE THE PRS OF INDIVIDUAL TCRs

CD8$^+$ T cells play a major role in the pathogenesis of autoimmunity, hematological disease, and transplant rejection, as described above. In the future, the ability to de-convolute the PRS of pathogenically relevant TCRs will allow us to dissect the underlying mechanisms of common CD8$^+$ T-cell mediated disease. This information can then be used to inform the rational design of

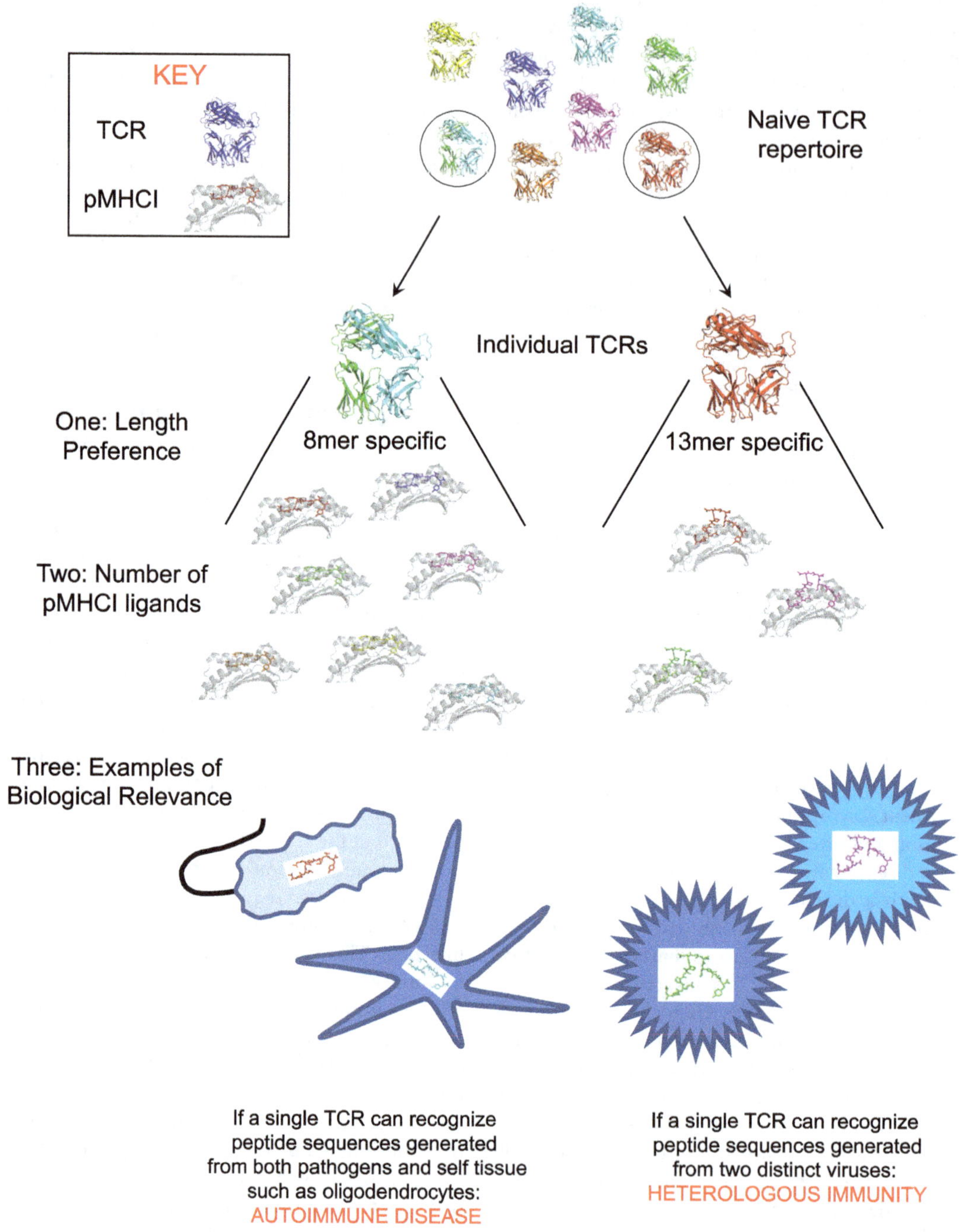

FIGURE 1 | The peptide recognition signature of every TCR consists of three components. The figure depicts the three components of the peptide recognition signature. *One: peptide length preference:* this finding implies that effective CD8+ T-cell immunity can only be achieved if "length-matched" antigen-specific CD8+ T-cell clonotypes are mobilized during an immune response, *two: number of peptides recognized at the preferred peptide length:* which can be very large (up to $\sim 10^6$). The ability of individual TCRs to recognize multiple pMHCI is essential for the provision of effective immune coverage against the multitude of foreign pMHCI that can be encountered, and; *three: sequence of the recognized peptides (which dictates the biological relevance of the peptide recognition signature):* the ability to be able to recognize both pathogen and self-derived pMHCI could be the basis for "molecular mimicry," which is the widely hypothesized cause of autoimmune disease. Evidence for this phenomenon exists in animal models of autoimmunity but convincing data in human disease is still lacking. By way of an example, the figure depicts the ability of the same TCR to recognize peptide sequences generated from both environmental pathogens and oligodendrocytes. Alternatively, if a TCR can respond to naturally processed and presented peptide sequences from more than one pathogen then this will allow a single TCR to provide immunity to more than one infection. It has been suggested that this phenomenon (often referred to as "heterologous immunity") is extremely important for the provision of effective immunity. By way of an example, the figure depicts the ability of the same TCR to recognize naturally processed and presented peptide sequences from two different viruses.

novel therapeutic strategies. As such there is a pressing need to design approaches that can be used to achieve this goal. There have been some elegant attempts to develop an approach that allows the identification of ligands recognized by $CD8^+$ T-cell populations of potential pathogenic significance (15, 53, 54). However, an appreciation that every TCR is characterized by a unique PRS will facilitate this analysis. Firstly, it will be necessary to define the peptide length preference of the individual TCR of interest so that appropriate ligand hunting tools can be selected, such as length-matched peptide libraries. Secondly, the number of peptides that can be recognized by the individual TCR may influence the approach that is being used. For example, highly cross-reactive TCRs will be more challenging than those that exhibit a more focused phenotype. And finally, tools to identify the origin of the peptide sequences (i.e., pathogen versus self protein) will be essential. Emphasis should be placed on developing an approach that is rapid and can be scaled up to allow the analysis of large numbers of TCRs in a short space of time. If this can be achieved, then the ability to de-convolute PRSs across the normal and diseased repertoire is expected to yield large but very important databases of information for the future.

CONCLUDING REMARKS

In summary, based on recently generated data, I suggest that every TCR in the naive repertoire is characterized by a unique PRS; all of which overlap to provide effective immune coverage against all possible foreign-MHCI-bound peptides that could be encountered. A comprehensive study to examine how the PRS of individual TCRs varies across the normal TCR repertoire will allow us to determine how a relatively limited number of TCRs can recognize the multitude of 8–14 amino acid length peptides that can be encountered in complex with MHCI, and thereby define the system requirements for effective $CD8^+$ T-cell immunity. In addition, approaches that can be used to de-convolute the PRSs of individual pathogenically relevant TCRs are essential if we are to gain an understanding of the mechanisms that underlie common $CD8^+$ T-cell mediated diseases.

ACKNOWLEDGMENTS

Linda Wooldridge is a WT Clinical Intermediate Fellow (grant WT079848MA). I would like to thank Professor David Price for his critical reading of this article and Dave K. Cole for his assistance with **Figure 1**.

REFERENCES

1. Rudolph MG, Stanfield RL, Wilson IA. How TCRs bind MHCs, peptides, and coreceptors. *Annu Rev Immunol* (2006) **24**:419–66. doi:10.1146/annurev.immunol.23.021704.115658
2. Burrows SR, Rossjohn J, McCluskey J. Have we cut ourselves too short in mapping CTL epitopes? *Trends Immunol* (2006) **27**:11–6. doi:10.1016/j.it.2005.11.001
3. Theobald M, Biggs J, Hernandez J, Lustgarten J, Labadie C, Sherman LA. Tolerance to p53 by A2.1-restricted cytotoxic T lymphocytes. *J Exp Med* (1997) **185**:833–41. doi:10.1084/jem.185.5.833
4. Blake N, Lee S, Redchenko I, Thomas W, Steven N, Leese A, et al. Human CD8+ T cell responses to EBV EBNA1: HLA class I presentation of the (Gly-Ala)-containing protein requires exogenous processing. *Immunity* (1997) **7**:791–802. doi:10.1016/S1074-7613(00)80397-0
5. Missale G, Redeker A, Person J, Fowler P, Guilhot S, Schlicht HJ, et al. HLA-A31- and HLA-Aw68-restricted cytotoxic T cell responses to a single hepatitis B virus nucleocapsid epitope during acute viral hepatitis. *J Exp Med* (1993) **177**:751–62. doi:10.1084/jem.177.3.751
6. Green KJ, Miles JJ, Tellam J, Van Zuylen WJ, Connolly G, Burrows SR. Potent T cell response to a class I-binding 13-mer viral epitope and the influence of HLA micropolymorphism in controlling epitope length. *Eur J Immunol* (2004) **34**:2510–9. doi:10.1002/eji.200425193
7. Yewdell JW, Reits E, Neefjes J. Making sense of mass destruction: quantitating MHC class I antigen presentation. *Nat Rev Immunol* (2003) **3**:952–61. doi:10.1038/nri1250
8. Blum JS, Wearsch PA, Cresswell P. Pathways of antigen processing. *Annu Rev Immunol* (2013) **31**:443–73. doi:10.1146/annurev-immunol-032712-095910
9. Mason D. A very high level of crossreactivity is an essential feature of the T-cell receptor. *Immunol Today* (1998) **19**:395–404. doi:10.1016/S0167-5699(98)01299-7
10. Arstila TP, Casrouge A, Baron V, Even J, Kanellopoulos J, Kourilsky P. A direct estimate of the human alphabeta T cell receptor diversity. *Science* (1999) **286**:958–61. doi:10.1126/science.286.5441.958
11. Hemmer B, Fleckenstein BT, Vergelli M, Jung G, McFarland H, Martin R, et al. Identification of high potency microbial and self ligands for a human autoreactive class II-restricted T cell clone. *J Exp Med* (1997) **185**:1651–9. doi:10.1084/jem.185.9.1651
12. Hausmann S, Martin M, Gauthier L, Wucherpfennig KW. Structural features of autoreactive TCR that determine the degree of degeneracy in peptide recognition. *J Immunol* (1999) **162**: 338–44.
13. Kissler S, Anderton SM, Wraith DC. Cross-reactivity and T-cell receptor antagonism of myelin basic protein-reactive T cells is modulated by the activation state of the antigen presenting cell. *J Autoimmun* (2002) **19**:183–93. doi:10.1006/jaut.2002.0614
14. Nino-Vasquez JJ, Allicotti G, Borras E, Wilson DB, Valmori D, Simon R, et al. A powerful combination: the use of positional scanning libraries and biometrical analysis to identify cross-reactive T cell epitopes. *Mol Immunol* (2004) **40**:1063–74. doi: 10.1016/j.molimm.2003.11.005
15. Crawford F, Huseby E, White J, Marrack P, Kappler JW. Mimotopes for alloreactive and conventional T cells in a peptide-MHC display library. *PLoS Biol* (2004) **2**:E90. doi:10.1371/journal.pbio.0020090
16. Lee JK, Stewart-Jones G, Dong T, Harlos K, Di Gleria K, Dorrell L, et al. T cell cross-reactivity and conformational changes during TCR engagement. *J Exp Med* (2004) **200**:1455–66. doi:10.1084/jem.20041251
17. Kan-Mitchell J, Bajcz M, Schaubert KL, Price DA, Brenchley JM, Asher TE, et al. Degeneracy and repertoire of the human HIV-1 Gag p17(77-85) CTL response. *J Immunol* (2006) **176**:6690–701.
18. Ishizuka J, Grebe K, Shenderov E, Peters B, Chen Q, Peng Y, et al. Quantitating T cell cross-reactivity for unrelated peptide antigens. *J Immunol* (2009) **183**:4337–45. doi:10.4049/jimmunol.0901607
19. Houghten RA, Pinilla C, Blondelle SE, Appel JR, Dooley CT, Cuervo JH. Generation and use of synthetic peptide combinatorial libraries for basic research and drug discovery. *Nature* (1991) **354**:84–6. doi:10.1038/354084a0
20. Pinilla C, Appel JR, Judkowski V, Houghten RA. Identification of B cell and T cell epitopes using synthetic peptide combinatorial libraries. *Curr Protoc Immunol* (2012) Chapter 9:Unit9.5. doi:10.1002/0471142735.im0905s99
21. Rubio-Godoy V, Dutoit V, Zhao Y, Simon R, Guillaume P, Houghten R, et al. Positional scanning-synthetic peptide library-based analysis of self- and pathogen-derived peptide cross-reactivity with tumor-reactive Melan-A-specific CTL. *J Immunol* (2002) **169**:5696–707.
22. Hiemstra HS, van Veelen PA, Willemen SJ, Benckhuijsen WE, Geluk A, de Vries RR, et al. Quantitative determination of TCR cross-reactivity using peptide libraries and protein databases. *Eur J Immunol* (1999) **29**:2385–91. doi:10.1002/(SICI)1521-4141(199908)29:08<2385::AID-IMMU2385>3.3.CO;2-2

23. Maynard J, Petersson K, Wilson DH, Adams EJ, Blondelle SE, Boulanger MJ, et al. Structure of an autoimmune T cell receptor complexed with class II peptide-MHC: insights into MHC bias and antigen specificity. *Immunity* (2005) **22**:81–92. doi:10.1016/S1074-7613(04)00378-4
24. Wilson DB, Wilson DH, Schroder K, Pinilla C, Blondelle S, Houghten RA, et al. Specificity and degeneracy of T cells. *Mol Immunol* (2004) **40**:1047–55. doi:10.1016/j.molimm.2003.11.022
25. Wooldridge L, Ekeruche-Makinde J, van den Berg HA, Skowera A, Miles JJ, Tan MP, et al. A single autoimmune T cell receptor recognizes more than a million different peptides. *J Biol Chem* (2012) **287**:1168–77. doi:10.1074/jbc.M111.289488
26. Kosmrlj A, Read EL, Qi Y, Allen TM, Altfeld M, Deeks SG, et al. Effects of thymic selection of the T-cell repertoire on HLA class I-associated control of HIV infection. *Nature* (2010) **465**:350–4. doi:10.1038/nature08997
27. Gillespie GM, Kaul R, Dong T, Yang HB, Rostron T, Bwayo JJ, et al. Cross-reactive cytotoxic T lymphocytes against a HIV-1 p24 epitope in slow progressors with B*57. *AIDS* (2002) **16**:961–72. doi:10.1097/00002030-200205030-00002
28. Turnbull EL, Lopes AR, Jones NA, Cornforth D, Newton P, Aldam D, et al. HIV-1 epitope-specific CD8+ T cell responses strongly associated with delayed disease progression cross-recognize epitope variants efficiently. *J Immunol* (2006) **176**:6130–46.
29. Chen H, Ndhlovu ZM, Liu D, Porter LC, Fang JW, Darko S, et al. TCR clonotypes modulate the protective effect of HLA class I molecules in HIV-1 infection. *Nat Immunol* (2012) **13**:691–700. doi:10.1038/ni.2342
30. Ekeruche-Makinde J, Miles JJ, van den Berg HA, Skowera A, Cole DK, Dolton G, et al. Peptide length determines the outcome of TCR/peptide-MHCI engagement. *Blood* (2013) **121**:1112–23. doi:10.1182/blood-2012-06-437202
31. Ernst B, Lee DS, Chang JM, Sprent J, Surh CD. The peptide ligands mediating positive selection in the thymus control T cell survival and homeostatic proliferation in the periphery. *Immunity* (1999) **11**:173–81. doi:10.1016/S1074-7613(00)80092-8
32. Starr TK, Daniels MA, Lucido MM, Jameson SC, Hogquist KA. Thymocyte sensitivity and supramolecular activation cluster formation are developmentally regulated: a partial role for sialylation. *J Immunol* (2003) **171**:4512–20.
33. Kirberg J, Berns A, von Boehmer H. Peripheral T cell survival requires continual ligation of the T cell receptor to major histocompatibility complex-encoded molecules. *J Exp Med* (1997) **186**:1269–75. doi:10.1084/jem.186.8.1269
34. Seddon B, Zamoyska R. TCR signals mediated by Src family kinases are essential for the survival of naive T cells. *J Immunol* (2002) **169**:2997–3005.
35. Skipper JC, Gulden PH, Hendrickson RC, Harthun N, Caldwell JA, Shabanowitz J, et al. Mass-spectrometric evaluation of HLA-A*0201-associated peptides identifies dominant naturally processed forms of CTL epitopes from MART-1 and gp100. *Int J Cancer* (1999) **82**:669–77. doi:10.1002/(SICI)1097-0215(19990827)82:5<669::AID-IJC9>3.0.CO;2-#
36. Ekeruche-Makinde J, Clement M, Cole DK, Edwards ES, Ladell K, Miles JJ, et al. T-cell receptor-optimized peptide skewing of the T-cell repertoire can enhance antigen targeting. *J Biol Chem* (2012) **287**:37269–81. doi:10.1074/jbc.M112.386409
37. Rosenberg SA, Dudley ME. Adoptive cell therapy for the treatment of patients with metastatic melanoma. *Curr Opin Immunol* (2009) **21**:233–40. doi:10.1016/j.coi.2009.03.002
38. Melenhorst JJ, Eniafe R, Follmann D, Molldrem J, Kirby M, El Ouriaghli F, et al. T-cell large granular lymphocyte leukemia is characterized by massive TCRBV-restricted clonal CD8 expansion and a generalized overexpression of the effector cell marker CD57. *Hematol J* (2003) **4**:18–25. doi:10.1038/sj.thj.6200212
39. Mustjoki S, Ekblom M, Arstila TP, Dybedal I, Epling-Burnette PK, Guilhot F, et al. Clonal expansion of T/NK-cells during tyrosine kinase inhibitor dasatinib therapy. *Leukemia* (2009) **23**:1398–405. doi:10.1038/leu.2009.46
40. Babbe H, Roers A, Waisman A, Lassmann H, Goebels N, Hohlfeld R, et al. Clonal expansions of CD8(+) T cells dominate the T cell infiltrate in active multiple sclerosis lesions as shown by micromanipulation and single cell polymerase chain reaction. *J Exp Med* (2000) **192**:393–404. doi:10.1084/jem.192.3.393
41. Skulina C, Schmidt S, Dornmair K, Babbe H, Roers A, Rajewsky K, et al. Multiple sclerosis: brain-infiltrating CD8+ T cells persist as clonal expansions in the cerebrospinal fluid and blood. *Proc Natl Acad Sci U S A* (2004) **101**:2428–33. doi:10.1073/pnas.0308689100
42. Gonzalez-Quintial R, Baccala R, Pope RM, Theofilopoulos AN. Identification of clonally expanded T cells in rheumatoid arthritis using a sequence enrichment nuclease assay. *J Clin Invest* (1996) **97**:1335–43. doi:10.1172/JCI118550
43. Risitano AM, Kook H, Zeng W, Chen G, Young NS, Maciejewski JP. Oligoclonal and polyclonal CD4 and CD8 lymphocytes in aplastic anemia and paroxysmal nocturnal hemoglobinuria measured by V beta CDR3 spectratyping and flow cytometry. *Blood* (2002) **100**:178–83. doi:10.1182/blood-2002-01-0236
44. Felix NJ, Allen PM. Specificity of T-cell alloreactivity. *Nat Rev Immunol* (2007) **7**:942–53. doi:10.1038/nri2200
45. Issa F, Schiopu A, Wood KJ. Role of T cells in graft rejection and transplantation tolerance. *Expert Rev Clin Immunol* (2010) **6**:155–69. doi:10.1586/eci.09.64
46. MacDonald WA, Chen Z, Gras S, Archbold JK, Tynan FE, Clements CS, et al. T cell allorecognition via molecular mimicry. *Immunity* (2009) **31**:897–908. doi:10.1016/j.immuni.2009.09.025
47. Amir AL, van der Steen DM, Hagedoorn RS, Kester MG, van Bergen CA, Drijfhout JW, et al. Allo-HLA reactive T cells inducing graft versus host disease are single peptide specific. *Blood* (2011) **118**:6733–42. doi:10.1182/blood-2011-05-354787
48. D'Orsogna LJ, Nguyen TH, Claas FH, Witt C, Mifsud NA. Endogenous-peptide-dependent alloreactivity: new scientific insights and clinical implications. *Tissue Antigens* (2013) **81**:399–407. doi:10.1111/tan.12115
49. Obst R, Netuschil N, Klopfer K, Stevanovic S, Rammensee HG. The role of peptides in T cell alloreactivity is determined by self-major histocompatibility complex molecules. *J Exp Med* (2000) **191**:805–12. doi:10.1084/jem.191.5.805
50. Welsh RM, Selin LK. No one is naive: the significance of heterologous T-cell immunity. *Nat Rev Immunol* (2002) **2**:417–26.
51. Selin LK, Cornberg M, Brehm MA, Kim SK, Calcagno C, Ghersi D, et al. CD8 memory T cells: cross-reactivity and heterologous immunity. *Semin Immunol* (2004) **16**:335–47. doi:10.1016/j.smim.2004.08.014
52. Wucherpfennig KW, Sethi D. T cell receptor recognition of self and foreign antigens in the induction of autoimmunity. *Semin Immunol* (2011) **23**:84–91. doi:10.1016/j.smim.2011.01.007
53. Zhao Y, Gran B, Pinilla C, Markovic-Plese S, Hemmer B, Tzou A, et al. Combinatorial peptide libraries and biometric score matrices permit the quantitative analysis of specific and degenerate interactions between clonotypic TCR and MHC peptide ligands. *J Immunol* (2001) **167**:2130–41.
54. Siewert K, Malotka J, Kawakami N, Wekerle H, Hohlfeld R, Dornmair K. Unbiased identification of target antigens of CD8+ T cells with combinatorial libraries coding for short peptides. *Nat Med* (2012) **18**:824–8. doi:10.1038/nm.2720

6

Analysis, isolation, and activation of antigen-specific CD4+ and CD8+ T cells by soluble MHC-peptide complexes

Julien Schmidt[1†], Danijel Dojcinovic[2†], Philippe Guillaume[2] and Immanuel Luescher[1]*

[1] Ludwig Center, University of Lausanne, Epalinges, Switzerland
[2] TCMetrix Sàrl, Epalinges, Switzerland

Edited by:
Bruno Laugel, Cardiff University, UK

Reviewed by:
Edward John Collins, The University of North Carolina at Chapel Hill, USA
Salvatore Valitutti, INSERM, France

***Correspondence:**
Immanuel Luescher, Ludwig Center, University of Lausanne, Chemin des Boveresses 155, 1066 Epalinges, Switzerland
e-mail: immanuel.luescher@unil.ch

[†]Julien Schmidt and Danijel Dojcinovic have contributed equally to this work.

T cells constitute the core of adaptive cellular immunity and protect higher organisms against pathogen infections and cancer. Monitoring of disease progression as well as prophylactic or therapeutic vaccines and immunotherapies call for conclusive detection, analysis, and sorting of antigen-specific T cells. This is possible by means of soluble recombinant ligands for T cells, i.e., MHC class I-peptide (pMHC I) complexes for CD8+ T cells and MHC class II-peptide (pMHC II) complexes for CD4+ T cells and flow cytometry. Here we review major developments in the development of pMHC staining reagents and their diverse applications and discuss perspectives of their use for basic and clinical investigations.

Keywords: T cells, T cell receptor, tetramers, MHC, flow cytometry, coreceptor

INTRODUCTION

TCRαβ+ thymus derived T lymphocytes constitute the core of adaptive cellular immunity in higher organisms and play essential roles in their protection against pathogen infection and neoplastic transformations (1). CD8+ T cells differentiate to cytotoxic T lymphocytes (CTL) capable of efficient killing of cells displaying pMHC I complexes containing 8–10 residues long peptides, derived from a pathogen or cancer (2). CD8αβ coreceptor of CTL substantially enhances their antigen recognition, namely by strengthening the pMHC I ligand binding and bringing CD8-associated $p56^{lck}$ to the TCR/CD3 complex, thus promoting TCR signal induction (3). In most cancer vaccines and immunotherapies, tumor antigen-specific CD8+ T cells take center stage (4, 5). Antigen-specific CD8+ T cells can be reliably detected, analyzed, and sorted by means of soluble pMHC oligomers (6, 7). Peptide-MHC complexes have limited life spans at 37°C and therefore MHC I molecules provide a dynamic display of endogenously produced peptides. pMHC complexes can be obtained by refolding of denatured heavy and light (β2m) chains in the presence of a peptide of interest (8). This procedure is simple, inexpensive, and yields highly pure pMHC complexes. Because the peptides bind to MHC I molecules in a canonical manner, in which both termini are firmly anchored in well-defined positions, these complexes are homogenous and structurally well-defined (9).

On the other hand, CD4+ T cells differentiate from a common precursor (TH0) in different types of effector cells, such as T help cells (Th1, Th2), or regulatory T cells (Treg). Efforts to detect antigen-specific CD4+ T cells by soluble pMHC II multimers fared less well than their class I counterparts for diverse reasons. MHC II molecules consist of non-covalently linked alpha and beta chains, both of which are transmembrane spanning proteins and their variable domains (alpha 1 and beta 1) form an open ended peptide binding groove that accommodates exogenous peptide usually 10–15 residues long (10). In contrast to MHC I, MHC II molecules, in particular HLA II molecules, are stable without a peptide, which allows loading of "empty" MHC II molecules with a peptide of interest (11). Newly synthesized MHC II molecules associate with invariant chain (li), which assists their refolding, prevents binding of endogenous peptides in the endoplasmic reticulum, and directs them to the endosomal/lysosomal pathway where they are loaded with peptides generated from exogenous antigens by lysosomal proteolytic activity (12). To prepare soluble recombinant MHC II molecules, their transmembrane and cytoplasmic domains are replaced by leucine zippers to prevent dissociation of the alpha and beta chains (13). With a few exceptions pMHC II complexes cannot be obtained in good yields by refolding and/or by mammalian expressions systems, but can be well expressed by insect expression systems, such as Drosophila S2 cells or SF9 cells infected with baculo virus (14, 15). While binding of soluble pMHC I complexes to CD8+ T cells is greatly strengthened by CD8, CD4 does not stabilize pMHC II binding to CD4+ T cells (16). Together with the fact that CD4+ T cells usually express lower affinity than CD8+ T cells, this accounts for frequent poor pMHC II tetramer staining and missing of a substantial fraction of antigen-specific CD4+ T cells; this is often aggravated by poor reagent quality, namely incomplete or disperse peptide loading (17).

CHRONOLOGICAL OVERVIEW OF SOLUBLE pMHC CLASS I COMPLEXES AND THEIR USE FOR T CELL ANALYSIS

Soluble recombinant pMHC complexes are valuable tools for investigations, analysis, and isolation of antigen-specific T cells (**Figure 1**). The smallest pMHC complex is a monomer, which according to SPR studies binds recombinant TCR with dissociation constants (K_D) in the range of 1–1000 μM, and dissociation kinetic rates in the range of 1–1500 s (18), which precludes analysis by flow cytometry or fluorescence microscopy.

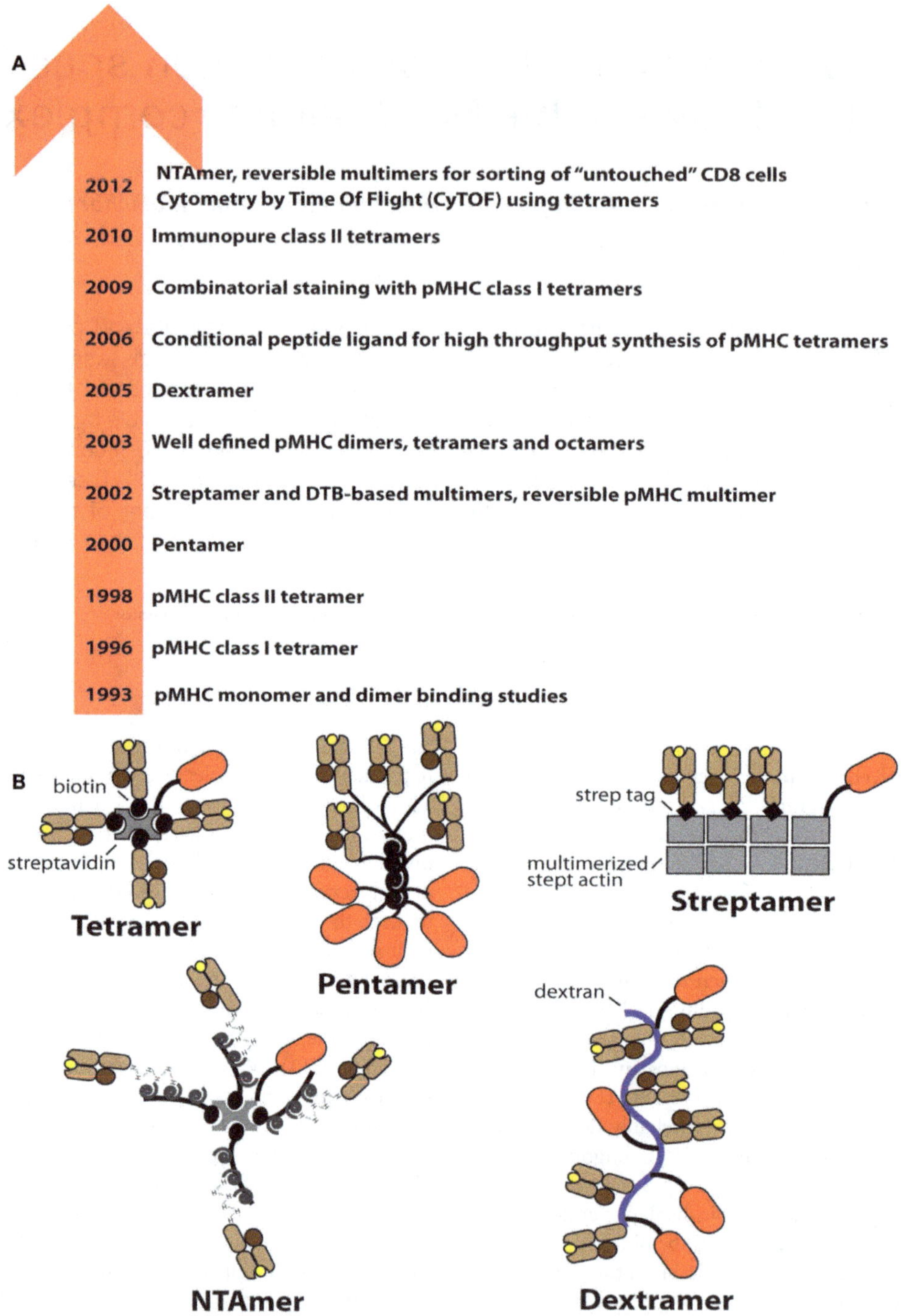

FIGURE 1 | Evolution of soluble pMHC complexes and their applications for T cell analysis and sorting. **(A)** Chronological listing of milestones in the use of pMHC complexes for the detection and analysis of antigen-specific CD8+ and CD4+ T cells. **(B)** Cartoons of the most frequently used pMHC oligomers; the red oval represents PE.

Nevertheless, the binding and dissociation of monomeric pMHC complexes was extensively studied on CD8+ CTL by means of TCR photoaffinity labeling (19, 20). These studies revealed that coordinate binding of CD8 to TCR-associated pMHC I complexes greatly strengthens pMHC I binding, mainly by decreasing the TCR–pMHC dissociation (3). It is noteworthy that although pMHC binding data measured by SPR are markedly different than those measured on living CD8+ T cells, they correlate well with CD8+ T cell activation. The likely explanation for this is that intercellular TCR–pMHC interactions precede

CD8 co-engagement, i.e., CD8 is recruited to sufficiently stable TCR–pMHC complexes (21).

Also in 1993 pMHC I dimers were described, with the capacity to fully activate $CD8^+$ CTL clones, whereas monomers were inactive (22). The ability of pMHC I and later also pMHC II dimers to inhibit antigen-specific T cells *in vitro* and *in vivo* was shown to be a promising means to block autoimmunity (23, 24). Peptide-MHC dimers built on chemical linkers were described only many years later (see below).

In 1996 the first pMHC I "tetramer" was described and its usefulness demonstrated for the detection and analysis of virus-specific $CD8^+$ T cells (25). The subunit pMHC I monomers carry a biotinylation sequence peptide (BSP) C-terminal of the alpha3 domain that is amenable to biotinylation with the biotin transferase BirA (26). Reaction of biotinylated pMHC I monomers with phycoerythrin-streptavidin (PE-SA) (or allophycocyanin-SA) typically results in mixtures of pMHC I conjugates of different stoichiometry and relative orientations and hence are better termed multimers (27). Our analysis indicated that such multimers contained species carrying up to 12 pMHC I monomer (unpublished results). Real tetramers can be prepared by using "tetra-grade" PE-SA and exhibit substantially reduced staining (see below).

In 1998 the first pMHC II multimers were described (28), which performed less well than their pMHC I counterparts, often exhibiting erratic, unreliable staining performance and according to one study approximately half of all antigen-specific $CD4^+$ T cells, especially self-antigens-specific ones, are not detected by conventional multimers (29). Only in 2010 molecular defined pMHC II multimers were described and their superior staining performance demonstrated (30, 31) (**Figure 1**).

In 2000 "Pentamers" (by ProImmune) were introduced that comprise five pMHC I complexes and five PE. Despite a lower valency compared to conventional multimers, the staining performance of both reagents seems to be similar (32). In 2002 meeting the increasing need for sorting of antigen-specific $CD8^+$ T cells namely for *in vitro* studies or adoptive cell transfer experiments, reversible multimers, based on biotin analogs, were introduced, which allow sorting of untouched $CD8^+$ T cells (33, 34). A third type of reversible multimers, the NTAmers, based on multivalent Ni^{2+}-NTA-His-tag complexes, followed nearly a decade later (35). In 2003 well-defined homologous pMHC dimers, tetramers, and octamers were described that contained linkers of defined lengths and configurations (36, 37). Binding and activation studies on cloned murine CTL and on $CD8^+$ T cells from melanoma patients revealed that the binding avidity and $CD8^+$ T cell activation critically depends not only on the valence, but also on pMHC–pMHC distances and configurations (38). In 2005 Dextramers (by Immudex) were introduced, which consist of long dextran fibers conjugated with multiple PE and pMHC I molecules (39) (**Figure 1**). While these studies contributed to improve analysis of antigen-specific T cells by means of pMHC oligomers, only recent developments have substantially increased their usefulness for comprehensive immune monitoring. For example an original new strategy allowing production of a wealth of different pMHC I complexes was introduced in 2006, i.e., the UV irradiation induced peptide exchange on pMHC I complexes containing a photoreactive peptide (40). This technique is useful especially for combinatorial multimer staining, independently established by two groups in 2009 (41, 42). Combinatorial multimer staining allows parallel detection of multiple specificities, which provides more information on precious, often small blood samples. One strategy uses binary color coding, i.e., antigen-specificity is defined by a unique combination of two colors (41), whereas the other strategy uses all possible color combinations, which affords higher number of color combinations, but also stronger reduction in fluorescence intensity (42). Three years later CyTOF was introduced, i.e., cytometry combined by time of flight measurements (43). The cells are labeled with lanthanide labeled pMHC multimers, resolved in a cytometer, converted in plasma, and its lanthanide content analyzed by mass spectrometry. Presently about 30 channels, i.e., different mass tags, are available, which provides more possibilities for parallel detection than flow cytometry (44). In 2012 also NTAmers were described, which are pMHC multimers built on NTA-Ni^{2+}-His-tag interactions that are nearly as stable as biotin–SA bonds, but upon addition of imidazole instantly decay in their constituents. By using Cy5 labeled pMHC molecules, NTAmers allow measurements of pMHC monomer dissociation kinetics on $CD8^+$ T cells (**Figure 4**).

WELL-DEFINED SOLUBLE pMHC COMPLEXES: TOOLS TO STUDY $CD8^+$ T CELLS LIGAND BINDING AND ACTIVATION

While most soluble pMHC complexes used for detection and isolation of antigen-specific T cells are heterogeneous, complexes of defined valence, configuration, and pMHC–pMHC distances were made and tested on $CD8^+$ T cells, which provided valuable insights on how they bind and are activated by pMHC complexes (**Figure 2**).

pMHC I MONOMERS

Due to the weak and transient nature of pMHC monomer binding to $CD8^+$ (and $CD4^+$) T cells, on cells binding studies require special techniques, such as TCR photoaffinity labeling (3, 19, 45, 46). To this end CTL clones were derived from mice immunized with a photoreactive derivative of the malaria circum sporozoite peptide $PbCS_{252-260}$ [SYIPSAEK(ABA)I, ABA: 4-azido-benzoic acid] that specifically recognize this peptide derivative. These binding studies on living $CD8^+$ T cells revealed that the coreceptor CD8αβ strongly strengthens TCR–pMHC interaction by coordinate binding to TCR-associated pMHC molecules (3). This increase in binding avidity varies in the range of 4- to 20-fold, depending of the clone and temperature and was mainly accounted for by decreased TCR–pMHC dissociation kinetics (45–47). The kinetics of pMHC monomer binding on living CTL exhibited a prominent temperature dependence, namely a dramatic decreases of dissociation rates with decreasing temperatures and biphasic association binding kinetics at 37°C, but not in the cold (3). Soluble monomeric complexes do not activate $CD8^+$ T cells unless these are adhered to a substrate; however, it was demonstrated that peptides of soluble pMHC monomers can be transferred to $CD8^+$ T cells CTL-associated MHC I molecules by an unknown mechanism and that this can engender CTL–CTL interactions (48, 49).

pMHC DIMERS

The first pMHC dimers described were fusion proteins consisting of pMHC monomers fused to IgG and provided initial new

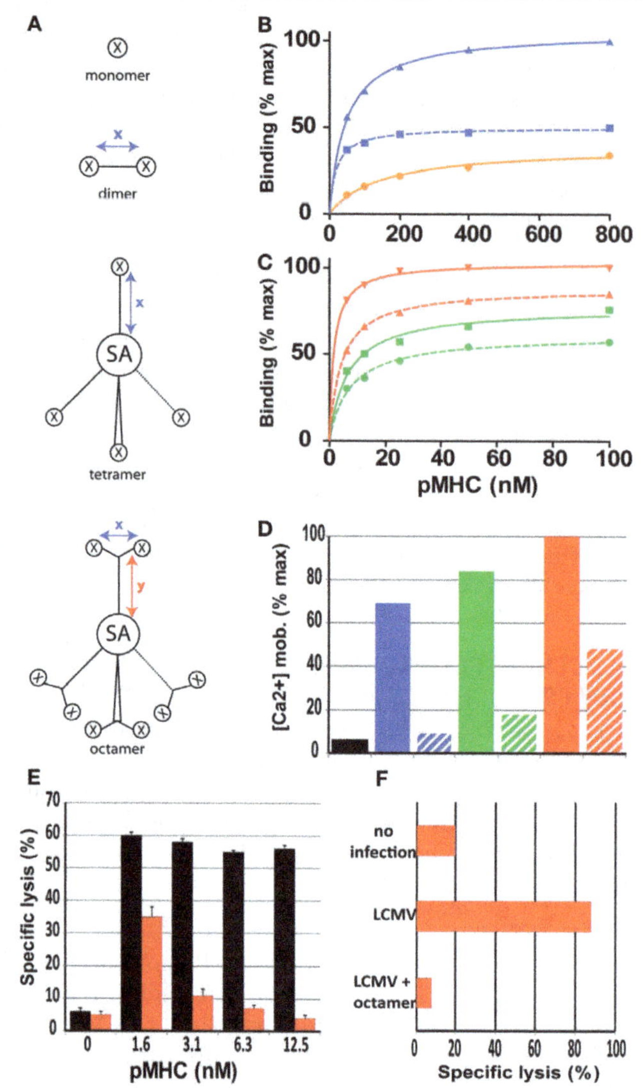

FIGURE 2 | Role of valence and spacer distances of soluble pMHC complexes on binding and activation of CD8⁺ T cells. **(A)** Cartoons of mono, di, tetra, and octamer pMHC complexes, in which *x* and *y* indicate maximal spacer distances in Å, X a pMHC monomer and SA streptavidin. The spacer distances for the pMHC dimers varies from 18 to 90 Å. **(B)** Relative binding on CD8⁺ T cells of monomer (black), short dimer (blue), and long dimer (dotted blue). **(C)** Same as **(B)** with short tetramer (green), long tetramer (dotted green), short octamer (red), and long octamer (dotted red). Short distances are <20 Å and long distances are >80 Å. **(D)** Relative activation (Ca^{2+} mobilization) of CD8⁺ T cells after binding of the represented pMHC complexes. **(E)** Specific lysis of target cells (GP33 peptide sensitized P815/Db cells) was assessed following incubation with LCMV d8 CD8⁺ CTL in the presence of Db/GP33 monomer (black bars) or Db/GP33 long octamer (red bars). **(F)** Specific lysis of GP33 peptide sensitized P815/Db cells was assessed in LCMV infected mice that were or were not (LCMV) injected previously with octamer. Presented data were derived from Ref. (36–38).

insights in pMHC dimer binding to $CD8^+$ T cells, namely that naïve, effector, and memory T cells exhibits substantially different binding and activation/inactivation properties (24, 50). More recently soluble pMHC I and II dimers were prepared that contain synthetic linkers of different length and flexibility (37). Testing of homologous K^d/PbCS(ABA) dimers containing linkers of 12–130 Å showed that the binding avidity (K_D) and the maximal binding (B_{max}) were maximal for very short cross-linkers and gradually decreased with the spacer length of the linker to nearly 50% reduced K_D and B_{max} values at ≥80 Å (37) (**Figure 2B**). Dimers containing short flexible linkers very strongly activated CTL, which frequently induced CTL death via irreversible mitochondrial damages (38) (**Figure 2D**). By contrast dimers containing >80 Å long, rigid linkers induced no significant CTL activation and were able to inhibit CTL activation (36). Moreover, pMHC I (and II) mixed dimers were used to investigate the role of endogenous pMHC complexes for T cell activation. Antigen-specific T cell activation can be triggered by just a few cognate complexes, but for this high sensitivity, endogenous complexes are needed that although unable to trigger T cells by themselves, can substantially boost T cell activation by a few cognate pMHC complexes (51, 52). Conceptually it was proposed that such mixed pMHC dimers, or by analogy vicinal pMHC complexes on antigen presenting cells, promote coreceptor/lck association with TCR/CD3 and/or promote initial TCR/coreceptor co-aggregation on which T cell activation relies (53).

pMHC TETRAMERS AND OCTAMERS

Conventional "tetramers" obtained by reacting biotinylated pMHC monomers with PE (or APC) labeled streptavidin are heterogenous, and unable to dissociate completely from $CD8^+$ T cells (54). True tetrameric pMHC complexes can be prepared based on tetra-grade PE-SA or SA labeled with low molecular weight fluorochromes, e.g., Cy dyes. Real tetramers typically exhibit substantially lower binding avidities and fluorescence intensities, even when PE is used as in the conventional multimers. Moreover, as noted for pMHC dimers, tetramers containing short flexible linkers connecting pMHC to SA avidly bound to cloned CTL and vigorously activated these, whereas those containing long (>80 Å) rigid linkers bound less avidly, barely activated CTL and were able to antagonize CTL activation (36) (**Figures 2C,D**).

Finally octameric complexes were prepared by reacting Cy5-SA with Y shaped dimers in which two pMHC complexes were connected via short flexible or long rigid linkers to a biotin containing stem (36). Octamers composed of dimers with short inter pMHC distances avidly bound to and activated cloned CTL, whereas those consisting of dimers containing long rigid linkers bound less avidly and barely activated CTL. Owing to their high valence even octamers containing long rigid linkers exhibited avid binding to CTL and were able to efficiently inhibit CTL killing *in vitro* and *in vivo* and hence constitute a novel type of $CD8^+$ T cell antagonists (36) (**Figures 2C–F**). Moreover, comparative binding studies on Melan-A-specific $CD8^+$ T cell clones derived from a melanoma patient with A2/Melan-A dimers, tetramers, octamers containing linkers of different length and flexibility revealed striking differences depending on the state of $CD8^+$ T cell differentiation (55). In particular dimeric complexes containing a short linker avidly and selectively stained a population of incompletely differentiation, dysfunctional $CD8^+$ T cells, that are typically observed in advanced melanoma patients, but never in healthy individuals (55).

SOLUBLE pMHC COMPLEXES BUILT ON Ni^{2+}-NTA–HIS-TAG CHELATE COMPLEXES

THE MAKE AND NATURE OF REVERSIBLE pMHC COMPLEXES

Conventional BSP multimers are prepared by using the biotin–streptavidin irreversible tandem. Although for some applications this irreversible binding is desirable, for T cell staining it is not as multimers can bind and strongly activate those cells, leading sometimes to their death (**Figure 3A**). Nitrilotriacetic acid (NTA) at neutral aqueous solutions chelates bivalent cations, e.g., Ni^{2+}, which in turn binds vicinal side chains of histidines. While the monomeric interaction is in the micro-molar range, picomolar dissociation constants were obtained for linear tetra-NTA compounds binding to pMHC molecules containing a C-terminal tandem His-tag ($2xHis_6$) (35). While these coordination complexes are stable, also at elevated temperatures, they decay within a few seconds upon addition of free imidazole.

SORTING OF ANTIGEN-SPECIFIC T CELLS BY REVERSIBLE SOLUBLE pMHC COMPLEXES

Although CTL are highly cytotoxic cells, they are remarkably susceptible to cell death, which can be induced by soluble pMHC complexes, e.g., directly by Fas/FasL mediated cytotoxicity, mitochondrial damages due to excessive CTL activation, or indirectly by fratricide caused by transfer of peptide from soluble to CTL-associated MHC molecules (37, 56). To prevent this and functional alterations, three types of reversible pMHC multimers have been described (**Figure 3B**) that allow sorting of "untouched" antigen-specific $CD8^+$ (and $CD4^+$) T cells (33–35, 57). Because T cell activation and signaling takes place at physiological temperatures, but not in the cold and pMHC monomers rapidly dissociate from T cells, they are stained with the multimers and sorted by FACS or MACS in the cold and cell-associated reagents are removed before culturing the sorted cells at 37°C. Two reversible multimers are built on altered biotin–SA scaffolds (33, 34, 57). The first ones, called streptamers, which are commercially available from IBA Life Science, consist of pMHC complexes containing C-terminal one or two streptags, i.e., a linear peptide sequence that mimics biotin and fluorescence labeled streptactin, a SA mutant that more avidly binds sterptags than SA. Because the binding of one streptag to streptactin is weak (micromolar range), it is advantageous to use a tandem streptag for improved stability. While streptamers (containing two streptags) in the cold are stable, decay becomes appreciable at 20°C, which risks to affect their shelf life, especially when brief periods of warming up cannot be excluded. The other type of reversible multimer contains desthiobiotin (DTB) in place of biotin, a biotin derivative with greatly weakened binding to SA (33). As the streptamer, these multimers can be readily dissociated by addition of free biotin. These reagents are only stable in the cold and readily decay at elevated temperatures, which can be reduced when using two DTB per pMHC entity. A third type of reversible pMHC multimers are NTAmer which being built on Ni^{2+}-NTA–His-tag chelates complexes, rapidly decay upon addition of free imidazole (35). NTAmers built on NTA_4-Ni^{2+}-tandem His_6-tag are nearly as stable as biotin–SA multimers and therefore are by far more stable than the other reversible multimers, especially at elevated temperatures (**Figure 3C**). As described below, multimer staining of antigen-specific $CD4^+$ T cells is greatly improved at elevated temperatures (18°C) and therefore for their sorting NTAmers are recommended.

Sorting of antigen-specific $CD8^+$ CTL with Streptamers or NTAmers yielded fully functional CTL, whereas when conventional tetramers were used their cytotoxicity and proliferation was impaired (35, 57, 58). The cloning efficiency of NTAmer sorted CTL was approximately twofold higher as compared to cloning with conventional, irreversible multimers. Analysis of CTL clones revealed that those preferentially lost by sorting with conventional multimers exhibited high physical and functional avidity, which is adverse in view of studies showing that high avidity CTL mediate superior tumor control (59) (**Figures 3D,E**). The use of reversible multimers thus is strongly recommended especially for sorting of antigen-specific T cells used in immunotherapy.

ADDITIONAL APPLICATIONS FOR NTA-BASED REVERSIBLE SCAFFOLDS

PE-NTAmers allow detection of low avidity antigen-specific T cells

Previous pMHC binding studies on $CD8^+$ T cells have revealed that the binding avidity substantially increases at decreasing pMHC–pMHC distances. In SA (and avidin derivatives) pMHC built complexes the minimal inter distance is in excess of the distance of their biotin binding sites (about 30 Å). By means of site-specific alkylation, we conjugated PE with linear NTA peptides and reacted this derivative with tandem His-tag carrying pMHC complexes [(35) and unpublished data, **Figures 4A–C**]. Phycoerythrin, a saddle shaped molecule, about fourfold larger than SA and with an abundance of surface lysines that permit the preparation of PE–pMHC conjugates with smaller pMHC–pMHC distances than in conventional multimers. The maximal degree of conjugation is 12–16 pMHC complexes per PE, but the maximal binding affinities were observed with conjugates containing 8–10 pMHC complexes per PE. Additionally these PE–pMHC NTAmers are molecularly better defined than conventional multimers, as they contain only one central PE, whereas conventional multimers contain higher order conjugates. In accordance with this, PE–pMHC NTAmer binding exhibit clear saturation and greatly increased binding avidity compared to conventional pMHC multimers and therefore can detect low avidity T cells that are missed by conventional staining reagents (**Figure 4D**). Conclusive detection of low avidity T cells is one of the formidable challenges in T cell monitoring, namely in cancer research where tumor antigen-specific T cells tend to be low avidity due to deletion of high affinity specificities by negative selection (60) and for $CD4^+$ T cells, on which multimer binding is not strengthened by the coreceptor.

NTAmers allow pMHC monomer dissociation kinetic measurements

NTAmer are not only substantially more stable than other reversible pMHC multimers, but their induced dissociation is also more rapid and therefore can be used to measure accurate pMHC monomer dissociation kinetics on living $CD8^+$ T cells (35). To this end NTAmers are prepared with Cy5 labeled monomers. $CD8^+$ T cells are stained in the cold and the cell-associated PE and Cy5 fluorescences are measured before and after addition of imidazole (**Figure 4E**). After very rapid disintegration of the NTAmer,

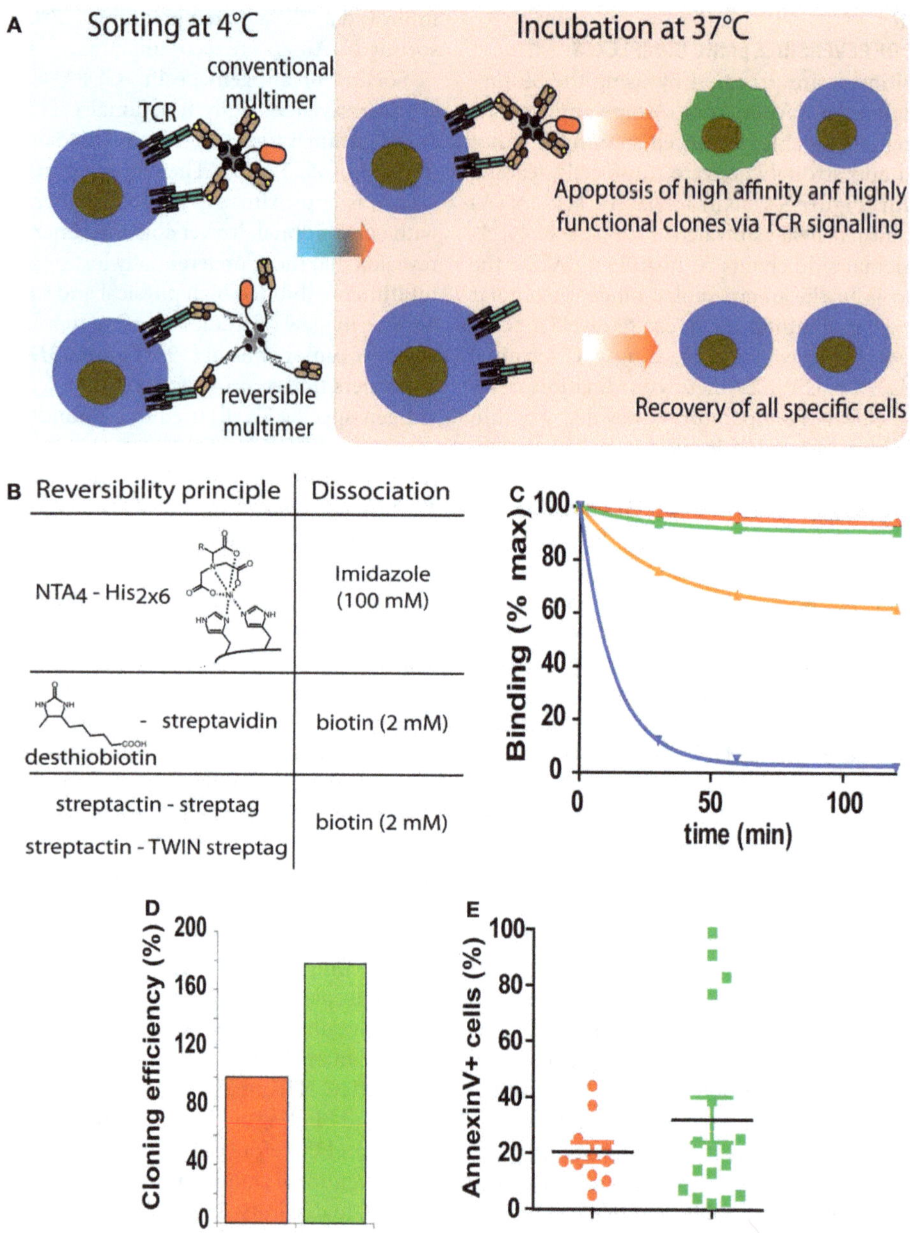

FIGURE 3 | Sorting of antigen-specific T cells with reversible pMHC multimers. (A) Cartoon illustrating the principle of sorting of "untouched" T cells. After cell staining and sorting, reversible, but not conventional multimers can be removed and the T cells cultured at 37°C in the absence of potentially harmful pMHC complexes. **(B)** Representation of the three types of reversible bonds used for the preparation of pMHC oligomers and agent used to provoke dissociation. **(C)** Flu matrix$_{58-66}$ peptide stimulated PBMC were stained at 4°C with A2/Flu multimers containing conventional irreversible (red), NTA$_4$-His (green), streptactin-streptag (orange), or desthiobiotin–streptavidin (blue) scaffolds, washed and cell-associated fluorescence measured after different periods of incubation at 20°C. **(D)** Alternatively cells labeled with BSP (red) or NTAmer were FACS sorted and cloned by limiting dilution. Hundred percent refers to the number of clones obtained from BSP multimer sorted cells. **(E)** Randomly chosen clones were incubated with BSP multimer at 37°C, stained with AnnexinV, and analyzed by flow cytometry. Presented data were derived from (35).

reflected by rapid disappearance of PE fluorescence, pMHC monomer dissociation from cells can be determined by from the decrease of cell-associated Cy5 fluorescence. While dissociation kinetics with pMHC multimers tend to be inaccurate due to incomplete dissociation and heterogenous composition, pMHC monomer dissociation reaches baseline and is more accurate (**Figures 4F,G**). This technique is less sensitive than SPR measurements, and inaccurate in the case of rapid kinetics, but provides information on pMHC–TCR interactions on cells, namely in the presence of CD8. Comparison of data obtained on a wide range of TCR-transduced cells, with NTAmers or directly by SPR showed a good correlation (unpublished data).

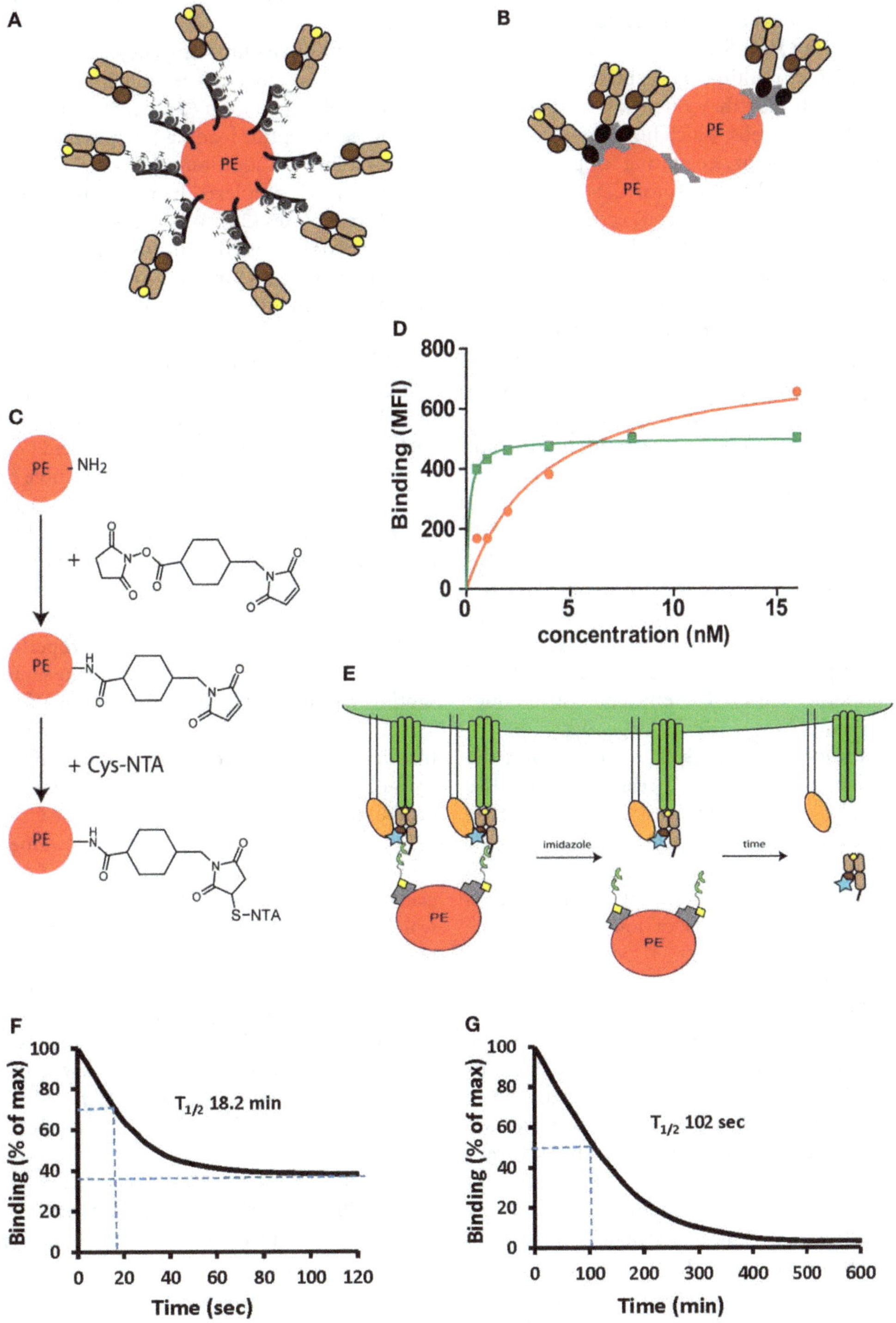

FIGURE 4 | Peptide-MHC oligomers built on switchable Ni^{2+}-NTA-His-tag chelate complexes. **(A,B)** Cartoons illustrating conventional BSP multimers pMHC **(B)** and reversible monomers directly coupled on PE via the NTA strategy **(A)**, where PE designates phycoerythrin. **(C)** The structure of a phycoerythrin molecule is shown in which lysine side chains reacted with a maleimido-*N*-hydroxysuccinimide ester and the resulting maleimido-PE will subsequently reacted with thio-NTA derivative. **(D)** Room temperature isotherms were shown for HLA-A2-Flu matrix$_{58-66}$ BSP multimers (red circles) or PE-NTAmer (green squares) as assessed on Flu peptide stimulated PBMC. **(E)** Cartoon illustrating the two-step dissociation of PE labeled pMHC NTAmer from T cells. Imidazole induced rapid decay of cell-associated NTAmers and disappearance of PE fluorescence, followed by slower dissociation of Cy5 labeled blue monomers from the cells. **(F)** Cloned Flu matrix-specific CD8^{+} T cells were stained in the cold with conventional A2/Flu$_{58-66}$ PE multimers, washed and cell-associated PE fluorescence measured by flow cytometry after the indicated periods of time. **(G)** Alternatively the cells were labeled with PE-NTAmers containing Cy5 conjugated A2/Flu$_{58-66}$ monomers and the monomer dissociation from the cells was assessed by flow cytometry as illustrated in **(E)**. The inserted numbers indicate the dissociation half-lives $T_{1/2}$. Presented data were derived from (33) and (35).

IMPROVED DETECTION AND ANALYSIS OF ANTIGEN-SPECIFIC CD4+ T CELLS BY MOLECULARLY DEFINED MHC CLASS II MULTIMERS

The performance of pMHC II multimers lags behind the one of pMHC I multimers, in particular they often fail to detect low avidity antigen-specific $CD4^+$ T cells, which limits integral analysis of $CD4^+$ T cell responses. Factor accounting for poor pMHC II multimer staining include (i) the coreceptor CD4, unlike CD8 fails to increase the pMHC binding avidity, (ii) certain types glycosylation and sialylation of $CD4^+$ T cell molecules, (iii) lower affinity of MHC class II-peptide restricted TCRs, (iv) conformational diversity of pMHC complexes, and (v) poor quality of pMHC II multimers (61). While refolding of pMHC I complexes provides highly pure monomers, production of pMHC II monomers by loading of "empty" MHC II molecules with peptides of interest does not and therefore the corresponding pMHC multimers contain a reduced fraction of active monomeric complexes. The fraction of correctly loaded pMHC II monomers depends on the peptide and the MHC class II allele and can be well below 50% (62, 63). Tethering the peptide on the MHC II beta chain does not circumvent this caveat. Different strategies were described that allow isolation of molecularly defined pMHC II monomers. Peptide-MHC II tetramers containing defined fractions of cognate and non-cognate monomers were used to investigate the dependence of pMHC II tetramer staining of $CD4^+$ T cells on pMHC II monomer purity. The efficiency of tetramer staining of antigen-specific $CD4^+$ T cells dependents on the tetramer's monomer purity; it decreases dramatically with the monomer purity for low avidity $CD4^+$ T cells, but much less for high affinity cells. This explains why most successful pMHC II tetramer staining reported thus far concerns pathogen-specific $CD4^+$ T cells and not tumor antigen-specific ones, which typically are of low avidity. The use of molecularly defined pMHC II tetramers permits conclusive analysis of low avidity $CD4^+$ T cells (64).

PEPTIDE-MHC II PRODUCTION

Soluble recombinant MHC II molecules typically consist of alpha and beta chain where transmembrane and cytoplasmic domains of which have been replaced by acidic and basic leucine zippers (10). With very few exceptions soluble MHC II molecules are expressed in insect cells, either stably in *Drosophila* Schneider cells or transiently in sf9 cells using baculo virus (11, 61). Because in insect cells there is no MHC II-peptide loading apparatus, nor any retention mechanisms, they are typically secreted in "empty" form, i.e., without a nominal peptide cargo (12). These soluble MHC II molecules are purified usually be means of affinity chromatography using anti-MHC II antibody columns (65). Even though this provides highly pure MHC II proteins, the conditions used for elution, such as extreme pH, are prone to cause partial denaturation, which is an important factor for incomplete peptide loading of "empty" MHC molecules. In order to circumvent this, soluble pMHC molecules have been made containing a C-terminal His-tag, which allows gentle affinity purification at neutral pH on chelating columns, e.g., NTA or IDA columns. Loading of peptides of interest onto "empty" pMHC molecules is usually accomplished at reduced pH and elevated temperatures (e.g., pH 5.5–6, 30–37°C for 24–72 h) and is on faith, i.e., without knowledge of the extent of loading.

The peptide loading efficiency can be assessed by means of a peptide tag, usually an N-terminal one, such as His-tag, dinitrophenyl (DNP), or biotin (31, 66, 67). Such studies indicated that the degree of peptide loading can vary over a wide range and get as low as 10–20%. In addition peptide tags allow isolation of correctly loaded pMHC complexes, henceforth referred to as immunopure pMHC complexes (31). While this is attractive it renders the synthesis of pMHC class II multimers more tedious; importantly, the addition peptide tags may affect $CD4^+$ T cell antigen recognition as suggested by observations that peptide truncations can have significant effects on $CD4^+$ T cell antigen recognition (68–70). Therefore the use of conditional peptide tags would be desirable and could be prepared similarly as conditional peptide ligands, namely by linking it to the peptide via a photocleavable residue such as 2-[2-nitro-phenyl]-propionic acid (71, 72).

An alternative strategy to prepare soluble pMHC monomers is by tethering a peptide of interest to the N-terminus of the beta chain via a long and flexible linker (10). This method allows the preparation of murine pMHC class II monomers and tetramers, which are difficult to obtain via peptide loading, as "empty" mouse MHC II molecules are unstable. It is important to note that tethered on peptides may or may not be properly nested in the MHC II's binding groove and that therefore the same concerns of denaturation, namely those related to immunoaffinity chromatography are applicable as mentions above. Moreover, it has been reported that depending on peptide truncations and linker length the tethered on peptides may bind in different registers and hence be differently recognized by antigen-specific $CD4^+$ T cells (30, 62).

A major shortcoming of pMHC II tetramers is that they fail to stain a fraction of antigen-specific $CD4^+$ T cells (29). This is especially a concern for tumor and self-antigen-specific $CD4^+$ T cells, which tend to be of low avidity, due to deletion of high affinity cells by thymic negative selection and much less for pathogen-specific $CD4^+$ T cells (29). This shortcoming curtails the usefulness of pMHC II tetramers especially in research related to cancer or autoimmunity (63, 73), because these fields of research become increasingly more important, we review in the following sections studies related to improving pMHC class II staining performance especially on low avidity $CD4^+$ T cells.

ON THE USE OF PEPTIDE TAGS TO ASSESS MHC II-PEPTIDE LOADING AND TO ISOLATE IMMUNOPURE MONOMERS

In order to be able to measure peptide loading and to purify correctly loaded pMHC II complexes, several peptide tags have been described; for example: (1) An N-terminal dinitrophenyl (DNP) residue, allowing ELISA detection and isolation of DNP–pMHC complexes by means of anti-DNP mAb. This technique is expensive and addition of DNP renders poorly (**Figure 5A**) soluble peptide completely water insoluble (74). (2) N-terminal His_6-peptide tags have been used that allow detection and isolation of specific pMHC complexes by means of chelators, such as Ni^{2+}-NTA or IDA (31, 75). Advantages of this strategy include facile peptide synthesis and improved solubility of peptides and inexpensive availability of chelators for affinity chromatography and ELISA applications. Disadvantages include (i) losses due to inadequate binding affinity,

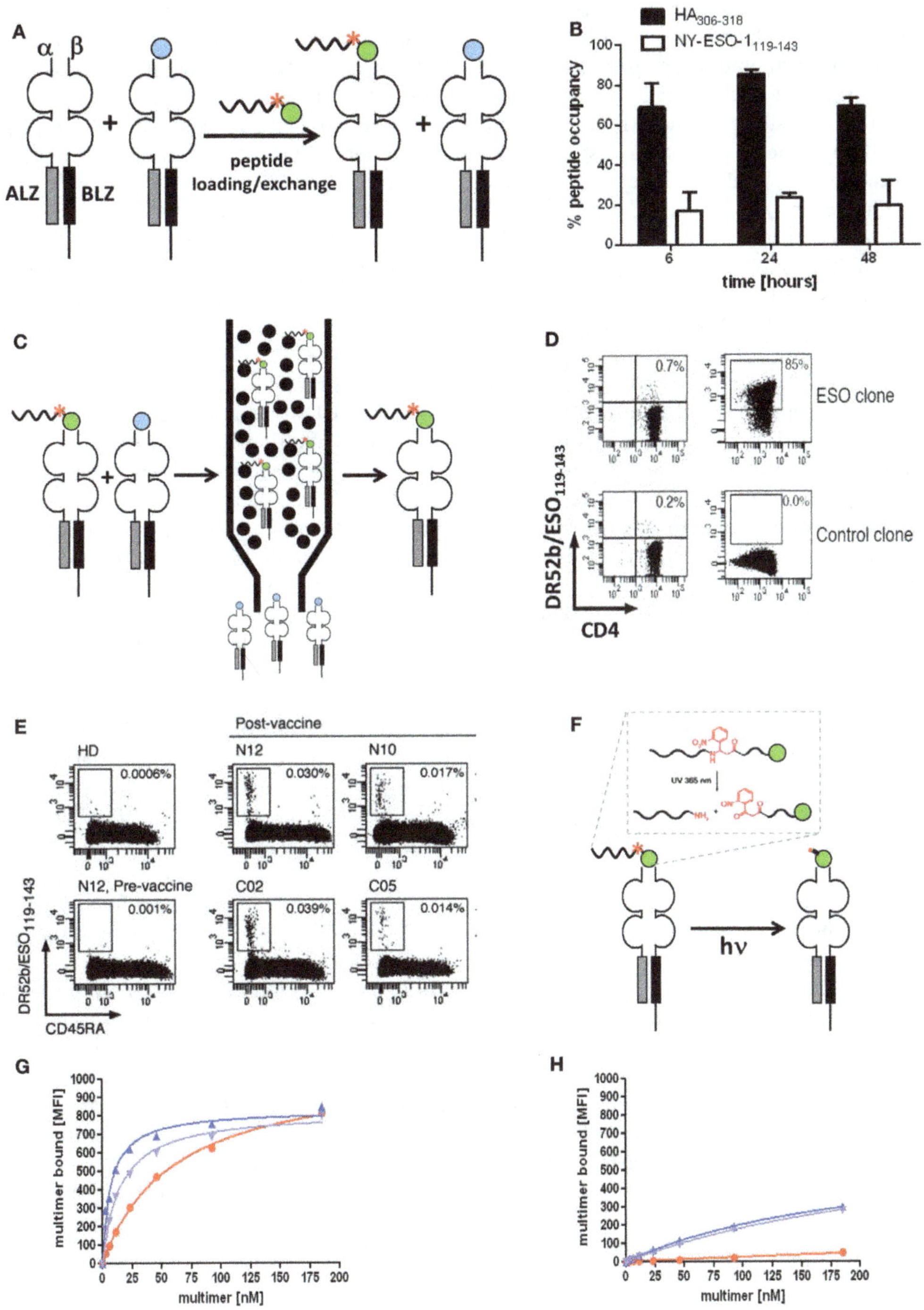

FIGURE 5 | Molecularly defined pMHC class II multimers detect low avidity CD4+ T cells. (A,C,F) Cartoons illustrating the use of photocleavable (red asterisk) peptide tags to discriminate pMHC II complexes containing the peptide of interest (green ball) or irrelevant peptides (blue ball) **(A)**, to affinity purify correctly loaded complexes **(C)** and to remove the peptide tag, either His_6 or desthiobiotin that is linked to the peptide via a β-nitrophenylglycine residue, which can be cleft by UV irradiation. **(B)** "Empty" HLA-DR4 was incubated for 6, 24, and 48 h at 37°C at pH 6, 32°C for 4 h with His_6-$HA_{306-318}$ (black bars) or His_6-NY-ESO-$1_{119-143}$ (white bars). Peptide occupancy was calculated as (amount of His_6-peptide bound to the DR4)/(amount of total DR4). After gel-filtration the peptide occupancy was determined by ELISA using affinity-purified complexes as reference (100%). **(D)** Staining of DR52b/NY-ESO-$1_{119-143}$-specific (top) or an irrelevant (SSX2-specific) CD4+ T cell clone (bottom) were stained with 5.6 nM of conventional (left) and "immunopure" DR52b/NY-ESO-$1_{119-143}$ multimers (right) at 37°C for 1 h and analyzed by flow cytometry. **(E)** *Ex vivo* CD4+ T cells from PBMC of a DR52b+ healthy donors (HD) or of DR52b melanoma patients either pre- or post-NY-ESO-1 vaccination were stained as in E plus anti-CD45RA antibody and analyzed by flow cytometry. **(G,H)** The 37°C binding isotherms of "immunopure" DR4/$HA_{306-318}$ (blue) and conventional multimers (red) on the DR4/$HA_{306-318}$-specific clones 9 **(G)** or 8 **(H)**. The immunopure multimers contained [dark blue or not (light blue)] the N-terminal His_6-tag that was used for affinity purification. Presented data were derived from (31).

(ii) backgrounds due to non-specific co-ligation, and (iii) incompatibility with multimer formation based on His-tag-NTA chelate complexes (35). (3) Biotin or desthiobiotin tag can be used for the detection of specifically peptide loaded pMHC II-peptide complexes. Disadvantages of these strategies include: (i) incompatibility with tetramer formation by means of biotin and streptavidin; (ii) for affinity purification of specially peptide loaded pMHC complexes, biotin binding tends to be too strong and DTB binding too weak (unpublished data); and (iii) aggravation of peptide solubility problems by addition of biotin.

Previous studies with His_6 or Cy5.5 tagged peptides revealed that peptide loading to "empty" HLA-DR4 and DR52b molecules is remarkably variable. As shown in **Figure 5B** the viral Flu HA peptide bound to over 80% of "empty" DR4 molecules, whereas the tumor antigen NY-ESO-1 peptide bound to only 20%. Similar striking differences were observed for other viral and tumor antigen derived epitopes on "empty" DR4, DR52b, and DP4 molecules, with the viral peptides typically being the better binders. It may be speculated that viruses that are older than adaptive immunity of mammals, like the influenza virus, actively participated in the evolutionary shaping of the MHC locus.

By means of an N-terminal His_6-peptide tag and IDA chromatography immunopure DR52b/NY-ESO-$1_{119-143}$ monomers were produced and with these PE labeled multimers, which exhibited dramatically improved staining a cloned ESO-specific $CD4^+$ T cells as compared to conventional DR52b/NY-ESO-$1_{119-143}$ multimers (**Figures 5A,C–E**) (31). More importantly, these immunopure multimer allowed detection and detailed phenotypic and repertoire analysis of DR52b/NY-ESO-$1_{119-143}$ specific $CD4^+$ T cell in PBMC from melanoma patients post, but not pre vaccination with NY-ESO-1 protein. In view of numerous reports indicating that residues flanking the peptide binding core sequence can sensibly affect their interaction with MHC class II molecules, we established a procedure to remove the peptide tag after affinity purification. To this end we used photocleavable 2-[2-nitro-phenyl]-propionic acid to link the His_6-peptide tag to the $HA_{306-318}$ peptide, which allowed removing this tag by UV irradiation at nanometers (**Figure 5F**). The photocleavage is rapid (~4 min using a 45 W mercury fluorescence lamp emitting at (365 ± 40 nm) and nearly quantitative (~90%) (data not shown). We then used this technique to prepare immunopure DR4/$HA_{306-318}$ multimers and compared their staining of cloned, flu-specific $CD4^+$ T cells before and after removal of the His_6-peptide tag. The multimer staining on one clone was modestly higher when the His_6-tag was present, but was unaffected on another clone, indicating that this tag may affect pMHC II binding and/or recognition on some, but not other $CD4^+$ T cell clones. What this experiment also shows is that the immunopure multimers bind significantly more avidly than the conventional multimer and that this difference is especially notable on low avidity clones, which are not significantly detected by the normal multimers (**Figures 5G,H**).

DETECTION LIMITS OF pMHC II MULTIMERS AND HOW THEY CAN BE INCREASED

A major shortcoming of pMHC II multimers is their failure to detect some antigen-specific $CD4^+$ T cells. Studies using 2D binding assays it has been shown that a substantial fraction of antigen-specific $CD4^+$ T cells responding in functional assays are not detected by tetramer staining, but are visible in a 2D binding assay (29). Interestingly comparison of $CD4^+$ T cells specific for a self versus viral antigens showed that the proportion of tetramer undetectable $CD4^+$ T cells is higher for the latter than the former. This is consistent with the view that for self-antigens $CD4^+$ T cells expressing high affinity TCR are deleted by negative thymic selection (76). It is important to note that the vast majority of tumor antigens are self-antigens and that therefore tumor antigen-specific $CD4^+$ (and $CD8^+$) T cell responses tend to be in average of lower avidity than viral specific $CD4^+$ T cells.

While on $CD8^+$ T cells pMHC binding is substantially strengthened by coordinate binding of CD8 to TCR-associated pMHC complexes, CD4 does not significantly contribute to pMHC binding (10). In addition, pMHC I complexes obtained by refolding all contain the peptide of interest; because this is not the case for pMHC II complexes obtained by loading of empty MHC II molecules, $CD4^+$ T cell tetramer staining can be compromised by incomplete peptide loading. To investigate this, tetramers were prepared that contained defined proportions of immunopure cognate and non-cognate pMHC monomers. Using binominal distribution the average contents of cognate pMHC II monomer, dimer, trimer, and tetramer were calculated for different ratios of cognate/non-cognate complexes used to make the tetramer (**Figure 6A**); from these four different binding curves can be calculated for the scenarios that a tetramer can stain a $CD4^+$ T cell when it contains (1) one, two, three, or four or (2) two, three, or four or (3) three and four or (4) only four cognate monomers (**Figure 6B**). Staining of seven randomly chosen DR4-restricted Flu $HA_{306-318}$ specific $CD4^+$ T cell clones (**Figure 6C**) with tetramers containing graded fractions of cognate, immunopure DR4-$HA_{306-318}$ monomer, showed that such binding curves are found, i.e., that clones can be grouped in different discrete avidity ranges (**Figures 6D–F**). Importantly, this shows that low avidity $CD4^+$ T cells will not be detected by tetramer staining, unless these contain only cognate pMHC monomers (**Figure 6F**). In view of the fact that pMHC II tetramer staining risks to miss a substantial fraction of antigen-specific $CD4^+$ T cells, the use of immunopure tetramers is highly recommended in order to detect low avidity cells (**Figures 6G,H**).

The tetramer staining efficiency also critically depends on $CD4^+$ T cells surface glycosylation and pretreatment of cells with a broadly active neuraminidase (e.g., from *Vibrio cholerae*) can increase tetramer staining by nearly 100% (77, 78). Testing on 37 Flu-specific Th1 clones we found increases of tetramer staining upon desialylation in the range of 20–95% (unpublished data).

CONCLUSION

Wide ranges of soluble pMHC I-peptide oligomers have been prepared and used to analyze, activate, inactivate, and sort antigen-specific $CD8^+$ T cells. Well-defined pMHC dimers, tetramers, and octamers containing linkers of defined length and flexibility were instrumental in dissecting mechanisms governing pMHC binding by $CD8^+$ T cells and the ensuing cell activation and eventual cell death. Reversible multimeric pMHC complexes emerged as useful reagents to sort "untouched" $CD8^+$ T cells; of particular

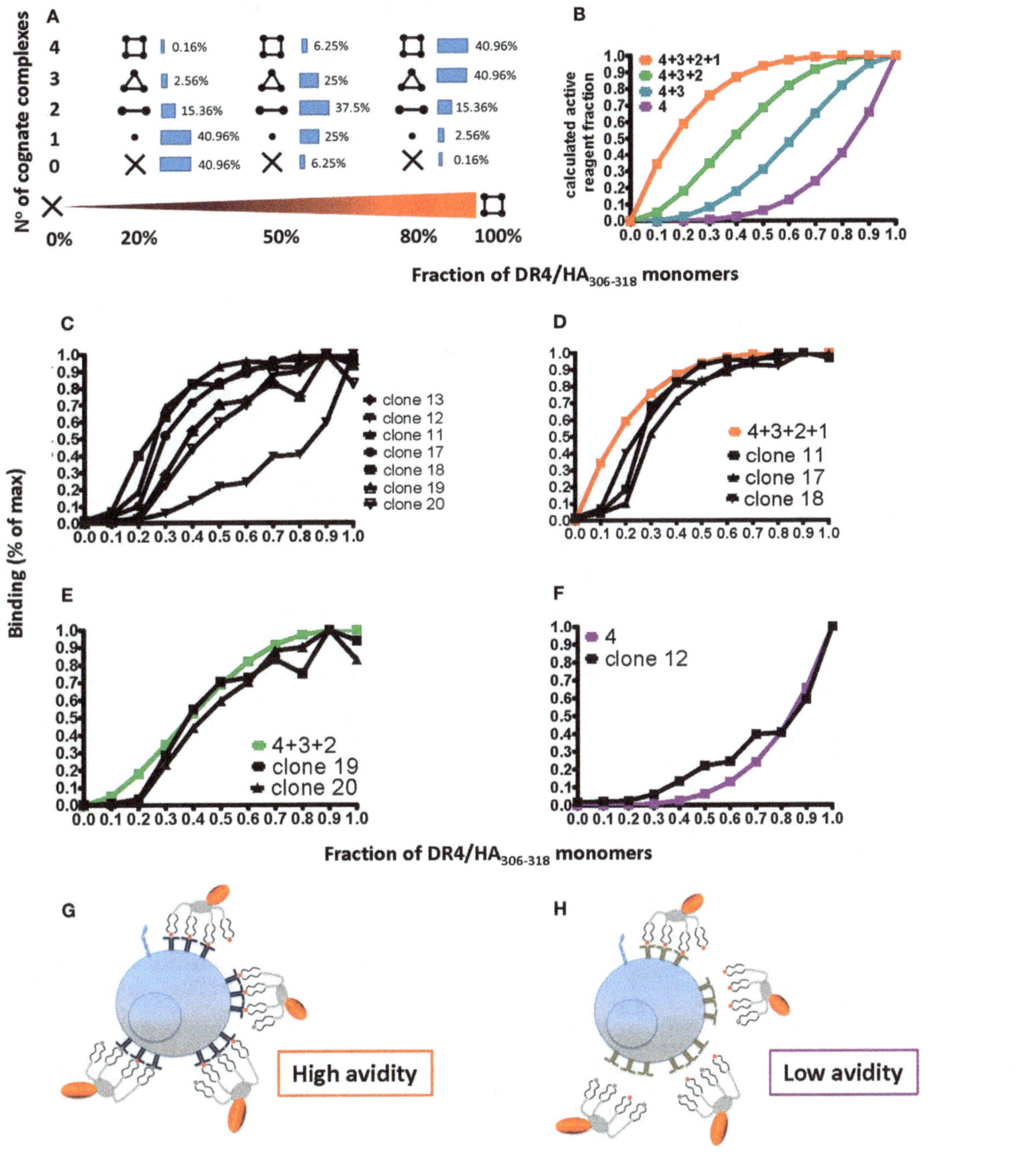

FIGURE 6 | Degree of peptide loading determines the avidity detection threshold on pMHC II multimer detection. (A,B) Cognate ($DR4/HA_{306-318}$) and irrelevant (DR4/CLIP) pMHC II monomers were mixed in different ratios (*x*-axis; fractions of one) and reacted with streptavidin–PE to make tetramers. For 0, 20, 50, 80, and 100% of cognate monomers the compositions of tetramers containing $X = 0$, 1, 2, 3, or 4 cognate monomers were calculated according to the binominal distribution and expressed in %, indicated by the inserted numbers **(A)**, with 100% being the sum of each row; alternatively it was plotted on the *y*-axis as fraction of 1 against the fraction of cognate/non-cognate complexes (*x*-axis) for the indicated four avidity levels T cell binding (red: all four complexes bind; green: three; blue: two; and purple: one). **(C)** Seven $DR4/HA_{306-318}$-specific $CD4^+$ T cell clones were incubated with 18.5 nM DR4 tetramers with DR4 tetramers containing the indicated factions of $HA_{306-318}$ and CLIP peptides (*x*-axis; fraction of one) for 1 h at 37°C and cell-associated fluorescence assessed by flow cytometry and expressed in % of maximal binding (*y*-axis). **(D–F)** From these binding isotherms those observed on the clones 11, 17, and 18 match the high avidity binding curve (in red) **(D)**, those recorded on the clones 19 and 20, match the green curve **(E)** and the one measured on the clone 12 the purple curve **(F)**. **(G,H)** The cartoon representation of high **(G)** and low avidity **(H)** $CD4^+$ T cells as defined by their ability to bind mixed tetramers.

interest were "switchable" NTAmer that additionally allowed measurement of pMHC monomer dissociation kinetics on living cells and detection of low avidity T cells. Detection of antigen-specific $CD4^+$ T cells by pMHC II multimers overall was more challenging and prone to miss significant fractions of cells, namely low avidity $CD4^+$ T cells; detection of these cells was dramatically improved by using molecularly defined multimers.

ACKNOWLEDGMENTS

We are indebted Profs. Perdro Romero, Danila Valmori, Maha Ayyoub, Daniel Speiser, and Drs. Petra Baumgartner, Nathalie Rufer, and Michael Hebeisen for competent collaborations, and Anne Wilson for expert assistance in flow cytometry. Financial support by SFN Grants 310030-12533/1 and 3100-61'946.00 are greatly acknowledged.

REFERENCES

1. Alam R, Gorska M. 3. Lymphocytes. *J Allergy Clin Immunol* (2003) **111**:S476–85. doi:10.1067/mai.2003.121
2. Fooksman DR, Vardhana S, Vasiliver-Shamis G, Liese J, Blair DA, Waite J, et al. Functional anatomy of T cell activation and synapse formation. *Annu Rev Immunol* (2010) **28**:79–105. doi:10.1146/annurev-immunol-030409-101308
3. Luescher IF, Vivier E, Layer A, Mahiou J, Godeau F, Malissen B, et al. CD8 modulation of T-cell antigen receptor-ligand interactions on living cytotoxic T lymphocytes. *Nature* (1995) **373**:353–6. doi:10.1038/373353a0
4. Cavallo F, Offringa R, van der Burg SH, Forni G, Melief CJ. Vaccination for treatment and prevention of cancer in animal models. *Adv Immunol* (2006) **90**:175–213. doi:10.1016/S0065-2776(06)90005-4
5. Nakamura Y, Watchmaker P, Urban J, Sheridan B, Giermasz A, Nishimura F, et al. Helper function of memory CD8+ T cells: heterologous CD8+ T cells support the induction of therapeutic cancer immunity. *Cancer Res* (2007) **67**:10012–8. doi:10.1158/0008-5472.CAN-07-1735
6. Guillaume P, Dojcinovic D, Luescher IF. Soluble MHC-peptide complexes: tools for the monitoring of T cell responses in clinical trials and basic research. *Cancer Immun* (2009) **9**:7.
7. Wooldridge L, Lissina A, Cole DK, van den Berg HA, Price DA, Sewell AK. Tricks with tetramers: how to get the most from multimeric peptide-MHC. *Immunology* (2009) **126**:147–64. doi:10.1111/j.1365-2567.2008.02848.x
8. Garboczi DN, Hung DT, Wiley DC. Hla-A2-peptide complexes – refolding and crystallization of molecules expressed in *Escherichia coli* and complexed with single antigenic peptides. *Proc Natl Acad Sci U S A* (1992) **89**:3429–33. doi:10.1073/pnas.89.8.3429
9. Cockfield SM, Halloran PF. A view from the groove: peptide binding by MHC molecules and the implications for regional immune responses. *Reg Immunol* (1989) **2**:266–72.
10. Fremont DH, Hendrickson WA, Marrack P, Kappler J. Structures of an MHC class II molecule with covalently bound single peptides. *Science* (1996) **272**:1001–4. doi:10.1126/science.272.5264.1001
11. Frayser M, Sato AK, Xu L, Stern LJ. Empty and peptide-loaded class II major histocompatibility complex proteins produced by expression in *Escherichia coli* and folding in vitro. *Protein Expr Purif* (1999) **15**:105–14. doi:10.1006/prep.1998.0987
12. Sadegh-Nasseri S, Stern LJ, Wiley DC, Germain RN. MHC class II function preserved by low-affinity peptide interactions preceding stable binding. *Nature* (1994) **370**:647–50. doi:10.1038/370647a0
13. Kalandadze A, Galleno M, Foncerrada L, Strominger JL, Wucherpfennig KW. Expression of recombinant HLA-DR2 molecules. Replacement of the hydrophobic transmembrane region by a leucine zipper dimerization motif allows the assembly and secretion of soluble DR alpha beta heterodimers. *J Biol Chem* (1996) **271**:20156–62. doi:10.1074/jbc.271.33.20156
14. Niemiec PK, Read LR, Sharif S. Synthesis of chicken major histocompatibility complex class II oligomers using a baculovirus expression system. *Protein Expr Purif* (2006) **46**:390–400. doi:10.1016/j.pep.2005.09.001
15. Khandekar SS, Brauer PP, Naylor JW, Chang HC, Kern P, Newcomb JR, et al. Affinity and kinetics of the interactions between an alphabeta T-cell receptor and its superantigen and class II-MHC/peptide ligands. *Mol Immunol* (1997) **34**:493–503. doi:10.1016/S0161-5890(97)00044-8
16. Huppa JB, Axmann M, Mortelmaier MA, Lillemeier BF, Newell EW, Brameshuber M, et al. TCR-peptide-MHC interactions in situ show accelerated kinetics and increased affinity. *Nature* (2010) **463**:963–7. doi:10.1038/nature08746
17. Sherman MA, Weber DA, Spotts EA, Moore JC, Jensen PE. Inefficient peptide binding by cell-surface class II MHC molecules. *Cell Immunol* (1997) **182**:1–11. doi:10.1006/cimm.1997.1219
18. Boniface JJ, Rabinowitz JD, Wulfing C, Hampl J, Reich Z, Altman JD, et al. Initiation of signal transduction through the T cell receptor requires the multivalent engagement of peptide/MHC ligands [corrected]. *Immunity* (1998) **9**:459–66. doi:10.1016/S1074-7613(00)80629-9
19. Luescher IF, Cerottini JC, Romero P. Photoaffinity labeling of the T cell receptor on cloned cytotoxic T lymphocytes by covalent photoreactive ligand. *J Biol Chem* (1994) **269**:5574–82.
20. Luescher IF, Romero P, Kuznetsov D, Rimoldi D, Coulie P, Cerottini JC, et al. HLA photoaffinity labeling reveals overlapping binding of homologous melanoma-associated gene peptides by HLA-A1, HLA-A29, and HLA-B44. *J Biol Chem* (1996) **271**:12463–71. doi:10.1074/jbc.271.21.12463
21. Jiang N, Huang J, Edwards LJ, Liu B, Zhang Y, Beal CD, et al. Two-stage cooperative T cell receptor-peptide major histocompatibility complex-CD8 trimolecular interactions amplify antigen discrimination. *Immunity* (2011) **34**:13–23. doi:10.1016/j.immuni.2010.12.017
22. Dal Porto J, Johansen TE, Catipovic B, Parfiit DJ, Tuveson D, Gether U, et al. A soluble divalent class I major histocompatibility complex molecule inhibits alloreactive T cells at nanomolar concentrations. *Proc Natl Acad Sci U S A* (1993) **90**:6671–5. doi:10.1073/pnas.90.14.6671
23. Casares S, Hurtado A, McEvoy RC, Sarukhan A, von Boehmer H, Brumeanu TD. Down-regulation of diabetogenic CD4+ T cells by a soluble dimeric peptide-MHC class II chimera. *Nat Immunol* (2002) **3**:383–91. doi:10.1038/ni770
24. O'Herrin SM, Slansky JE, Tang Q, Markiewicz MA, Gajewski TF, Pardoll DM, et al. Antigen-specific blockade of T cells in vivo using dimeric MHC peptide. *Mian Yi Xue Za Zhi* (2001) **167**:2555–60.
25. Altman JD, Moss PA, Goulder PJ, Barouch DH, McHeyzer-Williams MG, Bell JI, et al. Phenotypic analysis of antigen-specific T lymphocytes. *Science* (1996) **274**:94–6. doi:10.1126/science.274.5284.94
26. O'Callaghan CA, Byford MF, Wyer JR, Willcox BE, Jakobsen BK, McMichael AJ, et al. BirA enzyme: production and application in the study of membrane receptor-ligand interactions by site-specific biotinylation. *Anal Biochem* (1999) **266**:9–15. doi:10.1006/abio.1998.2930
27. Hugues S, Malherbe L, Filippi C, Glaichenhaus N. Generation and use of alternative multimers of peptide/MHC complexes. *J Immunol Methods* (2002) **268**:83–92. doi:10.1016/S0022-1759(02)00202-8
28. Gutgemann I, Fahrer AM, Altman JD, Davis MM, Chien YH. Induction of rapid T cell activation and tolerance by systemic presentation of an orally administered antigen. *Immunity* (1998) **8**:667–73. doi:10.1016/S1074-7613(00)80571-3
29. Sabatino JJ Jr, Huang J, Zhu C, Evavold BD. High prevalence of low affinity peptide-MHC II tetramer-negative effectors during polyclonal CD4+ T cell responses. *J Exp Med* (2011) **208**:81–90. doi:10.1084/jem.20101574
30. Landais E, Romagnoli PA, Corper AL, Shires J, Altman JD, Wilson IA, et al. New design of MHC class II tetramers to accommodate fundamental principles of antigen presentation. *Mian Yi Xue Za Zhi* (2009) **183**:7949–57. doi:10.4049/jimmunol.0902493
31. Ayyoub M, Dojcinovic D, Pignon P, Raimbaud I, Schmidt J, Luescher I, et al. Monitoring of NY-ESO-1 specific CD4+ T cells using molecularly defined MHC class II/His-tag-peptide tetramers. *Proc Natl Acad Sci U S A* (2010) **107**:7437–42. doi:10.1073/pnas.1001322107
32. Leisner C, Loeth N, Lamberth K, Justesen S, Sylvester-Hvid C, Schmidt EG, et al. One-pot, mix-and-read peptide-MHC tetramers. *PLoS ONE* (2008) **3**:e1678. doi:10.1371/journal.pone.0001678

33. Guillaume P, Baumgaertner P, Angelov GS, Speiser D, Luescher IF. Fluorescence-activated cell sorting and cloning of bona fide CD8+ CTL with reversible MHC-peptide and antibody Fab' conjugates. *Mian Yi Xue Za Zhi* (2006) **177**:3903–12.
34. Knabel M, Franz TJ, Schiemann M, Wulf A, Villmow B, Schmidt B, et al. Reversible MHC multimer staining for functional isolation of T-cell populations and effective adoptive transfer. *Nat Med* (2002) **8**:631–7. doi:10.1038/nm0602-631
35. Schmidt J, Guillaume P, Irving M, Baumgaertner P, Speiser D, Luescher IF. Reversible major histocompatibility complex I-peptide multimers containing Ni(2+)-nitrilotriacetic acid peptides and histidine tags improve analysis and sorting of CD8(+) T cells. *J Biol Chem* (2011) **286**:41723–35. doi:10.1074/jbc.M111.283127
36. Angelov GS, Guillaume P, Cebecauer M, Bosshard G, Dojcinovic D, Baumgaertner P, et al. Soluble MHC-peptide complexes containing long rigid linkers abolish CTL-mediated cytotoxicity. *Mian Yi Xue Za Zhi* (2006) **176**:3356–65.
37. Cebecauer M, Guillaume P, Mark S, Michielin O, Boucheron N, Bezard M, et al. CD8+ cytotoxic T lymphocyte activation by soluble major histocompatibility complex-peptide dimers. *J Biol Chem* (2005b) **280**:23820–8. doi:10.1074/jbc.M500654200
38. Cebecauer M, Guillaume P, Hozak P, Mark S, Everett H, Schneider P, et al. Soluble MHC-peptide complexes induce rapid death of CD8+ CTL. *Mian Yi Xue Za Zhi* (2005a) **174**:6809–19.
39. Batard P, Peterson DA, Devevre E, Guillaume P, Cerottini JC, Rimoldi D, et al. Dextramers: new generation of fluorescent MHC class I/peptide multimers for visualization of antigen-specific CD8+ T cells. *J Immunol Methods* (2006) **310**:136–48. doi:10.1016/j.jim.2006.01.006
40. Rodenko B, Toebes M, Hadrup SR, van Esch WJ, Molenaar AM, Schumacher TN, et al. Generation of peptide-MHC class I complexes through UV-mediated ligand exchange. *Nat Protoc* (2006) **1**:1120–32. doi:10.1038/nprot.2006.121
41. Hadrup SR, Bakker AH, Shu CJ, Andersen RS, van Veluw J, Hombrink P, et al. Parallel detection of antigen-specific T-cell responses by multidimensional encoding of MHC multimers. *Nat Methods* (2009) **6**:520–6. doi:10.1038/nmeth.1345
42. Newell EW, Klein LO, Yu W, Davis MM. Simultaneous detection of many T-cell specificities using combinatorial tetramer staining. *Nat Methods* (2009) **6**:497–9. doi:10.1038/nmeth.1344
43. Chen G, Weng NP. Analyzing the phenotypic and functional complexity of lymphocytes using CyTOF (cytometry by time-of-flight). *Cell Mol Immunol* (2012) **9**:322–3. doi:10.1038/cmi.2012.16
44. Newell EW, Sigal N, Bendall SC, Nolan GP, Davis MM. Cytometry by time-of-flight shows combinatorial cytokine expression and virus-specific cell niches within a continuum of CD8+ T cell phenotypes. *Immunity* (2012) **36**:142–52. doi:10.1016/j.immuni.2012.01.002
45. Kessler B, Hudrisier D, Cerottini JC, Luescher IF. Role of CD8 in aberrant function of cytotoxic T lymphocytes. *J Exp Med* (1997a) **186**:2033–8. doi:10.1084/jem.186.12.2033
46. Kessler BM, Bassanini P, Cerottini JC, Luescher IF. Effects of epitope modification on T cell receptor-ligand binding and antigen recognition by seven H-2Kd-restricted cytotoxic T lymphocyte clones specific for a photoreactive peptide derivative. *J Exp Med* (1997b) **185**:629–40. doi:10.1084/jem.185.4.629
47. Hudrisier D, Kessler B, Valitutti S, Horvath C, Cerottini JC, Luescher IF. The efficiency of antigen recognition by CD8+ CTL clones is determined by the frequency of serial TCR engagement. *Mian Yi Xue Za Zhi* (1998) **161**:553–62.
48. Ge Q, Stone JD, Thompson MT, Cochran JR, Rushe M, Eisen HN, et al. Soluble peptide-MHC monomers cause activation of CD8+ T cells through transfer of the peptide to T cell MHC molecules. *Proc Natl Acad Sci U S A* (2002) **99**:13729–34. doi:10.1073/pnas.212515299
49. Schott E, Bertho N, Ge Q, Maurice MM, Ploegh HL. Class I negative CD8 T cells reveal the confounding role of peptide-transfer onto CD8 T cells stimulated with soluble H2-Kb molecules. *Proc Natl Acad Sci U S A* (2002) **99**:13735–40. doi:10.1073/pnas.212515399
50. Schneck JP, Slansky JE, O'Herrin SM, Greten TF. Monitoring antigen-specific T cells using MHC-Ig dimers. In: Coligan JE, Bierer BE, Margulies DH, Shevach EM, Strober W, editors. *Current Protocols in Immunology*, Chap. 17. New York: Wiley & Sons (2001). Unit 17.2.
51. Juang J, Ebert PJ, Feng D, Garcia KC, Krogsgaard M, Davis MM. Peptide-MHC heterodimers show that thymic positive selection requires a more restricted set of self-peptides than negative selection. *J Exp Med* (2010) **207**:1223–34. doi:10.1084/jem.20092170
52. Krogsgaard M, Li QJ, Sumen C, Huppa JB, Huse M, Davis MM. Agonist/endogenous peptide-MHC heterodimers drive T cell activation and sensitivity. *Nature* (2005) **434**:238–43. doi:10.1038/nature03391
53. Doucey MA, Goffin L, Naeher D, Michielin O, Baumgartner P, Guillaume P, et al. CD3 delta establishes a functional link between the T cell receptor and CD8. *J Biol Chem* (2003) **278**:3257–64. doi:10.1074/jbc.M208119200
54. Dutoit V, Guillaume P, Ayyoub M, Hesdorffer CS, Luescher IF, Valmori D. Decreased binding of peptides-MHC class I (pMHC) multimeric complexes to CD8 affects their binding avidity for the TCR but does not significantly impact on pMHC/TCR dissociation rate. *Mian Yi Xue Za Zhi* (2003) **170**:5110–7.
55. Guillaume P, Baumgaertner P, Neff L, Rufer N, Wettstein P, Speiser DE, et al. Novel soluble HLA-A2/MELAN-A complexes selectively stain a differentiation defective subpopulation of CD8+ T cells in patients with melanoma. *Int J Cancer* (2010) **127**:910–23. doi:10.1002/ijc.25099
56. Xu XN, Purbhoo MA, Chen N, Mongkolsapaya J, Cox JH, Meier UC, et al. A novel approach to antigen-specific deletion of CTL with minimal cellular activation using alpha3 domain mutants of MHC class I/peptide complex. *Immunity* (2001) **14**:591–602. doi:10.1016/S1074-7613(01)00133-9
57. Neudorfer J, Schmidt B, Huster KM, Anderl F, Schiemann M, Holzapfel G, et al. Reversible HLA multimers (Streptamers) for the isolation of human cytotoxic T lymphocytes functionally active against tumor- and virus-derived antigens. *J Immunol Methods* (2007) **320**:119–31. doi:10.1016/j.jim.2007.01.001
58. Schmitt A, Tonn T, Busch DH, Grigoleit GU, Einsele H, Odendahl M, et al. Adoptive transfer and selective reconstitution of streptamer-selected cytomegalovirus-specific CD8+ T cells leads to virus clearance in patients after allogeneic peripheral blood stem cell transplantation. *Transfusion* (2011) **51**:591–9. doi:10.1111/j.1537-2995.2010.02940.x
59. Pittet MJ, Rubio-Godoy V, Bioley G, Guillaume P, Batard P, Speiser D, et al. Alpha 3 domain mutants of peptide/MHC class I multimers allow the selective isolation of high avidity tumor-reactive CD8 T cells. *Mian Yi Xue Za Zhi* (2003) **171**:1844–9.
60. Aleksic M, Liddy N, Molloy PE, Pumphrey N, Vuidepot A, Chang KM, et al. Different affinity windows for virus and cancer-specific T-cell receptors: implications for therapeutic strategies. *Eur J Immunol* (2012) **42**:3174–9. doi:10.1002/eji.201242606
61. Kwok WW. Challenges in staining T cells using HLA class II tetramers. *Clin Immunol* (2003) **106**:23–8. doi:10.1016/S1521-6616(02)00018-9
62. Cecconi V, Moro M, Del Mare S, Dellabona P, Casorati G. Use of MHC class II tetramers to investigate CD4+ T cell responses: problems and solutions. *Cytometry A* (2008) **73**:1010–8. doi:10.1002/cyto.a.20603
63. Vollers SS, Stern LJ. Class II major histocompatibility complex tetramer staining: progress, problems, and prospects. *Immunology* (2008) **123**:305–13. doi:10.1111/j.1365-2567.2007.02801.x
64. Poli C, Raffin C, Dojcinovic D, Luescher I, Ayyoub M, Valmori D. MHC class II/ESO tetramer-based generation of in vitro primed anti-tumor T-helper lines for adoptive cell therapy of cancer. *Haematologica* (2013) **98**:316–22. doi:10.3324/haematol.2012.071712
65. Maus MV, Riley JL, Kwok WW, Nepom GT, June CH. HLA tetramer-based artificial antigen-presenting cells for stimulation of CD4+ T cells. *Clin Immunol* (2003) **106**:16–22. doi:10.1016/S1521-6616(02)00017-7
66. Day CL, Seth NP, Lucas M, Appel H, Gauthier L, Lauer GM, et al. Ex vivo analysis of human memory CD4 T cells specific for hepatitis C virus using MHC class II tetramers. *J Clin Invest* (2003) **112**:831–42. doi:10.1172/JCI18509
67. Ye M, Kasey S, Khurana S, Nguyen NT, Schubert S, Nugent CT, et al. MHC class II tetramers containing influenza hemagglutinin and EBV EBNA1 epitopes detect reliably specific CD4(+) T cells in healthy volunteers. *Hum Immunol* (2004) **65**:507–13. doi:10.1016/j.humimm.2004.02.019

68. Carson RT, Desai DD, Vignali KM, Vignali DA. Immunoregulation of Th cells by naturally processed peptide antagonists. *Mian Yi Xue Za Zhi* (1999) **162**: 1–4.
69. Carson RT, Vignali KM, Woodland DL, Vignali DA. T cell receptor recognition of MHC class II-bound peptide flanking residues enhances immunogenicity and results in altered TCR V region usage. *Immunity* (1997) **7**:387–99. doi:10.1016/S1074-7613(00)80360-X
70. Sant'Angelo DB, Robinson E, Janeway CA Jr., Denzin LK. Recognition of core and flanking amino acids of MHC class II-bound peptides by the T cell receptor. *Eur J Immunol* (2002) **32**:2510–20. doi:10.1002/1521-4141(200209)32:9<2510::AID-IMMU2510>3.0.CO;2-Q
71. Toebes M, Coccoris M, Bins A, Rodenko B, Gomez R, Nieuwkoop NJ, et al. Design and use of conditional MHC class I ligands. *Nat Med* (2006) **12**:246–51. doi:10.1038/nm1360
72. Grotenbreg GM, Nicholson MJ, Fowler KD, Wilbuer K, Octavio L, Yang M, et al. Empty class II major histocompatibility complex created by peptide photolysis establishes the role of DM in peptide association. *J Biol Chem* (2007) **282**: 21425–36. doi:10.1074/jbc.M702844200
73. Gebe JA, Falk BA, Rock KA, Kochik SA, Heninger AK, Reijonen H, et al. Low-avidity recognition by CD4+ T cells directed to self-antigens. *Eur J Immunol* (2003) **33**:1409–17. doi:10.1002/eji.200323871
74. Schubert DA, Gordo S, Sabatino JJ Jr, Vardhana S, Gagnon E, Sethi DK, et al. Self-reactive human CD4 T cell clones form unusual immunological synapses. *J Exp Med* (2012) **209**:335–52. doi:10.1084/jem.20111485
75. Nag B, Mukku PV, Arimilli S, Kendrick T, Deshpande SV, Sharma SD. Separation of complexes of major histocompatibility class II molecules and known antigenic peptide by metal chelate affinity chromatography. *J Immunol Methods* (1994) **169**:273–85. doi:10.1016/0022-1759(94)90271-2
76. Palmer E. Negative selection – clearing out the bad apples from the T-cell repertoire. *Nat Rev Immunol* (2003) **3**:383–91. doi:10.1038/nri1085
77. Reddy J, Bettelli E, Nicholson L, Waldner H, Jang MH, Wucherpfennig KW, et al. Detection of autoreactive myelin proteolipid protein 139-151-specific T cells by using MHC II (IAs) tetramers. *Mian Yi Xue Za Zhi* (2003) **170**:870–7.
78. Massilamany C, Gangaplara A, Chapman N, Rose N, Reddy J. Detection of cardiac myosin heavy chain-alpha-specific CD4 cells by using MHC class II/IA(k) tetramers in A/J mice. *J Immunol Methods* (2011) **372**:107–18. doi:10.1016/j.jim.2011.07.004

An altered gp100 peptide ligand with decreased binding by TCR and CD8α dissects T cell cytotoxicity from production of cytokines and activation of NFAT

Niels Schaft[1]*, Miriam Coccoris[1], Joost Drexhage[1], Christiaan Knoop[1], I. Jolanda M. de Vries[2], Gosse J. Adema[2] and Reno Debets[1]*

[1] Laboratory of Experimental Tumor Immunology, Department Medical Oncology, Erasmus MC Cancer Institute, Rotterdam, Netherlands
[2] Department Tumor Immunology, Nijmegen Center for Molecular Life Sciences, Radboud University Nijmegen Medical Center, Nijmegen, Netherlands

Edited by:
Bruno Laugel, Cardiff University School of Medicine, UK

Reviewed by:
Edward John Collins, The University of North Carolina at Chapel Hill, USA
Koji Yasutomo, University of Tokushima, Japan
Chihiro Motozono, Kinki University School of Medicine, Japan

***Correspondence:**
Niels Schaft, Department of Dermatology, Universitätsklinikum Erlangen, Hartmannstraße 14, 91052 Erlangen, Germany
e-mail: niels.schaft@uk-erlangen.de;
Reno Debets, Laboratory of Experimental Tumor Immunology, Department of Medical Oncology, Erasmus MC Cancer Institute, Dr. Molewaterplein 50, 3015GE Rotterdam, Netherlands
e-mail: j.debets@erasmusmc.nl

Altered peptide ligands (APLs) provide useful tools to study T cell activation and potentially direct immune responses to improve treatment of cancer patients. To better understand and exploit APLs, we studied the relationship between APLs and T cell function in more detail. Here, we tested a broad panel of $gp100_{280-288}$ APLs with respect to T cell cytotoxicity, production of cytokines, and activation of Nuclear Factor of Activated T cells (NFAT) by human T cells gene-engineered with a gp100-HLA-A2-specific TCRαβ. We demonstrated that gp100-specific cytotoxicity, production of cytokines, and activation of NFAT were not affected by APLs with single amino acid substitutions, except for an APL with an amino acid substitution at position 3 (APL A3), which did not elicit any T cell response. A gp100 peptide with a double amino acid mutation (APL S4S6) elicited T cell cytotoxicity and production of IFNγ, and to a lesser extent TNFα, IL-4, and IL-5, but not production of IL-2 and IL-10, or activation of NFAT. Notably, T cell receptor (TCR)-mediated functions showed decreases in sensitivities for S4S6 versus gp100 wild-type (wt) peptide, which were minor for cytotoxicity but at least a 1000-fold more prominent for the production of cytokines. TCR-engineered T cells did not bind A3-HLA-A2, but did bind S4S6-HLA-A2 although to a lowered extent compared to wt peptide-HLA-A2. Moreover, S4S6-induced T cell function demonstrated an enhanced dependency on CD8α. Taken together, most gp100 APLs functioned as agonists, but A3 and S4S6 peptides acted as a null ligand and partial agonist, respectively. Our results further suggest that TCR-mediated cytotoxicity can be dissected from production of cytokines and activation of NFAT, and that the agonist potential of peptide mutants relates to the extent of binding by TCR and CD8α. These findings may facilitate the design of APLs to advance the study of T cell activation and their use for therapeutic applications.

Keywords: activation of nuclear factor of activated T cells, altered peptide ligands, cytokine production, cytotoxicity, human T lymphocytes, T cell receptor

INTRODUCTION

T lymphocytes are potent mediators of anti-tumor immune responses. In fact, T cell receptor (TCR) genes derived from anti-tumor T lymphocytes have been successfully used to redirect other, non-tumor-specific T lymphocytes to tumor cells, and have shown promising clinical activities in the treatment of tumor-bearing patients (1, 2). Adoptive T cell therapy to tumors is based on the ability of TCRs to selectively recognize antigens, i.e., peptides that are presented by Major Histocompatibility Complex (MHC) molecules. The clinical use of TCR-engineered T lymphocytes directed against the human leukocyte antigen (HLA)-A2-restricted antigens MART-1, gp100, or NY-ESO-1 resulted in objective responses in patients with metastatic melanoma up to 45% (3, 4). Importantly, the avidity and antigen reactivity of parental T cell clones, used as a source for TCR genes, are preserved by TCR gene transfer (5–7). Moreover, cytotoxic responses of TCR-engineered T cells toward a panel of gp100 peptide mutants are identical to those of parental CTL clones (7).

Studies with mutated peptides, so called altered peptide ligands (APLs), have eloquently demonstrated that T cell recognition of antigen is flexible and that binding of different APLs can result in distinct and selective T cell signaling and functions (8, 9). APLs can be classified depending on the T cell responses they elicit; e.g., agonists induce the full range of T cell activation such as proliferation, cytokine secretion, and cytotoxic killing; partial agonists sub-optimally activate T cells and cause a selective pattern of effector functions; null agonists do not activate T cells; whereas antagonists specifically inhibit T cell activation induced by the wild-type (wt) peptide [reviewed in (10, 11)]. Interestingly, melanoma cells can process and present antagonistic APLs themselves, thereby potentially providing cues that prevent maximal intra-tumoral T cell activation and facilitate immune evasion (12). Immune suppression mediated by antagonistic peptide variants can be reversed by APLs with highly agonist properties that are able to sensitize T cells and yield resistance against effects of inhibitory APLs (12, 13). Importantly, APLs have already been used in immunotherapeutic strategies with the intent to more effectively skew immune responses against autoimmune diseases, infectious diseases, and cancer [reviewed in (10)].

Numerous APLs have been designed for cancer epitopes and include, amongst others, MUC1-HLA-A2 (14), HER1-HLA-A2 (15), HER2-HLA-A2 (16), HER2-HLA-A24 (17), MelanA-HLA-A2 (18), gp100-HLA-A2 [epitopes 154, 209, and 280 (19)], TRP2-HLA-A2 (20), PSA-HLA-A2 (21), and NY-ESO1-HLA-A2 (22). Such APLs have principally been designed to improve the binding affinity of peptide to the MHC molecule, allowing induction of improved T cell responses against wt epitope. For example, MelanA-HLA-A2-specific T cell responses have rapidly and reproducibly been induced with the highly immunogenic APL with a Leucine at anchor position 2 (L2) (18, 23). However, enhanced immunogenicity of APLs may not necessarily be accompanied by the induction of a curative T cell response specific for the native epitope in patients with cancer. In fact, the modified MelanA epitope may alter TCR binding and prime T cells with different TCRs compared to the wt peptide (24). Indeed in patients with melanoma, T cells elicited by APL L2 demonstrated higher frequencies but weaker functional T cell avidity toward the native epitope (25). This is not necessarily a general finding as gp100 APLs ($gp100_{154-162}$ A8 and $gp100_{280-288}$ V9) were clinically equally effective when compared to wt peptides when used in combination with a DC vaccine (26). Collectively, however, these studies challenge the value and clinical applicability of APLs. Further and detailed studies into APLs and their effects on various T cell parameters are needed to gain a better understanding of the perimeters of T cell specificity and sensitivity. In addition, a correct definition of agonist and potential antagonist properties of APLs will allow successful translation of selected APLs to clinical settings. It is noteworthy that besides the setting of vaccination, where the frequency of the relevant TCR may be insufficient, the clinical potential of APLs may be extended to the setting of adoptive T cell therapy, which ensures a high frequency of the expected TCR in patients.

Here, we have used a panel of $gp100_{280-288}$ APLs and explored APL characteristics in relation to T cell recognition and different T cell responses. To this end, we have transferred a defined TCR, i.e., a gp100-HLA-A2-specific TCR, into human T cells, and tested the effect of individual and double amino acid substitutions of the wt gp100 peptide on T cell responses. Analyses of gp100 APLs revealed that all single amino acid mutants retain their agonistic properties, except for the A3 mutant and double amino acid S4S6 mutant that acted as a null ligand and partial agonist, respectively. Findings showed that TCR-mediated cytotoxicity can be dissected from production of cytokines and activation of nuclear factor of activated T cells (NFAT), and suggest that the agonist potential of APLs relates to the extent a peptide mutant is bound by TCR and CD8α.

MATERIALS AND METHODS

CELLS AND REAGENTS

Peripheral blood lymphocytes (PBL) from healthy donors were isolated by centrifugation through Ficoll-Isopaque (density = 1.077 g/cm^3; Pharmacia Biotech, Uppsala, Sweden). Obtaining and handling of human samples, such as PBL, were according to national and institutional guidelines and approved by the Erasmus MC Cancer Institute's ethical committee. Primary human T lymphocytes were cultured as described elsewhere (7). The TAP-deficient TxB cell hybrid and HLA-A2-positive T2, and the gp100-positive, HLA-A2-positive melanoma cell line FM3 were maintained in DMEM (Gibco BRL, Paisley, Scotland, UK) supplemented with 10% Bovine Calf Serum (BCS: Hyclone, Logan, UT, USA) and the antibiotics streptomycin (100 μg/ml) and penicillin (100 U/ml). The HLA-A2-positive melanoma cell lines BLM and BLMgp100 (the latter transfected with human gp100-encoding cDNA) were cultured as described previously (27, 28). The Jurkat T cell clone E6.1 was expanded in RPMI 1640 medium supplemented with L-glutamine, 10% BCS, and antibiotics.

PEPTIDES AND PEPTIDE-MHC MULTIMERS

Peptides used in this study were: the $gp100_{280-288}$ wt peptide YLEPGPVTA, the gp100 APLs A1–A8, G9, and S4S6, indicating an Alanine, Glycine, or Serine substitution at the indicated amino acid position of the wt peptide, and an irrelevant HLA-A2-binding EBV BMLF-1 wt peptide (GLCTLVAML). Peptide preparations were synthesized as described earlier (7) and found to be >90% pure as analyzed by analytical HPLC. MHC class I binding of peptides was analyzed via stabilization of HLA-A2 on T2 cells, as described previously (29, 30). The gp100 wt peptide, the gp100 APLs A3 and S4S6, and the BMFL-1 wt peptide were used to generate peptide-HLA-A2 monomers (Sanquin Blood Supply Foundation, Amsterdam, Netherlands). Multimers of peptide and HLA-A2 were freshly prepared by incubating streptavidin^{PE} and the corresponding soluble monomers at a 1:4 molar ratio for 1 h at 4°C as described elsewhere (31).

CLONING AND TRANSFER OF TCR GENES

Genes encoding $gp100_{280-288}$-HLA-A2-specific TCRαβ were PCR-amplified from CTL clone 296 (CTL-296) and cloned into the retroviral vector bullet, as described previously (7). Primary human T lymphocytes of healthy donors, pre-activated with anti-CD3 mAbs were transduced with TCR-positive retroviruses produced by the packaging cell line Phoenix-Amp (32, 33). A retroviral vector encoding human CD8α (34) was used to transduce Jurkat T cells prior to transfer of TCR genes (35). Transduction with Mock genes served as a negative control.

FLOW CYTOMETRY AND CELL-SORTING

T cells were analyzed for TCR transgene expression by flow cytometry using either PE-conjugated anti-TCRVβ27 mAb (Beckman-Coulter, Marseille, France) (nomenclature of TCRV regions according to http://imgt.org) or PE-conjugated gp100 wt peptide-HLA-A2 complexes (ProImmune Ltd., Oxford, UK), as described previously (7, 35). In short, 0.1–0.5 × 10^6 T cells were incubated with mAb on ice for 30 min or peptide-MHC complexes (see Peptides and Peptide-MHC Multimers) at room temperature for 1 h, washed, fixed (1% PFA). T cells were gated according to forward and sideward scatter properties using a FACSCalibur (Becton Dickinson, Alphen a/d Rijn, Netherlands) equipped with CellQuest software (BD Biosciences). Binding of peptide-MHC was analyzed within viable gate of TCR-engineered T cells with marker set at <1% positive binding for non-stained TCR-engineered T cells. TCR-engineered T cells were MACS-enriched using gp100 wt peptide-HLA-A2 multimers and anti-PE MACS MicroBeads according to the manufacturer's instructions (Miltenyi Biotec, Bergisch Gladbach, Germany).

CYTOTOXICITY ASSAY

Cytotoxic activity of T cells was assayed in standard 6 h ^{51}Cr-release assays using the following target cells: T2 cells pulsed with 1 μM or titrated amounts of either gp100 wt peptide, gp100 APLs, BMLF-1 wt peptide, or the melanoma cell lines BLM, BLMgp100, or FM3. Antigen-specificity was confirmed by addition of anti-TCRVβ27 mAb or mouse immunoglobulin (mIg; Jackson ImmunoResearch Laboratories, West Grove, PA, USA) (both at 1 μg/ml final), and the contribution of CD8 interactions was studied by addition of anti-CD8α mAb (clone 4H8, 10 μg/ml final, Sanquin Blood Supply Foundation) to T cells 30 min before cultivation with target cells. To inhibit NK cell activity during the cytotoxicity assay, an excess of non-labeled K562 cells was added to target cells prior to assay. The percentage of specific ^{51}Cr-release was determined as follows: [(test counts − spontaneous counts)/(maximum counts − spontaneous counts)] × 100% (36).

CYTOKINE MEASUREMENTS

To quantify the production of cytokines, 6×10^4 T cells were cultured in the presence of 2×10^4 T2 cells pulsed with titrated amounts of peptide for 18 h. Supernatants were harvested, and levels of IL-2, IL-4, IL-5, IL-10, IFNγ, and TNFα were determined via Cytokine Bead Array (CBA kit; BD Biosciences), according to the manufacturer's instructions. In some experiments, CBA data were supplemented with ELISAs (Sanquin Blood Supply Foundation), which were performed according to the manufacturer's instructions. As a positive control, T cells were stimulated with PMA and PHA.

NFAT REPORTER GENE ASSAY

Reporter gene assays for NFAT were performed as described in detail elsewhere (35). In short, exponentially growing TCR/CD8-co-transduced Jurkat T cells (5×10^6) were electroporated with a construct containing Firefly Luciferase coupled to six response elements of NFAT [FLuc-NFAT(RE)6]. Twenty hours post-transfection, Jurkat T cells were transferred to round-bottom 96-well plates at 2×10^5 cells/well and co-incubated with target cells at 10^5 cells per well for 6 h in RPMI 1640 medium supplemented with 1% BCS at 37°C and 5% CO_2. FM3 cells were pre-incubated O/N with IFNγ (PeproTech, NJ, USA, 10 ng/ml) and IL-1β (PeproTech, 30 ng/ml), and co-cultivation of these melanoma cells with Jurkat T cells was performed in the presence of anti-CD28 mAb (clone 15E8, 2 μg/ml, Sanquin Blood Supply Foundation). As a positive control for activation of NFAT, T cells were stimulated with PMA and ionomycin. Following stimulation, cells were lysed and luciferase activities were determined. Luciferase activities were expressed relative to a non-stimulated condition (medium only, which was set to 1.0; **Figure 1**) or in absolute light units corrected for a non-stimulated condition (LU corrected for medium only; **Figure 5**).

PRESENTATION OF THE DATA

All assays, i.e., cytotoxicity, cytokine production, and NFAT activation assays have at least three data points of which mean values (with all values within 15% of mean) were used for graphical presentation. For each graph the experiment as a whole was repeated several times (as indicated) and data of a representative experiment was shown (the latter based on the mean value of triplicate data points per experiment).

RESULTS

SINGLE AMINO ACID SUBSTITUTIONS OF THE gp100 wt PEPTIDE DO NOT AFFECT T CELL FUNCTIONS EXCEPT FOR E3 TO A SUBSTITUTION, WHICH RESULTS IN A NULL LIGAND

In order to study gp100 peptide requirements of various TCR-mediated responses, both primary human T cells and Jurkat T cells were retrovirally transduced with TCR α and β genes that originated from the gp100/HLA-A2-specific CTL clone 296, and MACsorted for high and equal levels of TCR expression. Flow cytometry with TCRVβ mAb showed that gp100 TCR expression levels were about 90% [mean fluorescence intensity (MFI): 103] and 93% (MFI: 214) for primary human T lymphocytes and Jurkat T cells, respectively (data not shown). CD8 expression on primary human T cells was >50% and Jurkat T cells were co-transduced with the human CD8α gene (expression level: 100%; MFI: 590) (data not shown). Antigen-specific responses of TCR-engineered T cells were validated at the level of T cell cytotoxicity, production of TNFα, and activation of NFAT. **Figure 1A** demonstrates that TCR-transduced primary human T lymphocytes were able to lyse gp100-positive, HLA-A2-positive but not gp100-negative, HLA-A2-positive melanoma cell lines. The antigen-specificity of this response was further confirmed by the use of anti-TCRVβ mAb (**Figure 1A**). In addition, **Figures 1B,C** demonstrate that TCR-transduced human T lymphocytes produced TNFα and activated the transcription factor NFAT in an antigen-specific manner. Mock-transduced T cells did not show cytotoxic reactivities, TNFα production, and NFAT activation in response to any of the tumor cell lines tested. Data shown in **Figure 1** confirm previous data from our group (7, 35) and further validate the antigen-specificity and use of the CTL296-derived TCRαβ for our *in vitro* analyses of APLs.

Using APLs with single amino acid substitutions, we studied the same three T cell responses with the following observations. *First*, all APLs ($n = 9$) sensitized T2 target cells for TCR-mediated lysis, except for APL with an E to A substitution at position 3 (i.e., APL A3) (**Figure 2A**). *Second*, although quantities of TNFα produced varied depending on the peptide used, all APLs, except for APL A3, induced production of this cytokine (**Figure 2B**). *Third*, again all APLs induced a clear activation of NFAT, except for APL A3 (**Figure 2C**). Mock-transduced T cells did not respond upon stimulation with any of the APLs tested, neither did TCR-transduced T cells respond to stimulation with BMLF-1 wt peptide (data not shown and **Figure 2**). Observations presented in **Figure 2** extend earlier data showing that the cytotoxic responses of the parental CTL-296 versus gp100 APL with single amino acid mutations are preserved following TCR gene transfer into human T cells (7).

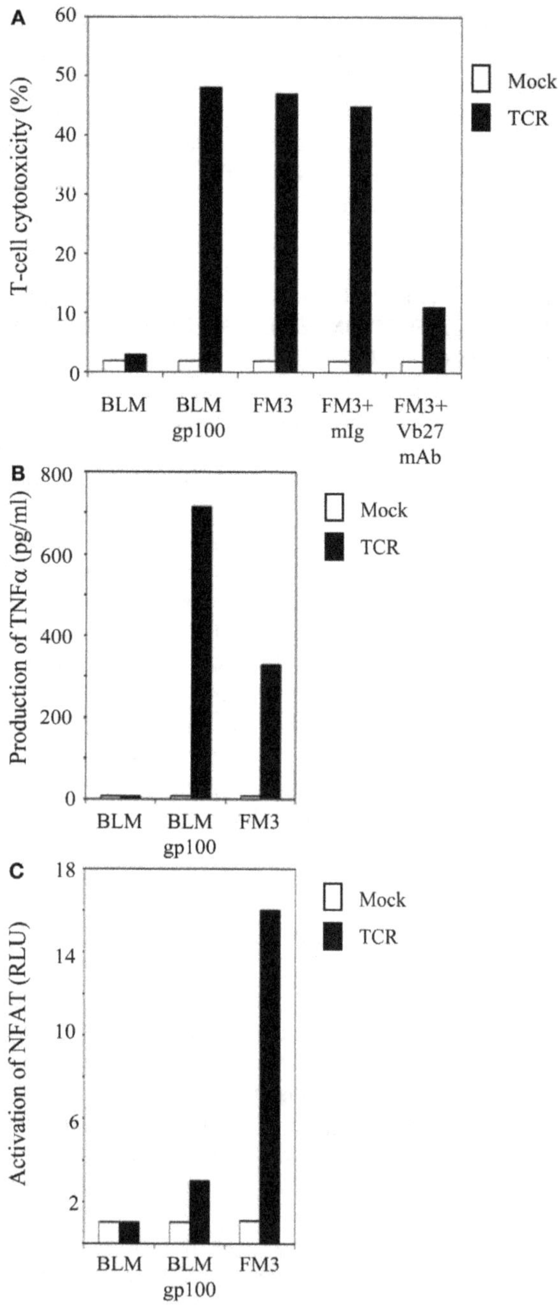

FIGURE 1 | T cells gene-engineered with a gp100/HLA-A2-specific TCR demonstrate antigen-specific reactivity against melanoma cells. **(A)** TCR-transduced human T cells lyse gp100-positive, HLA-A2-positive melanoma cells. Primary human T cells transduced with TCR (black bars) or Mock genes (white bars) were tested in a 6 h ^{51}Cr-release assay with the following target cells: the gp100-negative, HLA-A2-positive melanoma cell line BLM and the gp100-positive, HLA-A2-positive melanoma cell lines BLMgp100 and FM3. The effector to target cell ratio was 30:1. Inhibition studies were performed with T cells and FM3 target cells using anti-TCRVβ27 mAb (Vb27) or mIg. Specific lysis was calculated, and results of one (out of three) representative experiment are shown. **(B)** TCR-transduced human T cells produce TNFα in response to gp100-positive, HLA-A2-positive melanoma cells.

(Continued)

FIGURE 1 | Continued
T cells and melanoma cells as described in **(A)** were co-cultivated for 18 h at an effector to target cell ratio of 3:1, after which TNFα levels (in pg/ml) were determined in supernatants by ELISA. Results of one (out of three) representative experiment are shown. **(C)** TCR-transduced human T cells activate NFAT in response to gp100-positive, HLA-A2-positive melanoma cells. Jurkat T cells transduced with TCR (black bars) or Mock genes (white bars) were transfected with an NFAT reporter construct and subsequently co-cultivated for 6 h with the same target cells as described in **(A)** at an effector to target cell ratio of 2:1. Luciferase activities were determined in cell lysates and expressed relative to medium only [in Relative Light Units (RLU)]. Medium stimulations of TCR- and Mock-transduced Jurkat T cells were 0.024 and 0.018, respectively, and were both set to 1.0. Results of one (out of two) representative experiment are shown.

A P4 AND P6 TO S SUBSTITUTION VARIANT OF THE gp100 wt PEPTIDE FUNCTIONS AS A PARTIAL AGONIST AND DISSECTS T CELL CYTOTOXICITY FROM PRODUCTION OF CYTOKINES AND ACTIVATION OF NFAT

Next to the gp100 APLs with single amino acid substitutions, we generated an APL with a double amino acid mutation. The rationale behind designing this APL was to experimentally address whether replacement of both Proline amino acids, which are characterized by a rigid backbone, would affect and perhaps enhance T cell functions. Since Prolines at positions 4 and 6 in the wt gp100 peptide (YLEPGPVTA), when individually replaced by Alanine, did not alter function of T cells, we next replaced both Prolines by Serines, which are characterized by a more flexible backbone. This S4S6 peptide, when tested in the same set of assays as described above, was able to induce a cytotoxic T cell response and production of low levels of TNFα, but was not able to induce activation of NFAT in human T cells (**Figures 2A–C**).

Findings with gp100 APLs suggest that APLs A1, A2, A4, A5, A6, A7, A8, G9 act as full agonists; APL A3 acts as a null ligand; and APL S4S6 acts as a partial agonist (**Figure 2**). To verify whether APLs A3 and S4S6 present a true null ligand and partial agonist, respectively, we performed extensive peptide dose-response studies. Results of repeated experiments were highly consistent and showed that APL A3 did not elicit T cell cytotoxicity (**Figure 3**), production of cytokines (**Figure 4**), and activation of NFAT (**Figure 5**) when tested over a 7-log range of peptide concentrations (10^{-5}–10^{-12} M peptide). APL S4S6, however, induced decreased T cell cytotoxicity (**Figure 3**), an extremely lowered production of cytokines (**Figure 4**), but no activation of NFAT (**Figure 5**). When looking at wt peptide, we noted that over a large range of concentrations, T cell responses were comparable in all three assays, arguing that results with APLs are not due to differences in assay sensitivities. In example, wt peptide induced maximal T cell cytotoxicity, IFNγ production as well as NFAT activation over a 4-log range (10^{-5}–10^{-8} M peptide), whereas these T cell responses became suboptimal from 10^{-9} to 10^{-10} M peptide onward, and were negligible from 10^{-10} to 10^{-11} M or lower. Instead, quantities of S4S6 peptide that were able to induce maximal T cell cytotoxicity were 10–100-fold higher when compared to wt peptide (**Figure 3**). With respect to cytokines, wt peptide selectively induced levels of IFNγ, and to a lesser extent TNFα, IL-2, IL-4, and IL-5, but

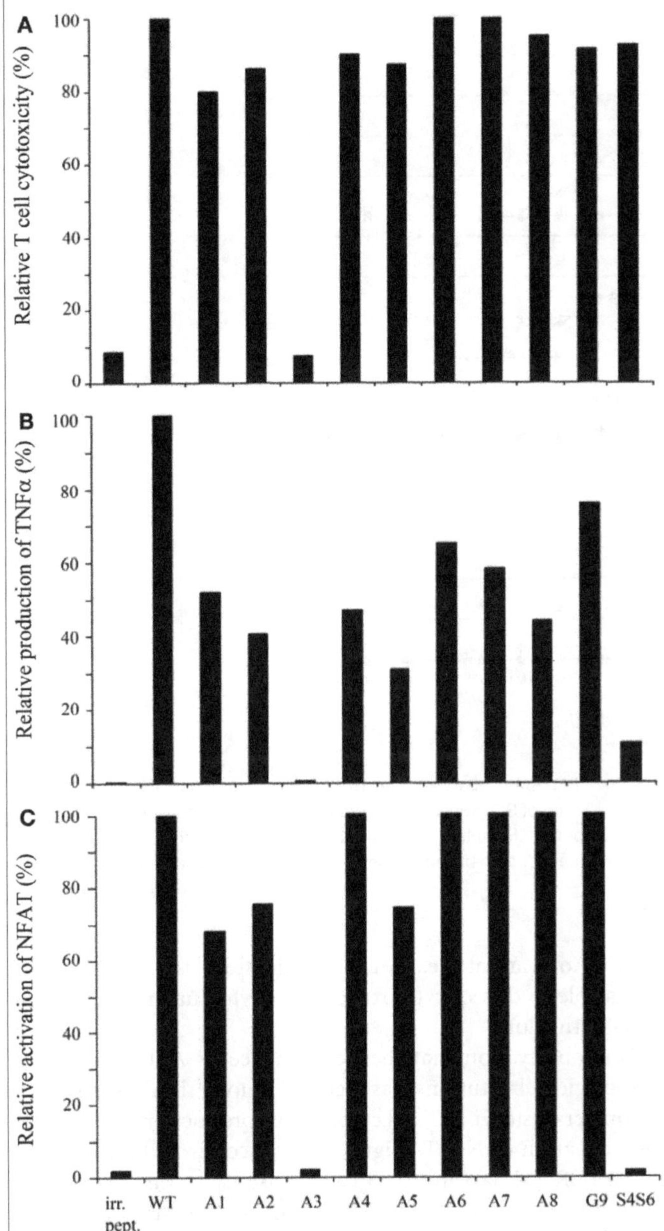

FIGURE 2 | gp100 APLs with single amino acid substitutions function as full agonists except for APL A3, which functions as a null ligand. Human T cells transduced with gp100/HLA-A2 TCR genes were tested in **(A)** ^{51}Cr-release, **(B)** TNFα production, and **(C)** NFAT reporter gene assays. Target cells used were T2 cells that were pre-incubated with 1 μM of gp100 wt peptide (wt), gp100 APLs A1–A8, and G9, or BMLF-1 wt peptide (irr. pept.). gp100 APLs are encoded as indicated in the Section "Materials and Methods." In the ^{51}Cr-release, TNFα production, and NFAT reporter gene assays, the effector to target cell ratios were 15:1, 3:1, and 2:1, respectively. T cell responses in all three assays are expressed relative to T2 target cells pulsed with gp100 wt peptide (specific lysis: 80%; production of TNFα: 1015 pg/ml; and activation of NFAT: 34.73 RLU, all set to 100%). Mock-transduced human T cells did not show activity in response to gp100 APLs (data not shown). Results of one (out of three) representative experiment are shown based on the mean value of triplicate data points. Note the null responses of the gp100 APL A3.

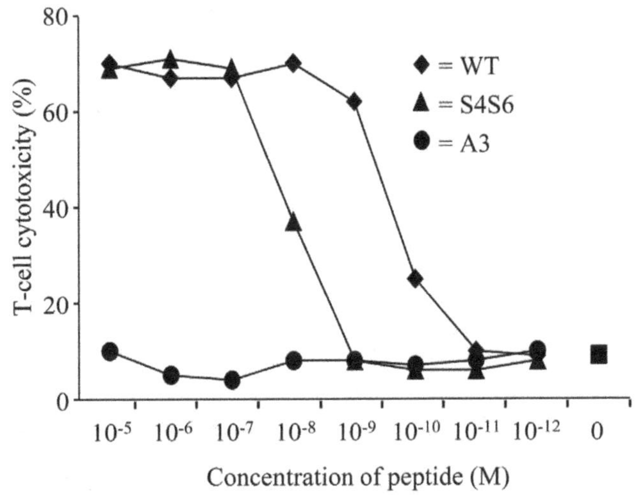

FIGURE 3 | The gp100 APL S4S6 is able to induce T cell cytotoxicity. TCR-engineered T cells were tested in a ^{51}Cr-release assay. T2 target cells were either non-loaded or loaded with titrated amounts of gp100 wt peptide (wt) or APLs A3 and S4S6 (range: 10^{-5}–10^{-12} M peptide). T cell cytotoxicity was assayed after 6 h with an effector to target cell ratio of 30:1, after which specific lysis was calculated. Results of one (out of two) representative experiment are shown based on the mean value of triplicate data points.

not IL-10 (**Figure 4**). S4S6 peptide, however, triggered maximal production of IFNγ at concentrations that were 10^5–10^6-fold higher when compared to wt peptide (**Figure 4**). Production of IL-4 and IL-5 upon stimulation with S4S6 peptide was only detectable at the highest peptide concentrations used (at most 750 pg/ml when stimulating with 10^{-5} M peptide) (**Figure 4**). Using TNFα ELISAs, in our experience more sensitive than CBA, we again only observed detectable production of TNFα at the highest peptide concentrations used (at most 500 pg/ml when stimulating with 10^{-5} M peptide) (data not shown). Lastly, activation of NFAT was not observed for S4S6 peptide independent of the peptide concentration tested (**Figure 5**).

APL S4S6-INDUCED T CELL FUNCTIONS SHOW ENHANCED DEPENDENCY ON CD8

In an effort to explain our results with APLs A3 and S4S6, we examined their ability to bind to HLA-A2, their ability to bind (when complexed to HLA-A2) to the gp100 TCR, and to what extent T cell function, in case of S4S6, relies on the co-receptor CD8α.

To study HLA-A2 binding of APLs, we performed an HLA-A2 stabilization assay using T2 cells. This assay showed that APLs A3 and S4S6 bind as efficient to HLA-A2 as does wt peptide (i.e., stabilization factors at 50 μM were 1.29, 1.14, and 1.25 for A3, S4S6, and wt peptide, respectively). The only APLs within our panel that bound significantly less to HLA-A2 are those that harbored a non-conservative mutation in one of the anchoring residues (i.e., APLs A2 and G9, but not V9, having stabilization factors at 50 μM of 0.00, 0.13, and 1.27, respectively). The abilities of APLs A3 and S4S6 to be stably bound by HLA-A2 allowed the synthesis of peptide-MHC multimers and detection of their

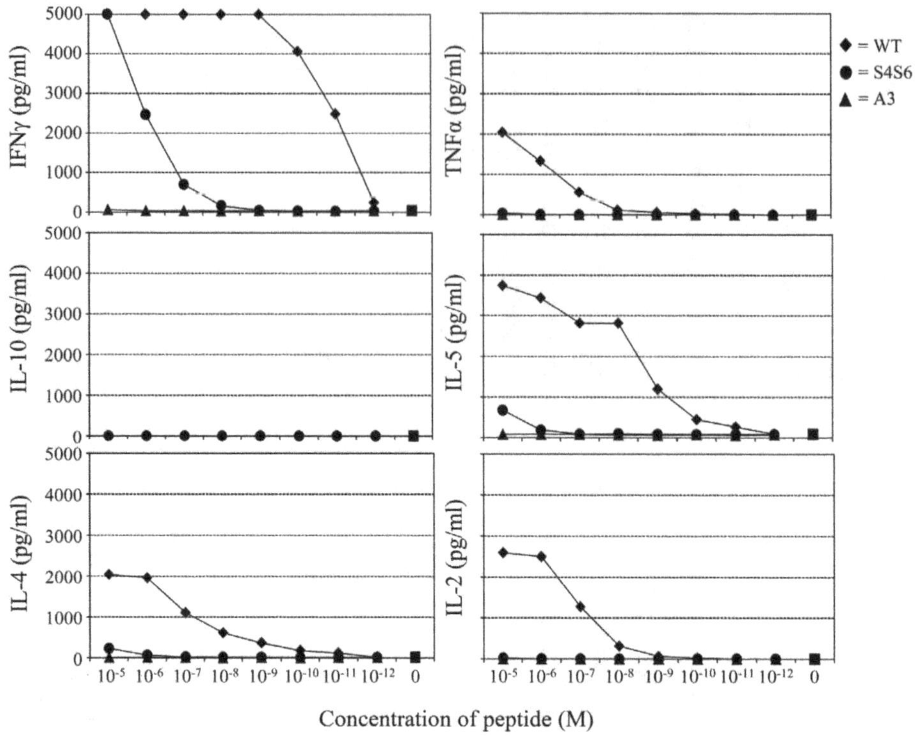

FIGURE 4 | The gp100 APL S4S6 induces a changed cytokine production profile. TCR-engineered T cells were tested for the production of IFNγ, TNFα, IL-2, IL-4, IL-5, and IL-10 using a Cytokine Bead Array (CBA). T2 target cells were either non-loaded or loaded with titrated amounts of gp100 wt peptide (wt) or APLs A3 and S4S6 (range: 10^{-5}–10^{-12} M peptide). Following an 18 h co-cultivation at an effector to target cell ratio of 3:1, supernatants were collected and measured for cytokine content. Results of one (out of three) representative experiment are shown based on the mean value of triplicate data points.

binding by TCR-engineered T cells by flow cytometry. When analyzing the binding of titrated amounts of peptide-HLA-A2 multimers, we observed that neither A3-HLA-A2, nor (the negative control) BMLF-1-HLA-A2 were bound by T cells (**Figure 6**). In contrast, S4S6-HLA-A2 was bound by T cells, although to a lower extent than wt peptide-HLA-A2 (**Figure 6**). Finally, we established the contribution of CD8α to S4S6-induced T cell functions, to which end we have tested T cell cytotoxicity in the presence of a CD8α blocking antibody (**Figure 7**). Anti-CD8α antibody fully neutralized gp100 TCR-mediated cytotoxicity upon stimulation with S4S6 peptide, whereas decrease in cytolytic activity was negligible upon stimulation with wt peptide (**Figure 7**; right versus left panels).

DISCUSSION

In this study, we have characterized peptide requirements for T cell cytotoxicity, production of cytokines, and activation of NFAT. To this end, TCRαβ genes originating from the $gp100_{280-288}$-HLA-A2-specific 296 CTL clone were transferred in human T cells, and receptor-mediated responses were tested versus gp100-positive and -negative melanoma cells (**Figure 1**) and a broad panel of gp100 APLs (**Figure 2**). We observed that APLs with single amino acid substitutions functioned as agonists. The E to A peptide mutant (i.e., APL A3) is an exception to this observation since it functions as a null ligand. The P to S double amino acid substitution variant (i.e., APL S4S6) functions as a partial agonist and is able to dissect cytotoxicity from cytokine production and NFAT activation.

Our observation that the performance of APLs with single amino acid substitutions was identical among the different T cell parameters tested, i.e., T cell cytotoxicity, production of cytokines, and activation of NFAT (**Figure 2**), was confirmed for a second gp100 TCR. Primary human T cells transduced with TCRαβ genes derived from the $gp100_{280-288}$-HLA-A2-specific MPD CTL clone (37) showed cytolytic responses which were in complete accordance with TNFα production upon stimulation with APLs with single amino acid mutations [(7), and data not shown]. In case of the CTL-296-derived TCR, APL A3 behaved as a null agonist with respect to T cell cytotoxicity, production of cytokines, and activation of NFAT (**Figure 2**). This non-responsiveness is not caused by less efficient presentation of A3 peptide since the binding capacity of this mutant to HLA-A2 molecules is in the same range as that of the wt peptide. Rather, the non-responsiveness is caused by the TCR's inability to bind A3-HLA-A2 complexes (**Figure 6**). The classification of APL A3 as a null agonist, and not as a potentially weak or partial agonist, is justified by the observation that peptide concentrations over a 7-log range did not affect T cell activities (**Figures 3–5**). In addition, we were unable to show an inhibitory effect of excess A3 peptide on wt peptide-induced responses in TCR-transduced human T cells, suggesting that this

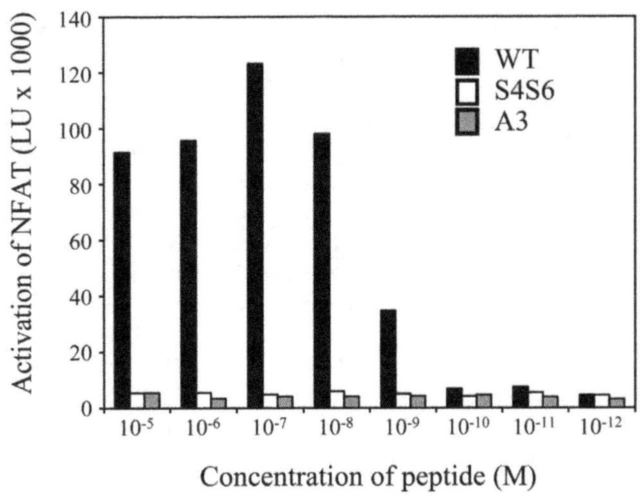

FIGURE 5 | The gp100 APL S4S6 is not able to induce activation of NFAT. TCR-engineered Jurkat T cells were transfected with NFAT reporter and β-galactosidase constructs and subsequently co-cultured with T2 target cells that were either non-loaded or loaded with titrated amounts of gp100 wt peptide (wt) or APLs A3 and S4S6 (range: 10^{-5}–10^{-12} M peptide). Following a 6 h co-cultivation at an effector to target cell ratio of 2:1, lysates were collected and measured for luciferase activities [depicted as light units (LU) corrected for medium only]. Results of one (out of two) representative experiment are shown based on the mean value of triplicate data points.

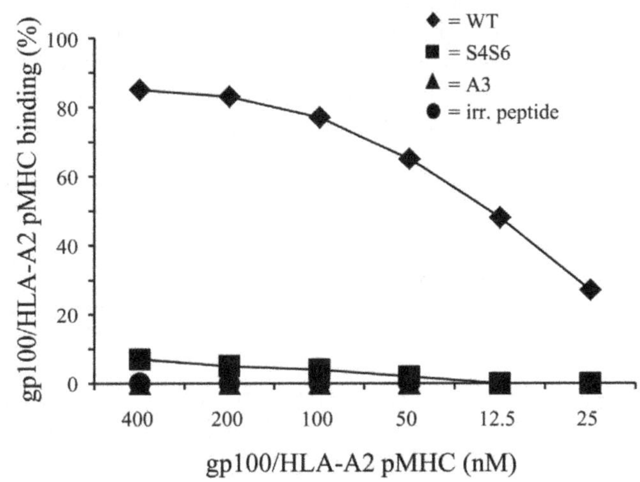

FIGURE 6 | Differential T cell responsiveness toward gp100 APLs is related to TCR's ability to bind gp100/HLA-A2 complexes. TCR-engineered T cells were stained with titrated amounts of PE-conjugated peptide-MHC multimers (range: 400–12,5 nM peptide-MHC complexes) and analyzed via flow cytometry. The gp100-HLA-A2 multimers comprise either gp100 wt peptide or APLs A3 and S4S6. The BMLF-1-HLA-A2 multimer served as a negative control. Binding of peptide-MHC multimers is analyzed as described in Section "Flow Cytometry and Cell-Sorting" and indicated in percentage. Percentages correspond to marker-positive T cells. Results of one (out of two) representative experiment are shown based on the mean value of triplicate data points.

peptide variant is not acting as an antagonist (data not shown). The possibility that APL A3 acts as a supra-agonist, i.e., a null ligand that enhances the reactivation of memory CTL responses (38), is currently under investigation.

Altered peptide ligand S4S6 was classified as a partial agonist since it was able to induce cytotoxicity, production of only selected cytokines, but not activation of NFAT when compared to wt peptide (**Figures 3–5**). When using titrated amounts of peptide we demonstrated that 10–100-fold more S4S6 peptide was needed to induce cytotoxicity when compared to wt peptide (**Figure 3**). The decreased sensitivity of TCR-mediated cytotoxicity was relatively minor and at least a 1000-fold less when compared to the decreased sensitivities of TCR-mediated cytokine production and NFAT activation for S4S6 versus wt peptide (see below). Induction of cytotoxic activity is considered an early T cell response and generally requires small amounts of antigenic peptide and hardly any TCR down-regulation. Cytolytic proteins, e.g., perforin and granzymes, are pre-synthesized and thereby lower the threshold to trigger their release, which may explain the success of partial agonists to induce cytotoxicity (39–43). S4S6 peptide induced the production of IFNγ and to a lesser extent of IL-4, IL-5, and TNFα, but not IL-2 and IL-10 (**Figure 4**) or the activation of NFAT (**Figure 5**). In fact, TCR-mediated production of IFNγ required 10^5–10^6-fold higher concentrations of S4S6 when compared to wt peptide, and production of IL-4, IL-5, and TNFα required $>10^6$-fold higher concentrations of S4S6, whereas production of IL-2, IL-10, and activation of NFAT could not even be measured at the highest concentration of S4S6 tested. These findings are in line with the notion that *de novo* synthesis of cytokines, which in

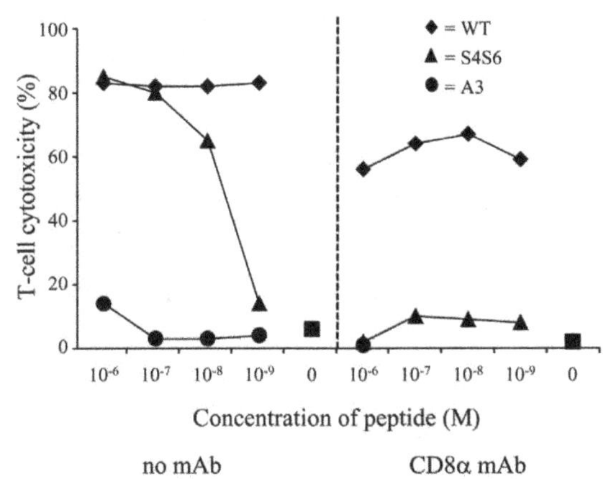

FIGURE 7 | The gp100 APL S4S6 renders the gp100/HLA-A2-specific TCR CD8 dependent. TCR-engineered T cells were tested in a ^{51}Cr-release assay as described in legend to **Figure 3** either without or with blocking anti-CD8 mAb (left and right panels, respectively). T2 cells were either non-loaded or loaded with titrated amounts of gp100 wt peptide (wt) or APLs A3 and S4S6 (range: 10^{-6}–10^{-9} M peptide). Results of one (out of two) representative experiment are shown based on the mean value of triplicate data points.

many cases depends on NFAT activation, generally requires higher amounts of antigenic peptide and a much stronger TCR signal, i.e., high levels of TCR occupancy and TCR down-regulation (43). Production of cytokines and activation of NFAT, considered late T cell responses, may therefore not be triggered by a partial agonist.

Partially agonistic peptides can selectively stimulate some T cell effector functions by inducing a pattern of signal transduction that is qualitatively different from the pattern induced by any concentration of the native peptide (9, 44–46). Partial agonistic signaling patterns are characterized by differential phosphorylation of TCR subunits, recruitment but no activation of ZAP-70, activation of MAP kinases (although for a shortened time period) and/or phenotypically distinct Ca^{2+} fluxes (11, 47, 48). A shortened period of MAP kinase activation and/or weakened Ca^{2+} flux could explain the observed lack of NFAT activation in T cells following stimulation with S4S6 peptide. Translocation of NFAT is reported to take place during "the TCR and co-receptor microclustering stage" in the formation of an immunological synapse (49). It would be interesting to find out whether S4S6 peptide would allow for TCR engagement but not proceeding to TCR microclustering and/or its coalescence into a central synapse. Another property of APL S4S6 may include its potential ability to induce T cell anergy. This state of T cell hyporesponsiveness is generally induced by triggering the TCR in the absence of sufficient T cell co-stimulation or in the presence of proficient T cell co-inhibition, and accompanied by the expression of anergy-associated genes, which subsequently contributes to impaired TCR signaling (50). Although there exist multiple forms of anergy, and it is mainly studied in CD4 T cells, the induction of anergy-associated genes appears to depend on the activation of NFAT. Hence, we argue that APL S4S6, because of its inability to activate NFAT, does not contribute to an anergic state of T cells.

The partial T cell responsiveness induced by APL S4S6 is not related to an altered ability of S4S6 peptide to bind to HLA-A2, but rather to a substantially decreased ability of the gp100 TCR to bind S4S6-HLA-A2 complexes (**Figure 6**). The new Serine residues, although not affecting binding to HLA-A2, apparently changed peptide-MHC conformation such that TCR chains showed a decreased fit for APL S4S6. Interestingly, APLs A2 and G9 with non-conservative amino acid substitutions at one of the peptide anchor positions to bind to HLA-A2 showed a significantly lowered stabilization of HLA-A2, yet were clearly able to induce cytotoxicity, TNFα production, and activation of NFAT (**Figure 2**). This apparent discrepancy most likely suggests that the CTL-296-derived TCR is of high affinity and that only a few peptide-loaded MHC class I molecules are needed to induce T cell activation. This would, in turn, further argue in favor of a dominant role for the interaction between peptide-MHC and TCR when compared to the interaction between peptide and MHC. Since the CD8α co-receptor can contribute to the stability of TCR:pMHC interactions and may, at least in part, compensate for a lowered affinity of a TCR for peptide-MHC (51, 52), we addressed whether S4S6 and wt peptide differed with respect to the CD8α-dependency of T cell cytotoxicity. In line with a decreased recognition by gp100 TCR, we observed that T cell responses toward APL S4S6 showed an enhanced involvement of CD8α (**Figure 7**). These observations extend those of Laugel and colleagues, who reported that T cell activation induced by strong, but not weak or partial agonists, does occur without CD8 co-activation (52). In fact, our results with APL S4S6 may suggest that the agonist potential of peptide mutants relates to the extent of binding by TCR and CD8α, a hypothesis that should be tested for multiple partial agonists.

Taken together, we have studied a novel panel of APLs in the context of TCR-engineered T cells and identified $gp100_{280-288}$ APLs that act either as full agonists, a null ligand, or a partial agonist. In addition, our findings dissected T cell cytotoxicity from T cell cytokine production and NFAT activation and revealed that early T cell responses may require less peptide-MHC when compared to late T cell responses. Notably, our data suggest that partial agonists show a decreased binding by TCR and an enhanced dependency on CD8α, which may represent a novel mechanism behind the properties of partial agonists. Building on the current report, further design and testing of additional APLs may be necessary to advance the therapeutic application of APLs.

ACKNOWLEDGMENTS

This work was supported by a Dutch Cancer Society grant (DDHK 1996-1253). We thank Dr. J. W. Drijfhout for peptide synthesis and Mrs. C. Groot-van Ruijven for her technical assistance.

REFERENCES

1. Coccoris M, Straetemans T, Govers C, Lamers C, Sleijfer S, Debets R. T cell receptor (TCR) gene therapy to treat melanoma: lessons from clinical and preclinical studies. *Expert Opin Biol Ther* (2010) **10**:547–62. doi:10.1517/14712591003614756
2. Rosenberg SA. Raising the bar: the curative potential of human cancer immunotherapy. *Sci Transl Med* (2012) **4**:127s8. doi:10.1126/scitranslmed.3003634
3. Johnson LA, Morgan RA, Dudley ME, Cassard L, Yang JC, Hughes MS, et al. Gene therapy with human and mouse T cell receptors mediates cancer regression and targets normal tissues expressing cognate antigen. *Blood* (2009) **114**:535–46. doi:10.1182/blood-2009-03-211714
4. Robbins PF, Morgan RA, Feldman SA, Yang JC, Sherry RM, Dudley ME, et al. Tumor regression in patients with metastatic synovial cell sarcoma and melanoma using genetically engineered lymphocytes reactive with NY-ESO-1. *J Clin Oncol* (2011) **29**:917–24. doi:10.1200/JCO.2010.32.2537
5. Morgan RA, Dudley ME, Yu YY, Zheng Z, Robbins PF, Theoret MR, et al. High efficiency TCR gene transfer into primary human lymphocytes affords avid recognition of melanoma tumor antigen glycoprotein 100 and does not alter the recognition of autologous melanoma antigens. *J Immunol* (2003) **171**:3287–95.
6. Rubinstein MP, Kadima AN, Salem ML, Nguyen CL, Gillanders WE, Nishimura MI, et al. Transfer of TCR genes into mature T cells is accompanied by the maintenance of parental T cell avidity. *J Immunol* (2003) **170**:1209–17.
7. Schaft N, Willemsen RA, de Vries J, Lankiewicz B, Essers BW, Gratama JW, et al. Peptide fine specificity of anti-glycoprotein 100 CTL is preserved following transfer of engineered TCR alpha beta genes into primary human T lymphocytes. *J Immunol* (2003) **170**:2186–94.
8. Kersh GJ, Allen PM. Essential flexibility in the T cell recognition of antigen. *Nature* (1996) **380**:495–8. doi:10.1038/380495a0
9. Sloan-Lancaster J, Allen PM. Altered peptide ligand-induced partial T cell activation: molecular mechanisms and role in T cell biology. *Annu Rev Immunol* (1996) **14**:1–27. doi:10.1146/annurev.immunol.14.1.1
10. Katsara M, Minigo G, Plebanski M, Apostolopoulos V. The good, the bad and the ugly: how altered peptide ligands modulate immunity. *Expert Opin Biol Ther* (2008) **8**:1873–84. doi:10.1517/14712590802494501

11. Uhlin M, Masucci M, Levitsky V. Is the activity of partially agonistic MHC:peptide ligands dependent on the quality of immunological help? *Scand J Immunol* (2006) **64**:581–7. doi:10.1111/j.1365-3083.2006.01850.x
12. Carrabba MG, Castelli C, Maeurer MJ, Squarcina P, Cova A, Pilla L, et al. Suboptimal activation of CD8(+) T cells by melanoma-derived altered peptide ligands: role of Melan-A/MART-1 optimized analogues. *Cancer Res* (2003) **63**:1560–7.
13. Madrenas J, Germain RN. Variant TCR ligands: new insights into the molecular basis of antigen-dependent signal transduction and T cell activation. *Semin Immunol* (1996) **8**:83–101. doi:10.1006/smim.1996.0011
14. Mitchell MS, Lund TA, Sewell AK, Marincola FM, Paul E, Schroder K, et al. The cytotoxic T cell response to peptide analogs of the HLA-A*0201-restricted MUC1 signal sequence epitope, M1.2. *Cancer Immunol Immunother* (2007) **56**:287–301. doi:10.1007/s00262-006-0191-1
15. Keogh E, Fikes J, Southwood S, Celis E, Chesnut R, Sette A. Identification of new epitopes from four different tumor-associated antigens: recognition of naturally processed epitopes correlates with HLA-A*0201-binding affinity. *J Immunol* (2001) **167**:787–96.
16. Tanaka Y, Amos KD, Joo HG, Eberlein TJ, Goedegebuure PS. Modification of the HER2/NEU-derived tumor antigen GP2 improves induction of GP2-reactive cytotoxic T lymphocytes. *Int J Cancer* (2001) **94**:540–4. doi:10.1002/ijc.1508
17. Mimura K, Kono K, Southwood S, Fikes J, Takahashi A, Miyagawa N, et al. Substitution analog peptide derived from HER-2 can efficiently induce HER-2-specific, HLA-A24 restricted CTLs. *Cancer Immunol Immunother* (2006) **55**:1358–66. doi:10.1007/s00262-006-0123-0
18. Valmori D, Fonteneau JF, Lizana CM, Gervois N, Lienard D, Rimoldi D, et al. Enhanced generation of specific tumor-reactive CTL in vitro by selected Melan-A/MART-1 immunodominant peptide analogues. *J Immunol* (1998) **160**:1750–8.
19. Parkhurst MR, Salgaller ML, Southwood S, Robbins PF, Sette A, Rosenberg SA, et al. Improved induction of melanoma-reactive CTL with peptides from the melanoma antigen gp100 modified at HLA-A*0201-binding residues. *J Immunol* (1996) **157**:2539–48.
20. Tang Y, Lin Z, Ni B, Wei J, Han J, Wang H, et al. An altered peptide ligand for naive cytotoxic T lymphocyte epitope of TRP-2(180-188) enhanced immunogenicity. *Cancer Immunol Immunother* (2007) **56**:319–29. doi:10.1007/s00262-006-0195-x
21. Terasawa H, Tsang KY, Gulley J, Arlen P, Schlom J. Identification and characterization of a human agonist cytotoxic T-lymphocyte epitope of human prostate-specific antigen. *Clin Cancer Res* (2002) **8**:41–53.
22. Chen JL, Dunbar PR, Gileadi U, Jager E, Gnjatic S, Nagata Y, et al. Identification of NY-ESO-1 peptide analogues capable of improved stimulation of tumor-reactive CTL. *J Immunol* (2000) **165**:948–55.
23. Parker KC, Bednarek MA, Hull LK, Utz U, Cunningham B, Zweerink HJ, et al. Sequence motifs important for peptide binding to the human MHC class I molecule, HLA-A2. *J Immunol* (1992) **149**:3580–7.
24. Cole DK, Edwards ES, Wynn KK, Clement M, Miles JJ, Ladell K, et al. Modification of MHC anchor residues generates heteroclitic peptides that alter TCR binding and T cell recognition. *J Immunol* (2010) **185**:2600–10. doi:10.4049/jimmunol.1000629
25. Speiser DE, Baumgaertner P, Voelter V, Devevre E, Barbey C, Rufer N, et al. Unmodified self antigen triggers human CD8 T cells with stronger tumor reactivity than altered antigen. *Proc Natl Acad Sci U S A* (2008) **105**:3849–54. doi:10.1073/pnas.0800080105
26. Lesterhuis WJ, Schreibelt G, Scharenborg NM, Brouwer HM, Gerritsen MJ, Croockewit S, et al. Wild-type and modified gp100 peptide-pulsed dendritic cell vaccination of advanced melanoma patients can lead to long-term clinical responses independent of the peptide used. *Cancer Immunol Immunother* (2011) **60**:249–60. doi:10.1007/s00262-010-0942-x
27. Bakker AB, Schreurs MW, de Boer AJ, Kawakami Y, Rosenberg SA, Adema GJ, et al. Melanocyte lineage-specific antigen gp100 is recognized by melanoma-derived tumor-infiltrating lymphocytes. *J Exp Med* (1994) **179**:1005–9. doi:10.1084/jem.179.3.1005
28. Kawakami Y, Eliyahu S, Delgado CH, Robbins PF, Sakaguchi K, Appella E, et al. Identification of a human melanoma antigen recognized by tumor-infiltrating lymphocytes associated with in vivo tumor rejection. *Proc Natl Acad Sci U S A* (1994) **91**:6458–62. doi:10.1073/pnas.91.14.6458
29. Nijman HW, Houbiers JG, van der Burg SH, Vierboom MP, Kenemans P, Kast WM, et al. Characterization of cytotoxic T lymphocyte epitopes of a self-protein, p53, and a non-self-protein, influenza matrix: relationship between major histocompatibility complex peptide binding affinity and immune responsiveness to peptides. *J Immunother Emphasis Tumor Immunol* (1993) **14**:121–6. doi:10.1097/00002371-199308000-00007
30. van der Burg SH, Ras E, Drijfhout JW, Benckhuijsen WE, Bremers AJ, Melief CJ, et al. An HLA class I peptide-binding assay based on competition for binding to class I molecules on intact human B cells. Identification of conserved HIV-1 polymerase peptides binding to HLA-A*0301. *Hum Immunol* (1995) **44**:189–98. doi:10.1016/0198-8859(95)00105-0
31. Govers C, Berrevoets C, Treffers-Westerlaken E, Broertjes M, Debets R. Magnetic-activated cell sorting of TCR-engineered T cells using tCD34 as a gene marker, but not pMHC multimers, results in significant numbers of functional CD4 and CD8 T cells. *Hum Gene Ther Methods* (2012): doi:10.1089/hgtb.2012.074. [Epub ahead of print].
32. Lamers CH, Willemsen RA, van Elzakker P, van Krimpen BA, Gratama JW, Debets R. Phoenix-ampho outperforms PG13 as retroviral packaging cells to transduce human T cells with tumor-specific receptors: implications for clinical immunogene therapy of cancer. *Cancer Gene Ther* (2006) **13**:503–9. doi:10.1038/sj.cgt.7700916
33. Schaft N, Lankiewicz B, Drexhage J, Berrevoets C, Moss DJ, Levitsky V, et al. T cell re-targeting to EBV antigens following TCR gene transfer: CD28-containing receptors mediate enhanced antigen-specific IFNgamma production. *Int Immunol* (2006) **18**:591–601. doi:10.1093/intimm/dxh401
34. Willemsen RA, Sebestyen Z, Ronteltap C, Berrevoets C, Drexhage J, Debets R. CD8 alpha coreceptor to improve TCR gene transfer to treat melanoma: down-regulation of tumor-specific production of IL-4, IL-5, and IL-10. *J Immunol* (2006) **177**:991–8.
35. Schaft N, Lankiewicz B, Gratama JW, Bolhuis RL, Debets R. Flexible and sensitive method to functionally validate tumor-specific receptors via activation of NFAT. *J Immunol Methods* (2003) **280**:13–24. doi:10.1016/S0022-1759(03)00067-X
36. Weijtens M, Willemsen R, Hart E, Bolhuis R. A retroviral vector system 'STITCH' in combination with an optimized single chain antibody chimeric receptor gene structure allows efficient gene transduction and expression in human T lymphocytes. *Gene Ther* (1998) **5**:1195–203. doi:10.1038/sj.gt.3300696
37. Bakker AB, Marland G, de Boer AJ, Huijbens RJ, Danen EH, Adema GJ, et al. Generation of antimelanoma cytotoxic T lymphocytes from healthy donors after presentation of melanoma-associated antigen-derived epitopes by dendritic cells in vitro. *Cancer Res* (1995) **55**:5330–4.
38. Micheletti F, Canella A, Vertuani S, Marastoni M, Tosi L, Volinia S, et al. Supra-agonist peptides enhance the reactivation of memory CTL responses. *J Immunol* (2000) **165**:4264–71.
39. Bachmann MF, Oxenius A, Speiser DE, Mariathasan S, Hengartner H, Zinkernagel RM, et al. Peptide-induced T cell receptor down-regulation on naive T cells predicts agonist/partial agonist properties and strictly correlates with T cell activation. *Eur J Immunol* (1997) **27**:2195–203. doi:10.1002/eji.1830270912
40. Griffiths GM, Mueller C. Expression of perforin and granzymes in vivo: potential diagnostic markers for activated cytotoxic cells. *Immunol Today* (1991) **12**:415–9. doi:10.1016/0167-5699(91)90145-J
41. Hollsberg P, Weber WE, Dangond F, Batra V, Sette A, Hafler DA. Differential activation of proliferation and cytotoxicity in human T cell lymphotropic virus type I Tax-specific CD8 T cells by an altered peptide ligand. *Proc Natl Acad Sci U S A* (1995) **92**:4036–40. doi:10.1073/pnas.92.9.4036
42. Itoh Y, Hemmer B, Martin R, Germain RN. Serial TCR engagement and down-modulation by peptide:MHC molecule ligands: relationship to the quality of individual TCR signaling events. *J Immunol* (1999) **162**:2073–80.
43. Valitutti S, Muller S, Dessing M, Lanzavecchia A. Different responses are elicited in cytotoxic T lymphocytes by different levels of T cell receptor occupancy. *J Exp Med* (1996) **183**:1917–21. doi:10.1084/jem.183.4.1917

44. Chau LA, Bluestone JA, Madrenas J. Dissociation of intracellular signaling pathways in response to partial agonist ligands of the T cell receptor. *J Exp Med* (1998) **187**:1699–709. doi:10.1084/jem.187.10.1699
45. Hemmer B, Stefanova I, Vergelli M, Germain RN, Martin R. Relationships among TCR ligand potency, thresholds for effector function elicitation, and the quality of early signaling events in human T cells. *J Immunol* (1998) **160**:5807–14.
46. Wei CH, Beeson C, Masucci MG, Levitsky V. A partially agonistic peptide acts as a selective inducer of apoptosis in CD8+ CTLs. *J Immunol* (1999) **163**:2601–9.
47. Kim JR, Irie A, Tsukamoto H, Nishimura Y. A role of kinase inactive ZAP-70 in altered peptide ligand stimulated T cell activation. *Biochem Biophys Res Commun* (2006) **341**:19–27. doi:10.1016/j.bbrc.2005.12.143
48. Madrenas J. Differential signalling by variant ligands of the T cell receptor and the kinetic model of T cell activation. *Life Sci* (1999) **64**:717–31. doi:10.1016/S0024-3205(98)00381-6
49. Krummel MF, Davis MM. Dynamics of the immunological synapse: finding, establishing and solidifying a connection. *Curr Opin Immunol* (2002) **14**:66–74. doi:10.1016/S0952-7915(01)00299-0
50. Abe BT, Macian F. Uncovering the mechanisms that regulate tumor-induced T cell anergy. *Oncoimmunology* (2013) **2**:e22679. doi:10.4161/onci.22679
51. Cole DK, Laugel B, Clement M, Price DA, Wooldridge L, Sewell AK. The molecular determinants of CD8 co-receptor function. *Immunology* (2012) **137**:139–48. doi:10.1111/j.1365-2567.2012.03625.x
52. Laugel B, van den Berg HA, Gostick E, Cole DK, Wooldridge L, Boulter J, et al. Different T cell receptor affinity thresholds and CD8 coreceptor dependence govern cytotoxic T lymphocyte activation and tetramer binding properties. *J Biol Chem* (2007) **282**:23799–810. doi:10.1074/jbc.M700976200

8

Re-directing CD4+ T cell responses with the flanking residues of MHC class II-bound peptides: the core is not enough

Christopher J. Holland[1], **David K. Cole**[1*†] **and Andrew Godkin**[1,2*†]

[1] Institute of Infection and Immunity, Cardiff University School of Medicine, Cardiff, UK
[2] Department of Integrated Medicine, University Hospital of Wales, Cardiff, UK

Edited by:
Bruno Laugel, Cardiff University, UK

Reviewed by:
Balbino Alarcon, Consejo Superior de Investigaciones Cientificas, Spain
Daniel M Altmann, Imperial College, UK

***Correspondence:**
David K. Cole and Andrew Godkin, Cardiff University School of Medicine, The Henry Wellcome Building, Cardiff, CF14 4XN, UK
e-mail: coledk@cf.ac.uk, godkinaj@cardiff.ac.uk

† David K. Cole and Andrew Godkin have contributed equally to this work.

Recombinant αβ T cell receptors, expressed on T cell membranes, recognize short peptides presented at the cell surface in complex with MHC molecules. There are two main subsets of αβ T cells: CD8+ T cells that recognize mainly cytosol-derived peptides in the context of MHC class I (pMHC-I), and CD4+ T cells that recognize peptides usually derived from exogenous proteins presented by MHC class II (pMHC-II). Unlike the more uniform peptide lengths (usually 8–13mers) bound in the MHC-I closed groove, MHC-II presented peptides are of a highly variable length. The bound peptides consist of a core bound 9mer (reflecting the binding motif for the particular MHC-II type) but with variable peptide flanking residues (PFRs) that can extend from both the N- and C-terminus of the MHC-II binding groove. Although pMHC-I and pMHC-II play a virtually identical role during T cell responses (T cell antigen presentation) and are very similar in overall conformation, there exist a number of subtle but important differences that may govern the functional dichotomy observed between CD8+ and CD4+ T cells. Here, we provide an overview of the impact of structural differences between pMHC-I and pMHC-II and the molecular interactions with the T cell receptor including the functional importance of MHC-II PFRs. We consider how factors such as anatomical location, inflammatory milieu, and particular types of antigen presenting cell might, in theory, contribute to the quantitative (i.e., pMHC ligand frequency) as well as qualitative (i.e., variable PFR) nature of peptide epitopes, and hence offer a means of control and influence of a CD4+ T cell response. Lastly, we review our recent findings showing how modifications to MHC-II PFRs can modify CD4+ T cell antigen recognition. These findings may have novel applications for the development of CD4+ T cell peptide vaccines and diagnostics.

Keywords: modified peptide, peptide flanking residue, peptide-major histocompatibility complex class II, T cell receptor, T cell repertoire, vaccine, crystal structure, MHC processing

INTRODUCTION

T cell immunity is mediated primarily by the membrane bound T cell receptor (TCR) that interacts with peptide epitopes presented by major histocompatibility molecules (pMHC) (1). This interaction governs T cell specificity and leads to downstream T cell activation. Classical MHC exists in two forms: MHC class I (MHC-I) and MHC class II (MHC-II), which differ in both their subunit composition and functional expression pattern. MHC-I presents peptides derived mainly from endogenous cytosolic proteins and is expressed upon the cell surface of most nucleated cells allowing cognate CD8+ T cells to scan cells for intracellular infections or abnormal proteins in cancerous cells (2, 3). In contrast, MHC-II is expressed mainly upon antigen presenting cells (APCs) e.g., dendritic cells and macrophages, that patrol the extracellular space, actively endocytosing potentially immunogenic proteins that are proteolysed and complexed with MHC-II (pMHC-II). Activated APCs enter the lymphatic system and travel to secondary lymphoid nodes allowing naive CD4+ T cells to interrogate cell surface expressed pMHC-II enabling CD4+ T cell activation and initiation of immune responses (3–5).

PEPTIDES PRESENTED BY MHC-I AND MHC-II HAVE DISTINCT STRUCTURAL CHARACTERISTICS

In spite of the differing subunit compositions of the two MHC classes, they are structurally very similar (**Figures 1A,B**). The peptide binding groove, in both cases, is comprised of two anti-parallel α-helices that form a channel in which the peptide can bind in an extended conformation, and eight anti-parallel β-sheets that provide specific peptide binding pockets in the base of the groove (**Figures 1C,D**) (3, 6). Peptides are selected according to their ability to bind to these MHC allele specific pockets within the floor of the peptide binding groove using peptide anchor residues. All of the currently available structural data suggest the TCRs bind to both pMHC-I and II with a fixed polarity (TCRα chain over the N-terminus of the peptide and the TCRβ chain over the C-terminus) and make similar interactions with the bound peptide and MHC surface (**Figures 1E,F**). Thus, the overall mechanism by which TCRs interact with MHC-I and II to initiate T cell activation is closely matched.

Despite these similarities, MHC-I and II present peptides in a distinct manner that is governed by the composition of the

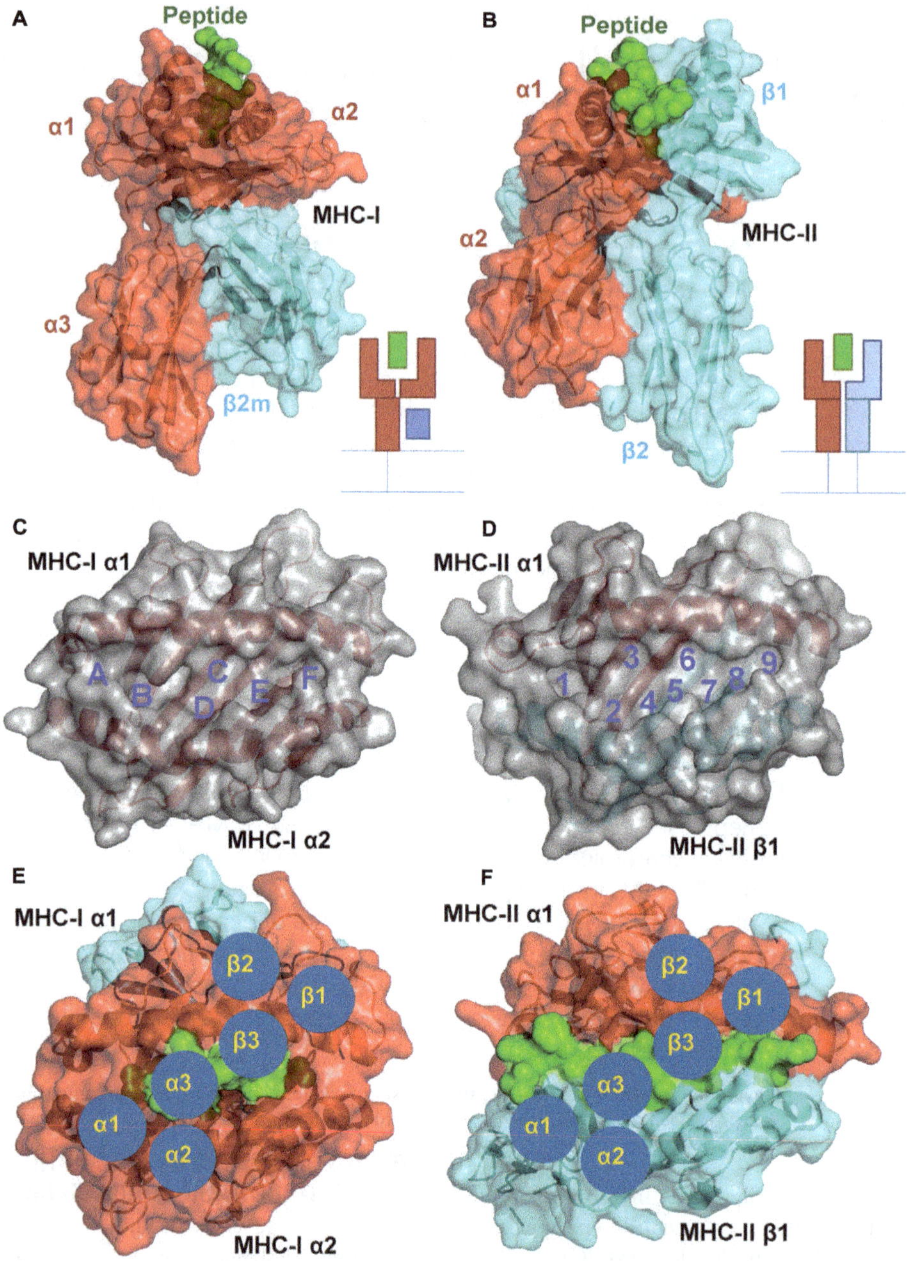

FIGURE 1 | A structural comparison of pMHC-I and pMHC-II. Although the subunit compositions of MHC-I (PDB: 1ZHL) **(A)** and MHC-II (PDB: 1KG0) **(B)** are different, the structural conformation they assume is very similar, illustrating their shared role in presenting antigenic peptides (green) to T cells. **(A)** MHC-I is comprised of three α-chain domains (1, 2, and 3 in red) and β2m (cyan), whereas **(B)** MHC-II is comprised of a two domain α-chain (red) and a two domain β-chain (cyan). A top down view of the MHC-I **(C)** and MHC-II **(D)** demonstrates the two molecules form similar peptide binding grooves comprised of two anti-parallel α-helices that form a channel in which the peptide can bind in an extended conformation, and eight anti-parallel β-sheets that provide specific peptide binding pockets in the base of the groove. These pockets are lined with polymorphic residues that define the size and chemical characteristics of each pocket, and therefore the specific peptide binding motif and register that can be accommodated by different MHC alleles. TCR binding to pMHC-I **(E)** and pMHC-II **(F)** is also conserved. The three complementarity determining loops (CDRs) of the TCR (blue circles) bind in a very similar overall orientation with the TCR α-chain over the N-terminus of the peptide and the TCR β-chain over the C-terminus

MHC peptide binding groove. The closed conformation of the MHC-I $\alpha_1\alpha_2$ binding grove (**Figure 2A**) restricts peptide length to ~8–13 amino acids (most commonly 9 or 10mers) (3, 7). In contrast, the MHC-II $\alpha_1\beta_1$ binding groove comprises an *open-ended* conformation (**Figure 2B**) that allows variable length peptides to bind. The core binding 9mer contains the motif for binding to the particular MHC-II heterodimer, but eluted and sequenced peptides often reveal families of processed peptides ~12–20 amino

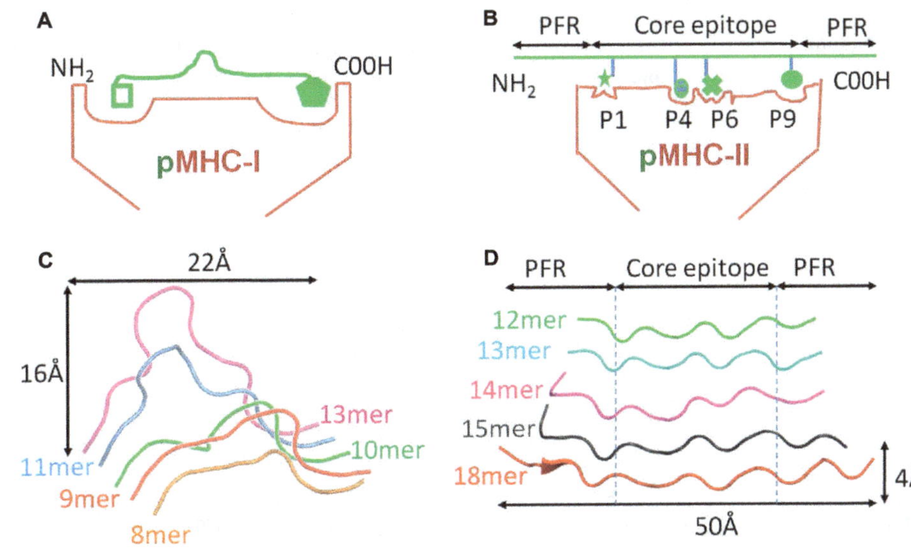

FIGURE 2 | Comparison of peptide conformations presented by MHC-I and MHC-II. Cartoon cross sections of the pMHC-I **(A)** and pMHC-II **(B)** binding grooves, show the key anchor sites in the floor of each groove determine which peptide can associate and the conformation it can assume. **(C)** The structural database of pMHC-I complexes shows that peptides presented by a MHC-I molecules (represented as ribbon cartoons) generally assume a central bulged conformation. As peptide length increases, the "closed" nature of the pMHC-I binding groove forces the central residues of the peptide up out of the groove to accommodate the extra residues. **(D)** In contrast, the pMHC-II binding groove is "open" enabling longer peptide to extend out of the groove at form peptide flanking regions. Thus, peptides presented by MHC-II molecules (represented as ribbon cartoons) generally assume a much flatter conformation in the MHC-II binding groove, irrespective of the length of the peptide presented.

acids (referred to as nested sets) sharing the core binding region (3, 8, 9). MHC-I-restricted peptides usually bind to the MHC surface using anchor residues located at, or near, the N- and C-termini of the peptide. Depending on the length of the peptide, this binding mode squeezes the central peptide residues up so that they extend out the groove (central bulge), exposing peptide side chains for direct interaction with the TCR (3, 10). Longer MHC-I peptides can only be accommodated by forming a larger central bulge, which presumably constrains the length of the peptide beyond a certain threshold (**Figure 2C**; **Table 1**).

MHC-II restricted peptides contain a central binding motif of nine "core" amino acids that bind to the MHC-II groove via an extensive hydrogen bond network between the MHC-II groove and the peptide backbone (**Figure 2B**). Peptide side chains also form contacts with allelic specific pockets of the MHC-II binding groove. These pockets, usually P1, P4, P6, and P9, are lined with polymorphic residues that define the size and chemical characteristics of each pocket, and therefore the specific peptide binding motif and register that can be accommodated by different MHC-II alleles (**Figure 1D**) (11, 12). Amino acids that are outside of the "core" peptide region can extend out of the open MHC-II binding groove forming so called "peptide flanking regions" (PFRs) at both the N- and C-terminus (**Figure 2D**; **Table 1**). Thus, although pMHC-I and pMHC-II are similar in their overall structure and function, the nature of peptide presentation is generally distinct (e.g., bulged versus flat peptides). These differences present different challenges for TCR binding at the atomic level. For example, the flat binding surface and lack of a central peptide bulge may enable MHC-II restricted TCRs to adopt a more flexible binding mode compared to MHC-I restricted TCRs. In support of this notion, the structures of a number of TCR-MHC-II complexes have shown that, although the binding mode can be very similar to the classical diagonal TCR-MHC binding mode (13–17), some MHC-II restricted TCR bind with highly unorthodox conformations (18, 19).

MHC-II RESTRICTED TCRS HAVE WEAKER BINDING AFFINITY COMPARED TO PMHC-I RESTRICTED TCRs

Biophysical studies have shown that TCR/pMHC affinity is relatively weak ($K_D = 100$ nM–270 μM), with fast kinetics, compared to antibody binding (usually nM–pM affinity) (20, 21). We have recently shown that TCR/pMHC-I binding affinities are, on average, fives times stronger compared to equivalent TCR/pMHC-II interactions (i.e., viral pMHC-I restricted TCRs versus viral pMHC-II restricted TCRs) (**Figures 3A,B**), which has limited the usefulness of pMHC-II multimers for the identification, isolation and detection of antigen specific $CD4^+$ T cells. This distinction in affinity was mainly due to a significantly faster on-rate for TCR/pMHC-I binding compared to that of TCR/pMHC-II, while the off-rate or half-lives of all of the TCR/pMHC interactions were relatively conserved, possibly indicating a more important role for off-rate in determining T cell activation. The consistent difference in binding affinity between TCRs restricted to either pMHC-I or pMHC-II is extraordinary when considering that the same pools of genes, on chromosome 9, encode the human TCR for both types of αβ T cell (22). The TCR itself is expressed before positive selection, at which point immature T cells express both the CD4 and CD8 co-receptors (double positive). Once positively selected, immature thymocytes become single positive for either CD4 or CD8 (22). Until this point, the thymocyte, which has

Table 1 | Comparison of peptide conformations presented by MHC-I and MHC-II.

MHC	Protein	Peptide length (mer)	Peptide Sequence	Height (Å)	Width (Å)	PDB (Ref)
HLA-B*3501	HIV-1 NEF_{75-82}	8	VPLRPMTY	4	21	1A1N (56)
HLA-A*0201	Flu A $Matrix_{58-66}$	9	GILGFVFTL	6	22	1HHI (57)
HLA-A*0201	MART-1_{26-35}	10	EAAGIGILTV	8	22	2GT9 (58)
HLA-B*3501	$EBV_{407-417}$	11	HPVGEADYFEY	13	22	2FZ3 (59)
HLA-B*3501	M-CSF_{4-17}	14	LPAVVGLSPGEQEY	16	22	1XH3 (60)
DRB1*0401, DRA1*0101	Collagen II $_{261-273}$	12	AYMRADAAAGGA	4	35	2SEB (61)
DRB1*0101, DRA1*0101	$HA_{306-318}$	13	PKYVKQNTLKLAT	4	37	1DLH (12)
DRB1*1501, DRA1*0101	MBP_{85-99}	14	ENPVVHFFKNIVTP	4	42	1BX2 (62)
DRB1*0101, DRA1*0101	MART-$1_{100-114}$	15	APPAYEKLSAEQSPP	4	44	3L6F (63)
DRB1*0101, DRA1*0101	$CLIP_{102-120}$	19	KPVSKMRMATPLLMQALPM	4	50	3PDO (64)

already developed antigen specificity through its TCR, can theoretically have either cell fate (23). Considering these shared genetic and developmental processes, it is possible that the differences in MHC restricted TCR binding is conferred by the variations in the "antigenic landscape" of pMHC-I versus pMHC-II.

As discussed above, peptides presented by MHC-I molecules generally assume a central bulged conformation, often requiring conformational adjustments in the binding regions of the TCR during ligand engagement (**Figure 2C**) (24–26). An extreme example of this observation is a 13mer Epstein-Barr virus derived peptide presented by HLA-B*3508 which forms a "superbulge" extending nearly 20Å out of the MHC-I binding groove (26). In contrast, MHC-II presented peptides generally assume a much flatter conformation in the MHC-II binding groove (13, 14) (**Figure 2D**). The presence of a solvent exposed central bulge for MHC-I peptide presentation may represent a structurally advantageous feature for TCR binding, providing an anchor point that can guide the TCR into the correct binding orientation to engage its cognate ligand (**Figure 3A**). Conversely, the flat, and relatively featureless surface of pMHC-II confers no dominant structural feature for the TCR to "latch" onto, and may reduce the chance of a productive TCR/pMHC-II interaction occurring (explaining the slower on-rate and weaker affinity compared to TCR/pMHC-I interactions) (**Figure 3B**). This notion is consistent with our recent observation that a MHC-II restricted TCR underwent minimal conformational adjustments during binding compared to most MHC-I restricted TCRs (27). The immunological significance of these topological and biophysical distinctions between MHC-I and MHC-II is still unclear. However, the difference in binding affinity between MHC restricted TCRs may represent a biophysical characteristic that relates to cellular function.

MHC-II ANTIGEN PROCESSING GENERATES VARIABLE LENGTH PEPTIDES

The "flat" surface of pMHC-II may contribute to the reduced affinity of MHC-II restricted TCRs. However, a striking difference in the peptides bound to MHC-II is the presence of non-bound PFRs, which may be available to interact with adjacent membrane proteins on the same or different cells. These PFRs can vary in length generating nested sets of peptides that are presented on the surface of APCs (28, 29). One consequence of having a longer PFR is an increased binding affinity of peptides to the MHC-II (30–33), and therefore an increased probability of a meaningful interaction with a cognate T cell.

These variable PFRs are generated by proteolytic processes during the exogenous antigen processing pathway that has been reviewed in detail elsewhere (34, 35). Briefly, extracellular protein antigens are endocytosed by tissue resident APCs (**Figure 4A**). The pH of the endosome containing potential antigens progressively decreases, activating proteases which cleave captured proteins (**Figure 4B**). Newly synthesized MHC-II molecules reside in the endoplasmic reticulum (ER) in complex with a stabilizing chaperon, calnexin. To prevent premature peptide association with the MHC-II binding groove by ER derived proteins, the groove is "plugged" with a protein known as the MHC-II associated invariant chain (I_i) (36) (**Figure 4C**). Exocytic vesicles containing precursor Ii:MHC-II complexes then combine with endosomes containing exogenous peptide fragments forming the MHC-II compartment (**Figure 4D**). The acidic pH of the MHC-II compartment and presence of the chaperon, HLA-DM (37), allows peptide exchange between the class II-associated invariant-chain peptide (CLIP) and high affinity complementary peptides proteolysed in the endosomal compartment. Peptide selection, that presumably plays a strong role in determining the characteristics of PFRs, is also facilitated by HLA-DM in a process termed "peptide-editing" which ensures that only stable MHC-II peptide complexes are expressed and transported to the cell surface for potential TCR interactions (38, 39) (**Figure 4E**). Structural modeling of HLA-DM association with pMHC-II indicated that peptide editing was achieved through conformational changes around pocket 1 (P1) of the binding groove, a pocket crucial for the stability of the peptide-MHC-II complex (40). Such conformational changes induced by HLA-DM were thought to weaken the hydrogen bond network between the bound peptide and MHC-II molecule and facilitate peptide release (41). A recent co-complex structure of HLA-DM with HLA-DRα*0101; β*0101 (HLA-DR1) has confirmed this experimentally, revealing that HLA-DM binding induced a conformational change in the α-helix of the DRα chain in the peptide binding groove (42). This change enabled two HLA-DR1 residues, DRα phenylalanine 51 and DRβ phenylalanine 89, to

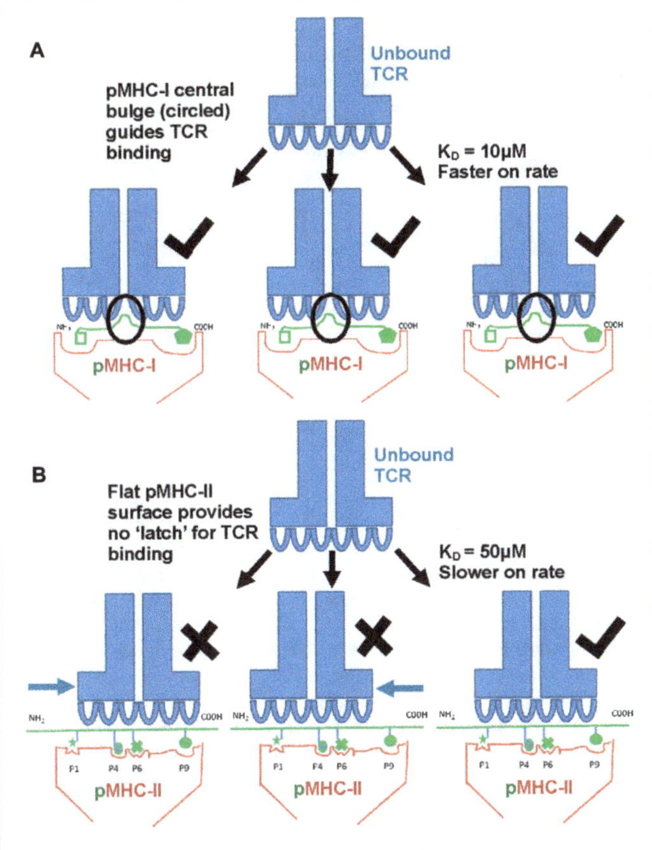

FIGURE 3 | TCRs bind with stronger affinity to pMHC-I compared to pMHC-II. Biophysical studies have shown that TCR/pMHC-I binding affinities are, on average, five times stronger compared to equivalent TCR/pMHC-II interactions (i.e., viral pMHC-I restricted TCRs versus viral pMHC-II restricted TCRs) because of faster on-rate for TCR/pMHC-I binding compared to that of TCR/pMHC-II. These differences could be due to the structural differences in peptide presentation between MHC-I and MHC-II. **(A)** Cartoon of TCR binding to pMHC-I. The presence of a solvent exposed central bulge for MHC-I peptide presentation may represent a structurally advantageous feature for TCR binding, providing an anchor point that can guide the TCR into the correct binding orientation to engage its cognate ligand. **(B)** Cartoon of TCR binding to the flatter surface of pMHC-II. This relatively featureless surface provides no dominant structural feature for the TCR to "latch" onto, and may reduce the chance of a productive TCR/pMHC-II interaction occurring (explaining the slower on-rate and weaker affinity compared to TCR/pMHC-I interactions).

bind to, and stabilize, the P1 binding pocket of the MHC-II binding groove, presumably blocking the association of weakly binding peptides. Thus, only the association of high affinity peptides with MHC-II results in displacement of these residues, enabling a revision in the conformation of MHC-II and the dissociation of HLA-DM (40, 42).

It is possible that the proteolytic events that occur before peptide-MHC-II loading govern the final pool of peptides available for selection during MHC-II peptide loading. However, it has also been suggested that the final pMHC-II, loaded with exogenous peptide, can be modified further in a process termed peptide trimming, whereby the length of the PFRs can be edited (**Figure 4F**) (43, 44). These processes demonstrate a remarkable degree of complexity and control during MHC-II peptide selection that is still not fully understood. The antigen processing by cellular proteases and the generation of pMHC-II may also be influenced by cell extrinsic factors such as inflammatory cytokines, e.g., IFNs (45), as well as cell intrinsic factors reflecting the type/subtype of APC (46, 47). The cellular machinery involved in antigen processing and presentation is different between cell types (48), hence the determinants resulting from protein digestion may vary depending on cell type or subtype (e.g., B cell versus macrophage; $CD8^+$ versus $CD8^-$ dendritic cells etc); and context (e.g., inflamed versus non-inflamed tissues, anatomical location). It is conceivable that a range of determinants presented in a lymph node may differ from those presented at the primary site of infection in both a quantitative fashion, i.e., the number of pMHC-II complexes per cell, and qualitative fashion i.e., length and type of PFRs and hence offer a local control of $CD4^+$ T cell responses accordingly.

MODULATING $CD4^+$ T CELL RESPONSES VIA ALTERED PEPTIDE FLANKING RESIDUES

There is convincing evidence that PFRs can modulate T cell function (49). A study of a HIV-I p24 (GAG) epitope, presented by HLA-DR1, revealed that antigen specific T cell activation was enhanced with longer flanking residues. Structural analyzes showed that the C-terminal flank could form a hairpin turn, raising the possibility that MHC-II PFRs may form more complex conformations that could directly impinge on TCR binding (50). Thus, the open ended nature of the MHC-II binding groove, that allows long peptides to extend beyond the binding region at both the N- and C-terminus (**Figures 2** and **3**), may play a direct role during T cell antigen recognition. In support of this notion, it has been demonstrated that removal of C-terminus PFRs from the immunodominant epitope in hen egg $lysosome_{52–61}$ (HEL) significantly altered the immunogenicity of the epitope, reducing T cell sensitivity (9).

Our previous work, using sequence analysis of eluted peptide ligands from a range of allelic variants of MHC-II molecules, has identified allele-transcending enrichments in PFRs at the peptide C- and N-terminus (51, 52). These data show that a range of different modifications to PFRs could modulate specific $CD4^+$ T cell responses including amino acids with biochemically distinct side chains (52, 53). The identification of these PFR amino acid enrichment patterns suggests that they play a role during $CD4^+$ T cell activation and can modulate antigen recognition. Further studies using antigen specific $CD4^+$ T cell clones demonstrated that PFR modifications could enhance $CD4^+$ T cell activation (53). Although a wide range of different amino acid substitutions in PFRs could generate stronger $CD4^+$ T cell responses, we observed that basic residues at the peptide C-terminus, or acidic residues in the N-terminus, were most commonly enriched and generated enhanced $CD4^+$ T cell responses across different MHC-II alleles and different peptides. Studies focusing on the C-terminal PFRs, in which the basic amino acid, arginine was substituted into the C-terminal flank (at position 10 or 11) of known T cell epitopes from haemagglutinin (HA) and myelin basic protein (MBP), demonstrated that these alterations led to a significant increase in $CD4^+$ T cell responses (52, 53). Screening T cells which recognized

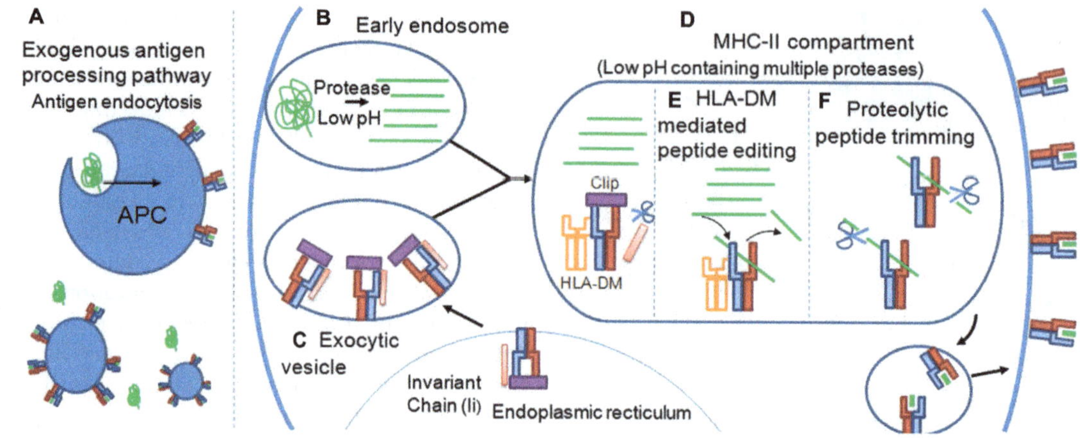

FIGURE 4 | Peptide flanking regions are determined during the MHC-II antigen processing pathway. (A) Extracellular protein antigens are endocytosed by tissue resident APCs. **(B)** The pH of the endosome containing potential antigens progressively decreases, activating proteases which cleave captured proteins. **(C)** Newly synthesized MHC-II molecules reside in the endoplasmic reticulum (ER) in complex with the MHC-II associated invariant chain (I_i), which "plugs" the MHC-II binding groove, preventing ER derived peptides from premature peptide association. **(D)** Exocytic vesicles containing precursor Ii:MHC-II complexes then combine with endosomes containing exogenous peptide fragments forming the MHC-II compartment. Formation of the MHC-II compartment results in proteolytic cleavage of the I_i chain leaving a 24 amino acid remnant called the class II-associated invariant-chain peptide (CLIP) within the binding groove of the MHC-II molecule. The acidic pH of the MHC-II compartment and presence of the chaperon, HLA-DM, allows peptide exchange between CLIP and high affinity complementary peptides proteolysed in the endosomal compartment. **(E)** Peptide selection, that presumably plays a strong role in determining the characteristics of PFRs, is also facilitated by HLA-DM in a process termed "peptide-editing" which ensures that only stable MHC-II peptide complexes are expressed and transported to the cell surface for potential TCR interactions. **(F)** The final pMHC-II, loaded with exogenous peptide, can also be modified further in a process termed peptide trimming that may play a role in governing PFR length. pMHC-II molecules are then transported to the cell surface for interrogation by CD4+ T cells.

this same MBP-derived epitope with a combinatorial library also revealed a preference for C-terminal basic residues (54).

However, in all of these examples, the mechanism for the effect of PFRs on T cell responsiveness had remained elusive. Two possibilities can be considered. Firstly, PFR modifications may alter the stability of pMHC-II molecules (a notion that has been experimentally observed (30–33), altering their expression levels at the surface of APCs. However, we have demonstrated that, although the substitution of basic residues in the C-terminus increased T cell activation, they actually reduced peptide/MHC binding (52). Secondly, if the TCR can directly contact the PFRs, then modifications in the PFR could alter TCR binding affinity and subsequent T cell activation. In order to investigate the second possibility, we conducted biophysical experiments by surface plasmon resonance using cloned TCRs specific for an influenza epitope ($HA_{305–320}$) presented by HLA-DR1 (53). The substitution of arginine into either position 10 (HA_{10R}) or 11 (HA_{11R}) of $HA_{306–318}$ generated approximately twofold increase in TCR binding affinity (**Figures 5A,B**). Intriguingly, analysis of the TCR clonotypic repertoire of peptide-expanded influenza-specific $CD4^+$ T cells from HLA-$DR1^+$ donors in response to $HA_{305-320}$ or arginine altered variants (HA_{10R} and HA_{11R}) demonstrated a marked alteration in TCR usage, with a striking focusing of the response when using the peptides which are known to increase TCR binding i.e., number of clonotypes for $HA > HA_{10R} > HA_{11R}$. The structure of DR1-$HA_{306–318}$ in complex with the MHC-II restricted TCR, HA1.7, has been solved by X-ray crystallography (55). This structure demonstrated that the TCR could not directly contact the short side chains of either Alanine at P10, or Threonine at P11 in the universal $HA_{306–318}$ epitope (**Figure 5C**). The closest proximity between the TCR and either P10 or P11 of the $HA_{306–318}$ peptide was over 8Å, which was beyond the limits for atomic contacts. However, structural modeling of the substitution of arginine, which has a long acidic side chain, at either P10 or P11 indicated this gap could be closed allowing additional interactions to form between the peptide and the TCR (**Figure 5D**) (53). These potential new contacts could offer an explanation for the stronger binding affinity between the HA1.7 TCR and the P10 or P11 substituted DR1-$HA_{306–318}$ epitope.

CONCLUSION

The function of classical MHC molecules is presentation of peptide epitopes to the cell mediated arm of adaptive immune response. However, the subtle differences that exist between the two classical forms of MHC, with respect to antigen processing and structural architecture, significantly alters the nature of the peptide each class of MHC can present upon the cell surface. In particular, the closed binding groove of MHC-I forces bound peptides to bulge in the center, compared to the open binding groove of MHC-II that allow PFRs to form. *In vitro* experiments using a variety of antigens in mice and human systems, including HA, GAG, MBP, and HEL, have demonstrated that the PFRs of an epitope can profoundly affect $CD4^+$ T cell function. Generation and selection of different PFRs might be governed according to the anatomical location, inflammatory milieu and particular types of APC involved during antigen processing. Thus, a key question that remains is whether particular changes in PFRs occur through a random, stochastic process, or whether changes are purposefully

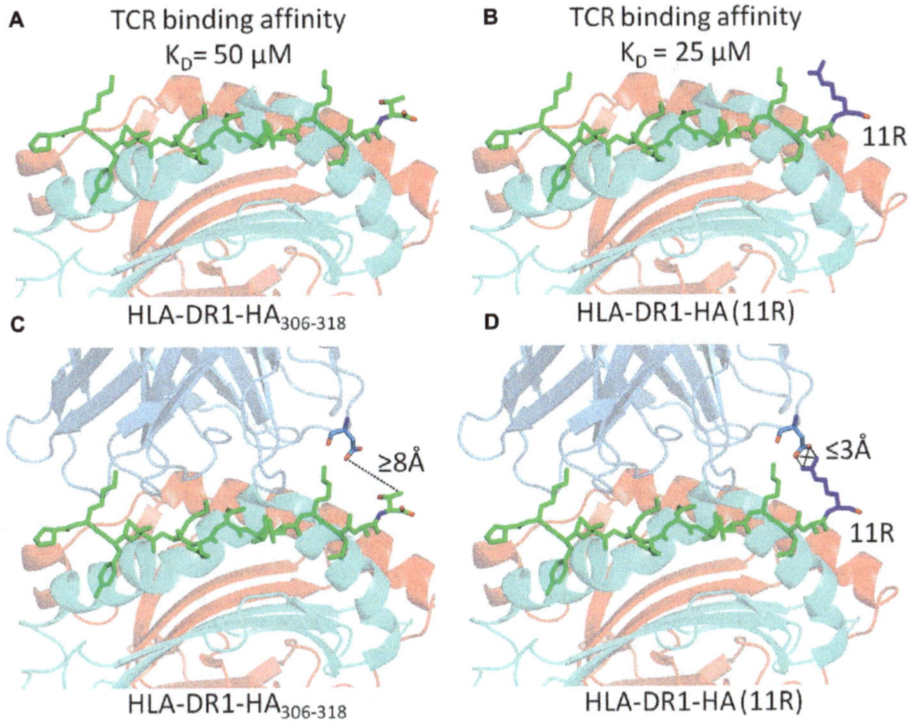

FIGURE 5 | Substitution of Arginine substitutions in the C-terminal flanking region of the native Flu1 peptide increases binding affinity. **(A,B)** Substitution of arginine at position 11 (blue) in the $HA_{305-320}$ epitope generates around a twofold increase in TCR binding affinity. **(C,D)** Cartoon representation of the interaction between the TCR and C-terminal PFR (modeled from PDB: 1FYT). **(C)** The TCR β-chain is beyond the limits for atomic contacts with $HA_{305-320}$ P11 (dotted line). **(D)** Modeling shows that a new interaction, possibly a salt bridge, could be formed between the TCR β-chain and arginine (blue) substituted at position 11 of the $HA_{305-320}$ peptide. This new interaction could explain the increase in affinity observed for cognate TCR binding to the $HA_{305-320}$ peptide and HA_{11R}.

intentioned to control or alter the nature of a specific immune response. Irrespective of the answer to this question, our recent data revealed that experimental PFR modifications could enhance TCR/pMHC-II affinities closer to the range typically observed for TCR/pMHC-I interactions. This exciting observation suggests that augmentation of pMHC-II antigens through C-terminal PFR modifications might be a useful strategy to enhance MHC-II restricted TCR binding affinity and $CD4^+$ T cell responsiveness, with attendant implications for vaccination and other immune system interventions.

ACKNOWLEDGMENTS

David K. Cole is a Wellcome Trust Research Career Development Fellow (WT095767).

REFERENCES

1. Katz DR. Antigen presentation, antigen-presenting cells and antigen processing. *Curr Opin Immunol* (1988) **1**:213–9. doi:10.1016/0952-7915(88)90004-0
2. Kumar V, Mcnerney ME. A new self: MHC-class-I-independent natural-killer-cell self-tolerance. *Nat Rev Immunol* (2005) **5**:363–74. doi:10.1038/nri1603
3. Rudolph MG, Stanfield RL, Wilson IA. How TCRs bind MHCs, peptides, and coreceptors. *Annu Rev Immunol* (2006) **24**:419–66. doi:10.1146/annurev.immunol.23.021704.115658
4. Garcia KC, Degano M, Speir JA, Wilson IA. Emerging principles for T cell receptor recognition of antigen in cellular immunity. *Rev Immunogenet* (1999) **1**:75–90.
5. Castellino F, Germain RN. Cooperation between CD4+ and CD8+ T cells: when, where, and how. *Annu Rev Immunol* (2006) **24**:519–40. doi:10.1146/annurev.immunol.23.021704.115825
6. Van Der Merwe PA, Davis SJ. Molecular interactions mediating T cell antigen recognition. *Annu Rev Immunol* (2003) **21**:659–84. doi:10.1146/annurev.immunol.21.120601.141036
7. Rammensee HG. Chemistry of peptides associated with MHC class I and class II molecules. *Curr Opin Immunol* (1995) **7**:85–96. doi:10.1016/0952-7915(95)80033-6
8. Altman JD, Moss PA, Goulder PJ, Barouch DH, Mcheyzer-Williams MG, Bell JI, et al. Phenotypic analysis of antigen-specific T lymphocytes. *Science* (1996) **274**:94–6. doi:10.1126/science.274.5284.94
9. Carson RT, Vignali KM, Woodland DL, Vignali DA. T cell receptor recognition of MHC class II-bound peptide flanking residues enhances immunogenicity and results in altered TCR V region usage. *Immunity* (1997) **7**:387–99. doi:10.1016/S1074-7613(00)80360-X
10. Rudolph MG, Luz JG, Wilson IA. Structural and thermodynamic correlates of T cell signaling. *Annu Rev Biophys Biomol Struct* (2002) **31**:121–49. doi:10.1146/annurev.biophys.31.082901.134423
11. Brown JH, Jardetzky TS, Gorga JC, Stern LJ, Urban RG, Strominger JL, et al. Three-dimensional structure of the human class II histocompatibility antigen HLA-DR1. *Nature* (1993) **364**:33–9. doi:10.1038/364033a0

12. Stern LJ, Brown JH, Jardetzky TS, Gorga JC, Urban RG, Strominger JL, et al. Crystal structure of the human class II MHC protein HLA-DR1 complexed with an influenza virus peptide. *Nature* (1994) **368**:215–21. doi:10.1038/368215a0
13. Hennecke J, Carfi A, Wiley DC. Structure of a covalently stabilized complex of a human alphabeta T-cell receptor, influenza HA peptide and MHC class II molecule, HLA-DR1. *EMBO J* (2000) **19**:5611–24. doi:10.1093/emboj/19.21.5611
14. Hennecke J, Wiley DC. Structure of a complex of the human alpha/beta T cell receptor (TCR) HA1.7, influenza hemagglutinin peptide, and major histocompatibility complex class II molecule, HLA-DR4 (DRA*0101 and DRB1*0401): insight into TCR cross-restriction and alloreactivity. *J Exp Med* (2002) **195**:571–81. doi:10.1084/jem.20011194
15. Li Y, Huang Y, Lue J, Quandt JA, Martin R, Mariuzza RA. Structure of a human autoimmune TCR bound to a myelin basic protein self-peptide and a multiple sclerosis-associated MHC class II molecule. *EMBO J* (2005) **24**:2968–79. doi:10.1038/sj.emboj.7600771
16. Deng L, Langley RJ, Brown PH, Xu G, Teng L, Wang Q, et al. Structural basis for the recognition of mutant self by a tumor-specific, MHC class II-restricted T cell receptor. *Nat Immunol* (2007) **8**:398–408. doi:10.1038/ni1447
17. Yin Y, Li Y, Kerzic MC, Martin R, Mariuzza RA. Structure of a TCR with high affinity for self-antigen reveals basis for escape from negative selection. *EMBO J* (2011) **30**:1137–48. doi:10.1038/emboj.2011.21
18. Hahn M, Nicholson MJ, Pyrdol J, Wucherpfennig KW. Unconventional topology of self peptide-major histocompatibility complex binding by a human autoimmune T cell receptor. *Nat Immunol* (2005) **6**:490–6. doi:10.1038/ni1187
19. Sethi DK, Schubert DA, Anders AK, Heroux A, Bonsor DA, Thomas CP, et al. A highly tilted binding mode by a self-reactive T cell receptor results in altered engagement of peptide and MHC. *J Exp Med* (2011) **208**:91–102. doi:10.1084/jem.20100725
20. Cole DK, Pumphrey NJ, Boulter JM, Sami M, Bell JI, Gostick E, et al. Human TCR-binding affinity is governed by MHC class restriction. *J Immunol* (2007) **178**:5727–34.
21. Bridgeman JS, Sewell AK, Miles JJ, Price DA, Cole DK. Structural and biophysical determinants of alphabeta T-cell antigen recognition. *Immunology* (2012) **135**:9–18. doi:10.1111/j.1365-2567.2011.03515.x
22. Sebzda E, Mariathasan S, Ohteki T, Jones R, Bachmann MF, Ohashi PS. Selection of the T cell repertoire. *Annu Rev Immunol* (1999) **17**:829–74. doi:10.1146/annurev.immunol.17.1.829
23. Jameson SC, Hogquist KA, Bevan MJ. Positive selection of thymocytes. *Annu Rev Immunol* (1995) **13**:93–126. doi:10.1146/annurev.iy.13.040195.000521
24. Miles JJ, El-Hassen D, Borg NA, Silins SL, Tynan FE, Burrows JM, et al. CTL recognition of a bulged viral peptide involves biased TCR selection. *J Immunol* (2005) **175**:3826–34.
25. Tynan FE, Borg NA, Miles JJ, Beddoe T, El-Hassen D, Silins SL, et al. High resolution structures of highly bulged viral epitopes bound to major histocompatibility complex class I. Implications for T-cell receptor engagement and T-cell immunodominance. *J Biol Chem* (2005) **280**:23900–9. doi:10.1074/jbc.M503060200
26. Tynan FE, Reid HH, Kjer-Nielsen L, Miles JJ, Wilce MC, Kostenko L, et al. A T cell receptor flattens a bulged antigenic peptide presented by a major histocompatibility complex class I molecule. *Nat Immunol* (2007) **8**:268–76. doi:10.1038/ni1432
27. Holland CJ, Rizkallah PJ, Vollers S, Calvo-Calle JM, Madura F, Fuller A, et al. Minimal conformational plasticity enables TCR cross-reactivity to different MHC class II heterodimers. *Sci Rep* (2012) **2**:629. doi:10.1038/srep00629
28. Chicz RM, Urban RG, Gorga JC, Vignali DA, Lane WS, Strominger JL. Specificity and promiscuity among naturally processed peptides bound to HLA-DR alleles. *J Exp Med* (1993) **178**:27–47. doi:10.1084/jem.178.1.27
29. Vignali DA, Urban RG, Chicz RM, Strominger JL. Minute quantities of a single immunodominant foreign epitope are presented as large nested sets by major histocompatibility complex class II molecules. *Eur J Immunol* (1993) **23**:1602–7. doi:10.1002/eji.1830230731
30. Nelson CA, Petzold SJ, Unanue ER. Identification of two distinct properties of class II major histocompatibility complex-associated peptides. *Proc Natl Acad Sci U S A* (1993) **90**:1227–31. doi:10.1073/pnas.90.4.1227
31. Nelson CA, Petzold SJ, Unanue ER. Peptides determine the lifespan of MHC class II molecules in the antigen-presenting cell. *Nature* (1994) **371**:250–2. doi:10.1038/371250a0
32. Sant'angelo DB, Robinson E, Janeway CA Jr., Denzin LK. Recognition of core and flanking amino acids of MHC class II-bound peptides by the T cell receptor. *Eur J Immunol* (2002) **32**:2510–20. doi:10.1002/1521-4141(200209)32:9<2510::AID-IMMU2510>3.0.CO;2-Q
33. O'brien C, Flower DR, Feighery C. Peptide length significantly influences in vitro affinity for MHC class II molecules. *Immunome Res* (2008) **4**:6. doi:10.1186/1745-7580-4-6
34. Mohan JF, Unanue ER. Unconventional recognition of peptides by T cells and the implications for autoimmunity. *Nat Rev Immunol* (2012) **12**:721–8. doi:10.1038/nri3294
35. Blum JS, Wearsch PA, Cresswell P. Pathways of antigen processing. *Annu Rev Immunol* (2013) **31**:443–73. doi:10.1146/annurev-immunol-032712-095910
36. Romagnoli P, Layet C, Yewdell J, Bakke O, Germain RN. Relationship between invariant chain expression and major histocompatibility complex class II transport into early and late endocytic compartments. *J Exp Med* (1993) **177**:583–96. doi:10.1084/jem.177.3.583
37. Weber DA, Evavold BD, Jensen PE. Enhanced dissociation of HLA-DR-bound peptides in the presence of HLA-DM. *Science* (1996) **274**:618–20. doi:10.1126/science.274.5287.618
38. Busch R, Doebele RC, Patil NS, Pashine A, Mellins ED. Accessory molecules for MHC class II peptide loading. *Curr Opin Immunol* (2000) **12**:99–106. doi:10.1016/S0952-7915(99)00057-6
39. Anders AK, Call MJ, Schulze MS, Fowler KD, Schubert DA, Seth NP, et al. HLA-DM captures partially empty HLA-DR molecules for catalyzed removal of peptide. *Nat Immunol* (2011) **12**:54–61. doi:10.1038/ni.1967
40. Painter CA, Negroni MP, Kellersberger KA, Zavala-Ruiz Z, Evans JE, Stern LJ. Conformational lability in the class II MHC 310 helix and adjacent extended strand dictate HLA-DM susceptibility and peptide exchange. *Proc Natl Acad Sci U S A* (2011) **108**:19329–34. doi:10.1073/pnas.1108074108
41. Narayan K, Chou CL, Kim A, Hartman IZ, Dalai S, Khoruzhenko S, et al. HLA-DM targets the hydrogen bond between the histidine at position beta81 and peptide to dissociate HLA-DR-peptide complexes. *Nat Immunol* (2007) **8**:92–100. doi:10.1038/ni1414
42. Pos W, Sethi DK, Call MJ, Schulze MS, Anders AK, Pyrdol J, et al. Crystal structure of the HLA-DM-HLA-DR1 complex defines mechanisms for rapid peptide selection. *Cell* (2012) **151**:1557–68. doi:10.1016/j.cell.2012.11.025
43. Manoury B, Hewitt EW, Morrice N, Dando PM, Barrett AJ, Watts C. An asparaginyl endopeptidase processes a microbial antigen for class II MHC presentation. *Nature* (1998) **396**:695–9. doi:10.1038/25379
44. Lippolis JD, White FM, Marto JA, Luckey CJ, Bullock TN, Shabanowitz J, et al. Analysis of MHC class II antigen processing by quantitation of peptides that constitute nested sets. *J Immunol* (2002) **169**:5089–97.
45. O'donnell PW, Haque A, Klemsz MJ, Kaplan MH, Blum JS. Cutting edge: induction of the antigen-processing enzyme IFN-gamma-inducible lysosomal thiol reductase in melanoma cells Is STAT1-dependent but CIITA-independent. *J Immunol* (2004) **173**:731–5.
46. Dudziak D, Kamphorst AO, Heidkamp GF, Buchholz VR, Trumpfheller C, Yamazaki S, et al. Differential antigen processing by dendritic cell subsets in vivo. *Science* (2007) **315**:107–11. doi:10.1126/science.1136080
47. Honke N, Shaabani N, Cadeddu G, Sorg UR, Zhang DE, Trilling M, et al. Enforced viral replication activates adaptive immunity and is essential for the control of a cytopathic virus. *Nat Immunol* (2012) **13**:51–7. doi:10.1038/ni.2169
48. Sercarz EE, Lehmann PV, Ametani A, Benichou G, Miller A, Moudgil K. Dominance and crypticity of T cell antigenic determinants. *Annu Rev Immunol* (1993) **11**:729–66. doi:10.1146/annurev.iy.11.040193.003501

49. Larsen SL, Pedersen LO, Buus S, Stryhn A. T cell responses affected by aminopeptidase N (CD13)-mediated trimming of major histocompatibility complex class II-bound peptides. *J Exp Med* (1996) **184**:183–9. doi:10.1084/jem.184.1.183
50. Zavala-Ruiz Z, Strug I, Walker BD, Norris PJ, Stern LJ. A hairpin turn in a class II MHC-bound peptide orients residues outside the binding groove for T cell recognition. *Proc Natl Acad Sci U S A* (2004) **101**:13279–84. doi:10.1073/pnas.0403371101
51. Godkin AJ, Davenport MP, Willis A, Jewell DP, Hill AV. Use of complete eluted peptide sequence data from HLA-DR and -DQ molecules to predict T cell epitopes, and the influence of the nonbinding terminal regions of ligands in epitope selection. *J Immunol* (1998) **161**:850–8.
52. Godkin AJ, Smith KJ, Willis A, Tejada-Simon MV, Zhang J, Elliott T, et al. Naturally processed HLA class II peptides reveal highly conserved immunogenic flanking region sequence preferences that reflect antigen processing rather than peptide-MHC interactions. *J Immunol* (2001) **166**:6720–7.
53. Cole DK, Gallagher K, Lemercier B, Holland CJ, Junaid S, Hindley JP, et al. Modification of the carboxy-terminal flanking region of a universal influenza epitope alters CD4(+) T-cell repertoire selection. *Nat Commun* (2012) **3**:665. doi:10.1038/ncomms1665
54. Hemmer B, Fleckenstein BT, Vergelli M, Jung G, Mcfarland H, Martin R, et al. Identification of high potency microbial and self ligands for a human autoreactive class II-restricted T cell clone. *J Exp Med* (1997) **185**:1651–9. doi:10.1084/jem.185.9.1651
55. Reinherz EL, Tan K, Tang L, Kern P, Liu J, Xiong Y, et al. The crystal structure of a T cell receptor in complex with peptide and MHC class II. *Science* (1999) **286**:1913–21. doi:10.1126/science.286.5446.1913
56. Smith KJ, Reid SW, Stuart DI, Mcmichael AJ, Jones EY, Bell JI. An altered position of the alpha 2 helix of MHC class I is revealed by the crystal structure of HLA-B*3501. *Immunity* (1996) **4**:203–13. doi:10.1016/S1074-7613(00)80429-X
57. Madden DR, Garboczi DN, Wiley DC. The antigenic identity of peptide-MHC complexes: a comparison of the conformations of five viral peptides presented by HLA-A2. *Cell* (1993) **75**:693–708. doi:10.1016/0092-8674(93)90490-H
58. Borbulevych OY, Insaidoo FK, Baxter TK, Powell DJ Jr., Johnson LA, Restifo NP, et al. Structures of MART-126/27-35 Peptide/HLA-A2 complexes reveal a remarkable disconnect between antigen structural homology and T cell recognition. *J Mol Biol* (2007) **372**:1123–36. doi:10.1016/j.jmb.2007.07.025
59. Miles JJ, Borg NA, Brennan RM, Tynan FE, Kjer-Nielsen L, Silins SL, et al. TCR alpha genes direct MHC restriction in the potent human T cell response to a class I-bound viral epitope. *J Immunol* (2006) **177**:6804–14.
60. Probst-Kepper M, Hecht HJ, Herrmann H, Janke V, Ocklenburg F, Klempnauer J, et al. Conformational restraints and flexibility of 14-meric peptides in complex with HLA-B*3501. *J Immunol* (2004) **173**:5610–6.
61. Dessen A, Lawrence CM, Cupo S, Zaller DM, Wiley DC. X-ray crystal structure of HLA-DR4 (DRA*0101, DRB1*0401) complexed with a peptide from human collagen II. *Immunity* (1997) **7**:473–81. doi:10.1016/S1074-7613(00)80369-6
62. Smith KJ, Pyrdol J, Gauthier L, Wiley DC, Wucherpfennig KW. Crystal structure of HLA-DR2 (DRA*0101, DRB1*1501) complexed with a peptide from human myelin basic protein. *J Exp Med* (1998) **188**:1511–20. doi:10.1084/jem.188.8.1511
63. Li Y, Depontieu FR, Sidney J, Salay TM, Engelhard VH, Hunt DF, et al. Structural basis for the presentation of tumor-associated MHC class II-restricted phosphopeptides to CD4+ T cells. *J Mol Biol* (2010) **399**:596–603. doi:10.1016/j.jmb
64. Gunther S, Schlundt A, Sticht J, Roske Y, Heinemann U, Wiesmuller KH, et al. Bidirectional binding of invariant chain peptides to an MHC class II molecule. *Proc Natl Acad Sci U S A* (2010) **107**:22219–24. doi:10.1073/pnas.1014708107

Increased peptide contacts govern high affinity binding of a modified TCR whilst maintaining a native pMHC docking mode

David K. Cole[1]*†, Malkit Sami[2†], Daniel R. Scott[3†], Pierre J. Rizkallah[1], Oleg Y. Borbulevych[3], Penio T. Todorov[2], Ruth K. Moysey[2,4], Bent K. Jakobsen[2], Jonathan M. Boulter[1$], Brian M. Baker[3]*† and Yi Li[2,5†]

[1] Cardiff University School of Medicine, Heath Park, Cardiff, UK
[2] Immunocore Limited, Oxon, UK
[3] Department of Chemistry and Biochemistry, University of Notre Dame, Notre Dame, IN, USA
[4] Oxford Nanopore Technologies Ltd., Oxford, UK
[5] Center for Infection and Immunity, Guangzhou Institutes of Biomedicine and Health, Chinese Academy of Sciences, Guangzhou, China

Edited by:
Bruno Laugel, Cardiff University School of Medicine, UK

Reviewed by:
Julian Dyson, Imperial College London, UK
Ed Palmer, University Hospital Basel, Switzerland
Chris O'Callaghan, University of Oxford, UK

***Correspondence:**
David K. Cole, Institute of Infection and Immunity, Cardiff University School of Medicine, Henry Wellcome Building, Heath Park, CF14 4XN Cardiff, UK
e-mail: coledk@cf.ac.uk;
Brian M. Baker, Department of Chemistry and Biochemistry, University of Notre Dame, 251 Nieuwland Science Hall, Notre Dame, IN 46556, USA
e-mail: brian-baker@nd.edu

† David K. Cole, Malkit Sami, Daniel R. Scott, Brian M. Baker and Yi Li have contributed equally to this work.

$ Deceased 14th May 2008

Natural T cell receptors (TCRs) generally bind to their cognate pMHC molecules with weak affinity and fast kinetics, limiting their use as therapeutic agents. Using phage display, we have engineered a high affinity version of the A6 wild-type TCR (A6wt), specific for the human leukocyte antigen (HLA-A*0201) complexed with human T cell lymphotropic virus type 1_{11-19} peptide (A2-Tax). Mutations in just 4 residues in the CDR3β loop region of the A6wt-TCR were selected that improved binding to A2-Tax by nearly 1000-fold. Biophysical measurements of this mutant TCR (A6c134) demonstrated that the enhanced binding was derived through favorable enthalpy and a slower off-rate. The structure of the free A6c134 TCR and the A6c134/A2-Tax complex revealed a native binding mode, similar to the A6wt/A2-Tax complex. However, concordant with the more favorable binding enthalpy, the A6c134 TCR made increased contacts with the Tax peptide compared with the A6wt/A2-Tax complex, demonstrating a peptide-focused mechanism for the enhanced affinity that directly involved the mutated residues in the A6c134 TCR CDR3β loop. This peptide-focused enhanced TCR binding may represent an important approach for developing antigen specific high affinity TCR reagents for use in T cell based therapies.

Keywords: human T leukocyte virus type 1, crystal structure, peptide-major histocompatibility complex, surface plasmon resonance, T cell, T cell receptor, A6 TCR, high affinity TCR

INTRODUCTION

$CD8^+$ αβ T cells recognize mainly intracellularly expressed antigens through an interaction mediated by the cell surface expressed T cell receptor (TCR). Intracellular proteins, processed by the proteasome into short peptides (generally 8–13 amino acids in length), are presented to $CD8^+$ T cells on the surface of almost all nucleated human cells by class I major histocompatibility complex proteins (pMHCI). TCR recognition of pMHCI initiates $CD8^+$ T cell activation and the adaptive immune response. The ability of $CD8^+$ T cells to scrutinize the intracellular environment provides an important mechanism to target aberrant disease epitopes that would be otherwise hidden from the immune system. Thus, $CD8^+$ T cells play an important role during viral infections (Miles et al., 2010), which typically elicit strong $CD8^+$ T cell responses, many of which have been well-characterized, including those to HTLV-1 (Bieganowska et al., 1999; Vine et al., 2004), although some viruses can escape $CD8^+$ T cell mediated clearance (Klenerman and Zinkernagel, 1998; Overbaugh and Bangham, 2001). Cancers too, as a result of their malignant transformation, have altered protein expression causing the presentation of tumor-associated peptide antigens (TAPAs) (Renkvist et al., 2001; Cole et al., 2009). However, although these TAPAs can elicit a host $CD8^+$ T cell response, this is often insufficient to cause tumor rejection (Blohm et al., 2002; Parkhurst et al., 2004). $CD8^+$ T cell responses are also integral to the initiation and progression of many autoimmune diseases, possibly through the unwanted recognition of self-peptide antigens (Bulek et al., 2012). The TCR/pMHC interaction, which governs $CD8^+$ T cell responses, is therefore an attractive therapeutic target in many varied diseases, particularly

Abbreviations: pMHC, peptide-major histocompatibility complex; RU, response unit; SPR, surface plasmon resonance.

in cases where a disease-associated peptide antigen "target" has been unambiguously established.

However, unlike antibodies that can undergo somatic hypermutation and bind with high affinity (K_D = nM–pM) and long half-lives (typically hours), TCRs are selected in the thymus to bind with weak affinity (K_D = 100 nM–270 μM) and short half-lives (typically seconds) (Cole et al., 2007; Bridgeman et al., 2012). Why TCRs are selected to bind within this weak affinity range is not fully understood, but may represent a balance between self-tolerance and a requirement for T cell cross-reactivity (Mason, 1998; Sewell, 2012; Wooldridge et al., 2012). However, the weak affinity and short half-lives of natural TCR/pMHC interactions imposes limitations on the use of TCRs for targeting cell surface expressed pMHCs, primarily because the short half-life is not adequate for the delivery of therapeutic interventions to target antigens. In order to overcome this limitation, we have recently implemented phage display to generate TCRs with an enhanced affinity for cognate antigen (Li et al., 2005; Dunn et al., 2006; Sami et al., 2007; Varela-Rohena et al., 2008; Liddy et al., 2012) that can be used to target cell surface expressed MHC molecules displaying any disease epitope of interest. Using this technique, we have generated several high affinity TCRs derived from the αβ TCR A6 (A6wt) that are specific for the HTLV-1_{11-19} peptide, presented by HLA-A*0201 (A2-Tax) (Li et al., 2005). High affinity TCRs generated using this method can be used for two distinct type of therapies. The first involves genetically reprograming host T cells so that they express a modified TCR (adoptive therapy) (Morgan et al., 2006; Varela-Rohena et al., 2008). The second involves using a soluble high affinity TCR to deliver a therapeutic payload intravenously (soluble therapy) (Liddy et al., 2012). The optimal TCR affinity for these two types of therapy, in terms for retaining specificity and reactivity, will probably be distinct and will likely be lower for adoptive therapy because of the polyvalent nature of T cell antigen recognition at the cell surface versus a soluble therapy in which the TCR reagent will likely require a longer half-life to effectively target intended disease markers. Understanding how these reagents function at the molecular level is key to determining these parameters and optimizing these types of T cell directed therapies.

Previous structural investigations of TCR/pMHC interactions have shown that TCRs bind with a relatively conserved diagonal orientation (Garboczi et al., 1996; Rudolph et al., 2006), with the α-chain focused toward the N-terminus of the peptide and the β-chain toward the C-terminus. Although exceptions occur (Burrows et al., 2010), this orientation enables the TCR complementarity determining region (CDR)2 loops to be positioned over mainly the MHC surface, the CDR3 loops to be positioned primarily over the peptide and the CDR1 loops positioned in between. This binding mode, and the low native TCR binding affinity, is presumably important for maintaining T cell specificity and antigen sensitivity, and is possibly important in T cell signaling (Adams et al., 2011). However, we have previously shown that just a small number of mutations in the TCR CDR loops can improve the low natural TCR/pMHC binding affinity dramatically (Li et al., 2005; Dunn et al., 2006; Hawse et al., 2012). Thus, it is likely that high affinity TCRs are generated in the thymus, but they are not selected for release into the periphery. In order to better understand the consequences of high affinity TCR interactions, and to provide further insight into: (1) how high affinity TCR binding is mediated and (2) what effects this binding is likely to have on TCR specificity, we solved the atomic structures of a high affinity TCR, A6c134, free, and in complex with A2-Tax. By comparing this structure with the previously published structures for the A6wt TCR (Garboczi et al., 1996; Scott et al., 2011), we provide a molecular explanation for the improved binding of this high affinity TCR.

RESULTS

DECONSTRUCTION OF HIGH AFFINITY A6 TCR VARIANTS SPECIFIC FOR A2-TAX

In order to generate a high affinity version of the A6wt TCR, we implemented phage display as previously described (Li et al., 2005). This process generated a number of high affinity TCRs, including the mutant A6c134 that varied from the A6wt TCR parental sequence at only four codons, all located within the CDR3β loop (**Table 1**). It has been previously determined that the A6wt TCR binds to A2-Tax with an affinity of ~1–3 μM and an off-rate ($t_{1/2}$) of ~7–10 s (Davis-Harrison et al., 2005; Armstrong and Baker, 2007; Cole et al., 2007). In contrast, the engineered high affinity A6c134 TCR bound to A2-Tax with an affinity of 4 nM (nearly 1000 times greater than the A6wt TCR, or $\Delta\Delta G^\circ = -3.96$ kcal/mol) and an off-rate ($t_{1/2}$) of 3900 s (>400 times longer than the A6wt TCR), as determined by surface plasmon resonance (SPR) (**Table 1**). A6c134 did not bind to other HLA-A2 restricted peptides that were used as negative controls in different SPR experiments, including as A2-ILAKFLHWL, A2-ELAGIGILTV, and A2-YLEPGPVTA demonstrating that A6c134 retained peptide specificity (data not shown). In order to investigate the molecular basis for how this high affinity was generated, we used reverse engineering to construct a range of A6wt-based TCRs containing different combinations of amino acids from the A6c134 CDR3β sequence and, conversely, a range of A6c134-based TCRs containing different combinations of amino acids from the A6wt CDR3β sequence (**Table 1**). All of these TCRs exhibited very similar on-rates, but showed marked differences in their off-rates (**Table 1**). In general, the mutations appeared to act cooperatively to enhance affinity. The mutation of the A6wt TCR from R_{102} to Q_{102} had only a small effect upon binding affinity and may have been selected because of the lower toxicity of the TCR to the TG1 phage host (Li et al., 2005).

A6c134 TCR BOUND TO A2-TAX USING A SIMILAR CONFORMATION TO THE A6wt TCR

In order to determine the structural basis of the high affinity binding for the A6c134 TCR, we solved the A6c134/A2-Tax complex structure to 2.74 Å. Molecular replacement was successful only in space group C121, consistent with the presence of one molecule of the complex per asymmetric unit, and the resolution was sufficiently high to show that the interface between the two molecules was well ordered and contained well defined electron density. The crystallographic R/R_{free} factors were 22 and 26%, within the accepted limits shown in the theoretically expected distribution (Tickle et al., 2000) (Table S1 in Supplementary Material). The overall buried surface area (BSA) of

Table 1 | Biophysical analysis of different combinations of "knock-in" and "knock-out" mutations (in bold type and underlined) of A6wt and A6c134 TCRs binding to A2-Tax.

Mutant	CDR3β	K_D	k_{on} ($s^{-1}M^{-1}$)	k_{off} (s^{-1})	$t_{1/2}$ (s)	ΔG° (kcal/mol)	ΔΔG° (kcal/mol)
A6wt	AGGR	3.2 μM	2.3×10^4	7.4×10^{-2}	9.3	−7.49	n/a
A6c134M	**M**GGR	1.9 μM	1.8×10^4	3.5×10^{-2}	20	−7.80	−0.31
A6c134S	A**S**GR	1.8 μM	2.3×10^4	4.1×10^{-2}	17	−7.83	−0.34
A6c134AE	A**SAE**	9.4 nM	2.3×10^4	5.2×10^{-4}	1320	−10.94	−3.45
A6c134E	**MSAE**	4.4 nM	5.5×10^4	2.2×10^{-4}	3120	−11.39	−3.90
A6c134R	**MSA**R	8 nM	1.9×10^4	1.5×10^{-4}	4500	−11.04	−3.55
A6c134	**MSAQ**	4 nM	4.5×10^4	1.8×10^{-4}	3900	−11.45	−3.96

Off-rates were determined by least squares fitting of single-component exponential decay equation to the decay curve following TCR binding to A2-Tax.
Half-lives were calculated using the equation $t_{1/2} = \ln 2/k_{off}$.
ΔΔG° = ΔG° of high affinity A6c134 variant binding to A2-Tax − ΔG° of A6wt binding to A2-Tax.

2445.4 Å (TCR/pMHC) was within the range observed for previously characterized TCR/pMHC interactions (Rudolph et al., 2006). The high affinity A6c134 TCR bound with a diagonal docking geometry to A2-Tax and showed one to one stoichiometry as previously reported of other TCR/pMHC complexes (Rudolph et al., 2006). We observed a high level of similarity between the A6wt/A2-Tax and A6c134/A2-Tax complexes, suggesting that overall conformation was unaffected by the mutations in A6c134. Importantly, the Tax peptide conformation was virtually identical in both complexes, discounting the possibility that structural changes in the peptide contributed to the high affinity observed (**Figures 1A,B**). Similarly, the architecture of the CDR loops was unaffected by the mutations in the A6c134 TCR (**Figure 1C**), and the crossing angle of both TCRs was identical at 34° (**Figure 1D**) and fell within the previously observed range (Rudolph et al., 2006). Thus, differences in binding affinity between the A6wt and A6c134 TCRs could not be explained by a large conformational change in geometry, consistent with observations in similar studies with other systems (Dunn et al., 2006; Sami et al., 2007; Madura et al., 2013).

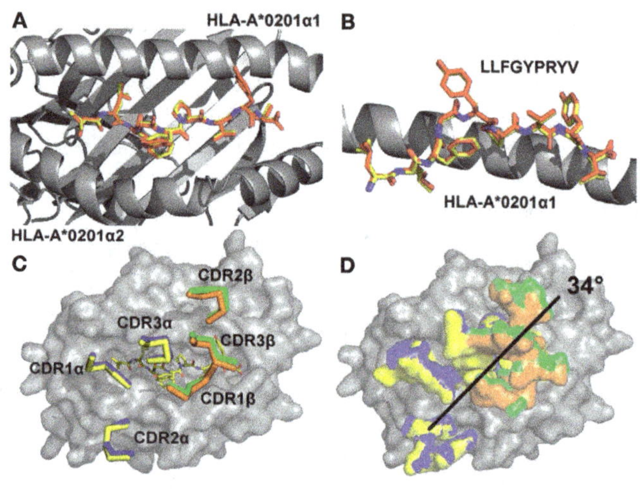

FIGURE 1 | The overall conformations of A6wt and A6c134 TCRs in complex with A2-Tax are similar. (A) Comparison of peptide conformation in the A6wt TCR (red sticks) and A6c134 TCR (yellow sticks) complex structures looking down on top of the MHC groove (gray sticks). **(B)** Comparison of peptide conformation in the A6wt TCR (red sticks) and A6c134 TCR (yellow sticks) complex structures looking from the side of the MHC groove (gray sticks). **(C)** Comparison of CDR loop conformation in the A6wt TCR (yellow and orange ribbons) and A6c134 TCR (blue and green ribbon) A2-Tax complex structures. **(D)** Crossing angle comparison of the A6wt TCR and A6c134 TCR in complex with A2-Tax. Colors as in C.

THE A6c134 TCR CDR LOOPS UNDERGO LARGE CONFORMATIONAL ADJUSTMENTS DURING A2-TAX ENGAGEMENT

We next solved the structure of the A6c134 TCR at 2 Å (Table S1 in Supplementary Material; **Figure 2**). The crystallographic R/R_{free} factors were 23.4 and 29.5%, consistent with the expected ratio range (Tickle et al., 2000). In many cases, although not all (Borbulevych et al., 2011b; Holland et al., 2012), TCR CDR loops have been shown to undergo numerous, and sometimes large, conformational changes upon pMHC binding (Armstrong et al., 2008b). Superposition of the free and the bound A6c134 TCR showed that, although the overall conformation of the TCR was virtually identical (**Figure 2A**), the CDR loops underwent substantial movements (**Figure 2B**). The CDR3 loops of both chains of the A6c134 TCR were poorly ordered and could not be fully resolved, indicating a large amount flexibility in this region of the TCR. Although the apex of the CDR3 loops could not be accurately located, the portions of the CDR3α and CDR3β loops that were visible underwent large hinge movements of ~5.9 and ~4.6 Å, respectively (**Figures 2C,D**). These changes were substantial compared to other structural studies in which the largest loop movement observed for a human MHCI restricted TCR was 5.6 Å (Kjer-Nielsen et al., 2002; Stewart-Jones et al., 2003). Interestingly, a nearly identical observation was made for A6wt TCR (Scott et al., 2011), for which the dynamics of the CDR3 loops were shown to have a large influence on the specificity and cross-reactivity of the TCR. This occurrence with A6c134 leads to the somewhat counterintuitive conclusion that substitution of the sequence AGGR with MSAQ in CDR3β does not greatly impact the overall dynamics of the loop, and leads us to suggest that the enhanced affinity of A6c134 was not attributable to "preorganization" of CDR3β, i.e., the MSAQ mutation did not alter the non-bound form of the A6c134 TCR to a conformation closer to that of the bound form. This conclusion is consistent with the observation that the binding of A6c134 to A2-Tax is characterized by a much more favorable enthalpy change along with a less favorable entropy change (as pre-organization would have resulted in a more favorable binding entropy) (Armstrong and Baker, 2007; Piepenbrink et al., 2009).

The CDR1 and CDR2 loops underwent a smaller rigid body shift and hinge movements of 2.5–4 Å (**Figures 2E–H**). On average, the A6c134 TCR CDR loops moved by 4.1 Å. Altogether, this degree of conformational plasticity is high compared to other TCRs (Armstrong et al., 2008b), and demonstrated that the A6c134 TCR undergoes a high degree of conformational melding during binding, as does the A6wt TCR (Borbulevych et al., 2011a). These movements enabled direct contacts between the A6c134 TCR and A2-Tax and resolved steric clashes that would have occurred between the unbound TCR and the MHC surface, as observed for the A6wt TCR (Scott et al., 2011).

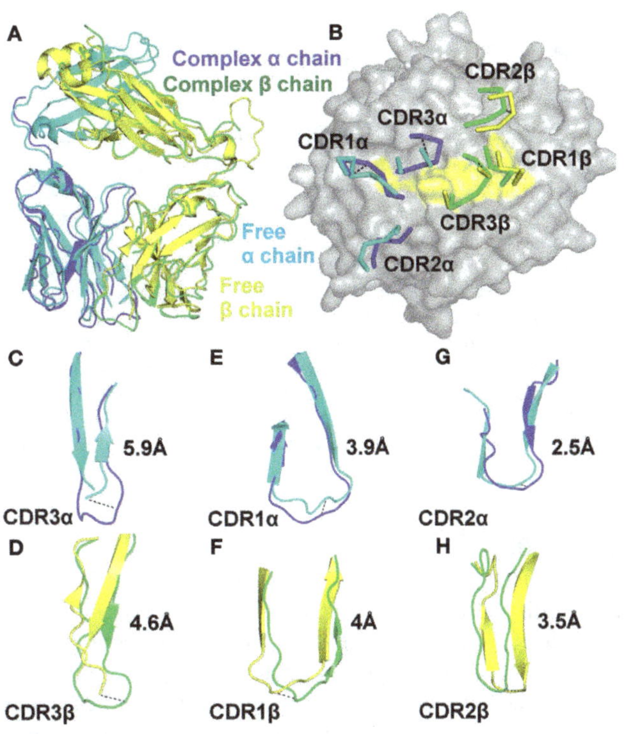

FIGURE 2 | The A6c134 TCR CDR loops undergo a large degree of conformational adjustment during binding to A2-Tax. Comparison of the conformations of the A6c134 TCR CDR1, CDR2, and CDR3 loops in the A6c134/A2-Tax complex versus A6c134 TCR free structures. **(A)** Superposition of the free (cyan and yellow cartoon) and complexed (blue and green cartoon) A6c134 TCR. **(B)** Superposition of the free (cyan and yellow lines) and complexed (blue and green lines) A6c134 TCR looking down on the A2-Tax surface (gray and yellow surface). **(C)** Superposition of the free (cyan cartoon) and complexed (blue cartoon) A6c134 TCR CDR3α loop. **(D)** Superposition of the free (yellow cartoon) and complexed (green cartoon) A6c134 TCR CDR3β loop. **(E)** Superposition of the free (cyan cartoon) and complexed (blue cartoon) A6c134 TCR CDR1α loop. **(F)** Superposition of the free (yellow cartoon) and complexed (green cartoon) A6c134TCR CDR1β loop. **(G)** Superposition of the free (cyan cartoon) and complexed (blue cartoon) A6c134 TCR CDR2α loop. **(H)** Superposition of the free (yellow cartoon) and complexed (green cartoon) A6c134TCR CDR2β loop. Loop moments at the apex, or region of greatest movement are shown.

THE HIGH AFFINITY BINDING OF THE A6c134 TCR WAS GOVERNED BY INCREASED PEPTIDE CONTACTS

As the overall free and bound conformations of A6wt and A6c134 were nearly identical, we decided to investigate differences in atomic interactions at the A6wt and A6c134 interfaces. The binding footprints of the A6wt and A6c134 TCRs on A2-Tax were similar, but not identical, resulting in the involvement of different peptide and MHC residues at the interface (**Figures 3A,B**). Although the A6c134 TCR α-chain contained no mutations, it utilized a different combination of TCR residues for binding A2-Tax compared with A6wt. As a result, the A6c134 TCR α-chain made a number of new and different contacts with A2-Tax compared with the A6wt TCR (Tables S2 and S3 in Supplementary Material; **Table 2**; **Figures 3C,D**). Thus, the mutations in the A6c134 TCR β-chain mediated a knock-on, or indirect effect resulting in a modified binding mode for the TCR α-chain.

In contrast with the A6c134 TCR α-chain, the A6c134 β-chain containing the mutated MSAQ motif formed a virtually identical footprint on A2-Tax compared to the A6wt TCR (**Figure 3D**). The A6c134 β-chain made a similar number of contacts with the MHC compared to the corresponding residues in the A6wt TCR (AGGR) (**Figures 4A,B**). This was reflected by the observation that the A6c134 TCR made only 11 more contacts with the MHC surface compared to the A6wt/A2-Tax complex. However, the A6c134 TCR made 26 extra contacts with the Tax peptide compared to the A6wt TCR, suggesting a TCR-peptide mediated mechanism for the enhanced affinity observed. This observation was also supported by the increase in shape complementarity index (Lawrence and Colman, 1993; Reinherz et al., 1999) (SC = 0.74) for the A6c134/A2-Tax complex compared to the A6wt/A2-Tax complex (SC = 0.63), and is consistent with the

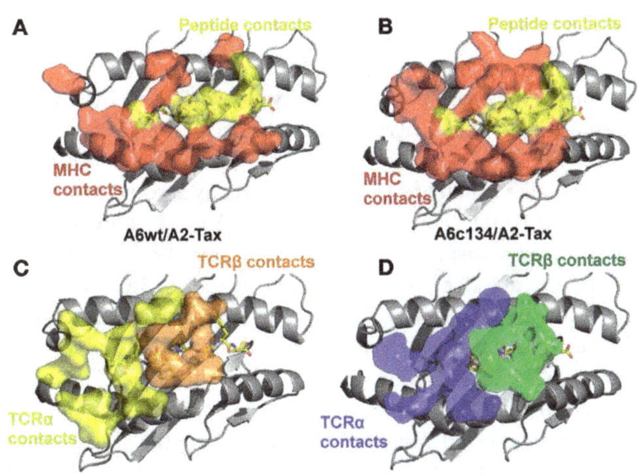

FIGURE 3 | The specific footprints made in the A6wt TCR/A2-Tax and A6c134 TCR/A2-Tax complex structures are unique. **(A)** MHC (red surface) and peptide (yellow surface) residues that are contacted by the A6wt TCR. **(B)** MHC (red surface) and peptide (yellow surface) residues that are contacted by the A6c134 TCR. **(C)** A6wt TCR residues (orange and yellow surface) that contact the pMHC. **(D)** A6c134 TCR residues (blue and green surface) that contact the pMHC. Although the overall contact footprint is similar, the A6c134 TCR makes new interactions with both the MHC surface and the peptide.

Table 2 | Direct contacts made by the A6wt TCR, or A6c134 TCR CDR3 loops.

	TCR	vdW (3.2–4 Å)	H-bonds (≤3.4 Å)
A6wt TCR CDR3α	Thr93	0	1
	Thr98	2	1
	Asp99	15	3
	Ser100	7	2
	Trp101	5	0
	Gly102	0	0
A6c134 TCR CDR3α	Thr93	1	0
	Thr98	2	1
	Asp99	15	2
	Ser100	12	2
	Trp101	9	0
	Gly102	3	0
A6wt TCR CDR3β	Arg95	0	1
	Leu98	14	1
	Ala99	0	0
	Gly100	1	0
	Gly101	6	2
	Arg102	14	1
	Pro103	5	0
A6c134 TCR CDR3β	Arg95	2	1
	Leu98	17	0
	Met99	4	0
	Ser100	6	0
	Ala101	17	1
	Gln102	7	0
	Pro103	11	0

Mutated residues are shown in red.

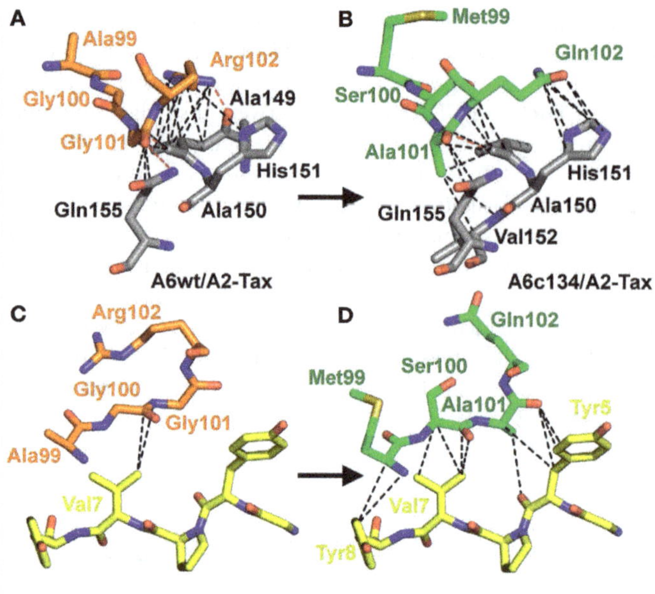

FIGURE 4 | Increased peptide contacts between A6c134 TCR and A2-Tax mediate the high affinity binding. Specific contacts (<4 Å) made by residues 99–102 in the TCR CDR3β-chain of either: AGGR (A6wt TCR) or MSAQ (A6c134 TCR). **(A)** Contacts (dotted lines) between the A6wt TCR CDR3β chain, residues 99–102 (AGGR) (shown in orange sticks) and the MHC (gray sticks). **(B)** Contacts (dotted lines) between the A6c134 TCR CDR3β chain, residues 99–102 (MSAQ) (shown in green sticks) and the MHC (gray sticks). **(C)** Contacts (dotted lines) between the A6wt TCR CDR3β chain, residues 99–102 (AGGR) (shown in orange sticks) and the peptide (yellow sticks). **(D)** Contacts (dotted lines) between the A6c134 TCR CDR3β chain, residues 99–102 (MSAQ) (shown in green sticks) and the peptide (yellow sticks). Contacts between the A6c134 and the MHC remain similar to the A6wt/A2-Tax complex whereas A6c134-peptide contacts are increased.

observation that the enhanced affinity of A6c134 was enthalpically driven as noted above (Armstrong and Baker, 2007; Piepenbrink et al., 2009).

Overall, the mutated MSAQ motif directly accounted for 11 of the 37 new contacts with the surface of A2-Tax (**Figures 4C,D**; **Table 2**). For instance; the A_{99}–M_{99} mutation generated 4 additional van der Waals contacts (**Figure 5A**), G_{100}–S_{100} generated an additional 5 additional van der Waals contacts (**Figure 5B**) and G_{101}–A_{101} generated 10 additional contacts (**Figure 5C**), with A2-Tax. Interestingly, the R_{102}–Q_{102} mutation resulted in the loss of seven van der Waals contacts and one hydrogen bond (**Figure 5D**). However, the overall affinity was stronger for A6c134 (MSAQ) compared to A6c134R (MSAR) suggesting that the R_{102}–Q_{102} mutation contributed indirectly to binding. Thus, 26 new contacts were generated through indirect interactions with non-mutated residues in the c134 TCR. The majority of these (21 new contacts) were made between non-mutated residues in the c134 TCR CDR3α and CDR3β loops demonstrating that the proximity of residues to the mutated MSAQ motif in the CDR3β loop was probably important for enabling the formation of these new interactions (**Table 2**).

DISCUSSION

Thymic selection generates T cells that express TCRs with a weak binding affinity ($K_D = 100$ nM–270 μM) for cognate antigen (Cole et al., 2007; Bridgeman et al., 2012). Presumably, this affinity range is important to ensure host protection against foreign invaders, whilst maintaining tolerance to self-antigens from a T cell repertoire of around 25 million (Arstila et al., 1999). In order to perform this function, growing evidence suggests that TCRs must be highly cross-reactive within the confines of MHC-restriction (Mason, 1998; Sewell, 2012; Wooldridge et al., 2012). We have previously shown that it is possible to enhance TCR binding affinity using phage display (Li et al., 2005). These engineered high affinity TCRs represent a potentially useful tool to target specific disease molecules, such as cancer (Liddy et al., 2012) or HIV (Varela-Rohena et al., 2008). However, how enhanced affinity affects TCR binding and specificity is not fully understood, and there are likely multiple mechanistic routes through which affinity can be enhanced. A greater understanding of such mechanisms is particularly important when developing T cell therapies that involve genetically modifying T cells with enhanced affinity TCRs or when using soluble high affinity TCR therapies, to limit potentially dangerous self-reactivity.

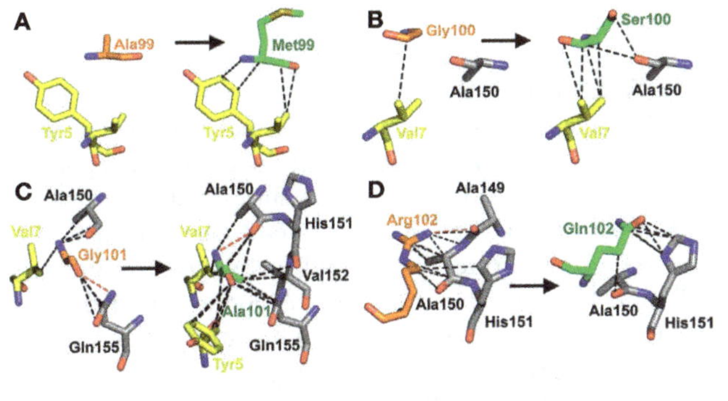

FIGURE 5 | The MSAQ motif (A6c134 TCR) makes an increased the number of contacts with A2-Tax compared to AGGR (A6wt TCR). (A) Differences in contacts made by A_{99} (A6wt TCR in orange sticks, left panel) compared to M_{99} (A6c134 TCR in green sticks, right panel). **(B)** Differences in contacts made by G_{100} (A6wt TCR in orange sticks, left panel) compared to S_{100} (A6c134 TCR in green sticks, right panel). **(C)** Differences in contacts made by Gly101 (A6wt TCR in orange sticks, left panel) compared to Ala101 (A6c134 TCR in green sticks, right panel). **(D)** Differences in contacts made by R_{102} (A6wt TCR in orange sticks, left panel) compared to Q_{102} (A6c134 TCR in green sticks, right panel). In all cases, VdW contacts are shown as black dotted lines (4 Å cut-off) and hydrogen bonds/salt bridges are shown as red dotted lines (3.4 Å cut-off). Peptide residues are shown as yellow sticks and MHC residues are shown as gray sticks.

In order to explore how TCR CDR3 loop mutations could influence TCR binding and enhance affinity, we generated a modified TCR with nearly 1000-fold enhanced binding affinity by mutating just four residues in the TCR CDR3β loop. Despite the enhanced binding affinity, the A6c134 TCR utilized a native binding mode with diagonal binding geometry as observed for other TCR/pMHC complexes (Rudolph et al., 2006). This observation is similar to other high affinity TCR structures that have been reported previously (Dunn et al., 2006; Sami et al., 2007; Madura et al., 2013). Furthermore, comparing the structures of the free and complexed A6c134 TCR demonstrated that the TCR CDR3 loops underwent a reduction in conformational flexibility upon ligand binding similar to that observed with the A6wt TCR. Thus, despite the mutation of two glycines in the CDR3β loop, high affinity binding did not seem to result from preorganization of the TCR binding site.

We observed that the total number of contacts across the interface was greater for A6c134/A2-Tax than for A6wt/A2-Tax. For instance, in the A6c134/A2-Tax complex, there were a total of 154 contacts, including 72 to peptide and 82 to the MHC. In the A6wt/A2-Tax complex, there were total of 117 contacts, including 46 to peptide and 71 to the MHC. Both the MHC and peptide were involved in generating these new contacts, and they were mediated by both mutated and non-mutated TCR residues. However, the majority of the new contacts arose from interactions between the peptide and the c134 TCR CDR3 loops. Thus, we concluded that higher affinity was mediated predominantly by new TCR-peptide interactions. This conclusion, that new contacts mediated the stronger binding affinity, is consistent with previous thermodynamic analyses, which showed that the A6c134 TCR bound to A2-Tax with a substantially more favorable enthalpy compared to the A6wt TCR ($\Delta\Delta H = -10$ kcal/mol) (Armstrong et al., 2008a; Piepenbrink et al., 2009).

Our generation of a high affinity TCR that contained mutations at only four residues in the CDR3β loop compared to the wt TCR sequence raises the question of why high affinity TCRs are not naturally selected in the thymus (Holler et al., 2003). Clearly, the structural framework of the TCR allows for high affinity binding, and the mutations we have identified fall within the rearranged gene segment of the TCR rather than the predefined germline encoded segments. Furthermore, the mutations in the TCR CDR3β chain generated an increase in peptide contacts within the boundaries of the native A6wt TCR binding mode and would thus be unlikely to alter MHC-restriction. Therefore, it seems very likely that high affinity TCR variants could be generated during the process of TCR rearrangement in the thymus. Yet such high affinity TCRs have not been observed during the peripheral immune response, implying that they are negatively selected (Holler et al., 2003). Presumably, this process is designed to limit self-reactivity. However, weaker affinity TCRs may also be selected to ensure a level of T cell cross-reactivity capable of fully protecting the host against all possible disease epitopes (Mason, 1998; Sewell, 2012; Wooldridge et al., 2012). In support of this notion, our data indicate that A6c134 and other high affinity TCRs can retain extremely high levels of specificity, and may be more specific than their wild-type parents (Laugel et al., 2005; Dunn et al., 2006; Madura et al., 2013). Generally, therapeutic TCRs do not need the capacity to be cross-reactive as they are designed to target a single disease epitope. This difference in desired function (immune response versus specific therapy) may represent an opportunity to improve the affinity of natural TCRs in a safe manner. Thus, our structural investigation of A6c134/A2-Tax, showing that the high affinity interaction was mediated by a native binding mechanism that was peptide-focused, may represent an important approach for developing antigen specific high affinity TCR reagents for use in T cell based therapies.

MATERIALS AND METHODS

PHAGE DISPLAY

Selection of high affinity A6wt TCR variants was performed as previously described (Li et al., 2005).

PROTEIN PURIFICATION

A2-Tax peptide-MHC complexes was prepared as previously described (Garboczi et al., 1992), by expressing HLA-A*0201 heavy-chain truncated at residue Pro-276 and β2 microglobulin separately in *E. coli* in the form of inclusion bodies, followed by *in vitro* refolding with synthetic peptide. pMHC for binding analysis was prepared similarly, but with the MHC fused to a biotinylation tag (Cull and Schatz, 2000) which was biotinylated *in vitro* by the BirA enzyme (O'callaghan et al., 1999). Disulfide-linked A6c134 TCR was prepared as previously described (Boulter et al., 2003; Li et al., 2005).

BINDING ANALYSIS BY SURFACE PLASMON RESONANCE (BIACORE™)

Binding analysis was performed on a Biacore™ 3000 machine using a CM-5 (research grade) chip as previously described (Cole et al., 2008; Miles et al., 2011). Streptavidin was immobilized on all flow cells using amine coupling to a level of >1000 RU (response units). Biotin tagged peptide-MHC was flowed over the streptavidin coated surface at a concentration of approximately 10 μg/ml until ~150 RU pHLA was bound. Control surfaces were coated with non-cognate pMHCs (A2-ILAKFLHWL, A2-ELAGIGILTV, and A2-YLEPGPVTA) or were left coated with streptavidin. Kinetic binding data were generated using the KINJECT program to inject 10 nM TCR over the flow cells. Data were analyzed using BIAevaluation™ software by kinetic fitting to calculate k_{on} and k_{off} rates. Binding affinities were calculated using the following equation: $K_D = k_{off}/k_{on}$.

CRYSTALLIZATION AND X-RAY DATA COLLECTION

A6c134/A2-Tax crystals were grown in MES 25 mM pH 6.5, 24% PEG 3350 and 10 mM NaCl; A6c134 free crystals were grown in MES 25 mM pH 6.5, 24% PEG 3350 and 10 mM NaCl. All crystals were soaked in 30% ethylene glycol before cryo-cooling. Data were collected at 100 K at the Advanced Photon Source at Argonne National Laboratory, USA. Reflection intensities were estimated with the XIA2 package (Winter, 2010) and the data were scaled, reduced, and analyzed with SCALA and the CCP4 package (Collaborative Computational Project, Number 4, 1994). Structures were solved with molecular replacement using PHASER (McCoy et al., 2007). Sequences were adjusted with COOT (Emsley and Cowtan, 2004) and the models refined with REFMAC5. Graphical representations were prepared with PYMOL (Delano, 2002). The reflection data and final model coordinates were deposited with the PDB database (A6c134/A2-Tax, PDB: 4FTV; A6c134 free, PDB: 4GRM).

ACKNOWLEDGMENTS

David K. Cole is a Wellcome Trust Research Career Development Fellow (WT095767). Pierre J. Rizkallah was supported by a RCUK Fellowship. Brian M. Baker is supported in part by grant GM067079 from the National Institute of General Medical Sciences, National Institutes of Health. Results shown in this report are derived from work performed at Argonne National Laboratory, Structural Biology Center at the Advanced Photon Source. Argonne is operated by UChicago Argonne, LLC, for the U.S. Department of Energy, Office of Biological and Environmental Research under contract DE-AC02-06CH11357.

SUPPLEMENTARY MATERIAL

The Supplementary Material for this article can be found online at http://www.frontiersin.org/T_Cell_Biology/10.3389/fimmu.2013.00168/abstract

Table S1 | Data collection and refinement statistics (molecular replacement).

Table S2 | Structural analysis of A6wt/A2-Tax contacts.

Table S3 | Structural analysis for A6c134/A2-Tax contacts (mutant residues in red).

REFERENCES

Adams, J. J., Narayanan, S., Liu, B., Birnbaum, M. E., Kruse, A. C., Bowerman, N. A., et al. (2011). T cell receptor signaling is limited by docking geometry to peptide-major histocompatibility complex. *Immunity* 35, 681–693. doi:10.1016/j.immuni.2011.09.013

Armstrong, K. M., and Baker, B. M. (2007). A comprehensive calorimetric investigation of an entropically driven T cell receptor-peptide/major histocompatibility complex interaction. *Biophys. J.* 93, 597–609. doi:10.1529/biophysj.107.104570

Armstrong, K. M., Insaidoo, F. K., and Baker, B. M. (2008a). Thermodynamics of T-cell receptor-peptide/MHC interactions: progress and opportunities. *J. Mol. Recognit.* 21, 275–287. doi:10.1002/jmr.896

Armstrong, K. M., Piepenbrink, K. H., and Baker, B. M. (2008b). Conformational changes and flexibility in T-cell receptor recognition of peptide-MHC complexes. *Biochem. J.* 415, 183–196. doi:10.1042/BJ20080850

Arstila, T. P., Casrouge, A., Baron, V., Even, J., Kanellopoulos, J., and Kourilsky, P. (1999). A direct estimate of the human alphabeta T cell receptor diversity. *Science* 286, 958–961. doi:10.1126/science.286.5441.958

Bieganowska, K., Hollsberg, P., Buckle, G. J., Lim, D. G., Greten, T. F., Schneck, J., et al. (1999). Direct analysis of viral-specific CD8+ T cells with soluble HLA-A2/Tax11-19 tetramer complexes in patients with human T cell lymphotropic virus-associated myelopathy. *J. Immunol.* 162, 1765–1771.

Blohm, U., Roth, E., Brommer, K., Dumrese, T., Rosenthal, F. M., and Pircher, H. (2002). Lack of effector cell function and altered tetramer binding of tumor-infiltrating lymphocytes. *J. Immunol.* 169, 5522–5530.

Borbulevych, O. Y., Piepenbrink, K. H., and Baker, B. M. (2011a). Conformational melding permits a conserved binding geometry in TCR recognition of foreign and self molecular mimics. *J. Immunol.* 186, 2950–2958. doi:10.4049/jimmunol.1003150

Borbulevych, O. Y., Santhanagopolan, S. M., Hossain, M., and Baker, B. M. (2011b). TCRs used in cancer gene therapy cross-react with MART-1/Melan-A tumor antigens via distinct mechanisms. *J. Immunol.* 187, 2453–2463. doi:10.4049/jimmunol.1101268

Boulter, J. M., Glick, M., Todorov, P. T., Baston, E., Sami, M., Rizkallah, P., et al. (2003). Stable, soluble T-cell receptor molecules for crystallization and therapeutics. *Protein Eng.* 16, 707–711. doi:10.1093/protein/gzg087

Bridgeman, J. S., Sewell, A. K., Miles, J. J., Price, D. A., and Cole, D. K. (2012). Structural and biophysical determinants of alphabeta T-cell antigen recognition. *Immunology* 135, 9–18. doi:10.1111/j.1365-2567.2011.03515.x

Bulek, A. M., Cole, D. K., Skowera, A., Dolton, G., Gras, S., Madura, F., et al. (2012). Structural basis for the killing of human beta cells by CD8(+) T cells in type 1 diabetes. *Nat. Immunol.* 13, 283–289. doi:10.1038/ni.2206

Burrows, S. R., Chen, Z., Archbold, J. K., Tynan, F. E., Beddoe, T., Kjer-Nielsen, L., et al. (2010). Hard wiring of T cell receptor specificity for the major histocompatibility complex is underpinned by TCR adaptability. *Proc. Natl. Acad. Sci. U.S.A.* 107, 10608–10613. doi:10.1073/pnas.1004926107

Cole, D. K., Dunn, S. M., Sami, M., Boulter, J. M., Jakobsen, B. K., and Sewell, A. K. (2008). T cell receptor engagement of peptide-major histocompatibility complex class I does not modify CD8 binding. *Mol. Immunol.* 45, 2700–2709. doi:10.1016/j.molimm.2007.12.009

Cole, D. K., Pumphrey, N. J., Boulter, J. M., Sami, M., Bell, J. I., Gostick, E., et al. (2007). Human TCR-binding affinity is governed by MHC class restriction. *J. Immunol.* 178, 5727–5734.

Cole, D. K., Yuan, F., Rizkallah, P. J., Miles, J. J., Gostick, E., Price, D. A., et al. (2009). Germ line-governed recognition of a cancer epitope by an immunodominant human T-cell receptor. *J. Biol. Chem.* 284, 27281–27289. doi:10.1074/jbc.M109.022509

Collaborative Computational Project, Number 4. (1994). The CCP4 suite: programs for protein crystallography. *Acta Crystallogr. D Biol. Crystallogr.* 50, 760–763. doi:10.1107/S0907444994003112

Cull, M. G., and Schatz, P. J. (2000). Biotinylation of proteins in vivo and in vitro using small peptide tags. *Meth. Enzymol.* 326, 430–440. doi:10.1016/S0076-6879(00)26068-0

Davis-Harrison, R. L., Armstrong, K. M., and Baker, B. M. (2005). Two different T cell receptors use different thermodynamic strategies to recognize the same peptide/MHC ligand. *J. Mol. Biol.* 346, 533–550. doi:10.1016/j.jmb.2004.11.063

Delano, W. L. (2002). *The PyMOL Molecular Graphics System.* San Carlos, CA: DeLano Scientific.

Dunn, S. M., Rizkallah, P. J., Baston, E., Mahon, T., Cameron, B., Moysey, R., et al. (2006). Directed evolution of human T cell receptor CDR2 residues by phage display dramatically enhances affinity for cognate peptide-MHC without increasing apparent cross-reactivity. *Protein Sci.* 15, 710–721. doi:10.1110/ps.051936406

Emsley, P., and Cowtan, K. (2004). Coot: model-building tools for molecular graphics. *Acta Crystallogr. D Biol. Crystallogr.* 60, 2126–2132. doi:10.1107/S0907444904019158

Garboczi, D. N., Ghosh, P., Utz, U., Fan, Q. R., Biddison, W. E., and Wiley, D. C. (1996). Structure of the complex between human T-cell receptor, viral peptide and HLA-A2. *Nature* 384, 134–141. doi:10.1038/384134a0

Garboczi, D. N., Hung, D. T., and Wiley, D. C. (1992). HLA-A2-peptide complexes: refolding and crystallization of molecules expressed in *Escherichia coli* and complexed with single antigenic peptides. *Proc. Natl. Acad. Sci. U.S.A.* 89, 3429–3433. doi:10.1073/pnas.89.8.3429

Hawse, W. F., Champion, M. M., Joyce, M. V., Hellman, L. M., Hossain, M., Ryan, V., et al. (2012). Cutting edge: evidence for a dynamically driven T cell signaling mechanism. *J. Immunol.* 188, 5819–5823. doi:10.4049/jimmunol.1200952

Holland, C. J., Rizkallah, P. J., Vollers, S., Calvo-Calle, J. M., Madura, F., Fuller, A., et al. (2012). Minimal conformational plasticity enables TCR cross-reactivity to different MHC class II heterodimers. *Sci. Rep.* 2, 629. doi:10.1038/srep00629

Holler, P. D., Chlewicki, L. K., and Kranz, D. M. (2003). TCRs with high affinity for foreign pMHC show self-reactivity. *Nat. Immunol.* 4, 55–62. doi:10.1038/ni863

Kjer-Nielsen, L., Clements, C. S., Brooks, A. G., Purcell, A. W., Mccluskey, J., and Rossjohn, J. (2002). The 1.5 A crystal structure of a highly selected antiviral T cell receptor provides evidence for a structural basis of immunodominance. *Structure* 10, 1521–1532. doi:10.1016/S0969-2126(02)00878-X

Klenerman, P., and Zinkernagel, R. M. (1998). Original antigenic sin impairs cytotoxic T lymphocyte responses to viruses bearing variant epitopes. *Nature* 394, 482–485. doi:10.1038/28860

Laugel, B., Boulter, J. M., Lissin, N., Vuidepot, A., Li, Y., Gostick, E., et al. (2005). Design of soluble recombinant T cell receptors for antigen targeting and T cell inhibition. *J. Biol. Chem.* 280, 1882–1892. doi:10.1074/jbc.M409427200

Lawrence, M. C., and Colman, P. M. (1993). Shape complementarity at protein/protein interfaces. *J. Mol. Biol.* 234, 946–950. doi:10.1006/jmbi.1993.1648

Li, Y., Moysey, R., Molloy, P. E., Vuidepot, A. L., Mahon, T., Baston, E., et al. (2005). Directed evolution of human T-cell receptors with picomolar affinities by phage display. *Nat. Biotechnol.* 23, 349–354. doi:10.1038/nbt1070

Liddy, N., Bossi, G., Adams, K. J., Lissina, A., Mahon, T. M., Hassan, N. J., et al. (2012). Monoclonal TCR-redirected tumor cell killing. *Nat. Med.* 18, 980–987. doi:10.1038/nm.2764

Madura, F., Rizkallah, P. J., Miles, K. M., Holland, C. J., Bulek, A. M., Fuller, A., et al. (2013). T-cell receptor specificity maintained by altered thermodynamics. *J. Biol. Chem.* doi:10.1074/jbc.M113.464560. [Epub ahead of print].

Mason, D. (1998). A very high level of crossreactivity is an essential feature of the T-cell receptor. *Immunol. Today* 19, 395–404. doi:10.1016/S0167-5699(98)01299-7

McCoy, A. J., Grosse-Kunstleve, R. W., Adams, P. D., Winn, M. D., Storoni, L. C., and Read, R. J. (2007). Phaser crystallographic software. *J. Appl. Crystallogr.* 40, 658–674. doi:10.1107/S0021889807021206

Miles, J. J., Bulek, A. M., Cole, D. K., Gostick, E., Schauenburg, A. J., Dolton, G., et al. (2010). Genetic and structural basis for selection of a ubiquitous T cell receptor deployed in Epstein-Barr virus infection. *PLoS Pathog.* 6:e1001198. doi:10.1371/journal.ppat.1001198

Miles, K. M., Miles, J. J., Madura, F., Sewell, A. K., and Cole, D. K. (2011). Real time detection of peptide-MHC dissociation reveals that improvement of primary MHC-binding residues can have a minimal, or no, effect on stability. *Mol. Immunol.* 48, 728–732. doi:10.1016/j.molimm.2010.11.004

Morgan, R. A., Dudley, M. E., Wunderlich, J. R., Hughes, M. S., Yang, J. C., Sherry, R. M., et al. (2006). Cancer regression in patients after transfer of genetically engineered lymphocytes. *Science* 314, 126–129. doi:10.1126/science.1129003

O'callaghan, C. A., Byford, M. F., Wyer, J. R., Willcox, B. E., Jakobsen, B. K., Mcmichael, A. J., et al. (1999). BirA enzyme: production and application in the study of membrane receptor-ligand interactions by site-specific biotinylation. *Anal. Biochem.* 266, 9–15. doi:10.1006/abio.1998.2930

Overbaugh, J., and Bangham, C. R. (2001). Selection forces and constraints on retroviral sequence variation. *Science* 292, 1106–1109. doi:10.1126/science.1059128

Parkhurst, M. R., Riley, J. P., Igarashi, T., Li, Y., Robbins, P. F., and Rosenberg, S. A. (2004). Immunization of patients with the hTERT:540-548 peptide induces peptide-reactive T lymphocytes that do not recognize tumors endogenously expressing telomerase. *Clin. Cancer Res.* 10, 4688–4698. doi:10.1158/1078-0432.CCR-04-0325

Piepenbrink, K. H., Borbulevych, O. Y., Sommese, R. F., Clemens, J., Armstrong, K. M., Desmond, C., et al. (2009). Fluorine substitutions in an antigenic peptide selectively modulate T-cell receptor binding in a minimally perturbing manner. *Biochem. J.* 423, 353–361. doi:10.1042/BJ20090732

Reinherz, E. L., Tan, K., Tang, L., Kern, P., Liu, J., Xiong, Y., et al. (1999). The crystal structure of a T cell receptor in complex with peptide and MHC class II. *Science* 286, 1913–1921. doi:10.1126/science.286.5446.1913

Renkvist, N., Castelli, C., Robbins, P. F., and Parmiani, G. (2001). A listing of human tumor antigens recognized by T cells. *Cancer Immunol. Immunother.* 50, 3–15. doi:10.1007/s002620000169

Rudolph, M. G., Stanfield, R. L., and Wilson, I. A. (2006). How TCRs bind MHCs, peptides, and coreceptors. *Annu. Rev. Immunol.* 24, 419–466. doi:10.1146/annurev.immunol.23.021704.115658

Sami, M., Rizkallah, P. J., Dunn, S., Molloy, P., Moysey, R., Vuidepot, A., et al. (2007). Crystal structures of high affinity human T-cell receptors bound to peptide major histocompatibility complex reveal native diagonal binding geometry. *Protein Eng. Des. Sel.* 20, 397–403. doi:10.1093/protein/gzm033

Scott, D. R., Borbulevych, O. Y., Piepenbrink, K. H., Corcelli, S. A., and Baker, B. M. (2011). Disparate degrees of hypervariable loop flexibility control T-cell receptor cross-reactivity, specificity, and binding mechanism. *J. Mol. Biol.* 414, 385–400. doi:10.1016/j.jmb.2011.10.006

Sewell, A. K. (2012). Why must T cells be cross-reactive? *Nat. Rev. Immunol.* 12, 669–677. doi:10.1038/nri3279

Stewart-Jones, G. B., Mcmichael, A. J., Bell, J. I., Stuart, D. I., and Jones, E. Y. (2003). A structural basis for immunodominant human T cell receptor recognition. *Nat. Immunol.* 4, 657–663. doi:10.1038/ni942

Tickle, I. J., Laskowski, R. A., and Moss, D. S. (2000). Rfree and the rfree ratio. II. Calculation of the expected values and variances of cross-validation statistics in macromolecular least-squares refinement. *Acta Crystallogr. D Biol. Crystallogr.* 56, 442–450. doi:10.1107/S0907444999016868

Varela-Rohena, A., Molloy, P. E., Dunn, S. M., Li, Y., Suhoski, M. M., Carroll, R. G., et al. (2008). Control of HIV-1 immune escape by CD8 T cells expressing enhanced T-cell receptor. *Nat. Med.* 14, 1390–1395. doi:10.1038/nm.1779

Vine, A. M., Heaps, A. G., Kaftantzi, L., Mosley, A., Asquith, B., Witkover, A., et al. (2004). The role of CTLs in persistent viral infection: cytolytic gene expression in CD8+ lymphocytes distinguishes between individuals with a high or low proviral load of human T cell lymphotropic virus type 1. *J. Immunol.* 173, 5121–5129.

Winter, G. (2010). Xia2: an expert system for macromolecular crystallography data reduction. *J. Appl. Cryst.* 43, 186–190. doi:10.1107/S0021889809045701

Wooldridge, L., Ekeruche-Makinde, J., Van Den Berg, H. A., Skowera, A., Miles, J. J., Tan, M. P., et al. (2012). A single autoimmune T cell receptor recognizes more than a million different peptides. *J. Biol. Chem.* 287, 1168–1177. doi:10.1074/jbc.M111.289488

10

Model T cells: a time-tested vehicle for gene therapy

Sid P. Kerkar *

Laboratory of Pathology, Center for Cancer Research, National Cancer Institute, National Institutes of Health, Bethesda, MD, USA

Edited by:
Bruno Laugel, Cardiff University School of Medicine, UK

Reviewed by:
David L. Wiest, Fox Chase Cancer Center, USA
Bruno Laugel, Cardiff University School of Medicine, UK

***Correspondence:**
Sid P. Kerkar, Laboratory of Pathology, Center for Cancer Research, National Cancer Institute, NIH Clinical Center, Room 2B38, Building 10, 10 Center Drive, Bethesda, MD 20892, USA
e-mail: kerkars@mail.nih.gov, spkerkar@yahoo.com

T lymphocytes first carried foreign genes safely into humans over two decades ago. Since these pioneering studies, scientific techniques to better understand the genomic landscape of cells has directly led to a more sophisticated appreciation of the diversity, functional complexity, and therapeutic potential of T cells. Through the use of mouse models, we now know the function of the many genes that are critical for T cells to recognize foreign, mutated, or self-antigens and the factors responsible for the lineage diversification of T cells that lead to inhibitory or stimulatory immune responses. This knowledge combined with well-established modalities to introduce genes into T cells allows for the design of effector and memory CD8 and CD4 T lymphocytes specific for viral, fungal, bacterial, parasitic, and tumor-antigens and to design regulatory lymphocytes specific for the self-antigens responsible for autoimmune and inflammatory diseases. Here, I review strategies for designing the ideal T cell by introducing genes controlling (1) the secretion of cytokines/chemokines and their receptors, (2) T-cell receptor specificity, (3) chimeric-antigen receptors that enable for the recognition of surface antigens in an MHC-independent fashion, (4) co-stimulatory/inhibitory surface molecules, and (5) disease defining single-gene factors.

Keywords: gene therapy, cancer, immunotherapy, T cells, inflammation, chimeric-antigen receptors, cytokines, severe combined immunodeficiency

INTRODUCTION

The Deoxyribonucleic acid (DNA) molecule, perhaps one of biology's greatest discoveries, helped unlock the secrets to the flow of genetic information that we now know forms the basis for the complexity of all life on earth. In the 1960s, the scientific community demonstrated for the first time that exogenous DNA could be taken up and ectopically expressed in mammalian cell lines (1). Shortly after, a growing understanding of viral reverse transcription processes and advances in recombinant DNA technologies paved the way for engineering viruses to carry therapeutic genes into cells (2).

Fast-forward 40 years and there now exists numerous viral and non-viral modalities to introduce therapeutic genes into cells. The most common viral vectors include retroviruses, adenovirus, and herpes simplex viral backbones with non-viral modalities centered on physical (DNA transfection/electroporation) or chemical (synthetic oligonucleotides, lipoplexes, nanoparticles) methods of delivery and transposon systems (3–6). Of these various modalities, gene therapy using retroviral based vectors is perhaps the most established methodology both in experimental models and in human clinical trials due to the ability to stably integrate genes into dividing cells (7–9).

In addition to the technologic advancements in gene therapy, a growing understanding of the genetic causes of human disease and the downstream function and network-like interactions between specific genes are enabling scientists to devise strategies to treat ailments once thought incurable (10, 11). While the *in vivo* delivery of genes targeting specific cell types remains a grand hope for the future, current methodologies readily enable for the stable introduction of foreign genes into cells *ex vivo*, allowing for the transfer of these cells back into patients (6).

T lymphocytes represent the ideal vehicle for carrying therapeutic genes into humans. T cells are easily obtained through peripheral blood draws or apheresis procedures and can be induced to divide robustly *ex vivo*, a characteristic that allows them to be highly permissible to retroviral introduction of ectopic genes (12). The first clinical trial to safely infuse a foreign gene into humans consisted of transducing tumor-infiltrating lymphocytes with a neomycin resistant gene that enabled for the detection of the transgene within a tumor biopsy several days following transfer (13). Today, the adoptive transfer of tumor-infiltrating lymphocytes combined with total-body irradiation, lymphodepleting chemotherapy, and high-dose IL-2 achieve response rates as high as 70% in patients with metastatic melanoma (14). The rapid development of gene therapy in this field promises to vastly improve current cellular therapies and opens the door to treat cancers of various histologies and wider arrays of human disease. Here, I discuss potential therapeutic genes that may improve current gene therapies, although rigorous pre-clinical testing and careful phase 1 clinical trials will be required for many of the suggestions in this review.

CYTOKINES, CHEMOKINES, AND THEIR RECEPTORS

The theory of immune surveillance in cancer is controversial but there exists reproducible scientific data pointing to the importance of interferon-gamma as a critical mediator for the elimination of malignantly transformed cells (15). Furthermore, there is a clear increase in the incidence of cancer in patients with HIV, Immunodeficiency syndromes triggered by mutations in genes such as GATA-2 (MonoMAC) and post-transplant patients receiving immune-suppressive drugs (16, 17).

Additional support for the importance of an immune response for cancer elimination can be garnered from clinical data with robust long-term follow up showing the ability of systemic IL-2, anti-CTLA-4 antibodies, and anti-PD-1/anti-PD-L1 antibodies, and the adoptive transfer of T lymphocytes to induce tumor regression in patients with metastatic melanoma and metastatic renal cell carcinoma (18, 19). Three major factors are important for an effective immune response against cancer: (1) overcoming suppressive factors induced by mutated cancer cells within the tumor microenvironment, (2) the quality of the T cells transferred, and (3) polymorphic factors of an individual's host immune response. Some of these factors can be readily modified by over-expressing cytokines, chemokines, and their receptors in transferred T cells, enabling lymphocytes to secrete supra-physiologic amounts of therapeutic immune-stimulatory molecules.

THE IL-12/IFN-γ/TH-1 AXIS

IL-12 is a hallmark inflammatory cytokine and is critical for driving an effective immunologic response against cancer and foreign pathogens (20). It is mainly produced by inflammatory cells such as dendritic cells, macrophages, and neutrophils and directly augments the functionality of multiple end effectors such as $CD4^+$ T cells, $CD8^+$ T cells, natural killer (NK) cells, and NKT cells (20). The anti-tumor effects of IL-12 are well documented (21). IL-12 enhances the ability of $CD8^+$ T cells to cause the regression of large established tumors by potently stimulating the production of high-levels of IFN-γ, resulting in an increase in the cross-presentation of tumor-antigens and the reversal of suppressive functions of myeloid-derived suppressor cells, alternatively activated macrophages, and dendritic cells (22). These changes subsequently lead to the collapse of the tumor stroma and the regression of large established masses (22, 23).

Unlike activated lymph nodes stimulated by pathogen-activated molecular patterns, sterile conditions within tumors lead to low levels of IL-12 secretion by innate immune cells. This lack of a danger signal within the tumor microenvironment results in a skewing away from a Th-1 type effector immune response. One attractive approach is to increase the levels of IL-12 directly at the point of T-cell/Tumor cell and T-cell/Antigen-presenting contact within tumors (24) (**Figure 1**). Several studies show that over-expressing a single-chain, functionally active IL-12 gene in tumor-antigen-specific lymphocytes significantly increases the levels of IL-12 to supra-physiological levels within tumors, leading to the regression of large established masses (25–28). This modification enables for therapeutic anti-tumor immunity with smaller numbers of T cells and does not require the use of systemic gamma-chain cytokines to support the transfer of cells *in vivo*. Currently, clinical trials are determining if the benefits of IL-12 gene therapy outweigh the many risks associated with a systemic increase in IL-12 and IFN-γ.

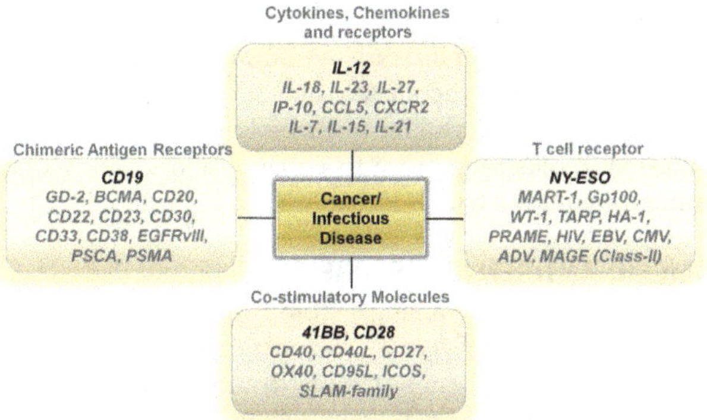

FIGURE 1 | Potential therapeutic gene therapies in T cells for Cancer and Infectious Diseases.

ADDITIONAL CYTOKINES, CHEMOKINES, AND CHEMOKINE RECEPTORS

The importance of gamma-chain cytokines in the proliferation and maintenance of memory T cells remains a critical and extremely important avenue of research for many investigators (29–32). However, clinical trials using TIL transduced with the IL-2 gene did not show a clinical benefit (33). Over-expressing the other gamma-chain cytokines such as IL-7, IL-15, or IL-21 in T cells may lead to better results. However, the constitutive expression of genes that drive T-cell proliferation carries the risk of causing an uncontrollable expansion of transferred T cells due to the stable integration of retrovirally transduced genes being expressed in every daughter cell (**Figure 1**). Designing viral vectors using a NFAT promoter for inducible gene expression upon T-cell receptor (TCR) ligation may provide an important degree of safety (26). Another strategy is to use adenoviral vectors or systems that only transiently express the genes that control T-cell memory formation.

Other potentially attractive cytokines include those within the IL-12 family, such as IL-23, and IL-27 (**Figure 1**). These cytokines may invoke beneficial downstream mechanisms for anti-tumor immunity without the heavy reliance on the induction of IFN-γ secretion. Furthermore, genetic polymorphisms within the human population may make certain individuals more likely to mount an anti-tumor response to one of the alternate members of the IL-12 family rather than IL-12 itself.

Another strategy that may turn out to be fruitful is the over-expression of chemokines and chemokine receptors in T cells (**Figure 1**). Melanomas can secrete chemokines such as CXCL1 and CXCL8 to aid in the recruitment of monocytes into local microenvironments and studies show that expressing the chemokine receptor CXCR2 on transferred T cells aids in the ability of T cells to infiltrate tumors and cause regression (34). This approach can be easily tailored to other tumor histologies depending on the chemokine secretion profile of the cancer. Additionally, over-expressing chemokines in T cells may also provide some benefit. Upon recognizing cognate antigens, T cells arrest their migration and accumulate at sites with productive antigen presentation. The over-expression of chemokines such as IP-10 or CCL5 in transferred T cells may enable antigen-specific T cells to secrete products that attract activated T cells to the local microenvironment they inhabit. This in turn may provide a positive feedback loop that enables for an increase in infiltrating antigen-specific T cells and an improved therapeutic outcome. Thus, the possibility to genetically alter the cytokine or chemokine profile of adoptively transferred T cells may prove to enhance and simplify current treatments requiring lymphodepletion and high-dose IL-2.

CHIMERIC-ANTIGEN RECEPTORS

The ability to generate a single fusion molecule that can bind surface antigens and trigger T-cell function holds great promise for the future of cell therapy. Chimeric-antigen receptors (CAR) are the latest form of gene therapy, where a single vector is constructed with a binding moiety recognizing a surface antigen [usually designed from a single-chain variable fragment (scFv) derived from a tumor-antigen-specific monoclonal antibody] (35–37). The beauty of CAR generated T cells is the ability to generate lymphocyte specificity in an MHC-independent fashion due to the ability to design receptors that recognize surface antigens. This is accomplished by cloning the sequences from the variable region of antibodies (many of which already exist) and adding T-cell signaling and co-stimulatory domains to the vector construct.

Early phase trials for CARs recognizing the antigen CD19, expressed on many B cell lymphomas and leukemias are showing promising results in adult and pediatric patients at multiple institutions (38–41). One of the major advantages of using CARs as the main platform for gene therapy is the ability to rapidly and clearly define the expression of the target protein. Often, the antibodies whose variable region is cloned into the CAR vector can also be used diagnostically to look for the expression of the desired target.

Other antigen targets that may be worthwhile exploring for CAR development includes GD-2 for neuroblastomas (42), CD20 (43), and CD22 for B cell lymphomas (44), BCMA (B cell maturation antigen) (45), and CD38 for multiple myeloma (46), CD23 for chronic lymphocytic leukemia/small lymphocytic lymphoma (CLL/SLL) (47), CD30 for Hodgkin's lymphoma and anaplastic large cell lymphomas (48), CD33 for acute myeloid leukemias (49), EGFRvIII for glioblastomas (50) and PSCA (51) and PSMA (52) for prostate adenocarcinomas (**Figure 1**).

T-CELL RECEPTORS

Although CAR-directed gene therapy remains a promising modality for the future, many cancers, especially carcinomas and sarcomas, do not possess known surface expression of unique non-shared antigens. Targeting surface proteins that may be expressed on normal tissue with CARs may cause serious end organ damage and toxicity. Gene therapy using high avidity TCR enables for the design of lymphocytes targeting epitopes from differentially expressed or mutated intra-nuclear and/or intra-cytoplasmic proteins such as transcription factors (22, 53). Emerging data now shows that tumor-infiltrating lymphocytes possess the ability to recognize mutated melanoma antigens (54, 55). This exciting finding opens up a large window of opportunity to develop effective TCR gene therapies. It is possible that in the future we may perform whole exome sequencing for every tumor for diagnostic purposes, enabling us to design TCR recognizing the most frequently mutated epitopes for different tumor histologies.

A great example of the success of TCR gene therapy was recently described with a clinical trial utilizing the NY-ESO TCR (56). This study led to significant tumor regression in four out of six patients with synovial sarcoma and five out of 11 patients with metastatic melanoma. Overall, the cancer-testis antigens represent an ideal set of target antigens due to their relatively low to negligible expression on normal tissue, except in the testis, where cells express low levels of MHC Class I. Identifying antigens with limited normal tissue distribution will be critical to extending TCR gene therapy to different types of cancer. Developing TCRs for breast, prostate, and thyroid cancer also seems reasonable since targeting of normal tissue in these organs might not be accompanied with serious life-threatening adverse events (**Figure 1**).

CO-STIMULATORY MOLECULES

Generating both a specific and a productive T-cell response requires not only appropriate signaling through the TCR but an additional secondary co-stimulatory signal. The most well studied co-stimulatory molecule is CD28, a disulfide linked homodimer that is constitutively expressed on naive T cells (57). CD28 engagement with CD80 and CD86 on antigen-presenting cells enables T cells to differentiate and become functionally activated (57). However, after initial antigen encounter and under altered cytokine conditions, T cells can lose or decrease their expression of CD28, leading to replicative senescence and functional anergy. The lack of CD28 signaling can also result in an impaired memory response and activation induced cell death (AICD) (58). One strategy to circumvent these physiological restraints is to constitutively over-express CD28 in T cells. Currently, second and third generation CAR constructs use the intracellular domain of CD28 to improve the persistence, function, and activity of CAR transduced T cells (59). Other important co-stimulatory molecules include 41BB, CD27, OX40, CD40, CD27, ICOS, Fas ligand, and the Slam family of proteins (60, 61). These molecules all have been implicated in tipping the balance in favor of generating a functional T-cell response and helping avoid AICD during antigen re-stimulation. The intracellular domains of 41BB, OX40, and CD27 are currently being incorporated into various CAR constructs that are being developed. Thus, it is possible that the constitutive over-expression of these various co-stimulatory molecules may aid in designing long lived, functionally active T cells that are resistant to cellular senescence (**Figure 1**).

SEVERE COMBINED IMMUNODEFICIENCY SYNDROMES

The first successful therapeutic gene therapy in humans in the early 1990s involved treating two children with severe combined immunodeficiency syndrome (SCID) caused by a genetic defect in the enzyme adenosine deaminase (SCID-ADA) (62). This syndrome resulted in defective T and B cells, leading to debilitating recurrent opportunistic infections. A normal/wild type ADA gene, enabling for the production of a functional enzyme, was introduced into T cells and infused back into the patient. The results were striking, and for the first time in these patients, there was evidence for IgM antibody production and the detection of tetanus antibody in the serum following immunization (62). In one patient, approximately 20% of the circulating lymphocytes still expressed the retrovirally inserted gene 10 years following transfer (63).

Although these initial results led to heightened optimism, attempts to develop gene therapies for SCID-X1, a disease characterized by a defective common gamma-c cytokine receptor subunit, by retroviral transfer of the corrected gene into CD34+ hematopoietic stem cells, led to the development of leukemias in some patients (64, 65). These setbacks sent shock waves through the scientific and medical communities. We now know that retroviral vectors can result in insertional mutagenesis, although this phenomenon still remains poorly understood (66). Five out of 20 patients treated in trials carried out in London and Paris developed leukemias secondary to the expansion of clones containing vector integration near proto-oncogenes such as *CCND* and *LMO2* (65).

Despite the clear dangers of gamma-retroviral gene transfer into hematopoietic stem cells, transferring genes into T cells *ex vivo* appears to be much more resistant to oncogenic transformation. There now exists robust long-term follow up for over a 100 patients treated on various gene therapy trials utilizing *ex vivo* retroviral insertion of genes into T cells with no evidence of malignant transformation (9). The mechanisms for the differences in oncogenesis between transducing hematopoietic stem cells versus T cells is not well understood. Perhaps introducing genes into more differentiated cells that contain a vastly different genetic and epigenetic landscape from stem cells leads to retroviral integration away from oncogenes.

Currently, gene therapists are continuing to try to improve safety through vector design. One strategy gaining support includes creating self inactivating gamma (SIN) retroviral vectors and lentiviral vectors by deleting the U3 region in the 3′ LTR (67). This modification generates a pro-virus with defective transcriptional activity at both the 5′ and 3′ LTR end regions, preventing the possibility of transcriptionally activating cellular oncogenes near the site of viral integration. Importantly, an internal promoter will need to be designed to drive the expression of the desired transgene within the SIN vector construct. Additionally safety measures include the genetic modification of shorter lived cell populations or the use of suicide genes (68).

The current progress in improving the safety of gene therapies is helping the field move forward. In regard to SCID, although mutations in the common gamma-c chain receptor is the most common cause of the disease, a broad range of single-gene mutations can result in a similar disease pattern of recurrent opportunistic infections (**Figure 2**). Theoretically, for all the various defects that may occur, introducing a correctly functioning gene *ex vivo* into T cells or hematopoietic stem cells/monocyte/dendritic cell populations may re-capitulate the early excitement seen in the SCID-ADA trials and build on the recent successes of gene therapy for cancer.

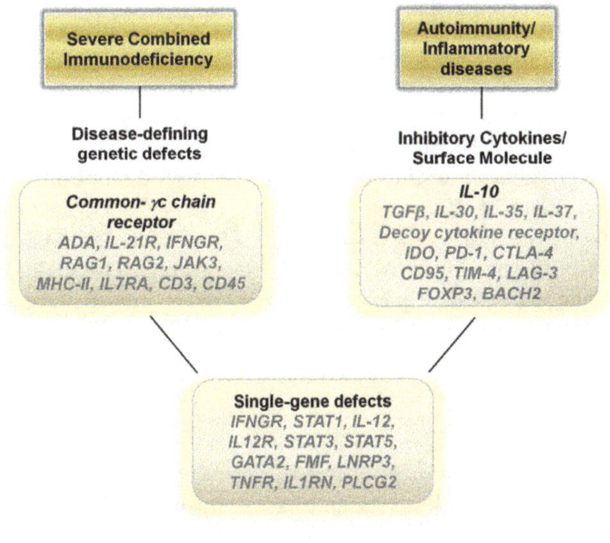

FIGURE 2 | Potential therapeutic genes to over-express in hematopoietic stem cells, monocytes, dendritic cells or T cells for autoimmune, inflammatory, and single-gene disorders.

AUTOIMMUNE AND INFLAMMATORY DISEASES

Although genetic modifications to stimulate the immune system is beneficial for battling infectious organisms and cancer, there also exists a set of devastating diseases that are caused by an over-zealous and unchecked immune response. The targeting of self-antigens under normal physiologic conditions can cause a range of serious ailments including type 1 diabetes, multiple sclerosis, rheumatoid arthritis, systemic lupus erythematosus, and autoimmune encephalomyelitis. Recently, a relatively new set of autoimmune diseases categorized as autoinflammatory diseases are beginning to be characterized such as familial Mediterranean fever (FMF), neonatal onset multisystem inflammatory disease (NOMID), tumor necrosis factor (TNF) receptor-associated periodic syndrome (TRAPS), deficiency of the Interleukin-1 receptor antagonist (DIRA) and Behcet's disease (69, 70). Additional inflammatory diseases that cause morbidity and mortality in a large number of patients include inflammatory bowel disease (Crohn's disease and ulcerative colitis), chronic granulomatous disease (CGD), and the various forms of vasculitis (71, 72).

In general, dampening the immune response is the ideal treatment for autoimmune and inflammatory diseases and current therapies revolve around the use of steroids, cytokine antagonists, or directly down regulating the immune system utilizing various modalities. Gene therapies may provide a viable biological alterative to directly blunt an over-active immune response. Over-expressing anti-inflammatory cytokines such as IL-10, TGF-β, IL-30, IL-35, or IL-37 in T cells or monocyte/dendritic cell populations *ex vivo* with a re-infusion of the modified cells may aid in decreasing inflammatory driven symptoms (**Figure 2**). Another alternative may be to construct a decoy cytokine receptor that contains the correct receptor sequence to enable for binding of pro-inflammatory cytokines such as IL-12 combined with a non-functioning cytoplasmic signal transducing sequence. Over-expressing these "dominant-negative" receptors would enable re-infused immune cells to function as sinks for the inflammatory cytokines responsible for the pathophysiology of the disease. Other genes that may aid in dampening the immune response include over-expressing indoleamine 2,3-dioxygenase in monocytes/dendritic cells or *CTLA-4*, *PD-1*, *CD95*, *LAG-3*, *FOXP3*, and *BACH2* in T cells (73) (**Figure 2**).

SINGLE-GENE DEFECTS

Although many human diseases are caused by complex genetic polymorphisms, perhaps the greatest potential for gene therapy is in the ability to treat diseases caused by single Mendelian gene defects. Mutations in genes such as *IFNGR1*, *STAT1*, *IL-12*, and *IL-12R* can lead to immune dysfunction and recurrent mycobacterial infections (74). Genetic disruptions also cause many of the autoinflammatory diseases, such as mutations in the *FMF* gene in FMF, the *LNRP3* gene in NOMID, the *TNFR* gene in TRAPs, and *IL1RN* gene in DIRA. Inserting the corrected sequence for these genes into hematopoietic cells or more safely into differentiated immune cells may result in dramatic improvements in the health of these patients (**Figure 2**).

CONCLUSION

T lymphocytes represent one of the first vehicles to carry therapeutic genes into humans, and its current use, centered on the adoptive transfer of T cells, is proving to be a promising cancer therapeutic modality. However, logistic hurdles still exist for the wider use of this technology due to costs associated with GMP quality viral production and the requirement of significant technologic infrastructure and expertise. Increased collaboration between industry and academia for developing gene therapies may help overcome current financial limitations by developing viable business models.

There exist over 4000 known single-gene disease causing disorders in addition to the innumerable genetic polymorphisms that increase susceptibilities for diseases. Gene therapy in T cells is paving the way for a broader application of this therapeutic modality in human disease. The ability to stably introduce functional genes into hematopoietic stem cells or differentiated cells *ex vivo* provides hope for the thousands of patients diagnosed with a wide range of devastating genetic diseases, highlighted by recent successes in childhood cerebral adrenoleukodystrophy (75) and hemophilia B (76). Gene therapy represents the ultimate form of personalized medicine, and in the future, it is conceivable to imagine that diseases that were once considered untreatable will be readily controlled or eradicated with a single specialized treatment.

ACKNOWLEDGMENTS

This research was supported by the Intramural Research Program of the NIH, National Cancer Institute, Center for Cancer Research. The author has no conflicting financial interests.

REFERENCES

1. Friedmann T. A brief history of gene therapy. *Nat Genet* (1992) **2**(2):93–8. doi:10.1038/ng1092-93
2. Varmus HE. Form and function of retroviral proviruses. *Science* (1982) **216**(4548):812–20. doi:10.1126/science.6177038
3. Kay MA, Glorioso JC, Naldini L. Viral vectors for gene therapy: the art of turning infectious agents into vehicles of therapeutics. *Nat Med* (2001) **7**(1):33–40. doi:10.1038/83324
4. Wolff JA, Budker V. The mechanism of naked DNA uptake and expression. *Adv Genet* (2005) **54**:3–20.
5. Gao X, Kim KS, Liu D. Non-viral gene delivery: what we know and what is next. *AAPS J* (2007) **9**(1):E92–104. doi:10.1208/aapsj0901009
6. Naldini L. Ex vivo gene transfer and correction for cell-based therapies. *Nat Rev Genet* (2011) **12**(5):301–15. doi:10.1038/nrg2985
7. Hwu P, Rosenberg SA. The genetic modification of T cells for cancer therapy: an overview of laboratory and clinical trials. *Cancer Detect Prev* (1994) **18**(1):43–50.
8. Brenner MK. Gene transfer and the treatment of haematological malignancy. *J Intern Med* (2001) **249**(4):345–58. doi:10.1046/j.1365-2796.2001.00807.x
9. Scholler J, Brady TL, Binder-Scholl G, Hwang WT, Plesa G, Hege KM, et al. Decade-long safety and function of retroviral-modified chimeric antigen receptor T cells. *Sci Transl Med* (2012) **4**(132):132ra153. doi:10.1126/scitranslmed.3003761
10. Rao MS, Collins FS. Steering a new course for stem cell research: NIH's intramural center for regenerative medicine. *Stem Cells Transl Med* (2012) **1**(1):15–7. doi:10.5966/sctm.2011-0032
11. Varmus H, Kumar HS. Addressing the growing international challenge of cancer: a multinational perspective. *Sci Transl Med* (2013) **5**(175):175cm172. doi:10.1126/scitranslmed.3005899
12. Kershaw MH, Westwood JA, Darcy PK. Gene-engineered T cells for cancer therapy. *Nat Rev Cancer* (2013) **13**(8):525–41. doi:10.1038/nrc3565
13. Rosenberg SA, Aebersold P, Cornetta K, Kasid A, Morgan RA, Moen R, et al. Gene transfer into humans – immunotherapy of patients with advanced melanoma, using tumor-infiltrating lymphocytes modified by retroviral gene transduction. *N Engl J Med* (1990) **323**(9):570–8. doi:10.1056/NEJM199008303230904
14. Restifo NP, Dudley ME, Rosenberg SA. Adoptive immunotherapy for cancer: harnessing the T cell response. *Nat Rev Immunol* (2012) **12**(4):269–81. doi:10.1038/nri3191
15. Dighe AS, Richards E, Old LJ, Schreiber RD. Enhanced in vivo growth and resistance to rejection of tumor cells expressing dominant negative IFN gamma receptors. *Immunity* (1994) **1**(6):447–56. doi:10.1016/1074-7613(94)90087-6
16. Rosenzweig SD, Holland SM. Recent insights into the pathobiology of innate immune deficiencies. *Curr Allergy Asthma Rep* (2011) **11**(5):369–77. doi:10.1007/s11882-011-0212-9
17. O'Shea JJ, Holland SM, Staudt LM. JAKs and STATs in immunity, immunodeficiency, and cancer. *N Engl J Med* (2013) **368**(2):161–70. doi:10.1056/NEJMra1202117
18. Mellman I, Coukos G, Dranoff G. Cancer immunotherapy comes of age. *Nature* (2011) **480**(7378):480–9. doi:10.1038/nature10673
19. Sharma P, Wagner K, Wolchok JD, Allison JP. Novel cancer immunotherapy agents with survival benefit: recent successes and next steps. *Nat Rev Cancer* (2011) **11**(11):805–12. doi:10.1038/nrc3153
20. Trinchieri G. Interleukin-12 and the regulation of innate resistance and adaptive immunity. *Nat Rev Immunol* (2003) **3**(2):133–46. doi:10.1038/nri1001
21. Colombo MP, Trinchieri G. Interleukin-12 in anti-tumor immunity and immunotherapy. *Cytokine Growth Factor Rev* (2002) **13**(2):155–68. doi:10.1016/S1359-6101(01)00032-6
22. Kerkar SP, Goldszmid RS, Muranski P, Chinnasamy D, Yu Z, Reger RN, et al. IL-12 triggers a programmatic change in dysfunctional myeloid-derived cells within mouse tumors. *J Clin Invest* (2011) **121**(12):4746–57. doi:10.1172/JCI58814
23. Kerkar SP, Leonardi AJ, van Panhuys N, Zhang L, Yu Z, Crompton JG, et al. Collapse of the tumor stroma is triggered by IL-12 induction of Fas. *Mol Ther* (2013) **21**(7):1369–77. doi:10.1038/mt.2013.58
24. Kerkar SP, Muranski P, Kaiser A, Boni A, Sanchez-Perez L, Yu Z, et al. Tumor-specific CD8+ T cells expressing interleukin-12 eradicate established cancers in lymphodepleted hosts. *Cancer Res* (2010) **70**(17):6725–34. doi:10.1158/0008-5472.CAN-10-0735
25. Chmielewski M, Kopecky C, Hombach AA, Abken H. IL-12 release by engineered T cells expressing chimeric antigen receptors can effectively Muster an antigen-independent macrophage response on tumor cells that have shut down tumor antigen expression. *Cancer Res* (2011) **71**(17):5697–706. doi:10.1158/0008-5472.CAN-11-0103
26. Zhang L, Kerkar SP, Yu Z, Zheng Z, Yang S, Restifo NP, et al. Improving adoptive T cell therapy by targeting and controlling IL-12 expression to the tumor environment. *Mol Ther* (2011) **19**(4):751–9. doi:10.1038/mt.2010.313
27. Chinnasamy D, Yu Z, Kerkar SP, Zhang L, Morgan RA, Restifo NP, et al. Local delivery of interleukin-12 using T cells targeting VEGF receptor-2 eradicates multiple vascularized tumors in mice. *Clin Cancer Res* (2012) **18**(6):1672–83. doi:10.1158/1078-0432.CCR-11-3050

28. Pegram HJ, Lee JC, Hayman EG, Imperato GH, Tedder TF, Sadelain M, et al. Tumor-targeted T cells modified to secrete IL-12 eradicate systemic tumors without need for prior conditioning. *Blood* (2012) **119**(18): 4133–41. doi:10.1182/blood-2011-12-400044
29. Gattinoni L, Lugli E, Ji Y, Pos Z, Paulos CM, Quigley MF, et al. A human memory T cell subset with stem cell-like properties. *Nat Med* (2011) **17**(10):1290–7. doi:10.1038/nm.2446
30. Hinrichs CS, Borman ZA, Gattinoni L, Yu Z, Burns WR, Huang J, et al. Human effector CD8+ T cells derived from naive rather than memory subsets possess superior traits for adoptive immunotherapy. *Blood* (2011) **117**(3):808–14. doi:10.1182/blood-2010-05-286286
31. Klebanoff CA, Gattinoni L, Palmer DC, Muranski P, Ji Y, Hinrichs CS, et al. Determinants of successful CD8+ T-cell adoptive immunotherapy for large established tumors in mice. *Clin Cancer Res* (2011) **17**(16):5343–52. doi:10.1158/1078-0432.CCR-11-0503
32. Muranski P, Borman ZA, Kerkar SP, Klebanoff CA, Ji Y, Sanchez-Perez L, et al. Th17 cells are long lived and retain a stem cell-like molecular signature. *Immunity* (2011) **35**(6):972–85. doi:10.1016/j.immuni.2011.09.019
33. Heemskerk B, Liu K, Dudley ME, Johnson LA, Kaiser A, Downey S, et al. Adoptive cell therapy for patients with melanoma, using tumor-infiltrating lymphocytes genetically engineered to secrete interleukin-2. *Hum Gene Ther* (2008) **19**(5):496–510. doi:10.1089/hum.2007.0171
34. Peng W, Ye Y, Rabinovich BA, Liu C, Lou Y, Zhang M, et al. Transduction of tumor-specific T cells with CXCR2 chemokine receptor improves migration to tumor and antitumor immune responses. *Clin Cancer Res* (2010) **16**(22):5458–68. doi:10.1158/1078-0432.CCR-10-0712
35. Lee DW, Barrett DM, Mackall C, Orentas R, Grupp SA. The future is now: chimeric antigen receptors as new targeted therapies for childhood cancer. *Clin Cancer Res* (2012) **18**(10):2780–90. doi:10.1158/1078-0432.CCR-11-1920
36. Riddell SR, Jensen MC, June CH. Chimeric antigen receptor – modified T cells: clinical translation in stem cell transplantation and beyond. *Biol Blood Marrow Transplant* (2013) **19**(1 Suppl):S2–5. doi:10.1016/j.bbmt.2012.10.021
37. Sadelain M, Brentjens R, Rivière I. The basic principles of chimeric antigen receptor design. *Cancer Discov* (2013) **3**(4):388–98. doi:10.1158/2159-8290.CD-12-0548
38. Kochenderfer JN, Yu Z, Frasheri D, Restifo NP, Rosenberg SA. Adoptive transfer of syngeneic T cells transduced with a chimeric antigen receptor that recognizes murine CD19 can eradicate lymphoma and normal B cells. *Blood* (2010) **116**(19):3875–86. doi:10.1182/blood-2010-01-265041
39. Kalos M, Levine BL, Porter DL, Katz S, Grupp SA, Bagg A, et al. T cells with chimeric antigen receptors have potent antitumor effects and can establish memory in patients with advanced leukemia. *Sci Transl Med* (2011) **3**(95):95ra73. doi:10.1126/scitranslmed.3002842
40. Porter DL, Levine BL, Kalos M, Bagg A, June CH. Chimeric antigen receptor-modified T cells in chronic lymphoid leukemia. *N Engl J Med* (2011) **365**(8):725–33. doi:10.1056/NEJMoa1103849
41. Brentjens RJ, Davila ML, Riviere I, Park J, Wang X, Cowell LG, et al. CD19-targeted T cells rapidly induce molecular remissions in adults with chemotherapy-refractory acute lymphoblastic leukemia. *Sci Transl Med* (2013) **5**(177):177ra138. doi:10.1126/scitranslmed.3005930
42. Mujoo K, Cheresh DA, Yang HM, Reisfeld RA. Disialoganglioside GD2 on human neuroblastoma cells: target antigen for monoclonal antibody-mediated cytolysis and suppression of tumor growth. *Cancer Res* (1987) **47**(4): 1098–104.
43. Till BG, Jensen MC, Wang J, Qian X, Gopal AK, Maloney DG, et al. CD20-specific adoptive immunotherapy for lymphoma using a chimeric antigen receptor with both CD28 and 4-1BB domains: pilot clinical trial results. *Blood* (2012) **119**(17):3940–50. doi:10.1182/blood-2011-10-387969
44. Haso W, Lee DW, Shah NN, Stetler-Stevenson M, Yuan CM, Pastan IH, et al. Anti-CD22-chimeric antigen receptors targeting B-cell precursor acute lymphoblastic leukemia. *Blood* (2013) **121**(7):1165–74. doi:10.1182/blood-2012-06-438002
45. Carpenter RO, Evbuomwan MO, Pittaluga S, Rose JJ, Raffeld M, Yang S, et al. B-cell maturation antigen is a promising target for adoptive T-cell therapy of multiple myeloma. *Clin Cancer Res* (2013) **19**(8):2048–60. doi:10.1158/1078-0432.CCR-12-2422
46. Mihara K, Bhattacharyya J, Kitanaka A, Yanagihara K, Kubo T, Takei Y, et al. T-cell immunotherapy with a chimeric receptor against CD38 is effective in eliminating myeloma cells. *Leukemia* (2012) **26**(2):365–7. doi:10.1038/leu.2011.205
47. Giordano Attianese GM, Marin V, Hoyos V, Savoldo B, Pizzitola I, Tettamanti S, et al. In vitro and in vivo model of a novel immunotherapy approach for chronic lymphocytic leukemia by anti-CD23 chimeric antigen receptor. *Blood* (2011) **117**(18):4736–45. doi:10.1182/blood-2010-10-311845
48. Di Stasi A, De Angelis B, Rooney CM, Zhang L, Mahendravada A, Foster AE, et al. T lymphocytes coexpressing CCR4 and a chimeric antigen receptor targeting CD30 have improved homing and antitumor activity in a Hodgkin tumor model. *Blood* (2009) **113**(25):6392–402. doi:10.1182/blood-2009-03-209650
49. Dutour A, Marin V, Pizzitola I, Valsesia-Wittmann S, Lee D, Yvon E, et al. In vitro and in vivo antitumor effect of anti-CD33 chimeric receptor-expressing EBV-CTL against CD33 acute myeloid leukemia. *Adv Hematol* (2012) **2012**:683065. doi:10.1155/2012/683065
50. Morgan RA, Johnson LA, Davis JL, Zheng Z, Woolard KD, Reap EA, et al. Recognition of glioma stem cells by genetically modified T cells targeting EGFRvIII and development of adoptive cell therapy for glioma. *Hum Gene Ther* (2012) **23**(10):1043–53. doi:10.1089/hum.2012.041
51. Morgenroth A, Cartellieri M, Schmitz M, Günes S, Weigle B, Bachmann M, et al. Targeting of tumor cells expressing the prostate stem cell antigen (PSCA) using genetically engineered T-cells. *Prostate* (2007) **67**(10):1121–31. doi:10.1002/pros.20608
52. Ma Q, Safar M, Holmes E, Wang Y, Boynton AL, Junghans RP. Anti-prostate specific membrane antigen designer T cells for prostate cancer therapy. *Prostate* (2004) **61**(1):12–25. doi:10.1002/pros.20073
53. Merhavi-Shoham E, Haga-Friedman A, Cohen CJ. Genetically modulating T-cell function to target cancer. *Semin Cancer Biol* (2012) **22**(1):14–22. doi:10.1016/j.semcancer.2011.12.006
54. Lu YC, Yao X, Li YF, El-Gamil M, Dudley ME, Yang JC, et al. Mutated PPP1R3B is recognized by T cells used to treat a melanoma patient who experienced a durable complete tumor regression. *J Immunol* (2013) **190**(12):6034–42. doi:10.4049/jimmunol.1202830
55. Robbins PF, Lu YC, El-Gamil M, Li YF, Gross C, Gartner J, et al. Mining exomic sequencing data to identify mutated antigens recognized by adoptively transferred tumor-reactive T cells. *Nat Med* (2013) **19**(6):747–52. doi:10.1038/nm.3161
56. Robbins PF, Morgan RA, Feldman SA, Yang JC, Sherry RM, Dudley ME, et al. Tumor regression in patients with metastatic synovial cell sarcoma and melanoma using genetically engineered lymphocytes reactive with NY-ESO-1. *J Clin Oncol* (2011) **29**(7): 917–24. doi:10.1200/JCO.2010.32.2537
57. Shahinian A, Pfeffer K, Lee KP, Kündig TM, Kishihara K, Wakeham A, et al. Differential T cell costimulatory requirements in CD28-deficient mice. *Science* (1993) **261**(5121):609–12. doi:10.1126/science.7688139
58. Radvanyi LG, Shi Y, Vaziri H, Sharma A, Dhala R, Mills GB, et al. CD28 costimulation inhibits TCR-induced apoptosis during a primary T cell response. *J Immunol* (1996) **156**(5):1788–98.
59. Kowolik CM, Topp MS, Gonzalez S, Pfeiffer T, Olivares S, Gonzalez N, et al. CD28 costimulation provided through a CD19-specific chimeric antigen receptor enhances in vivo persistence and antitumor efficacy of adoptively transferred T cells. *Cancer Res* (2006) **66**(22):10995–1004. doi:10.1158/0008-5472.CAN-06-0160
60. Paulos CM, Carpenito C, Plesa G, Suhoski MM, Varela-Rohena A, Golovina TN, et al. The inducible costimulator (ICOS) is critical for the development of human T(H)17 cells. *Sci Transl Med* (2010) **2**(55):55ra78. doi:10.1126/scitranslmed.3000448
61. Song DG, Ye Q, Poussin M, Harms GM, Figini M, Powell DJ Jr. CD27 costimulation augments the survival and antitumor activity of redirected human T cells in vivo. *Blood* (2012) **119**(3):696–706. doi:10.1182/blood-2011-03-344275
62. Blaese RM, Culver KW, Miller AD, Carter CS, Fleisher T, Clerici M, et al. T lymphocyte-directed

gene therapy for ADA-SCID: initial trial results after 4 years. *Science* (1995) **270**(5235):475–80. doi: 10.1126/science.270.5235.475
63. Muul LM, Tuschong LM, Soenen SL, Jagadeesh GJ, Ramsey WJ, Long Z, et al. Persistence and expression of the adenosine deaminase gene for 12 years and immune reaction to gene transfer components: long-term results of the first clinical gene therapy trial. *Blood* (2003) **101**(7):2563–9. doi:10.1182/blood-2002-09-2800
64. Cavazzana-Calvo M, Hacein-Bey S, de SaintBasile G, Gross F, Yvon E, Nusbaum P, et al. Gene therapy of human severe combined immunodeficiency (SCID)-X1 disease. *Science* (2000) **288**(5466):669–72. doi: 10.1126/science.288.5466.669
65. Fischer A, Hacein-Bey-Abina S, Cavazzana-Calvo M. Gene therapy of primary T cell immunodeficiencies. *Gene* (2013) **525**(2):170–73. doi:10.1016/j.gene.2013.03.092
66. Knight S, Collins M, Takeuchi Y. Insertional mutagenesis by retroviral vectors: current concepts and methods of analysis. *Curr Gene Ther* (2013) **13**(3):211–27. doi:10.2174/1566523211313030006
67. Romano G. Development of safer gene delivery systems to minimize the risk of insertional mutagenesis-related malignancies: a critical issue for the field of gene therapy. *ISRN Oncol* (2012) **2012**:616310. doi:10.5402/2012/616310
68. Di Stasi A, Tey SK, Dotti G, Fujita Y, Kennedy-Nasser A, Martinez C, et al. Inducible apoptosis as a safety switch for adoptive cell therapy. *N Engl J Med* (2011) **365**(18):1673–83. doi:10.1056/NEJMoa1106152
69. Aksentijevich I, Kastner DL. Genetics of monogenic autoinflammatory diseases: past successes, future challenges. *Nat Rev Rheumatol* (2011) **7**(8):469–78. doi:10.1038/nrrheum.2011.94
70. Park H, Bourla AB, Kastner DL, Colbert RA, Siegel RM. Lighting the fires within: the cell biology of autoinflammatory diseases. *Nat Rev Immunol* (2012) **12**(8):570–80. doi:10.1038/nri3261
71. Strober W, Fuss I, Mannon P. The fundamental basis of inflammatory bowel disease. *J Clin Invest* (2007) **117**(3):514–21. doi:10.1172/JCI30587
72. Roos D, Kuhns DB, Maddalena A, Roesler J, Lopez JA, Ariga T, et al. Hematologically important mutations: X-linked chronic granulomatous disease (third update). *Blood Cells Mol Dis* (2010) **45**(3):246–65. doi:10.1016/j.bcmd.2010.07.012
73. Roychoudhuri R, Hirahara K, Mousavi K, Clever D, Klebanoff CA, Bonelli M, et al. BACH2 represses effector programs to stabilize T(reg)-mediated immune homeostasis. *Nature* (2013) **498**(7455):506–10. doi:10.1038/nature12199
74. Milner JD, Holland SM. The cup runneth over: lessons from the ever-expanding pool of primary immunodeficiency diseases. *Nat Rev Immunol* (2013) **13**(9):635–48. doi:10.1038/nri3493
75. Cartier N, Hacein-Bey-Abina S, Bartholomae CC, Veres G, Schmidt M, Kutschera I, et al. Hematopoietic stem cell gene therapy with a lentiviral vector in X-linked adrenoleukodystrophy. *Science* (2009) **326**(5954):818–23. doi:10.1126/science.1171242
76. Nathwani AC, Tuddenham EG, Rangarajan S, Rosales C, McIntosh J, Linch DC, et al. Adenovirus-associated virus vector-mediated gene transfer in hemophilia B. *N Engl J Med* (2011) **365**(25):2357–65. doi:10.1056/NEJMoa1108046

11

TCR-engineered T cells meet new challenges to treat solid tumors: choice of antigen, T cell fitness, and sensitization of tumor milieu

Andre Kunert[1,2]*, Trudy Straetemans[1,2], Coen Govers[1,2], Cor Lamers[1,2], Ron Mathijssen[2], Stefan Sleijfer[2] and Reno Debets[1,2]*

[1] Laboratory of Experimental Tumor Immunology, Erasmus MC Cancer Institute, Rotterdam, Netherlands
[2] Department of Medical Oncology, Erasmus MC Cancer Institute, Rotterdam, Netherlands

Edited by:
Bruno Laugel, Cardiff University School of Medicine, UK

Reviewed by:
Gavin Bendle, University of Birmingham, UK
Anna Mondino, San Raffaele Scientific Institute, Italy

***Correspondence:**
Andre Kunert and Reno Debets, Department of Medical Oncology, Laboratory of Experimental Tumor Immunology, Erasmus MC Cancer Institute, Dr. Molewaterplein 50, Rotterdam 3015 GE, Netherlands
e-mail: a.kunert@erasmusmc.nl; j.debets@erasmusmc.nl

Adoptive transfer of T cells gene-engineered with antigen-specific T cell receptors (TCRs) has proven its feasibility and therapeutic potential in the treatment of malignant tumors. To ensure further clinical development of TCR gene therapy, it is necessary to target immunogenic epitopes that are related to oncogenesis and selectively expressed by tumor tissue, and implement strategies that result in optimal T cell fitness. In addition, in particular for the treatment of solid tumors, it is equally necessary to include strategies that counteract the immune-suppressive nature of the tumor micro-environment. Here, we will provide an overview of the current status of TCR gene therapy, and redefine the following three challenges of improvement: "choice of target antigen"; "fitness of T cells"; and "sensitization of tumor milieu." We will categorize and discuss potential strategies to address each of these challenges, and argue that advancement of clinical TCR gene therapy critically depends on developments toward each of the three challenges.

Keywords: antigens, inhibitory micro-milieu, solid tumors, T cell avidity, T cell co-stimulation, T cells, TCR affinity, TCR transgenes

TCR GENE THERAPY: CLINICAL POTENCY AND TOXICITIES

T cells possess distinct properties such as the ability to specifically recognize tumor antigens, serially kill tumor cells, self-replicate, form memory and induce a complete tumor response. It is because of these properties that the therapeutic use of T cells in certain types of cancer may be advantageous when compared to drugs, antibodies, or small molecule inhibitors.

T cell therapy intends to treat cancer by transferring autologous and *ex vivo* expanded T cells to patients. Therapy with tumor-infiltrating T lymphocytes (TILs) preceded by non-myeloablative lymphodepletion resulted in objective responses in about 50% of metastatic melanoma patients in two different medical centers (1, 2). Equally notable were the durable complete responses observed in these trials that ranged between 10 and 22% (ongoing for more than 3 years) (1, 2). Likewise, adoptive transfer of tumor-specific T cell clones generated from autologous peripheral T cells resulted in regression of individual metastases, and responses in 8 out of 10 melanoma patients (3). In addition, co-culture of peripheral T cells with artificial antigen-presenting cells (APC) loaded with tumor antigens resulted in T cells that were clinically effective in four out of seven evaluable melanoma patients (4). Response rates observed with T cell therapy are generally higher than those observed for other treatments of melanoma, such as chemotherapeutic drugs, high-dose cytokines, inhibitors of kinases, or antibodies against T cell co-inhibitory molecules. See **Table 1** for an overview of clinical outcomes of T cell therapies and other treatments of melanoma.

Despite its clinical successes, T cell therapy has its limitations in availability and generation of therapeutic T cells for a larger group of patients. Genetic introduction of T cell receptors (TCRs) or chimeric antigen receptors (CARs) into autologous T cells, termed gene-engineering of T cells, can provide an alternative that is more widely applicable and can potentially be extended to multiple types of cancer (5). Key preclinical achievements and clinical tests with TCR-engineered T cells, the focus of the current review, are depicted in **Figures 1A,B**, respectively. Therapeutic advances with CAR-engineered T cells is reviewed elsewhere (6). The principle of clinical TCR gene therapy is straightforward: transferral of TCRαβ genes into T cells; *ex vivo* expansion of T cells; and infusion of T cells into the patient. In this way, TCRα and β genes are used as "off the shelf" reagents to confer tumor reactivity to patients whose tumor expresses the appropriate antigen and HLA restriction element. At the moment of writing this review, eight clinical trials using TCR-engineered T cells have reported their results (see **Figure 1B** and **Table 2** for details), and at least another 10 trials using TCR-engineered T cells are open and actively recruiting patients or will recruit patients soon[1].

Most clinical TCRs tested so far were HLA-A2-restricted and directed against either melanoma-associated antigen recognized by T cells 1 (MART-1), glycoprotein (gp) 100, carcinoembryonic antigen (CEA), p53, melanoma-associated antigen (MAGE-)A3, or New York esophageal squamous cell carcinoma antigen (NY-ESO)1. Another TCR tested clinically was HLA-A1-restricted and

[1] www.clinicaltrials.gov

Table 1 | Overview of standard and experimental none-gene-based therapies for metastatic melanoma.

Therapy	Function	Type of trial	OR (%)[a]	CR (%)[a]	Reference
T CELL THERAPY					
Tumor-infiltrating lymphocytes (TILs)	Adoptive transfer of tumor-specific T cells	n.c.	52/93 **(56)**	20/93 **(22)**	(1)
		n.c.	15/31 **(48)**	3/31 **(10)**	(2)[b]
T cell clones		n.c.	8/10 **(80)**	n.r.	(3)
"Educated T cells"		n.c.	4/9 **(44)**	1/9 **(11)**	(4)
STANDARD THERAPY					
High-dose IL-2	Cytokine that induces T cell growth	n.c.	43/270 **(16)**	16/270 **(6)**	(178)
Dacarbazine (DTIC)	Drug that alkylates DNA	Phase III trial	18/149 **(12)**	4/149 **(3)**	(179)
Vemurafenib (PLX-4032)	Small molecule that inhibits BRAF kinase activity	Phase III trial	106/219 **(48)**	2/219 **(1)**	(180)
EXPERIMENTAL THERAPY					
Dabrafenib	Small molecule that blocks BRAF kinase activity	Phase III trial	29/54 **(54)**	n.r.	(181)
Dabrafenib + Trametinib	Small molecules that block BRAF and MEK kinase activities	Phase III trial	41/54 **(76)**	n.r.	(181)
Ipilimumab (MDX-010) + vaccination	Antibody that blocks T cell CTLA4	Phase III trial	39/137 **(28)**	3/137 **(2)**	(182)
Ipilimumab + DTIC		Phase III trial	34/252 **(14)**	26/252 **(10)**	(183)
Nivolumab (MDX-1106)[c]	Antibody that blocks T cell PD1	Phase I trial	5/39 **(13)**	1/39 **(3)**	(184)
		Phase I trial	26/94 **(28)**	n.r.	(185)
Nivolumab + Ipilimumab		Phase I trial	21/53 **(40)**	n.r.	(186)
Lambrolizumab (MK-3475)	Antibody that blocks T cell PD1	Phase I trial	51/135 **(38)**	n.r.	(187)
Anti-PD-L1 (MDX-1105)	Antibody that blocks tumor cell PDL1	Phase I trial	17/135 **(13)**	n.r.	(188)

[a] OR, objective responses; CR, complete responses; both according to Response Evaluation Criteria for Solid Tumors (RECIST). Number of patients with responses = before dash; total number of patients treated = after dash; percentage of responses = between brackets.

[b] Dr. Jacob Schachter, Cellular Therapy of Cancer Symposium, September 24–27th, Montpellier, France, 2010.

[c] This study included patients with metastatic melanoma, but also patients with renal cell carcinoma, colorectal cancer, prostate cancer, and non-small-cell lung cancer. BRAF, gene responsible for production of B-Raf-kinase; CTLA4, cytotoxic T-lymphocyte antigen 4; IL-2, Interleukin 2; n.c., not classified; n.r., none reported; mAb, monoclonal antibody; MAPK, mitogen-activated protein kinase; PD1, programed cell death 1 receptor; PDL1, programed cell death 1 ligand.

directed against MAGE-A3. Collectively, these trials have not only demonstrated feasibility but also demonstrated significant clinical responses in patients with metastatic melanoma, colorectal carcinoma, and synovial sarcoma (**Table 2**). Responses, although variable and tested in a cumulative number of about 80 patients (based on trials listed in **Table 2**), ranged from 12 to 67%. Notably, the finding that TCR gene-engineered T cells were able to traffic to the central nervous system and cause complete responses of brain metastasis in patients with melanoma was not only encouraging but also underscored the strength of T cell therapy toward metastasized and poorly accessible tumors (7). Clinical testing, however, also clearly demonstrated that therapy is currently hampered by treatment-related toxicity and a transient nature of tumor regression. Treatment-related toxicity became evident from studies with TCRs, in particular those of high-affinity, directed against antigens that are over-expressed on tumors but also expressed on healthy cells. Toxicities included severe but treatable inflammation of skin, eyes, ears (MART-1/HLA-A2; gp100/HLA-A2), and colon (CEA/HLA-A2). In addition, lethal neurological toxicities were observed in two patients when targeting MAGE-A3/HLA-A2, and lethal cardiac toxicities were observed in three patients when targeting MART-1/HLA-A2 (another epitope as above) or MAGE-A3/HLA-A1. The transient nature of tumor regression became evident from observations that anti-tumor responses are initially significant but not sustainable and ultimately incomplete in 80–90% of patients. **Table 2** offers an up-to-date and detailed overview of toxicities as well as clinical responses reported for TCR gene therapy trials.

Strategies that aim at preventing or limiting toxicities as well as tumor recurrences have already been developed, some of which need further preclinical testing and some of which have already been implemented in clinical trials. In this review, we have categorized these strategies along three renewed challenges, i.e., "choice of target antigen"; "fitness of T cells," and "sensitization of micromilieu for T cell therapy," as illustrated in **Figure 2.** We propose and will argue that optimizations along each or combinations of these challenges will contribute most significantly to the advancement of clinical TCR gene therapy.

CHOICE OF TARGET ANTIGEN

Ideally, target antigens are selectively expressed by tumor tissue and not healthy tissue, and hence not expected to evoke a response against self. At the same time, target antigens should have proficient immunogenicity to initiate an effective anti-tumor response.

SELECTIVE EXPRESSION

Tumor-associated antigens (TAAs) can generally be divided into four groups (8).

- Differentiation antigens: cell surface proteins that are expressed at different stages of tissue development or cell activation.

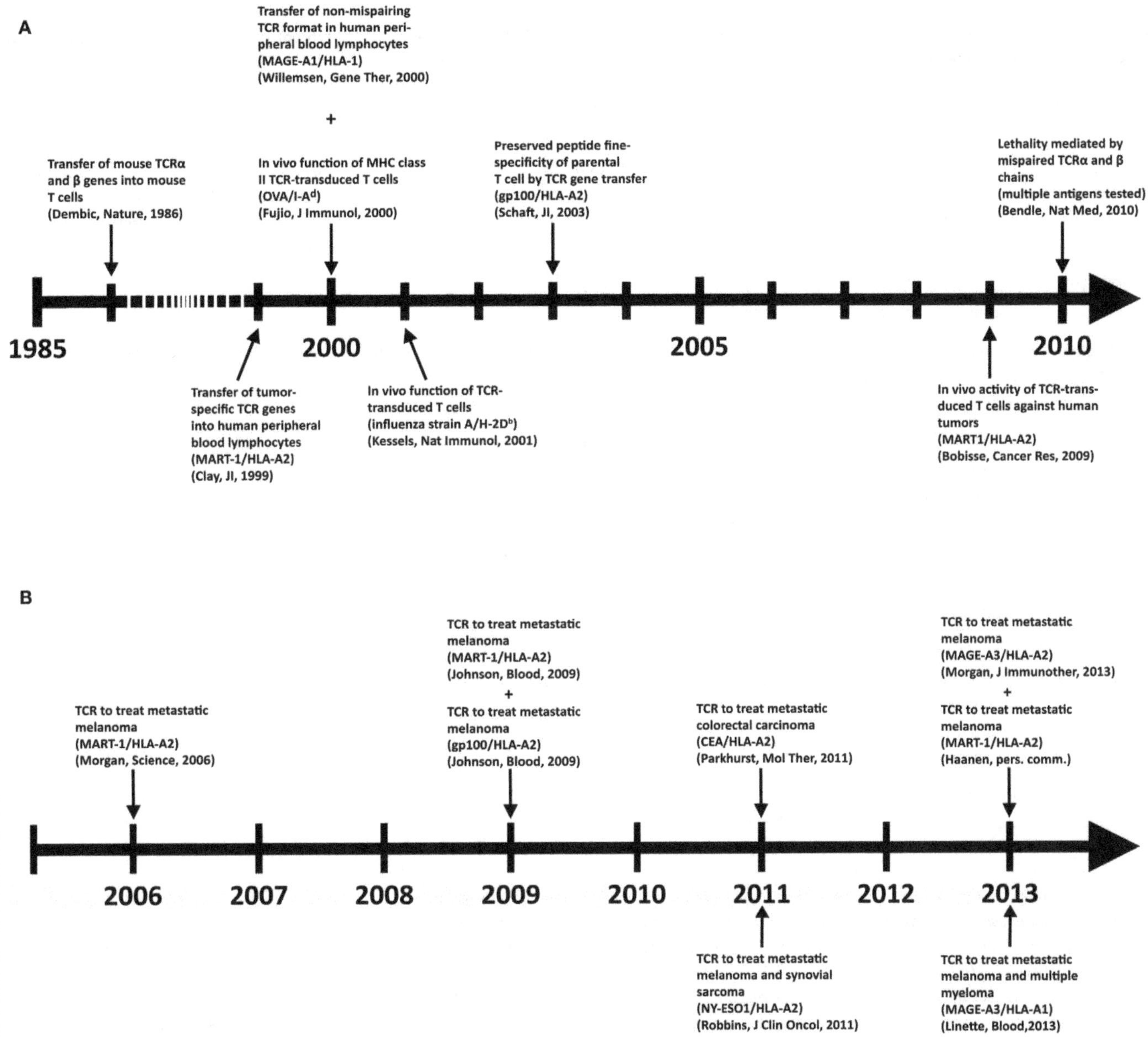

FIGURE 1 | Key achievements in the field of TCR gene therapy directed against solid tumors. **(A)** Timeline of selected preclinical findings that have contributed to the development of TCR gene therapy. **(B)** Timeline of clinical findings with TCR gene-engineered T cells. Details with respect to clinically used TCRs can be found in **Table 2**.

Expression of these antigens may discriminate tumor cells from surrounding healthy cells, but expression by healthy cells is not absent. Examples include MART-1, gp100, CEA, and tyrosinase related protein (TRP)1 and 2.

- Over-expressed antigens: cell surface proteins that are highly, but not selectively, expressed by tumor cells when compared to healthy cells. Examples include the epidermal growth factor receptor (HER)2 or survivin.
- Cancer Testis Antigens (CTAs): proteins that are expressed by tumors and a limited number of healthy and adult cell types. A defined number of CTAs may not be expressed by healthy adult cell types. Examples include MAGE-A1, MAGE-C2, and NY-ESO1.
- Neo-antigens: proteins that result from gene mutations or aberrations in tumor cells. These proteins are uniquely expressed by tumor cells but not healthy cells. Examples include mutated protein (p)53, B-Raf kinase, and cyclin-dependent kinase 4 (CDK4).

Looking at these four groups of TAAs, CTAs, and neo-antigens may represent the best available choices for therapy with TCR-engineered T cells. With respect to CTAs, over several hundreds

Table 2 | T cell receptor gene therapy trials – an update on efficacy and safety.

Target antigen (epitope)	Original T cell clone/lines	Tumor type	OR (%)	CR (%)	Toxicity (%)[a]	Type of toxicity	Reference
MART-1(AAG)/ HLA-A2	TIL clone DMF4 from responding patient	Metastatic melanoma	2/17 **(12)**	n.r.	0/17 **(0)**	n.r.	(189)
MART-1(AAG)/ HLA-A2	TIL clone DMF5 from responding patient with high *in vitro* avidity	Metastatic melanoma	6/20 **(30)**	n.r.	9/36 **(25)**	Severe melanocyte destruction in skin, eye, and ear (in some cases leading to uveitis and hearing loss)	(190)
gp100(KTW)/ HLA-A2	Splenocytes from immunized mouse	Metastatic melanoma	3/16 **(19)**	n.r.			
CEA(IMI)/ HLA-A2	Splenocytes from immunized mouse; TCR is affinity-enhanced	Metastatic colorectal carcinoma	1/3 **(33)**	n.r.	(3/3) **(100)**	Severe inflammation of colon	(191)
NY-ESO1(SLL)/ HLA-A2	T cell clone 1G4 from human subject; TCR is affinity-enhanced	Metastatic melanoma	5/11 **(45)**	2/11 **(18)**	0/11 **(0)**	n.r.	(192)
		Metastatic synovial sarcoma	4/6 **(67)**	0/6 **(0)**	0/6 **(0)**		
MAGE-A3(KVA)/ HLA-A2	Splenocytes from immunized mouse; TCR is affinity-enhanced	Metastatic melanoma	5/9 **(55)**	2/9 **(22)**	3/9 **(33)**	Changes in mental status, two patients fell into coma and subsequently died, one patient recovered	(29)
MART-1(ELA)/ HLA-A2	T cell clone 1D3 from human subject; TCR is codon-optimized and murinized	Metastatic melanoma	n.r.	n.r.	1/1 **(100)**	Lethal cardiac toxicity in one patient	b
MAGE-A3(EVD)/ HLA-A1	T cell clone a3a from human subject; TCR is affinity-enhanced	Metastatic melanoma and multiple myeloma	n.r.	n.r.	2/2 **(100)**	Lethal cardiac toxicity in two patients	(30)

OR, objective responses; CR, complete responses, both according to Response Evaluation Criteria for Solid Tumors (RECIST). Number of patients with responses = before dash; total number of patients = after dash; percentage of responses = between brackets.

[a]Number of patients with Serious Adverse Events (toxicity grading ≥3 according to National Cancer Institute common toxicity criteria) and total number of patients treated are put before and after dash, respectively.

[b]Dr. John Haanen, Cellular Therapy of Cancer Symposium, London, UK, February 27th–March 2nd, 2013.

CEA, carcinoembryonic antigen; gp, glycoprotein; HLA, human leukocyte antigen; MAGE, melanoma-associated antigen; MART, melanoma antigen recognized by T cells; n.r., none reported; NY-ESO1, New York esophageal squamous cell carcinoma 1.

of genes have been identified (see for a full description of CTAs[2]). Approximately 40 of these genes belong to multigene families that are located on the X-chromosome. A selected number of mostly X-chromosome-located CTAs may be of interest for T cell therapy. *First*, these antigens are not expressed by healthy tissues except testes and placentas (determined using RT-PCR), and these latter tissues do not express Major Histocompatibility (MHC) molecules and cannot be targeted by T cells (9). *Second*, CTAs are expressed by tumor tissues of various histological origins as a result of aberrant epigenetic regulation (9), and expression of CTAs has been associated with advanced stages of disease and unfavorable patient prognosis (10). Along these lines, there is evidence that MAGE proteins are related to oncogenesis as they suppress p53-dependent apoptosis and cause fibronectin-controlled increase in tumor cell proliferation and metastasis (11–15). *Third*, CTAs are immunogenic proteins that have been reported to induce both humoral and cell-mediated immune responses in patients without the concomitant induction of toxicities (10, 16, 17). Undeniably, current patient studies emphasize the need for careful identification of target CTAs. In one study, Robbins and colleagues demonstrated that a TCR directed against NY-ESO1/HLA-A2 showed significant anti-tumor responses in patients with metastatic melanoma and synovial sarcoma without detectable toxicities (**Table 2**). Unexpectedly, in another study using a TCR directed against MAGE-A3/HLA-A2, two patients with metastatic melanoma lapsed into coma and died. These adverse events were most likely caused by T cell recognition of rare neurons that were positive for MAGE-A12

[2]http://www.cta.lncc.br

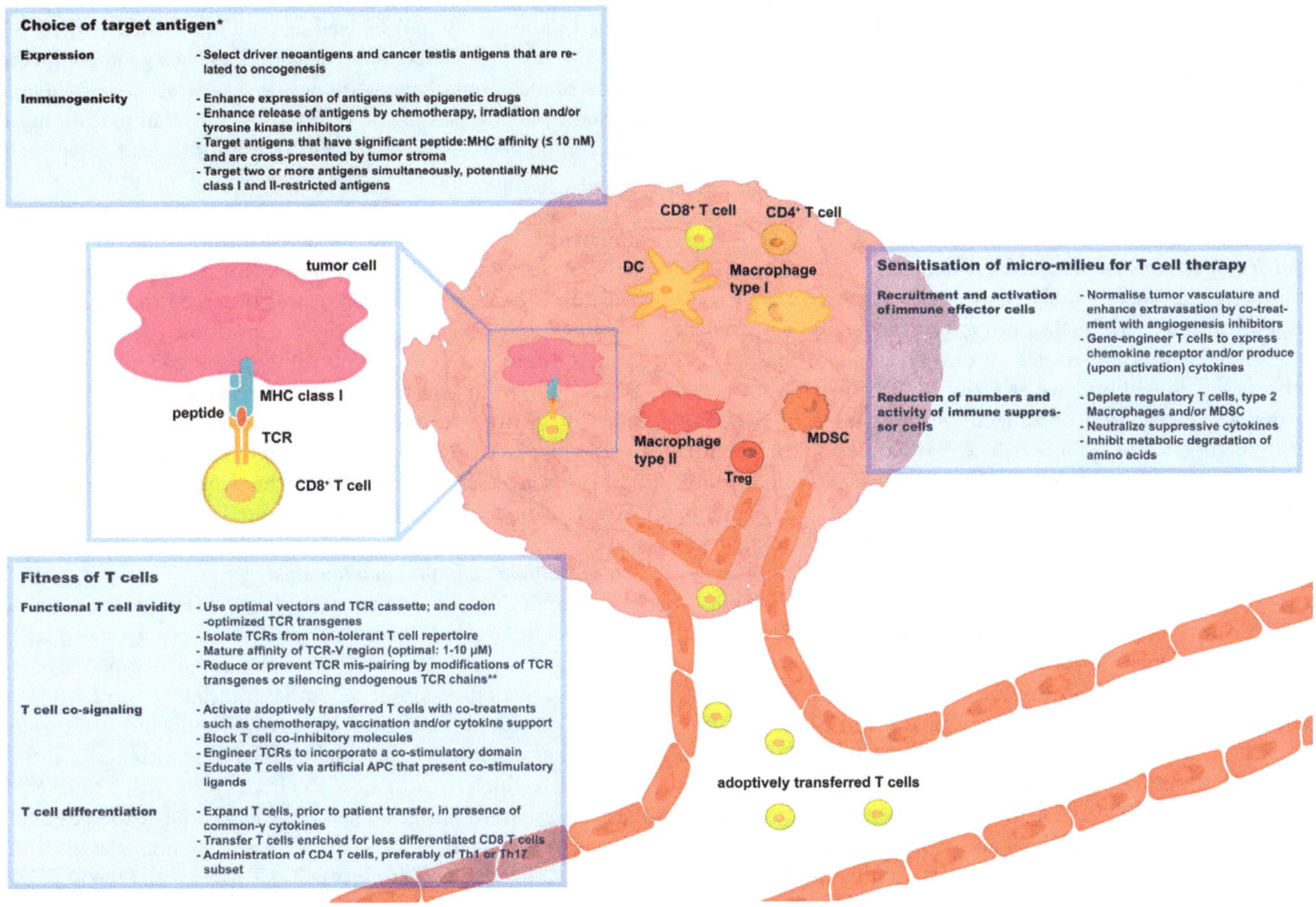

FIGURE 2 | Three challenges that determine the success rate of TCR gene therapy. In this figure, recent and successful strategies to improve TCR gene therapy have been categorized along three renewed challenges: "choice of target antigen"; "fitness of T cells"; and "sensitization of micro-milieu for T cell therapy." Boxes provide selected strategies that are discussed in more detail in Sections "Choice of Target Antigen," "Fitness of T cells," and "Sensitization of Micro-Milieu for T Cell Therapy." We propose that advancement of clinical TCR gene therapy is guided by the principles of these challenges. *Independent of choice of target antigen, it is recommended to perform stringent *in silico* analysis and preclinical tests to confirm that healthy cells do not express the target antigen prior to proceeding with the clinical testing of TCR-engineered T cells. **Strategies to reduce or prevent TCR mis-pairing do not only enhance T cell avidity but also reduce the potential risk of off-target toxicity. APC, antigen-presenting cells; DC, Dendritic cells; MDSC, myeloid-derived suppressor cells; Th, T helper cells; Treg, T regulatory cells.

and possibly MAGE-A9 antigens, which contain shared or highly similar epitopes compared to MAGE-A3 antigen (**Table 2**). In a third study, in which a TCR was used directed against MAGE-A3/HLA-A1, one patient with melanoma and one patient with myeloma suffered from cardiovascular toxicity and died. This toxicity was possibly caused by T cell recognition of a similar but not identical peptide from the muscle protein titin (so-called "off-target" toxicity, **Table 2**).

With respect to neo-antigens, the expression of these antigens may vary significantly among different patients, but their expression is unique to tumor tissues. In case a neo-antigen is the result of "driver mutations," the antigen may constitute an ideal target for T cell therapy. Driver mutations are related to oncogenesis, may be linked to known genes (~400), and may provide tumors with a selective growth advantage (18, 19). Nevertheless, it is important to realize that only 15% of up to 100,000 mutations that are encountered in tumor genomes are considered "driver" mutations (18, 20). Moreover, not all driver mutations may result in new immunogenic antigens. A quest for neo-antigen targets does not only require next-generation sequencing techniques to identify tumor-specific mutations (21), but also techniques to determine whether a neo-epitope can be presented by MHC and recognized by T cells (22, 23).

In short, we consider epitopes from selected (non-shared) CTA and neo-antigens as potentially safe T cell target antigens. However, no matter what the antigen, it is recommended to perform stringent *in silico* analysis and preclinical testing to confirm the antigen's absence from vital organs. Strategies used to identify titin as a cross-recognized peptide, such as amino acid scanning, gene database searches, and use of three-dimensional cell cultures, are potentially helpful in this respect (24). In addition, one could consider using suicide systems to deplete self-reactive T cells prior to proceeding with clinical testing (25–28). Although suicide genes provide the option to delete TCR-transduced T cells, it is questionable whether such a switch could counteract the fast kinetics of toxicity reported in the above-mentioned trials (29, 30).

IMMUNOGENICITY

The immunogenicity of an antigen, i.e., its ability to initiate immune responses, is determined by the level of its expression, how it is processed and presented, and how well it is recognized by T cells.

Level of expression and processing of antigens

Ideally, target antigens should be expressed at high levels by most if not all tumor cells. Such a property is generally restricted to those antigens that are related to oncogenesis and that tumors cannot easily do without (see Selective Expression). It is noteworthy that the production of antigens, such as those of MAGE-A family members and NY-ESO1, is enhanced and becomes more homogeneous within tumors by treatment with demethylation agents and/or histone deacetylases (31–34). In a phase II clinical study, in which hematological malignancies were targeted and which included treatments with epigenetic drugs, it was observed that T cell responses directed against CTA were enhanced with no evidence of adverse events (35). In addition, the production of antigens may depend on immune or intermediate proteasomes, rather than standard proteasomes, and on unconventional post-translational events such as reverse splicing and deamidation of proteins (36–38). Such processing of antigens, in particular when mediated by immune proteasomes, may benefit from local production of interferon (IFN)γ. Finally, the release and hence the availability of antigens may be enhanced via treatment-induced cell death following (co-treatments with) chemotherapy, irradiation, and/or therapy with tyrosine kinase inhibitors (39, 40).

Cross-presentation of antigens

Antigen cross-presentation may take part in the infiltration of antigen-specific CD8 T cells (41) and cause activation of T cells and subsequent stroma destruction, thereby preventing outgrowth of antigen-negative tumor cells. Recently, Engels and colleagues revealed that peptide:MHC affinities of 10 nM or less allowed for cross-presentation of antigens by stromal cells (42). Notably, using an experimental model in which mice transgenic for TCRs with different antigen specificities were used either as donors or recipients of T cells, they showed that the use of peptide targets that can be cross-presented result in complete anti-tumor responses. Destruction of tumor stroma, a bystander response that may put an advantage to T cells over drugs (43, 44), may require optimal T cell fitness (as measured by production of IFNγ) and IFNγ-mediated preservation of Fas expression by stromal cells (45).

Robustness of antigenicity

Loss of tumor antigen expression after infusion of T cells, and its impact on the recurrence of tumors, is an important yet controversial aspect. Decreased antigen expression has been proposed to be a consequence of molecular alterations in tumor cells, such as genetic and epigenetic changes in antigen genes, MHC genes, and genes related to antigen processing and presentation (46–48). Indeed, selective loss of antigen or HLA-A2 expression has been reported in primary and metastatic melanoma lesions in non-treated patients (49, 50) as well as patients treated with T cells (51, 52). Also, Landsberg and colleagues, using a gene-engineered model of melanoma, have eloquently demonstrated that a therapy-resistant phenotype may be directed by an inflammatory milieu and tumor necrosis factor (TNF)α's ability to lead to epithelial dedifferentiation and decreased expression of melanoma antigens (53). In contrast to these findings, there is increasing evidence to support the view that tumors progress without loss of T cell antigens. In various preclinical models, in which either skin, lung, or ovarium tumors were studied, it was observed that tumors progressed despite continued antigen expression (54–56). In these models, tumor progression was rather a consequence of reduced T cell infiltration and reduced T cell responsiveness. We postulate that in the setting of T cell therapy, loss of target antigen, whether by T cell-dependent selection or epigenetic silencing (57, 58), is *not* necessarily a driving mechanism in tumor recurrence (Straetemans et al., manuscript submitted).

Target multiple antigens simultaneously

In current TCR gene therapy trials, single MHC class I-restricted antigens are targeted. Preclinical studies have suggested that the targeting of two or more antigens enhances the therapeutic potential of T cells. For example, adoptive transfer of two CD8 T cell populations to simultaneously target ovalbumin and gp100, rather than either one antigen, resulted in delayed recurrence of tumors (59). Interestingly, treatment with viruses positive for three MHC class II-restricted antigens, i.e., neuroblastoma RAS, TRP1, and cytochrome c1, resulted in complete anti-tumor responses that were accompanied by significant CD4 T helper cell type 17 (Th17) responses (60). Since cooperation of CD4 and CD8 T cells appears important in the effector phase of an anti-tumor response and may contribute to the bystander elimination of tumor stroma (61), it may be worthwhile to simultaneously target MHC class I and II targets. With respect to human antigens, it is interesting to note that X-chromosome linked CTAs are coordinately expressed in tumor tissues (62), which may allow the simultaneous targeting of multiple CTAs.

FITNESS OF T CELLS

The responsiveness of T cells toward tumor antigen is generally tuned down, most likely at various levels. First, reactive T cells may be deleted during T cell development in the thymus; second, peripheral T cells may be susceptibility to anergy; and third, intra-tumoral T cells may require enhanced co-stimulation (63). To overcome such T cell tolerizing mechanisms one can optimize T cell fitness. Here, we define T cell fitness according to the following three T cell properties: functional T cell avidity, T cell co-signaling, and T cell differentiation.

FUNCTIONAL T CELL AVIDITY

Functional T cell avidity is considered as the ability of T cells to respond to a given concentration of cognate peptide antigen, and can be enhanced via strategies, often involving gene-engineering of TCRαβ transgenes, that either increase the level of cell surface expression of TCR chains or the TCR's affinity for peptide-MHC.

Expression level of TCR transgenes

One angle to enhance the surface expression of TCR transgenes is through optimization of the TCR gene transfer methodology, including choice of gene delivery method, use of optimal vector elements, and use of transgene cassettes [reviewed in Ref. (6, 64)]. Another angle to enhance the surface expression of TCR transgenes is through limitation or abolishment of TCR mis-pairing. TCR mis-pairing is the formation of TCR heterodimers that comprise one transgenic TCR chain and one endogenous TCR chain, and represents a phenomenon that is inherent to the generation of TCR-engineered T cells. Importantly, TCR mis-pairing dilutes the surface expression of the transgenic TCRαβ chains, and mis-paired TCRs are of unknown specificity and can yield self-reactive T cells. Although in clinical trials performed so far, no formal observations of toxicities mediated by TCR mis-pairing have been made, preclinical studies have clearly demonstrated that TCR mis-pairing has the potential to induce harmful recognition of self-antigens (65, 66). Strategies to promote preferential pairing between transgenic TCRα and TCRβ chains (and consequently prevent or reduce TCR mis-pairing) can be grouped according to those that depend on gene-engineering of TCR transgenes and those that do not. The first group of strategies are reviewed in Ref. (67). In short, these strategies include murinization of TCR (68), addition of cysteine amino acids to TCR (69, 70), mutations in TCR transmembrane and constant domains (71, 72), and equipment of TCR with a signaling cassette that replaces TCR transmembrane and intracellular domains with the CD3ζ accessory molecule (73, 74). More recently, a limited number of murine amino acids have been identified that are responsible for enhanced expression and preferential pairing of murinized TCRs (75, 76). Similar efforts to minimize the number of amino acids in a CD3ζ signaling cassette failed, and it was observed that properties of TCRs equipped with CD3ζ signaling cassettes are best preserved when incorporating a complete CD3ζ molecule (77). The other group of strategies includes technologies that enhance expression levels of CD3 molecules in T cells and those that interrupt expression of endogenous TCR chains. Co-transfer of CD3 and TCR genes into T cells resulted in higher levels of TCR expression and allowed T cells to respond to lower concentrations of antigen, and to infiltrate and eliminate tumors with faster kinetics (78). RNA interference techniques have been shown to specifically down-regulate the expression of endogenous but not transgenic TCR chains (79, 80). An alternative method encompasses the use of zinc finger nucleases and a sequential knock-out of endogenous TCRα and β chains, followed by introduction and sorting of TCRα and β transgenes (81). The latter method is relatively new and not yet widely or clinically applied, but holds promise to effectively address TCR mis-pairing.

Affinity-enhancement of TCRαβ transgenes

Affinity-enhancement of tumor-specific TCRs, and its exploitation, relies on the existence of a window for optimal TCR affinities. The existence of such a window is based on observations that TCRs specific for HLA-A2-restricted pathogens have K_D values that are generally about 10-fold lower when compared to TCRs specific for HLA-A2-restricted tumor-associated self-antigens (82). In support of this notion are the observations that a high-affinity MART-1/HLA-A2 TCR mediated improved objective response rates compared to a lower affinity MART-1/HLA-A2 TCR, and that an affinity-enhanced NY-ESO1 TCR mediated significant clinical responses (**Table 2**). Affinity-enhanced TCRs can be obtained through various routes. First, allo-reactive settings can be used to circumvent self-tolerance and yield T cells with a higher avidity when compared to T cells derived from autologous settings (=patients). Examples of such settings include *in vitro* generation of allo-HLA reactive, peptide-specific T cells (83–85), and immunization of mice transgenic for human-MHC or human TCR (86, 87). Second, TCR affinities can be enhanced by rationally designed mutations of the TCR's complementarity-determining regions (CDRs) (88, 89). Third, high-affinity TCR variants can be selected from a library of CDR mutants by yeast, phage, or T cell display (90–92). Although the affinity of TCRs significantly contributes to the functional avidity of T cells, recent studies warrant caution when therapeutically implementing this strategy. Clinical reports suggest that CDR mutations in TCRs directed against CEA/HLA-A2, MAGE-A3/HLA-A2, and MAGE-A3/HLA-A1, but not NY-ESO/HLA-A2, were possibly related to patient toxicities (**Table 2**). Investigations whether defined locations and types of mutations are more prone to lead to toxicities than others would most likely benefit further development of CDR-mutated TCRs. Also, preclinical reports suggest the existence of a functional ceiling with respect to TCR affinity (93, 94). In fact, studies with primary human T cells transduced with affinity-enhanced TCRs directed against NY-ESO1/HLA-A2 (93) or gp100/HLA-A2 (Govers et al., manuscript submitted) pointed to the existence of a K_D threshold of 1–5 μM, below which T cell function became compromised. The functional impairment of high avidity T cells in the presence of high levels of antigen, as is often the case in tumors, may be related to enhanced expression of the exhaustion marker programed cell death (PD1) and enhanced activity of its downstream sarcoma homology domain 2 phosphatase (SHP)1 (95, 96).

T CELL CO-SIGNALING

T cell co-signaling is directed by interactions between co-stimulatory or co-inhibitory molecules and their ligands and determines, in addition to interactions between TCR and peptide-MHC, the functional outcome of T cells [reviewed by Chen and Flies (97)]. The best characterized co-stimulatory and co-inhibitory molecules expressed by T cells are CD28 and cytotoxic T-lymphocyte associated protein (CTLA)4, respectively, which both interact with CD80 and CD86 ligands expressed by APCs. More recent examples of co-stimulatory and co-inhibitory molecules include inducible T cell co-stimulation (ICOS), 4-1BB, OX40, CD40, B and T-lymphocyte attenuator (BTLA), and PD1.

Tumors provide continuous stimulation with antigen often in the absence of co-stimulatory ligands, which may result in exhausted T cells with reduced proliferative capacity, reduced effector function (such as IFNγ production) (98), and up-regulated expression of T cell co-inhibitory molecules (99). Immunotherapy with monoclonal antibodies to block the T cell co-inhibitory molecules CTLA4, PD1, PDL1, or the combination of CTLA4 and PD1 showed clear clinical successes in the treatment of advanced melanoma (see **Table 1**). These clinical activities have provided an impetus for the development of blocking other co-inhibitory molecules and/or stimulation of co-stimulatory molecules (100–104). The beneficial outcome of targeting T cell co-signaling most likely relies on enhancement of infiltration of T effector cells (Teff) into tumor tissue and activation of Teff, as well as depletion of intra-tumoral T regulatory cells (Treg) (103–105). We would advocate explorative studies to test the combination of blocking T cell co-inhibitory molecules and adoptive transfer of Teff. In addition to this combination of immune therapies, two other approaches to implement T cell co-signaling in protocols of T cell therapy have already been clinically tested. First, TCR transgenes can be equipped with a signaling cassette that harbors a co-stimulatory molecule. Such a signaling cassette, designed in analogy to those used in co-stimulatory CARs (6), typically introduces accessory and co-stimulatory molecules to enhance the function of T cells expressing the TCR transgene. It is noteworthy that clinical trials using CARs containing CD28 or CD137 demonstrated significant objective responses in patients with B cell leukemia (106–108), and while CARs may evoke immune responses, these were directed against murine idiotypes, but never against boundaries between genetically introduced human molecules (109). According to this rationale, single and two-chain TCR genes have been coupled to a combination of CD28 and CD3 molecules and were shown to provide T cells with improved function *in vitro* (110, 111) (Govers et al., manuscript submitted). Second, T cells can be stimulated *ex vivo* with human artificial APC (aAPCs) that express co-stimulatory ligands (4, 112). In addition to co-stimulatory ligands, these aAPCs are mostly engineered to express HLA-A × 0201 and used to stimulate T cells in the presence of common-γ cytokines other than interleukin (IL)-2. These combined activations allow for the generation of HLA-A2-restricted, antigen-specific T cells with a less differentiated phenotype ($CD45RA^+$ $CD62L^+$) and superior T cell functions *in vivo* (112). In a clinical study, T cells educated with aAPC presenting CD80, CD83, and a MART-1 peptide, and cultured in the presence of IL-2 and IL-15, resulted in objective responses in patients with metastatic melanoma (**Table 1**). Notably, inclusion of T cell co-stimulation by either one of the two above-mentioned approaches relieved the requirement for patient preconditioning with chemotherapy and/or *in vivo* IL-2 administration (4, 106).

T CELL DIFFERENTIATION

The differentiation of naïve T cells into mature CD8 Teff or CD4 Th1 or Th17 cells is required for T cells to make full use of their functional attributes directed against tumor cells, such as cytotoxicity and production of IFNγ and TNFα. The differentiation of T cells is largely driven by environmental stimuli, with cytokines being well-studied examples of such stimuli (113, 114). Progression of T cells into a differentiated subset is not necessarily permanent, and in particular T helper cell subsets have shown plasticity and may change into another T helper cell subset (114). Differentiation of CD8 and CD4 T cells, although occurring according to similar principles, follow different routes and show different outcomes. Strategies to manipulate T cell differentiation to advance T cell therapy are discussed separately for both T cell subsets.

CD8 T cells

Naïve CD8 T cells can differentiate, depending on the quantity and quality of the initial antigenic and co-stimulatory stimuli, into stem-cell memory T cells, central memory T cells, effector memory T cells, or T effector cells (115). An important observation that came from preclinical studies was the inverse relationship between CD8 T cell differentiation and proliferation, and hence the inverse relationship between CD8 T cell differentiation and *in vivo* persistence and therapeutic activity (113). Two strategies have been reported to exploit this inverse relationship and improve adoptive T cell therapy. In one such strategy, as shortly mentioned in Section "T Cell Co-Signaling," T cells are exposed to common-γ cytokines other than IL-2 prior to adoptive T cell transfer. For example, treatments with either IL-7 + IL-15 or IL-15 + IL-21 generated gene-engineered T cells with a less differentiated CD8 T cell phenotype (i.e., central memory phenotype), prolonged peripheral persistence, and potent antigen reactivity (116, 117). In addition to soluble cytokines, Singh and colleagues reported on aAPC that express membrane-bound IL-15 and IL-21 and facilitate the generation of "young" T cells (112). In other reports, the anti-tumor efficacy of T cells was enhanced either via *in vivo* administration of IL-15 + IL-21 (118) or conjugation of nanoparticles, encapsulating these cytokines, to the surface of therapeutic T cells (119). In a second strategy, T cells are enriched for less differentiated T cell populations, i.e., based on CD62L expression, and subsequently used as recipient cells for gene transfer (120, 121). A recently identified population of "stem-cell memory" CD8 T cells, expressing high levels of CD95, IL2Rβ and demonstrating increased proliferative potential and ability to mediate anti-tumor responses, may represent a promising subset of T cells for gene-engineering and therapeutic application (122). In fact, Cieri and colleagues have set up a protocol to obtain and gene-modify stem-cell memory CD8 T cells, which includes the use of CD3/CD28 mAbs and IL-7 and IL-15 and could potentially be translated to a clinical setting (123).

CD4 T cells

Naïve CD4 T cells can differentiate into multiple subsets, including Th1, 2, 9, 17, 22, follicular helper and various Tregs, often defined by the expression of "signature cytokines" or typical functions, such as B cell activation or the down-modulation of T cell responses (124). With respect to anti-tumor responses, it appears that upon cell transfer Th1 and Th17 are the most potent CD4 T cell subsets (125, 126). Administration of CD4 T cells, and in particular Th1 cells, has been shown to prevent exhaustion of CD8 T cells, enhance tumor infiltration of CD8 T cells and result in effective tumor eradication (125, 127–130). More recently, it was discovered that adoptive transfer of Th17 cells effectively mediate rejection of TRP1-positive tumors in a TCR-transgenic mouse model (126). Furthermore, Th17 cells appear to be long-lived and their molecular signature resembles that of stem-cell memory CD8 T cells (131). Interestingly, the anti-tumor activity of Th17 cells depended on its (incomplete) differentiation and conversion into Th1 cells, resulting in a co-existence of Th17 and Th1 cells, and it may very well be this multi-potent aspect that provides a therapeutic advantage.

Collectively, these data argue in favor of a combined therapeutic use of CD8 T cells and Th1 or Th17 cells. To this end, CD4 T cells can be functionally endowed with MHC I-restricted TCR and/or CD8 via gene transfer (132–135). Alternatively, one could opt for strategies that induce *in vivo* conversion of CD4 T cells into Th1 cells, such as IL-12, IFNα, IFNγ, or blocking PD1 ligation (136–139). Also, metabolic signals, such as activation of T cell mammalian target of rapamycin (mTOR) and aerobic glycolysis can enhance differentiation toward IFNγ-producing T cells and may be exploited therapeutically (140, 141).

SENSITIZATION OF MICRO-MILIEU FOR T CELL THERAPY

Tumors, following initial regression upon treatment with T cells, most often become resistant to T cell therapy and recur. Recent understanding suggests that, at least in some tumors, therapy resistance may be part of a negative feedback loop that is initiated once an anti-tumor CD8 T cell has occurred (142). Therapy resistance is often characterized by a dis-balance between numbers and activation state of immune effectors cells versus those of suppressor cells. Strategies to manipulate numbers and activation state of immune cells are discussed separately for effector and suppressor cells.

RECRUITMENT AND ACTIVATION OF IMMUNE EFFECTOR CELLS

Immune effector cells that have been recognized for their contribution to an anti-tumor response are numerous and, in addition to CD4 and CD8 T cells, include natural killer (NK), natural killer T cells (NKT), macrophages, and neutrophils. Here we will focus on Teff and macrophages and how manipulation of the micro-milieu may enhance their recruitment and activation.

Enhance recruitment of T effector cells

Clinical studies have demonstrated an unfavorable prognostic value of a limited CD8 T cell infiltration in melanoma, colorectal and ovarium carcinomas (143–145). Vascular changes have been reported to contribute to arrested T cell infiltration and include insufficient vascular maturation and enhanced expression of endothelin B receptor, regulator of G-protein signaling 5 (Rgs5) and/or extracellular matrix components [reviewed in Ref. (146)]. Such changes may be targeted, as evidenced by angiostatic therapy in which antibodies directed against vascular endothelial growth factor (VEGF) or angiopoietin 2, or in which T cells gene-engineered with a CAR directed against VEGF receptor (VEGFR)2 resulted in enhanced T cell infiltration (147–149). In addition, drugs that inhibit angiogenesis or endothelin receptor B were able to enhance the expression of intercellular adhesion molecule (ICAM)1 on endothelial cells and to normalize T cell infiltration (150, 151). In various solid tumors, T cell infiltration appears to be facilitated by vessels that closely mimic high endothelial venules (HEV) and which may be part of ectopic lymphoid structures in tumor stroma (152, 153). A better understanding of the development of such HEV in tumor stroma may provide novel targets to improve T cell infiltration in tumors.

In addition to vascular changes, spontaneous cutaneous melanoma tumors in mice demonstrated a decreased mRNA expression of chemoattractants that contribute to recruitment of CD8 T cells, such as chemokine (CC motif) ligand (CCL)5 and chemokine (CXC motif) ligands (CXCL)9 and 10 (146). In a subset of patients with melanoma metastases, lack of chemoattractants coincides with limited migration of CD8 T cells and limited presence of lymphoid structures (154). Current findings from our laboratory suggest that a decreased expression of selected chemoattractants and adhesion molecules are related to a decreased infiltration of CD8 T cells and tumor relapse following T cell therapy (Straetemans et. al., manuscript submitted). Interestingly, Hong and colleagues have shown that the chemotherapeutic drugs dacarbazine, temozolomide, and cisplatin enhanced the expression of CCL5, CXCL9, and CXCL10 in patient melanoma, which in turn correlated with improved immune control of tumors (155). Vice versa, T cells when gene-engineered to express chemokine (CXC motif) receptor (CXCR)2 displayed enhanced trafficking toward tumor cells secreting the corresponding chemokine ligand CXCL1 (156). Also, in xenograft tumor models of mesothelioma and neuroblastoma, the genetic introduction of chemokine (CC motif) receptor (CCR)2 in T cells resulted in increased T cell infiltration in tumors secreting CCL2 and was associated with significantly increased anti-tumor activity (157, 158). Other molecules often present in the micro-milieu that, when targeted, resulted in enhanced T cell accumulation at the tumor site are indoleamine 2,3-dioxygenase (IDO) and reactive nitrogen species. Inhibition of IDO by a small molecule blocks tryptophan depletion, enhances T cell infiltration, and delays tumor growth (159). Reactive nitrogen species induce TIL unresponsiveness (160), nitration of the TCR complex (161), and modification of the chemokine CCL2 (162). Drugs affecting the local production of reactive nitrogen species restore TIL function and improve intra-tumoral T cell migration and an anti-tumor T cell response (160, 162). Taken together, the above studies show the drug-ability of molecules that are involved in T cell extravasation and T cell migration into tumor tissues, and advocate studies to combine such drugs with adoptive T cell therapy.

Enhance T cell effector functions

Early protocols of adoptive T cell therapy already demonstrated the beneficial effects of co-treatments such as chemotherapy, vaccination, and/or cytokine support on T cell activation [reviewed in Ref. (64)]. More recently, additional strategies that enhance anti-tumor functions of Teff have been reported. A first strategy became apparent from clinical success with additional T cell co-stimulation or blocking of T cell co-inhibition (see T Cell Co-Signaling and **Table 1**). A second strategy relates to the inhibition of T cell suppressive cytokines, such as transforming growth factor (TGF)β. For example, genetic introduction of a dominant-negative TGFβ receptor II in TCR-engineered T cells resulted in increased anti-tumor T cell responses in a spontaneous tumor model of prostate cancer (163). Another study tested the safety of mouse T cells engineered with this dominant-negative receptor, and could not detect spontaneous proliferation of these T cells *in vivo* (164). Genetic knockdown of negative regulators of T cell activation represents yet another strategy to enhance T cell activation. T cells with siRNA-mediated knockdown of casitas B-lineage lymphoma b (Cbl-b) displayed a lower threshold for T cell activation and, when adoptively transferred in mice with disseminated leukemia, resulted in enhanced anti-tumor effects (165). These latter findings warrant further testing of T cells with enhanced T cell activation, including tests that assess the safe use of these T cells.

Enhance recruitment and activation of macrophages

High numbers of macrophages with a tumor-promoting (M2) phenotype, but not those with a tumor-inhibiting (M1) phenotype, correlate with poor prognosis for patients with various cancers (166). When conjugated to a vascular homing peptide and targeted to tumors, TNFα resulted in a switch from M2 to M1 macrophages, which was accompanied by normalization of tumor vasculature and enhanced infiltration of CD8 T cells (167). Interestingly, T cells gene-engineered to release the cytokine IL-12 were shown to improve the therapeutic efficacy of T cells, an effect that is likely mediated by cells of the innate immune system (168, 169). T cells that express IL-12 under the control of the Nuclear Factor of Activated T cell (NFAT) promoter, and deliver IL-12 locally in the tumor environment upon encounter of cognate antigen, induce destruction of antigen-negative cancer cells with a prominent role for monocytes and monocyte-derived TNFα (168). Such findings are not necessarily restricted to IL-12 since IL-15, when provided locally into tumors, also enhanced the responsiveness of adoptively transferred T cells and facilitated the removal of antigen-negative tumor cells (170).

REDUCE NUMBERS AND ACTIVITY OF IMMUNE SUPPRESSOR CELLS

T regulatory cells, M2 macrophages, and myeloid-derived suppressor cells (MDSC) are among the major immune-suppressive cell types in the tumor micro-milieu. Immune suppressor cells can reduce T cell infiltration into the tumor and suppress local T cell responses by: release of reactive nitrogen and oxygen species (171); expression of IDO and arginase (159, 172); and production of cytokines such as TGFβ, IL-4, and IL-13 (173). Despite initial removal of these cells by administration of chemotherapeutic agents, the populations of MDSCs and Tregs may recover at a faster rate than CD4 and CD8 Teff (174). Furthermore, Jensen and colleagues demonstrated that therapeutic $CD4^+$ T eff can convert into a $Foxp3^+CD4^+$ Treg population (175). Various strategies have been reported to deplete or inactivate Tregs. These strategies include administration of anti-CD25 antibodies, combined intratumoral injection of anti-CTLA4 and OX40 mAbs, or blocking IDO (104, 176). Interestingly, blocking IDO may induce conversion from Treg to Th17 helper cells, which can further contribute to anti-tumor T cell responses (176). With respect to MDSCs, it is of interest to note that classical chemotherapeutic agents, such as docetaxel, are able to deplete these cells. Docetaxel-mediated depletion of MDSC, when combined with adoptive T cell therapy and dendritic cell vaccination, was shown to enhance anti-tumor responses (174). Alternatively, differentiation of MDSC into mature myeloid cells, which can be established upon administration of β-glucans (glucose monomers from cell walls), may also provide an angle to relieve immune suppression (177).

FUTURE PERSPECTIVES

By now, the feasibility of TCR gene therapy studies has been well established by the pioneering trials listed in **Figure 1B**, and is further enhanced by current optimizations and standardizations of protocols. TCR gene therapy, alike any cell-based therapy, requires specialized good manufacturing practice (GMP) and patient treatment facilities. Such facilities allow the generation and testing of virus batches and the gene processing and expansion of T cells, and are already integrated in multiple academic and private centers. Notably, parameters, such as time-lines and costs to manufacture a therapeutic T cell product, are considered competitive when compared to other clinical-grade products, such as antibodies. An ongoing EU project to treat metastatic esophagus-gastric cancer and melanoma with NY-ESO1 TCR-engineered T cells, in which we participate, shows that time-lines and costs to obtain a T cell product are about 2 weeks and 36 k€ per patient (13.5 k€ for production, quality testing, and test runs of virus batch; and 22.5 k€ for T cell processing), respectively. For comparison: estimated per patients costs of Ipilimumab (3 mg/kg every 3 weeks, 4 times) and Vemurafenib (0.96 g twice daily for 6 months), both registered treatments for metastasized melanoma in The Netherlands since 2012, are 84 and 57 k€ [Association of Health Insurances (CVZ), The Netherlands]. The next step, and allowing a more valid comparison, would be the testing of T cell therapy versus standard treatment of care in a randomized trial.

Clinical testing of TCR-engineered T cells, when looking at single trials, demonstrated impressive and unprecedented efficacy but at the same time is hampered by treatment-related toxicity and a transient nature of tumor regression (**Table 2**). There exists a multitude of strategies that are developed and tested toward advanced safety and efficacy of TCR gene therapy. Here, we have defined three challenges and have categorized recent and successful strategies along these three challenges, which have been schematically depicted in **Figure 2**. With respect to the first challenge, i.e., choice for target antigen, an important criterion is minimal or no expression of such an antigen by healthy tissues. In this respect, non-shared and tumor-restricted CTAs as well as neo-antigens should be considered as potentially safe target antigens. Advances in the isolation and characterization of anti-tumor T cells from individual patient samples may increase the number of CTAs and neo-antigens that may qualify as target antigens. T cell-based recognition of similar, but unrelated peptides should be excluded, and to this end it is strongly recommended to perform stringent *in silico* analysis and preclinical tests to confirm that cross-reactive antigens are absent in healthy tissue. In order to improve patient safety further, measures to allow directed killing of engineered T cells have been tested and should be considered, at least for novel TCRs tested in the near future. In addition to tumor-restricted expression, another criterion to choose target antigens is maximal immunogenicity. Peptide epitopes that are cross-presented or the targeting of a more than a single peptide have been reported to induce complete anti-tumor responses, and may represent examples to consider when selecting target antigens.

With respect to the second and third challenges, i.e., fitness of T cells and sensitization of tumor micro-milieu, we would like to propose a two-step treatment protocol. The first step represents the transfer of fit T cells. T cell fitness involves optimal T cell avidity, additional T cell co-signaling, and using T cells with a preferred differentiation stage. T cell avidity can be optimized by enhancement of TCR affinity, yet reported treatment-related toxicities warrant caution when using affinity-enhanced TCRs (**Table 2**) and recommend further studies to define rules of TCR binding of cognate versus non-cognate peptides. With respect to T cell co-signaling, antibodies that block T cell co-inhibitory molecules and T cells gene-engineered with co-stimulatory receptors have demonstrated clinical successes. The implementation of such strategies in T cell therapy protocols holds promise for future trials. Also, developments to obtain and gene-modify early differentiation stages of CD8 T cells, including stem-cell memory CD8 T cells, are at the brim of being translated to a clinical setting. Whatever the chosen route, an important measure for T cell fitness *in vivo* is the ability of these cells, whether it be CD8 T cells or certain subsets of CD4 T cells, to produce IFNγ and TNFα. The production of these cytokines not only determines T cell responsiveness, but also to what extent innate immune cells are recruited into the tumor and become activated to further improve an anti-tumor response and potentially avoid tumor relapse. The second step represents antagonism of an immune-suppressed milieu. Various strategies, such as antibodies or drugs to mediate angiostasis, chemotherapeutic agents to enhance intra-tumoral T cell infiltration, and local (T cell-mediated) delivery of cytokines, have proven beneficial to enhance the local ratio between effector and suppressor immune cells. Development of such a two-step protocol, together with the targeting of a selected antigen, is the way forward and expected to further enhance the success rate of TCR gene therapy to treat solid tumors.

REFERENCES

1. Dudley ME, Yang JC, Sherry R, Hughes MS, Royal R, Kammula U, et al. Adoptive cell therapy for patients with metastatic melanoma: evaluation of inten- sive myeloablative chemoradiation preparative regimens. *J Clin Oncol* (2008) **26**(32):5233–9. doi:10.1200/JCO.2008.16.5449
2. Besser MJ, Shapira-Frommer R, Treves AJ, Zippel D, Itzhaki O, Hershkovitz L, et al. Clinical responses in a phase II study using adoptive transfer of short-term cultured tumor infiltration lymphocytes in metastatic melanoma patients. *Clin Cancer Res* (2010) **16**(9):2646–55. doi:10.1158/1078-0432.CCR-10-0041
3. Yee C, Thompson JA, Byrd D, Riddell SR, Roche P, Celis E, et al. Adoptive T cell therapy using antigen-specific CD8+ T cell clones for the treatment of patients with metastatic melanoma: in vivo persistence, migration, and antitumor effect of transferred T cells. *Proc Natl Acad Sci U S A* (2002) **99**(25):16168–73. doi:10.1073/pnas.242600099
4. Butler MO, Friedlander P, Milstein MI, Mooney MM, Metzler G, Murray AP, et al. Establishment of antitumor memory in humans using in vitro-educated CD8+ T cells. *Sci Transl Med* (2011) **3**(80):80ra34. doi:10.1126/scitranslmed. 3002207
5. Park TS, Rosenberg SA, Morgan RA. Treating cancer with genetically engineered T cells. *Trends Biotechnol* (2011) **29**(11):550–7. doi:10.1016/j.tibtech. 2011.04.009
6. Gilham DE, Debets R, Pule M, Hawkins RE, Abken H. CAR-T cells and solid tumors: tuning T cells to challenge an inveterate foe. *Trends Mol Med* (2012) **18**(7):377–84. doi:10.1016/j.molmed.2012.04.009
7. Hong JJ, Rosenberg SA, Dudley ME, Yang JC, White DE, Butman JA, et al. Successful treatment of melanoma brain metastases with adoptive cell therapy. *Clin Cancer Res* (2010) **16**(19):4892–8. doi:10.1158/1078-0432.CCR-10-1507
8. Lucas S, Coulie PG. About human tumor antigens to be used in immunother- apy. *Semin Immunol* (2008) **20**(5):301–7. doi:10.1016/j.smim.2008.02.001
9. Hofmann O, Caballero OL, Stevenson BJ, Chen YT, Cohen T, Chua R, et al. Genome-wide analysis of cancer/testis gene expression. *Proc Natl Acad Sci U S A* (2008) **105**(51):20422–7. doi:10.1073/pnas.0810777105
10. Caballero OL, Chen YT. Cancer/testis (CT) antigens: potential targets for immunotherapy. *Cancer Sci* (2009) **100**(11):2014–21. doi:10.1111/j.1349-7006.2009.01303.x
11. Monte M, Simonatto M, Peche LY, Bublik DR, Gobessi S, Pierotti MA, et al. MAGE-A tumor antigens target p53 transactivation function through histone deacetylase recruitment and confer resistance to chemotherapeutic agents. *Proc Natl Acad Sci U S A* (2006) **103**(30):11160–5. doi:10.1073/pnas.0510834103
12. Yang B, O'Herrin SM, Wu J, Reagan-Shaw S, Ma Y, Bhat KM, et al. MAGE- A, mMage-b, and MAGE-C proteins form complexes with KAP1 and sup- press p53-dependent apoptosis in MAGE-positive cell lines. *Cancer Res* (2007) **67**(20):9954–62. doi:10.1158/0008-5472.CAN-07-1478
13. Liu W, Cheng S, Asa SL, Ezzat S. The melanoma-associated antigen A3 mediates fibronectin-controlled cancer progression and metastasis. *Cancer Res* (2008) **68**(19):8104–12. doi:10.1158/0008-5472.CAN-08-2132
14. Doyle JM, Gao J, Wang J, Yang M, Potts PR. MAGE-RING protein com- plexes comprise a family of E3 ubiquitin ligases. *Mol Cell* (2010) **39**(6):963–74. doi:10.1016/j.molcel.2010.08.029
15. Nardiello T, Jungbluth AA, Mei A, Diliberto M, Huang X, Dabrowski A, et al. MAGE-A inhibits apoptosis in proliferating myeloma cells through repression of Bax and maintenance of survivin. *Clin Cancer Res* (2011) **17**(13):4309–19. doi:10.1158/1078-0432.CCR-10-1820
16. Schuler-Thurner B, Schultz ES, Berger TG, Weinlich G, Ebner S, Woerl P, et al. Rapid induction of tumor-specific type 1 T helper cells in metasta- tic melanoma patients by vaccination with mature, cryopreserved, peptide- loaded monocyte-derived dendritic cells. *J Exp Med* (2002) **195**(10):1279–88. doi:10.1084/jem.20012100
17. Lurquin C, Lethé B, De Plaen E, Corbière V, Théate I, van Baren N, et al. Con- trasting frequencies of antitumor and anti-vaccine T cells in metastases of a melanoma patient vaccinated with a MAGE tumor antigen. *J Exp Med* (2005) **201**(2):249–57. doi:10.1084/jem.20041378
18. Stratton MR. Exploring the genomes of cancer cells: progress and promise. *Science* (2011) **331**(6024):1553–8. doi:10.1126/science.1204040
19. Lee W, Jiang Z, Liu J, Haverty PM, Guan Y, Stinson J, et al. The mutation spectrum revealed by paired genome sequences from a lung cancer patient. *Nature* (2010) **465**(7297):473–7. doi:10.1038/nature09004
20. Wood LD, Parsons DW, Jones S, Lin J, Sjöblom T, Leary RJ, et al. The genomic landscapes of human breast and colorectal cancers. *Science* (2007) **318**(5853):1108–13. doi:10.1126/science.1145720
21. Meyerson M, Gabriel S, Getz G. Advances in understanding cancer genomes through second-generation sequencing. *Nat Rev Genet* (2010) **11**(10):685–96. doi:10.1038/nrg2841
22. Heemskerk B, Kvistborg P, Schumacher TN. The cancer antigenome. *EMBO J*(2013) **32**(2):194–203. doi:10.1038/emboj.2012.333
23. Robbins PF, Lu YC, El-Gamil M, Li YF, Gross C, Gartner J, et al. Min- ing exomic sequencing data to identify mutated antigens recognized by adoptively transferred tumor-reactive T cells. *Nat Med* (2013) **19**(6):747–52. doi:10.1038/nm.3161
24. Cameron BJ, Gerry AB, Dukes J, Harper JV, Kannan V, Bianchi FC, et al. Identification of a Titin-derived HLA-A1-presented peptide as a cross-reactive target for engineered MAGE A3-directed T cells. *Sci Transl Med* (2013) **5**(197):197ra103. doi:10.1126/scitranslmed.3006034
25. Bonini C, Ferrari G, Verzeletti S, Servida P, Zappone E, Ruggieri L, et al. HSV-TK gene transfer into donor lymphocytes for control of allogeneic graft- versus-leukemia. *Science* (1997) **276**(5319):1719–24. doi:10.1126/science.276. 5319.1719
26. Di Stasi A, Tey SK, Dotti G, Fujita Y, Kennedy-Nasser A, Martinez C, et al. Inducible apoptosis as a safety switch for adoptive cell therapy. *N Engl J Med* (2011) **365**(18):1673–83. doi:10.1056/NEJMoa1106152
27. Kieback E, Charo J, Sommermeyer D, Blankenstein T, Uckert W. A safeguard eliminates T cell receptor gene-modified autoreactive T cells after adoptive transfer. *Proc Natl Acad Sci U S A* (2008) **105**(2):623–8. doi:10.1073/pnas. 0710198105
28. Marin V, Cribioli E, Philip B, Tettamanti S, Pizzitola I, Biondi A, et al. Comparison of different suicide-gene strategies for the safety improvement of genet- ically manipulated T cells. *Hum Gene Ther Methods*
29. Morgan RA, Chinnasamy N, Abate-Daga D, Gros A, Robbins PF, Zheng Z, et al. Cancer regression and neurological toxicity following anti-MAGE- A3 TCR gene therapy. *J Immunother* (2013) **36**(2):133–51. doi:10.1097/CJI. 0b013e3182829903
30. Linette GP, Stadtmauer EA, Maus MV, Rapoport AP, Levine BL, Emery L, et al. Cardiovascular toxicity and titin cross-reactivity of affinity-enhanced T cells in myeloma and melanoma. *Blood* (2013) **122**(6):863–71. doi:10.1182/blood- 2013-03-490565
31. Coral S, Sigalotti L, Altomonte M, Engelsberg A, Colizzi F, Cattarossi I, et al. 5-aza-2ʹ -deoxycytidine-induced expression of functional cancer testis antigens in human renal cell carcinoma: immunotherapeutic implications. *Clin Cancer Res* (2002) **8**(8):2690–5.
32. Chou J, Voong LN, Mortales CL, Towlerton AM, Pollack SM, Chen X, et al. Epigenetic modulation to enable antigen-specific T-cell therapy of colorectal cancer. *J Immunother* (2012) **35**(2):131–41. doi:10.1097/CJI. 0b013e31824300c7
33. Pollack SM, Li Y, Blaisdell MJ, Farrar EA, Chou J, Hoch BL, et al. NYESO-1/LAGE-1s and PRAME are targets for antigen specific T cells in chondrosarcoma following treatment with 5-Aza-2-deoxycitabine. *PLoS One* (2012) **7**(2):e32165. doi:10.1371/journal.pone.0032165
34. Wargo JA, Robbins PF, Li Y, Zhao Y, El-Gamil M, Caragacianu D, et al. Recog- nition of NY-ESO-1+ tumor cells by engineered lymphocytes is enhanced by improved vector design and epigenetic modulation of tumor antigen expres- sion. *Cancer Immunol Immunother* (2009) **58**(3):383–94. doi:10.1007/s00262-008-0562-x
35. Goodyear O, Agathanggelou A, Novitzky-Basso I, Siddique S, McSkeane T, Ryan G, et al. Induction of a CD8+ T-cell response to the MAGE cancer testis antigen by combined treatment with azacitidine and sodium valproate in patients with acute myeloid leukemia and myelodysplasia. *Blood* (2010) **116**(11):1908–18. doi:10.1182/blood-2009-11-249474

36. Skipper JC, Hendrickson RC, Gulden PH, Brichard V, Van Pel A, Chen Y, et al. An HLA-A2-restricted tyrosinase antigen on melanoma cells results from posttranslational modification and suggests a novel pathway for processing of membrane proteins. *J Exp Med* (1996) **183**(2):527–34. doi:10.1084/jem.183. 2.527
37. Dalet A, Robbins PF, Stroobant V, Vigneron N, Li YF, El-Gamil M, et al. An antigenic peptide produced by reverse splicing and double asparagine deami- dation. *Proc Natl Acad Sci U S A* (2011) **108**(29):E323–31. doi:10.1073/pnas. 1101892108
38. Guillaume B, Stroobant V, Bousquet-Dubouch MP, Colau D, Chapiro J, Parmentier N, et al. Analysis of the processing of seven human tumor antigens by intermediate proteasomes. *J Immunol* (2012) **189**(7):3538–47. doi:10.4049/jimmunol.1103213
39. Klebanoff CA, Khong HT, Antony PA, Palmer DC, Restifo NP. Sinks, suppressors and antigen presenters: how lymphodepletion enhances T cell-mediated tumor immunotherapy. *Trends Immunol* (2005) **26**(2):111–7. doi:10.1016/j.it. 2004.12.003
40. Blank CU, Hooijkaas AI, Haanen JB, Schumacher TN. Combination of targeted therapy and immunotherapy in melanoma. *Cancer Immunol Immunother* (2011) **60**(10):1359–71. doi:10.1007/s00262-011-1079-2
41. Walch JM, Zeng Q, Li Q, Oberbarnscheidt MH, Hoffman RA, Williams AL, et al. Cognate antigen directs CD8+ T cell migration to vascularized trans- plants. *J Clin Invest* (2013) **123**(6):2663–71. doi:10.1172/JCI66722
42. Engels B, Engelhard VH, Sidney J, Sette A, Binder DC, Liu RB, et al. Relapse or eradication of cancer is predicted by peptide-major histocompatibility complex affinity. *Cancer Cell* (2013) **23**(4):516–26. doi:10.1016/j.ccr.2013.03.018
43. Anders K, Buschow C, Herrmann A, Milojkovic A, Loddenkemper C, Kammer- toens T, et al. Oncogene-targeting T cells reject large tumors while oncogene inactivation selects escape variants in mouse models of cancer. *Cancer Cell* (2011) **20**(6):755–67. doi:10.1016/j.ccr.2011.10.019
44. Briesemeister D, Sommermeyer D, Loddenkemper C, Loew R, Uckert W, Blankenstein T, et al. Tumor rejection by local interferon gamma induction in established tumors is associated with blood vessel destruction and necrosis. *Int J Cancer* (2011) **128**(2):371–8. doi:10.1002/ijc.25350
45. Listopad JJ, Kammertoens T, Anders K, Silkenstedt B, Willimsky G, Schmidt K, et al. Fas expression by tumor stroma is required for cancer eradication. *Proc Natl Acad Sci U S A* (2013) **110**(6):2276–81. doi:10.1073/pnas.1218295110
46. Algarra I, Cabrera T, Garrido F. The HLA crossroad in tumor immunology. *Hum Immunol* (2000) **61**(1):65–73. doi:10.1016/S0198-8859(99)00156-1
47. Marincola FM, Jaffee EM, Hicklin DJ, Ferrone S. Escape of human solid tumors from T-cell recognition: molecular mechanisms and functional significance. *Adv Immunol* (2000) **74**:181–273. doi:10.1016/S0065-2776(08)60911-6
48. Seliger B, Maeurer MJ, Ferrone S. Antigen-processing machinery breakdown and tumor growth. *Immunol Today* (2000) **21**(9):455–64. doi:10.1016/S0167- 5699(00)01692-3
49. Maeurer MJ, Gollin SM, Martin D, Swaney W, Bryant J, Castelli C, et al. Tumor escape from immune recognition: lethal recurrent melanoma in a patient asso- ciated with downregulation of the peptide transporter protein TAP-1 and loss of expression of the immunodominant MART-1/Melan-A antigen. *J Clin Invest* (1996) **98**(7):1633–41. doi:10.1172/JCI118958
50. Wang Z, Marincola FM, Rivoltini L, Parmiani G, Ferrone S. Selective histo- compatibilityleukocyte antigen (HLA)-A2 loss caused by aberrant pre-mRNA splicing in 624MEL28 melanoma cells. *J Exp Med* (1999) **190**(2):205–15. doi:10.1084/jem.190.2.205
51. Khong HT, Wang QJ, Rosenberg SA. Identification of multiple antigens recog- nized by tumor-infiltrating lymphocytes from a single patient: tumor escape by antigen loss and loss of MHC expression. *J Immunother* (2004) **27**(3):184–90. doi:10.1097/00002371-200405000-00002
52. Mackensen A, Meidenbauer N, Vogl S, Laumer M, Berger J, Andreesen R. Phase I study of adoptive T-cell therapy using antigen-specific CD8+ T cells for the treatment of patients with metastatic melanoma. *J Clin Oncol* (2006) **24**(31):5060–9. doi:10.1200/JCO.2006.07.1100
53. Landsberg J, Kohlmeyer J, Renn M, Bald T, Rogava M, Cron M, et al. Melanomas resist T-cell therapy through inflammation-induced reversible dedifferentia- tion. *Nature* (2012) **490**(7420):412–6. doi:10.1038/nature11538
54. Scarlett UK, Rutkowski MR, Rauwerdink AM, Fields J, Escovar-Fadul X, Baird J, et al. Ovarian cancer progression is controlled by phenotypic changes in dendritic cells. *J Exp Med* (2012) **209**(3):495–506. doi:10.1084/jem.20111413
55. Ward PL, Koeppen HK, Hurteau T, Rowley DA, Schreiber H. Major histocom- patibility complex class I and unique antigen expression by murine tumors that escaped from CD8+ T-cell-dependent surveillance. *Cancer Res* (1990) **50**(13):3851–8.
56. DuPage M, Cheung AF, Mazumdar C, Winslow MM, Bronson R, Schmidt LM, et al. Endogenous T cell responses to antigens expressed in lung adenocarci- nomas delay
57. DuPage M, Mazumdar C, Schmidt LM, Cheung AF, Jacks T. Expression of tumour-specific antigens underlies cancer immunoediting. *Nature* (2012) **482**(7385):405–9. doi:10.1038/nature10803
58. Matsushita H, Vesely MD, Koboldt DC, Rickert CG, Uppaluri R, Magrini VJ, et al. Cancer exome analysis reveals a T-cell-dependent mechanism of cancer immunoediting. *Nature* (2012) **482**(7385):400–4. doi:10.1038/nature10755
59. Kaluza KM, Kottke T, Diaz RM, Rommelfanger D, Thompson J, Vile R. Adop- tive transfer of cytotoxic T lymphocytes targeting two different antigens lim- its antigen loss and tumor escape. *Hum Gene Ther* (2012) **23**(10):1054–64. doi:10.1089/hum.2012.030
60. Pulido J, Kottke T, Thompson J, Galivo F, Wongthida P, Diaz RM, et al. Using virally expressed melanoma cDNA libraries to identify tumor-associated anti- gens that cure melanoma. *Nat Biotechnol* (2012) **30**(4):337–43. doi:10.1038/ nbt.2157
61. Schietinger A, Philip M, Liu RB, Schreiber K, Schreiber H. Bystander killing of cancer requires the cooperation of CD4(+) and CD8(+) T cells during the effector phase. *J Exp Med* (2010) **207**(11):2469–77. doi:10.1084/jem.20092450
62. Gure AO, Chua R, Williamson B, Gonen M, Ferrera CA, Gnjatic S, et al. Cancer-testis genes are coordinately expressed and are markers of poor out- come in non-small cell lung cancer. *Clin Cancer Res* (2005) **11**(22):8055–62. doi:10.1158/1078-0432.CCR-05-1203
63. Cheung AF, Dupage MJ, Dong HK, Chen J, Jacks T. Regulated expres- sion of a tumor-associated antigen reveals multiple levels of T-cell toler- ance in a mouse model of lung cancer. *Cancer Res* (2008) **68**(22):9459–68. doi:10.1158/0008-5472.CAN-08-2634
64. Coccoris M, Straetemans T, Govers C, Lamers C, Sleijfer S, Debets R. T cell receptor (TCR) gene therapy to treat melanoma: lessons from clinical and preclinical studies. *Expert Opin Biol Ther* (2010) **10**(4):547–62. doi:10.1517/ 14712591003614756
65. Bendle GM, Linnemann C, Hooijkaas AI, Bies L, de Witte MA, Jorritsma A, et al. Lethal graft-versus-host disease in mouse models of T cell receptor gene therapy. *Nat Med* (2010) **16**(5):565–70. doi:10.1038/nm.2128
66. van Loenen MM, de Boer R, Amir AL, Hagedoorn RS, Volbeda GL, Willemze R, et al. Mixed T cell receptor dimers harbor potentially harmful neoreac- tivity. *Proc Natl Acad Sci U S A* (2010) **107**(24):10972–7. doi:10.1073/pnas. 1005802107
67. Govers C, Sebestyén Z, Coccoris M, Willemsen RA, Debets R. T cell receptor gene therapy: strategies for optimizing transgenic TCR pairing. *Trends Mol Med* (2010) **16**(2):77–87. doi:10.1016/j.molmed.2009.12.004
68. Cohen CJ, Zhao Y, Zheng Z, Rosenberg SA, Morgan RA. Enhanced antitumor activity of murine-human hybrid T-cell receptor (TCR) in human lympho- cytes is associated with improved pairing and TCR/CD3 stability. *Cancer Res* (2006) **66**(17):8878–86. doi:10.1158/0008-5472.CAN-06-1450
69. Kuball J, Dossett ML, Wolfl M, Ho WY, Voss RH, Fowler C, et al. Facilitating matched pairing and expression of TCR chains introduced into human T cells. *Blood* (2007) **109**(6):2331–8. doi:10.1182/blood-2006-05-023069
70. Thomas S, Xue SA, Cesco-Gaspere M, San José E, Hart DP, Wong V, et al. Targeting the Wilms tumor antigen 1 by TCR gene transfer: TCR variants improve tetramer binding but not the function of gene modified human T cells. *J Immunol* (2007) **179**(9):5803–10.
71. Haga-Friedman A, Horovitz-Fried M, Cohen CJ. Incorporation of transmem- brane hydrophobic mutations in the TCR enhance its surface expression and T cell functional avidity. *J Immunol* (2012) **188**(11):5538–46. doi:10.4049/jimmunol.1103020
72. Kuball J, Hauptrock B, Malina V, Antunes E, Voss RH, Wolfl M, et al. Increasing functional avidity of TCR-redirected T cells by removing defined N-glycosylation sites in the TCR constant domain. *J Exp Med* (2009) **206**(2):463–75. doi:10.1084/jem.20082487
73. Willemsen RA, Weijtens ME, Ronteltap C, Eshhar Z, Gratama JW, Chames P, et al. Grafting primary human T lymphocytes with cancer-specific chimeric single chain and two chain TCR. *Gene Ther* (2000) **7**(16):1369–77. doi:10. 1038/sj.gt.3301253
74. Sebestyén Z, Schooten E, Sals T, Zaldivar I, San José E, Alarcón B, et al. Human TCR that incorporate CD3zeta induce highly preferred pairing between TCRalpha and beta chains following gene transfer. *J Immunol* (2008) **180**(11):7736–46.
75. Sommermeyer D, Uckert W. Minimal amino acid exchange in human TCR constant regions fosters improved function of TCR gene-modified T cells. *J Immunol* (2010) **184**(11):6223–31. doi:10.4049/jimmunol.0902055
76. Bialer G, Horovitz-Fried M, Ya'Acobi S, Morgan RA, Cohen CJ. Selected murine residues endow human TCR with enhanced tumor recognition. *J Immunol* (2010) **184**(11):6232–41. doi:10.4049/jimmunol.0902047

77. Govers C, Sebestyén Z, Berrevoets C, Venselaar H, Debets R. T cell receptor fused to CD3ζ: transmembrane domain of CD3ζ prevents TCR mispairing, whereas complete CD3ζ directs functional TCR expression. *Open Gene Ther J*(2011) **4**:11–22. doi:10.2174/1875037001104010011
78. Ahmadi M, King JW, Xue SA, Voisine C, Holler A, Wright GP, et al. CD3 limits the efficacy of TCR gene therapy in vivo. *Blood* (2011) **118**(13):3528–37. doi:10.1182/blood-2011-04-346338
79. Ochi T, Fujiwara H, Okamoto S, An J, Nagai K, Shirakata T, et al. Novel adoptive T-cell immunotherapy using a WT1-specific TCR vector encoding silencers for endogenous TCRs shows marked antileukemia reactivity and safety. *Blood* (2011) **118**(6):1495–503. doi:10.1182/blood-2011-02-337089
80. Okamoto S, Mineno J, Ikeda H, Fujiwara H, Yasukawa M, Shiku H, et al. Improved expression and reactivity of transduced tumor-specific TCRs in human lymphocytes by specific silencing of endogenous TCR. *Cancer Res* (2009) **69**(23):9003–11. doi:10.1158/0008-5472.CAN-09-1450
81. Provasi E, Genovese P, Lombardo A, Magnani Z, Liu PQ, Reik A, et al. Editing T cell specificity towards leukemia by zinc finger nucleases and lentiviral gene transfer. *Nat Med* (2012) **18**(5):807–15. doi:10.1038/nm.2700
82. Aleksic M, Liddy N, Molloy PE, Pumphrey N, Vuidepot A, Chang KM, et al. Different affinity windows for virus and cancer-specific T-cell receptors: implications for therapeutic strategies. *Eur J Immunol* (2012) **42**(12):3174–9. doi:10.1002/eji.201242606
83. Sadovnikova E, Jopling LA, Soo KS, Stauss HJ. Generation of human tumor- reactive cytotoxic T cells against peptides presented by non-self HLA class I molecules. *Eur J Immunol* (1998) **28**(1):193–200. doi:10.1002/(SICI)1521-4141(199801)28:01<193::AID-IMMU193>3.3.CO;2-B
84. Savage P, Gao L, Vento K, Cowburn P, Man S, Steven N, et al. Use of B cell-bound HLA-A2 class I monomers to generate high-avidity, allo-restricted CTLs against the leukemia-associated protein Wilms tumor antigen. *Blood* (2004) **103**(12):4613–5. doi:10.1182/blood-2003-11-3903
85. Wilde S, Geiger C, Milosevic S, Mosetter B, Eichenlaub S, Schendel DJ. Genera- tion of allo-restricted peptide-specific T cells using RNA-pulsed dendritic cells: a three phase experimental procedure. *Oncoimmunology* (2012) **1**(2):129–40. doi:10.4161/onci.1.2.18216
86. Stanislawski T, Voss RH, Lotz C, Sadovnikova E, Willemsen RA, Kuball J, et al. Circumventing tolerance to a human MDM2-derived tumor antigen by TCR gene transfer. *Nat Immunol* (2001) **2**(10):962–70. doi:10.1038/ni1001-962
87. Li LP, Lampert JC, Chen X, Leitao C, Popovic J, Müller W, et al. Transgenic mice with a diverse human T cell antigen receptor repertoire. *Nat Med* (2010) **16**(9):1029–34. doi:10.1038/nm.2197
88. Robbins PF, Li YF, El-Gamil M, Zhao Y, Wargo JA, Zheng Z, et al. Single and dual amino acid substitutions in TCR CDRs can enhance antigen-specific T cell functions. *J Immunol* (2008) **180**(9):6116–31.
89. Zoete V, Michielin O. Comparison between computational alanine scanning and per-residue binding free energy decomposition for protein-protein asso- ciation using MM-GBSA: application to the TCR-p-MHC complex. *Proteins* (2007) **67**(4):1026–47. doi:10.1002/prot.21395
90. Holler PD, Chlewicki LK, Kranz DM. TCRs with high affinity for foreign pMHC show self-reactivity. *Nat Immunol* (2003) **4**(1):55–62. doi:10.1038/ni863
91. Li Y, Moysey R, Molloy PE, Vuidepot AL, Mahon T, Baston E, et al. Directed evolution of human T-cell receptors with picomolar affinities by phage display. *Nat Biotechnol* (2005) **23**(3):349–54. doi:10.1038/nbt1070
92. Chervin AS, Aggen DH, Raseman JM, Kranz DM. Engineering higher affin- ity T cell receptors using a T cell display system. *J Immunol Methods* (2008) **339**(2):175–84. doi:10.1016/j.jim.2008.09.016
93. Schmid DA, Irving MB, Posevitz V, Hebeisen M, Posevitz-Fejfar A, Sarria JC, et al. Evidence for a TCR affinity threshold delimiting maximal CD8 T cell function. *J Immunol* (2010) **184**(9):4936–46. doi:10.4049/jimmunol.1000173
94. Thomas S, Xue SA, Bangham CR, Jakobsen BK, Morris EC, Stauss HJ. Human T cells expressing affinity-matured TCR display accelerated responses but fail to recognize low density of MHC-peptide antigen. *Blood* (2011) **118**(2):319–29. doi:10.1182/blood-2010-12-326736
95. Brentville VA, Metheringham RL, Gunn B, Durrant LG. High avidity cyto- toxic T lymphocytes can be selected into the memory pool but they are exquisitely sensitive to functional impairment. *PLoS One* (2012) **7**(7):e41112. doi:10.1371/journal.pone.0041112
96. Hebeisen M, Baitsch L, Presotto D, Baumgaertner P, Romero P, Michielin O, et al. SHP-1 phosphatase activity counteracts increased T cell receptor affinity. *J Clin Invest* (2013) **123**(3):1044–56. doi:10.1172/JCI65325
97. Chen L, Flies DB. Molecularmechanisms of T cell co-stimulation and co- inhibition. *Nat Rev Immunol* (2013) **13**(4):227–42. doi:10.1038/nri3405
98. Zippelius A, Batard P, Rubio-Godoy V, Bioley G, Liénard D, Lejeune F, et al. Effector function of human tumor-specific CD8 T cells in melanoma lesions: a state of local functional tolerance. *Cancer Res* (2004) **64**(8):2865–73. doi:10.1158/0008-5472.CAN-03-3066
99. Wherry EJ. T cell exhaustion. *Nat Immunol* (2011) **12**(6):492–9. doi:10.1038/ ni.2035
100. Murphy TL, Murphy KM. Slow down and survive: enigmatic immunoregu- lation by BTLA and HVEM. *Annu Rev Immunol* (2010) **28**:389–411. doi:10. 1146/annurev-immunol-030409-101202
101. Ngiow SF, von Scheidt B, Akiba H, Yagita H, Teng MW, Smyth MJ. Anti-TIM3 antibody promotes T cell IFN-gamma-mediated antitumor immunity and suppresses established tumors. *Cancer Res* (2011) **71**(10):3540–51. doi:10.1158/0008-5472.CAN-11-0096
102. Fourcade J, Sun Z, Benallaoua M, Guillaume P, Luescher IF, Sander C, et al. Upregulation of Tim-3 and PD-1 expression is associated with tumor antigen- specific CD8+ T cell dysfunction in melanoma patients. *J Exp Med* (2010) **207**(10):2175–86. doi:10.1084/jem.20100637
103. Curran MA, Kim M, Montalvo W, Al-Shamkhani A, Allison JP. Combination CTLA-4 blockade and 4-1BB activation enhances tumor rejection by increas- ing T-cell infiltration, proliferation, and cytokine production. *PLoS One* (2011) **6**(4):e19499. doi:10.1371/journal.pone.0019499
104. Marabelle A, Kohrt H, Sagiv-Barfi I, Ajami B, Axtell RC, Zhou G, et al. Deplet- ing tumor-specific Tregs at a single site eradicates disseminated tumors. *J Clin Invest* (2013) **123**(6):2447–63. doi:10.1172/JCI64859
105. Simpson TR, Li F, Montalvo-Ortiz W, Sepulveda MA, Bergerhoff K, Arce F, et al. Fc-dependent depletion of tumor-infiltrating regulatory T cells co-defines the efficacy of anti-CTLA-4 therapy against melanoma. *J Exp Med* (2013) **210**(9):1695–710. doi:10.1084/jem.20130579
106. Kalos M, Levine BL, Porter DL, Katz S, Grupp SA, Bagg A, et al. T cells with chimeric antigen receptors have potent antitumor effects and can estab- lish memory in patients with advanced leukemia. *Sci Transl Med* (2011) **3**(95):95ra73. doi:10.1126/scitranslmed.3002842
107. Brentjens RJ, Rivière I, Park JH, Davila ML, Wang X, Stefanski J, et al. Safety and persistence of adoptively transferred autologous CD19-targeted T cells in patients with relapsed or chemotherapy refractory B-cell leukemias. *Blood* (2011) **118**(18):4817–28. doi:10.1182/blood-2011-04-348540
108. Kochenderfer JN, Dudley ME, Feldman SA, Wilson WH, Spaner DE, Maric I, et al. B-cell depletion and remissions of malignancy along with cytokine- associated toxicity in a clinical trial of anti-CD19 chimeric-antigen-receptor- transduced T cells. *Blood* (2012) **119**(12):2709–20. doi:10.1182/blood-2011- 10-384388
109. Lamers CH, Willemsen R, van Elzakker P, van Steenbergen-Langeveld S, Broert- jes M, Oosterwijk-Wakka J, et al. Immune responses to transgene and retro- viral vector in patients treated with ex vivo-engineered T cells. *Blood* (2011) **117**(1):72–82. doi:10.1182/blood-2010-07-294520
110. Aggen DH, Chervin AS, Schmitt TM, Engels B, Stone JD, Richman SA, et al. Single-chain ValphaVbeta T-cell receptors function without mispairing with endogenous TCR chains. *Gene Ther* (2012) **19**(4):365–74. doi:10.1038/gt.2011. 104
111. Schaft N, Lankiewicz B, Drexhage J, Berrevoets C, Moss DJ, Levitsky V, et al. T cell re-targeting to EBV antigens following TCR gene transfer: CD28- containing receptors mediate enhanced antigen-specific IFNgamma produc- tion. *Int Immunol* (2006) **18**(4):591–601. doi:10.1093/intimm/dxh401
112. Singh H, Figliola MJ, Dawson MJ, Huls H, Olivares S, Switzer K, et al. Repro- gramming CD19-specific T cells with IL-21 signaling can improve adoptive immunotherapyofB-lineage malignancies. *Cancer Res* (2011) **71**(10):3516–27. doi:10.1158/0008-5472.CAN-10-3843
113. Klebanoff CA, Gattinoni L, Torabi-Parizi P, Kerstann K, Cardones AR, Finkel- stein SE, et al. Central memory self/tumor-reactive CD8+ T cells confer supe- rior antitumor immunity compared with effector memory T cells. *Proc Natl Acad Sci U S A* (2005) **102**(27):9571–6. doi:10.1073/pnas.0503726102
114. Nakayamada S, Takahashi H, Kanno Y, O'Shea JJ. Helper T cell diversity and plasticity. *Curr Opin Immunol* (2012) **24**(3):297–302. doi:10.1016/j.coi.2012.01.014
115. Gattinoni L, Klebanoff CA, Restifo NP. Paths to stemness: building the ultimate antitumour T cell. *Nat Rev Cancer* (2012) **12**(10):671–84. doi:10.1038/nrc3322
116. Kaneko S, Mastaglio S, Bondanza A, Ponzoni M, Sanvito F, Aldrighetti L, et al. IL-7 and IL-15 allow the generation of suicide gene-modified allore- active self-renewing central memory human T lymphocytes. *Blood* (2009) **113**(5):1006–15. doi:10.1182/blood-2008-05-156059
117. Pouw N, Treffers-Westerlaken E, Kraan J, Wittink F, ten HagenT, Verweij J, et al. Combination of IL-21 and IL-15 enhances tumour-specific cytotoxicity and cytokine production

of TCR-transduced primary T cells. *Cancer Immunol Immunother* (2010) **59**(6):921–31. doi:10.1007/s00262-010-0818-0

118. Zeng R, Spolski R, Finkelstein SE, Oh S, Kovanen PE, Hinrichs CS, et al. Synergy of IL-21 and IL-15 in regulating CD8+ T cell expansion and function. *J Exp Med* (2005) **201**(1):139–48. doi:10.1084/jem.20041057

119. Stephan MT, Moon JJ, Um SH, Bershteyn A, Irvine DJ. Therapeutic cell engineering with surface-conjugated synthetic nanoparticles. *Nat Med* (2010) **16**(9):1035–41. doi:10.1038/nm.2198

120. Berger C, Jensen MC, Lansdorp PM, Gough M, Elliott C, Riddell SR. Adoptive transfer of effector CD8+ T cells derived from central memory cells establishes persistent T cell memory in primates. *J Clin Invest* (2008) **118**(1):294–305. doi:10.1172/JCI32103

121. Hinrichs CS, Borman ZA, Cassard L, Gattinoni L, Spolski R, Yu Z, et al. Adop- tively transferred effector cells derived from naive rather than central memory CD8+ T cells mediate superior antitumor immunity. *Proc Natl Acad Sci U S A* (2009) **106**(41):17469–74. doi:10.1073/pnas.0907448106

122. Gattinoni L, Lugli E, Ji Y, Pos Z, Paulos CM, Quigley MF, et al. A human mem- ory T cell subset with stem cell-like properties. *Nat Med* (2011) **17**(10):1290–7. doi:10.1038/nm.2446

123. Cieri N, Camisa B, Cocchiarella F, Forcato M, Oliveira G, Provasi E, et al. IL-7 and IL-15 instruct the generation of human memory stem T cells from naive precursors. *Blood* (2013) **121**(4):573–84. doi:10.1182/blood-2012-05-431718

124. Hirahara K, Poholek A, Vahedi G, Laurence A, Kanno Y, Milner JD, et al. Mechanisms underlying helper T-cell plasticity: implications for immune- mediated disease. *J Allergy Clin Immunol* (2013) **131**(5):1276–87. doi:10.1016/ j.jaci.2013.03.015

125. Nishimura T, Iwakabe K, Sekimoto M, Ohmi Y, Yahata T, Nakui M, et al. Distinct role of antigen-specific T helper type 1 (Th1) and Th2 cells in tumor eradica- tion in vivo. *J Exp Med* (1999) **190**(5):617–27. doi:10.1084/jem.190.5.617

126. Muranski P, Boni A, Antony PA, Cassard L, Irvine KR, Kaiser A, et al. Tumor- specific Th17-polarized cells eradicate large established melanoma. *Blood* (2008) **112**(2):362–73. doi:10.1182/blood-2007-11-120998

127. Hunziker L, Klenerman P, Zinkernagel RM, Ehl S. Exhaustion of cytotoxic T cells during adoptive immunotherapy of virus carrier mice can be pre- vented by B cells or CD4+ T cells. *Eur J Immunol* (2002) **32**(2):374–82. doi:10.1002/1521-4141(200202)32:2<374::AID-IMMU374>3.0.CO;2-9

128. Marzo AL, Kinnear BF, Lake RA, Frelinger JJ, Collins EJ, Robinson BW, et al. Tumor-specific CD4+ T cells have a major "post-licensing" role in CTL medi- ated anti-tumor immunity. *J Immunol* (2000) **165**(11):6047–55.

129. Antony PA, Piccirillo CA, Akpinarli A, Finkelstein SE, Speiss PJ, Surman DR, et al. CD8+ T cell immunity against a tumor/self-antigen is augmented by CD4+ T helper cells and hindered by naturally occurring T regulatory cells. *J Immunol* (2005) **174**(5):2591–601.

130. Gyobu H, Tsuji T, Suzuki Y, Ohkuri T, Chamoto K, Kuroki M, et al. Generation and targeting of human tumor-specific Tc1 and Th1 cells transduced with lentivirus containing a chimeric immunoglobulin T-cell receptor. *Cancer Res* (2004) **64**(4):1490–5. doi:10.1158/0008-5472.CAN-03-2780

131. Muranski P, Borman ZA, Kerkar SP, Klebanoff CA, Ji Y, Sanchez-Perez L, et al. Th17 cells are long lived and retain a stem cell-like molecular signature. *Immunity* (2011) **35**(6):972–85. doi:10.1016/j.immuni.2011.09.019

132. Kuball J, Schmitz FW, Voss RH, Ferreira EA, Engel R, Guillaume P, et al. Coop- eration of human tumor-reactive CD4+ and CD8+ T cells after redirection of their specificity by a high-affinity p53A2.1-specific TCR. *Immunity* (2005) **22**(1):117–29. doi:10.1016/j.immuni.2004.12.005

133. Willemsen R, Ronteltap C, Heuveling M, Debets R, Bolhuis R. Redirecting human CD4+ T lymphocytes to the MHC class I-restricted melanoma anti- gen MAGE-A1 by TCR alphabeta gene transfer requires CD8alpha. *Gene Ther* (2005) **12**(2):140–6. doi:10.1038/sj.gt.3302388

134. Morris EC, Tsallios A, Bendle GM, Xue SA, Stauss HJ. A critical role of T cell antigen receptor-transduced MHC class I-restricted helper T cells in tumor protection. *Proc Natl Acad Sci U S A* (2005) **102**(22):7934–9. doi:10.1073/pnas.0500357102

135. Willemsen RA, Sebestyén Z, Ronteltap C, Berrevoets C, Drexhage J, Debets R. CD8 alpha coreceptor to improve TCR gene transfer to treat melanoma: down- regulation of tumor-specific production of IL-4, IL-5, and IL-10. *J Immunol* (2006) **177**(2):991–8.

136. Mukasa R, Balasubramani A, Lee YK, Whitley SK, Weaver BT, Shibata Y, et al. Epigenetic instability of cytokine and transcription factor gene loci under- lies plasticity of the T helper 17 cell lineage. *Immunity* (2010) **32**(5):616–27. doi:10.1016/j.immuni.2010.04.016

137. Lighvani AA, Frucht DM, Jankovic D, Yamane H, Aliberti J, Hissong BD, et al. T-bet is rapidly induced by interferon-gamma in lymphoid and myeloid cells. *Proc Natl Acad Sci U S A* (2001) **98**(26):15137–42. doi:10.1073/pnas. 261570598

138. Afkarian M, Sedy JR, Yang J, Jacobson NG, Cereb N, Yang SY, et al. T-bet is a STAT1-induced regulator of IL-12R expression in naive CD4+ T cells. *Nat Immunol* (2002) **3**(6):549–57. doi:10.1038/ni794

139. Amarnath S, Mangus CW, Wang JC, Wei F, He A, Kapoor V, et al. The PDL1-PD1 axis converts human TH1 cells into regulatory T cells. *Sci Transl Med* (2011) **3**(111):111ra120. doi:10.1126/scitranslmed.3003130

140. Delgoffe GM, Kole TP, Zheng Y, Zarek PE, Matthews KL, Xiao B, et al. The mTOR kinase differentially regulates effector and regulatory T cell lineage com- mitment. *Immunity* (2009) **30**(6):832–44. doi:10.1016/j.immuni.2009.04.014

141. Chang CH, Curtis JD, Maggi LBJr, Faubert B, Villarino AV, O'Sullivan D, et al. Posttranscriptional control of T cell effector function by aerobic glycolysis. *Cell* (2013) **153**(6):1239–51. doi:10.1016/j.cell.2013.05.016

142. Spranger S, Spaapen RM, Zha Y, Williams J, Meng Y, Ha TT, et al. Up- regulation of PD-L1, IDO, and Tregs in the melanoma tumor microenvi- ronment is driven by CD8+ T cells. *Sci Transl Med* (2013) **5**(200):200ra116. doi:10.1126/scitranslmed.3006504

143. Galon J, Costes A, Sanchez-Cabo F, Kirilovsky A, Mlecnik B, Lagorce-Pagès C, et al. Type, density, and location of immune cells within human col- orectal tumors predict clinical outcome. *Science* (2006) **313**(5795):1960–4. doi:10.1126/science.1129139

144. Kalialis LV, Drzewiecki KT, Klyver H. Spontaneous regression of metastases from melanoma: review of the literature. *Melanoma Res* (2009) **19**(5):275–82. doi:10.1097/CMR.0b013e32832eabd5

145. Zhang L, Conejo-Garcia JR, Katsaros D, Gimotty PA, Massobrio M, Regnani G, et al. Intratumoral T cells, recurrence, and survival in epithelial ovarian cancer. *N Engl J Med* (2003) **348**(3):203–13. doi:10.1056/NEJMoa020177

146. Rahir G, Moser M. Tumor microenvironment and lymphocyte infiltration. *Cancer Immunol Immunother* (2012) **61**(6):751–9. doi:10.1007/s00262-012- 1253-1

147. Shrimali RK, Yu Z, Theoret MR, Chinnasamy D, Restifo NP, Rosenberg SA. Antiangiogenic agents can increase lymphocyte infiltration into tumor and enhance the effectiveness of adoptive immunotherapy of cancer. *Cancer Res* (2010) **70**(15):6171–80. doi:10.1158/0008-5472.CAN-10-0153

148. Mazzieri R, Pucci F, Moi D, Zonari E, Ranghetti A, Berti A, et al. Targeting the ANG2/TIE2 axis inhibits tumor growth and metastasis by impairing angiogen- esis and disabling rebounds of proangiogenic myeloid cells. *Cancer Cell* (2011) **19**(4):512–26. doi:10.1016/j.ccr.2011.02.005

149. Chinnasamy D, Yu Z, Theoret MR, Zhao Y, Shrimali RK, Morgan RA, et al. Gene therapy using genetically modified lymphocytes targeting VEGFR-2 inhibits the growth of vascularized syngenic tumors in mice. *J Clin Invest* (2010) **120**(11):3953–68. doi:10.1172/JCI43490

150. Dirkx AE, oude Egbrink MG, Castermans K, van derSchaft DW, Thijssen VL, Dings RP, et al. Anti-angiogenesis therapy can overcome endothelial cell anergy and promote leukocyte-endothelium interactions and infiltration in tumors. *FASEB J* (2006) **20**(6):621–30. doi:10.1096/fj.05-4493com

151. Buckanovich RJ, Facciabene A, Kim S, Benencia F, Sasaroli D, Balint K, et al. Endothelin B receptor mediates the endothelial barrier to T cell hom- ing to tumors and disables immune therapy. *Nat Med* (2008) **14**(1):28–36. doi:10.1038/nm1699

152. Martinet L, Garrido I, Filleron T, Le Guellec S, Bellard E, Fournie JJ, et al. Human solid tumors contain high endothelial venules: association with T- and B-lymphocyte infiltration and favorable prognosis in breast cancer. *Cancer Res* (2011) **71**(17):5678–87. doi:10.1158/0008-5472.CAN-11-0431

153. Cipponi A, Mercier M, Seremet T, Baurain JF, Théate I, van den Oord J, et al. Neogenesis of lymphoid structures and antibody responses occur in human melanoma metastases. *Cancer Res* (2012) **72**(16):3997–4007. doi:10.1158/0008-5472.CAN-12-1377

154. Harlin H, Meng Y, Peterson AC, Zha Y, Tretiakova M, Slingluff C, et al. Chemokine expression in melanoma metastases associated with CD8+ T-cell recruitment. *Cancer Res* (2009) **69**(7):3077–85. doi:10.1158/0008-5472.CAN- 08-2281

155. Hong M, Puaux AL, Huang C, Loumagne L, Tow C, Mackay C, et al. Chemotherapy induces intratumoral expression of chemokines in cutaneous melanoma, favoring T-cell infiltration and tumor control. *Cancer Res* (2011) **71**(22):6997–7009. doi:10.1158/0008-5472.CAN-11-1466

156. Kershaw MH, Wang G, Westwood JA, Pachynski RK, Tiffany HL, Marincola FM, et al. Redirecting migration of T cells to chemokine secreted from tumors by genetic modification with CXCR2. *Hum Gene Ther* (2002) **13**(16):1971–80. doi:10.1089/10430340260355374

157. Craddock JA, Lu A, Bear A, Pule M, Brenner MK, Rooney CM, et al. Enhanced tumor trafficking of GD2 chimeric antigen receptor T cells by expres- sion of the chemokine receptor CCR2b. *J Immunother* (2010) **33**(8):780–8. doi:10.1097/CJI.0b013e3181ee6675

158. Moon EK, Carpenito C, Sun J, Wang LC, Kapoor V, Predina J, et al. Expression of a functional CCR2 receptor enhances tumor localization and tumor eradi- cation by retargeted human T cells expressing a mesothelin-specific chimeric antibody receptor. *Clin Cancer Res* (2011) **17**(14):4719–30. doi:10.1158/1078- 0432.CCR-11-0351

159. Uyttenhove C, Pilotte L, Théate I, Stroobant V, Colau D, Parmentier N, et al. Evidence for a tumoral immune resistance mechanism based on tryptophan degradation by indoleamine 2,3-dioxygenase. *Nat Med* (2003) **9**(10):1269–74. doi:10.1038/nm934

160. Bronte V, Zanovello P. Regulation of immune responses by L-arginine metab- olism. *Nat Rev Immunol* (2005) **5**(8):641–54. doi:10.1038/nri1668

161. Nagaraj S, Gupta K, Pisarev V, Kinarsky L, Sherman S, Kang L, et al. Altered recognition of antigen is a mechanism of CD8+ T cell tolerance in cancer. *Nat Med* (2007) **13**(7):828–35. doi:10.1038/nm1609

162. Molon B, Ugel S, Del Pozzo F, Soldani C, Zilio S, Avella D, et al. Chemokine nitration prevents intratumoral infiltration of antigen-specific T cells. *J Exp Med* (2011) **208**(10):1949–62. doi:10.1084/jem.20101956

163. Zhang Q, Yang X, Pins M, Javonovic B, Kuzel T, Kim SJ, et al. Adoptive transfer of tumor-reactive transforming growth factor-beta-insensitive CD8+ T cells: eradication of autologous mouse prostate cancer. *Cancer Res* (2005) **65**(5):1761–9. doi:10.1158/0008-5472.CAN-04-3169

164. Lacuesta K, Buza E, Hauser H, Granville L, Pule M, Corboy G, et al. Assessing the safety of cytotoxic T lymphocytes transduced with a dominant negative transforming growth factor-beta receptor. *J Immunother* (2006) **29**(3):250–60. doi:10.1097/01.cji.0000192104.24583.ca

165. Stromnes IM, Blattman JN, Tan X, Jeevanjee S, Gu H, Greenberg PD. Abrogating Cbl-b in effector CD8(+) T cells improves the efficacy of adop- tive therapy of leukemia in mice. *J Clin Invest* (2010) **120**(10):3722–34. doi:10.1172/JCI41991

166. Lee HW, Choi HJ, Ha SJ, Lee KT, Kwon YG. Recruitment of mono- cytes/macrophages in different tumor microenvironments. *Biochim Biophys Acta* (2013) **1835**(2):170–9.

167. Johansson A, Hamzah J, Ganss R. Intratumoral TNFalpha improves immuno- therapy. *Oncoimmunology* (2012) **1**(8):1395–7. doi:10.4161/onci.20981

168. Chmielewski M, Kopecky C, Hombach AA, Abken H. IL-12 release by engi- neered T cells expressing chimeric antigen receptors can effectively Muster an antigen-independent macrophage response on tumor cells that have shut down tumor antigen expression. *Cancer Res* (2011) **71**(17):5697–706. doi:10.1158/0008-5472.CAN-11-0103

169. Kerkar SP, Muranski P, Kaiser A, Boni A, Sanchez-Perez L, Yu Z, et al. Tumor-specific CD8+ T cells expressing interleukin-12 eradicate established cancers in lymphodepleted hosts. *Cancer Res* (2010) **70**(17):6725–34. doi:10.1158/0008- 5472.CAN-10-0735

170. Liu RB, Engels B, Schreiber K, Ciszewski C, Schietinger A, Schreiber H, et al. IL-15 in tumor microenvironment causes rejection of large established tumors by T cells in a noncognate T cell receptor-dependent manner. *Proc Natl Acad Sci U S A* (2013) **110**(20):8158–63. doi:10.1073/pnas.1301022110

171. Grohmann U, Bronte V. Control of immune response by amino acid metabolism. *Immunol Rev* (2010) **236**:243–64. doi:10.1111/j.1600-065X.2010. 00915.x

172. Rodriguez PC, Hernandez CP, Quiceno D, Dubinett SM, Zabaleta J, Ochoa JB, et al. Arginase I in myeloid suppressor cells is induced by COX-2 in lung carcinoma. *J Exp Med* (2005) **202**(7):931–9. doi:10.1084/jem.20050715

173. Vesely MD, Kershaw MH, Schreiber RD, Smyth MJ. Natural innate and adap- tive immunity to cancer. *Annu Rev Immunol* (2011) **29**:235–71. doi:10.1146/ annurev-immunol-031210-101324

174. Kodumudi KN, Weber A, Sarnaik AA, Pilon-Thomas S. Blockade of myeloid- derived suppressor cells after induction of lymphopenia improves adop- tive T cell therapy in a murine model of melanoma. *J Immunol* (2012) **189**(11):5147–54. doi:10.4049/jimmunol.1200274

175. Jensen SM, Twitty CG, Maston LD, Antony PA, Lim M, Hu HM, et al. Increased frequency of suppressive regulatory T cells and T cell-mediated antigen loss results in murine melanoma recurrence. *J Immunol* (2012) **189**(2):767–76. doi:10.4049/jimmunol.1103822

176. Sharma MD, Hou DY, Liu Y, Koni PA, Metz R, Chandler P, et al. Indoleamine 2,3-dioxygenase controls conversion of Foxp3+ Tregs to TH17-like cells in tumor-draining lymph nodes. *Blood* (2009) **113**(24):6102–11. doi:10.1182/ blood-2008-12-195354

177. Tian J, Ma J, Ma K, Guo H, Baidoo SE, Zhang Y, et al. beta-Glucan enhances anti- tumor immune responses by regulating differentiation and function of mono- cytic myeloid-derived suppressor cells. *Eur J Immunol* (2013) **43**(5):1220–30. doi:10.1002/eji.201242841

178. Atkins MB, Lotze MT, Dutcher JP, Fisher RI, Weiss G, Margolin K, et al. High- dose recombinant interleukin 2 therapy for patients with metastatic melanoma: analysis of 270 patients treated between 1985 and 1993. *J Clin Oncol* (1999) **17**(7):2105–16.

179. Middleton MR, Grob JJ, Aaronson N, Fierlbeck G, Tilgen W, Seiter S, et al. Randomized phase III study of temozolomide versus dacarbazine in the treat- ment of patients with advanced metastatic malignant melanoma. *J Clin Oncol* (2000) **18**(1):158–66.

180. Chapman PB, Hauschild A, Robert C, Haanen JB, Ascierto P, Larkin J, et al. Improved survival with vemurafenib in melanoma with BRAF V600E muta- tion. *N Engl J Med* (2011) **364**(26):2507–16. doi:10.1056/NEJMoa1103782

181. Flaherty KT, Infante JR, Daud A, Gonzalez R, Kefford RF, Sosman J, et al. Com- bined BRAF and MEK inhibition in melanoma with BRAF V600 mutations. *NEnglJMed*(2012) **367**(18):1694–703. doi:10.1056/NEJMoa1210093

182. Hodi FS, O'Day SJ, McDermott DF, Weber RW, Sosman JA, Haanen JB, et al. Improved survival with ipilimumab in patients with metastatic melanoma. *N Engl J Med* (2010) **363**(8):711–23. doi:10.1056/NEJMoa1003466

183. Robert C, Thomas L, Bondarenko I, O'Day S, M D JW, Garbe C, et al. Ipilimumab plus dacarbazine for previously untreated metastatic melanoma. *N Engl J Med* (2011) **364**(26):2517–26. doi:10.1056/NEJMoa1104621

184. Brahmer JR, Drake CG, Wollner I, Powderly JD, Picus J, Sharfman WH, et al. Phase I study of single-agent anti-programmed death-1 (MDX-1106) in refrac- tory solid tumors: safety, clinical activity, pharmacodynamics, and immuno- logic correlates. *J Clin Oncol* (2010) **28**(19):3167–75. doi:10.1200/JCO.2009. 26.7609

185. Topalian SL, Hodi FS, Brahmer JR, Gettinger SN, Smith DC, McDermott DF, et al. Safety, activity, and immune correlates of anti-PD-1 antibody in cancer. *N Engl J Med* (2012) **366**(26):2443–54. doi:10.1056/NEJMoa1200690

186. Wolchok JD, Kluger H, Callahan MK, Postow MA, Rizvi NA, Lesokhin AM, et al. Nivolumab plus ipilimumab in advanced melanoma. *N Engl J Med* (2013) **369**(2):122–33. doi:10.1056/NEJMoa1302369

187. Hamid O, Robert C, Daud A, Hodi FS, Hwu WJ, Kefford R, et al. Safety and tumor responses with lambrolizumab (anti-PD-1) in melanoma. *N Engl J Med* (2013) **369**(2):134–44. doi:10.1056/NEJMoa1305133

188. Brahmer JR, Tykodi SS, Chow LQ, Hwu WJ, Topalian SL, Hwu P, et al. Safety and activity of anti-PD-L1 antibody in patients with advanced cancer. *N Engl J Med* (2012) **366**(26):2455–65. doi:10.1056/NEJMoa1200694

189. Morgan RA, Dudley ME, Wunderlich JR, Hughes MS, Yang JC, Sherry RM, et al. Cancer regression in patients after transfer of genetically engineered lymphocytes. *Science* (2006) **314**(5796):126–9. doi:10.1126/ science.1129003

190. Johnson LA, Morgan RA, Dudley ME, Cassard L, Yang JC, Hughes MS, et al. Gene therapy with human and mouse T-cell receptors mediates cancer regression and targets normal tissues expressing cognate antigen. *Blood* (2009) **114**(3):535–46. doi:10.1182/blood-2009-03-211714

191. Parkhurst MR, Yang JC, Langan RC, Dudley ME, Nathan DA, Feldman SA, et al. T cells targeting carcinoembryonic antigen can mediate regression of metastatic colorectal cancer but induce severe transient colitis. *Mol Ther* (2011) **19**(3):620–6. doi:10.1038/mt.2010.272

192. Robbins PF, Morgan RA, Feldman SA, Yang JC, Sherry RM, Dudley ME, et al. Tumor regression in patients with metastatic synovial cell sarcoma and melanoma using genetically engineered lymphocytes reactive with NY-ESO-1. *J Clin Oncol* (2011) **29**(7):917–24. doi:10.1200/JCO.2010.32.2537

12

Cellular plasticity of CD4+ T cells in the intestine

Verena Brucklacher-Waldert†, Edward J. Carr†, Michelle A. Linterman and Marc Veldhoen*

Laboratory for Lymphocyte Signalling and Development, The Babraham Institute, Cambridge, UK

Edited by:
Dragana Jankovic, National Institutes of Health, USA

Reviewed by:
John J. Miles, Queensland Institute of Medical Research, Australia
Sid P. Kerkar, National Institutes of Health, USA

***Correspondence:**
Marc Veldhoen, Laboratory for Lymphocyte Signalling and Development, The Babraham Institute, Babraham Research Campus, Cambridge CB22 3AT, UK
e-mail: marc.veldhoen@babraham.ac.uk

†Verena Brucklacher-Waldert and Edward J. Carr have contributed equally to this work.

Barrier sites such as the gastrointestinal tract are in constant contact with the environment, which contains both beneficial and harmful components. The immune system at the epithelia must make the distinction between these components to balance tolerance, protection, and immunopathology. This is achieved via multifaceted immune recognition, highly organized lymphoid structures, and the interaction of many types of immune cells. The adaptive immune response in the gut is orchestrated by CD4+ helper T (Th) cells, which are integral to gut immunity. In recent years, it has become apparent that the functional identity of these Th cells is not as fixed as initially thought. Plasticity in differentiated T cell subsets has now been firmly established, in both health and disease. The gut, in particular, utilizes CD4+ T cell plasticity to mold CD4+ T cell phenotypes to maintain its finely poised balance of tolerance and inflammation and to encourage biodiversity within the enteric microbiome. In this review, we will discuss intestinal helper T cell plasticity and our current understanding of its mechanisms, including our growing knowledge of an evolutionarily ancient symbiosis between microbiota and malleable CD4+ T cell effectors.

Keywords: T cells, plasticity, intestines, Th1 cells, Th17 cell

INTRODUCTION

The adult human gastrointestinal tract is the largest surface area of the body that contacts with the environment, covering 200–300 m^2 (1). This intestinal surface is constantly exposed to a diverse range of foreign antigens originating from microorganisms (both commensals and pathogens) and food antigens from the diet (2). Commensal microorganisms play an essential role in extracting nutrients from food that are otherwise inaccessible to the host [such as the metabolism of vitamin K by *E. coli* (3)], they are required for the development of the host's immune system and for the prevention of colonization of the gastrointestinal tract by pathogens. Mucosal pathogens, including viruses, fungi, parasites, and bacteria, can cause pathology either by local effects after mucosal colonization – such as inducing local inflammation or secreting toxins – or, through systemic infection after breeching mucosa. Microorganism-derived antigens, food-derived antigens, and airborne particles, can be potential immunogens. An inappropriate response to these immunogens at the mucosal surface can be detrimental, leading to local or systemic pathology that result in acute or chronic inflammation. Therefore, it is essential that the myriad of antigens present at the intestinal surface is dealt with appropriately to minimize potential danger and maximize host benefit. This protection is achieved by a flexible, multilayered system of physical, and immunological barriers within the gastrointestinal tract.

A central part of the complex host defense system is gut-associated lymphoid tissue (GALT). GALT is a system of highly organized immune structures strategically placed along the entire gastrointestinal tract, containing specialized micro-environments where gut-derived antigens are presented by professional antigen presenting cells (APCs) to lymphocytes [reviewed recently in Ref. (4)]. The broad antigenic sampling within the GALT facilitates the interaction between rare antigen-specific B and T cells leading to the initiation of an appropriate adaptive immune response (5). CD4+ T cells are critical players in the adaptive immune response within the GALT. Naïve T cells egress from the thymus as immature T cells with a broad range of T cell receptors (TCRs) and can be activated in the periphery following encounter with their specific antigen. T cell activation is initiated by ligation of the TCR by peptide–MHC class II complex in conjunction with co-stimulatory signals. During T cell priming, cytokine receptor ligation can skew activated T cells into a particular effector cell type (6). These cell types are commonly referred to lineages or subsets, with each being identified by selected expression of characteristic transcription factors and effector molecules (7). With the exception of thymically derived regulatory T cells (Tregs) [reviewed in Ref. (8)], thymic emigrants lack any predisposition to make effector molecules associated with a particular CD4+ T cell subset, and require signals in the periphery to skew their differentiation into a particular cell subset. Present understanding of T cell lineage commitment is dominated by single fate model, a process whereby a naive T cell differentiates along a terminal fixed expression program, in response to signals at the time of antigen encounter. However, this view has needed revision in light of findings from many groups, which together demonstrate that CD4+ T cell subset fate is not a permanent attribute, but rather a flexible, plastic, feature that can be modified to suit the requirements of the immune system at a particular point in space and time. Thus, the new paradigm of T cell differentiation encompasses the ability of CD4+ T cells to change between expression programs traditionally thought to be mutually exclusive terminal states of differentiation (9). This feature has been reported *in vivo* in several experimental systems, and intriguingly, is a prominent feature of CD4+ T cell biology within the GALT.

The detailed mechanisms underlying T cell plasticity within the GALT remains to be defined, but several factors that facilitate its occurrence have been proposed and can be divided into extrinsic and intrinsic pathways. In this review, we will summarize the recent literature on $CD4^+$ T cell plasticity in the gut, highlight possible underlying mechanisms and discuss its potential benefits for intestinal homeostasis and health.

$CD4^+$ T CELL DIFFERENTIATION IN THE GALT

The GALT contains one of the largest lymphoid cell population found anywhere in the body. GALT is distributed along the intestinal tract and is separated from the luminal content, containing about 100 trillion microorganisms (10) and many dietary products, by a single epithelial layer covered with an intricate network of glycoproteins; the mucous layers. The GALT provides three functions: provides antigenic samples from throughout the GI tract; optimizes the opportunities for naïve lymphocytes to encounter antigen, and finally supports the activated lymphocyte and its initial differentiation. A network of highly organized lymphoid structures comprise the GALT (**Figure 1**) – including mesenteric lymph nodes (mLNs), Peyer's patches (PPs), isolated lymphoid follicles (ILFs), cryptopatches (CPs), and fat-associated lymphoid tissues – as well as the loose connective tissue of the lamina propria (LP). Despite the numerous types of GALT, the organization of all GALT lymphoid tissues shares a basic cellular architecture that facilitates the interaction of APCs with lymphocytes and their subsequent activation and differentiation. However, the GALT tissues differ from each other both in function and in the physical distance to the intestinal lumen; CP and ILFs are located directly underneath the epithelial layer, PPs are further from the lumen and most distant are mLNs and fat-associated lymphoid tissues. The specialized functions of each the GALT tissues have been recently reviewed in Ref. (4), and therefore will not be discussed in detail in this review.

Naïve L-selectin-expressing $CD4^+$ T cells migrate from the blood through high endothelial venules (HEVs) to the PPs, CP, ILFs, and mLNs. In these inductive sites of the adaptive immune system, they encounter their cognate antigen presented by APCs on MHC class II. Naïve T cells that did not encounter their cognate antigen leave via efferent lymphatic vessels into the systemic circulation to continue their search for their cognate antigen. In PPs, CP, and ILFs, dendritic cells (DCs) receive antigens transported from the mucosal surface by specialized epithelial cells overlying these lymphoid structures, the microfold (M) cells, and Goblet cells [reviewed in Ref. (4)]. mLNs receive antigens via afferent lymphatics that are connected with the PPs, while fat-associated lymphoid tissues obtain antigen by lymphatic drainage directly from the intestine and from the peritoneal cavity (4).

After activation in the intestine $CD4^+$ T cells proliferate, shed L-selectin from their surface, increase surface expression of gut-specific adhesion molecules and differentiate into an effector T cell, of a particular subset. Antigen-experienced effector T cells usually leave via efferent lymphatic vessels and home to effector tissues such as the intestine after re-circulation in the blood, but

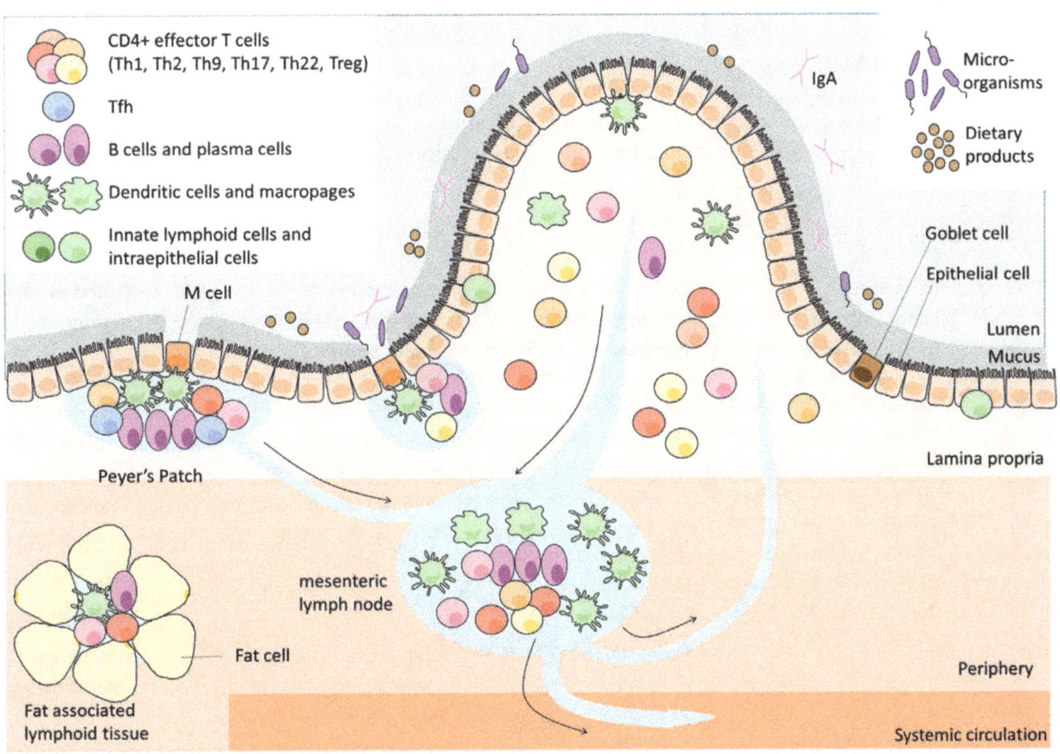

FIGURE 1 | Architecture of gut-associated lymphoid tissue.

some remain in the lymphoid organs to perform their specialized effector functions (11). Upon arriving in the intestine, effector T cells are likely to re-encounter their specific antigen presented by a diverse range of cells such as macrophages, B cells various types of DCs, and stromal and epithelial cells. This second antigen-specific interaction will trigger the T cells to execute their effector function.

It is the nature of antigen presentation and the surrounding micro-environment that largely seems to determine the outcome of CD4$^+$ T cell differentiation and the subsequent spectrum of T cell identities leaving the lymphoid structures (6). The CD4$^+$ T cell subsets currently recognized are: T helper cells of type-1 (Th1), Th2, Th9, Th17, Th22, Tregs, and follicular helper T cells (Tfh). Each subset is characterized by the potential to produce a defined set of mediators such as cytokines and chemokines, respond to particular stimuli via the expression of selected cytokine and chemokine receptors, largely driven by so called "master regulator" transcription factors (summarized in **Table 1**).

CD4$^+$ T CELL PLASTICITY

Plasticity of effector CD4$^+$ T cells has been increasingly recognized in recent years. Initially, there were single reports of observations of particular subsets behaving "non-typically," by the expression of transcription factors, cytokines, or both, of another subset. Together these various reports support a more nuanced view of Tfh differentiation, in place of the monolithic view of distinct, non-interchangeable lineages (12). T helper cells are able to acquire a mixed phenotype or to switch entirely to the transcription and cytokine profile of another lineage (**Table 2**). These hybrid cells or ex-Th lineage cells may either directly differentiate from naïve CD4$^+$ T cells or arise during secondary immunological challenge. Current data suggest that, within the gut, particular transitions between CD4$^+$ T helper cell subsets occur and are important for maintaining gastrointestinal homeostasis, as outlined below.

Th1/Th2 CELL PLASTICITY

T helper cells of type-1 cells are an abundant effector population in the gut responsible for protection against invading intracellular bacteria and viruses (31). In contrast, Th2 cells are absent in the intestine of laboratory mice and humans under healthy conditions (31, 32); not surprising in view of their role in coordinating host responses to helminths and the absence of these organisms in a healthy intestinal flora (31). Identification of Th1 and Th2 as distinct cell types was the first, time where CD4$^+$ T cell subsets were divided on the basis of phenotypic differences *in vitro* (33). It is therefore interesting that culture of T cells under mixed Th1 and Th2 conditions results in a continuum of cytokine expression, with some single positive IFNγ$^+$ or IL-4$^+$ and double positive cells, correlating with expression levels of Tbet and GATA-3 (34), the respective master transcription factors for the Th1 and Th2 subsets, demonstrating these cell fates are not a distinct as originally thought. Importantly, this finding is consistent with *in vivo* observations; during infections with *Heligmosomoides polygyrus*, a parasite that triggers a strong Th2 response, Th1/Th2 hybrid cells were observed (13). In the intestine, mLNs and spleen, these Th1/Th2 hybrid cells express simultaneously the Tbet and GATA-3 and not transcription factors of other subsets [retinoic acid (RA) receptor-related orphan nuclear receptor (ROR)γt or Bcl-6]. In addition, they express the Th1 cell-associated molecules CXCR3 and IFNγ concordantly with the Th2 cell-associated IL-33R, IL-4, IL-13, and IL-5. Furthermore, Th2 cells *in vivo* can express Tbet and IFNγ upon infection with lymphocytic choriomeningitis virus (LCMV), a potent Th1 skewing pathogen. These Th1/Th2 hybrid cells represent a stable phenotype, where attempts at reprogramming by stimulation under Th1 or Th2 polarizing conditions result in quantitative changes of Th1/Th2 cytokine production without fully extinguishing either. Upon transfer into wild-type mice, around 20% of LCMV-specific Th1/Th2 cells maintained their expression of GATA-3, IL-4, and IL-13 alongside Tbet and IFNγ

Table 1 | Effector CD4$^+$ T cells in the gut.

Cell type	Differentiation signals	Transcription factor (master transcription factor)	Cell surface and cytokine markers	Location in the gut under homeostatic conditions	Function in the gut
Th1	IL-12, IFNγ	*Tbet*, STAT1, STAT4, and Runx3	CXCR3, IFNγ	mLN, PP, CP, ILF, and LP	Responding to intracellular pathogens and assisting with viral infections
Th2	IL-4, IL-2	*GATA-3*, STAT6, and STAT5	IL-33R, IL-4, IL-13, and IL-5	Virtually absent	Responding to helminths
Th9	TGFβ, IL-4	PU.1	IL-9	Exact location to be determined	Involved in tumor immunology
Th17	IL-6, TGFβ, IL-1β, and (IL-23, IL-21)	*RORγt*, AhR, STAT3, Batf, Runx1, and RORα	CD161, IL-17A, IL-17F, and GM-CSF	mLN, PP, CP, ILF, and LP	Protect the host from infectious assault at mucosal site
Th22	IL-6, IL-13, and TNFα	AhR	CCR4, CCR6, CCR10, and IL-22	Exact location to be determined	Wound repair and induction of antimicrobials
Tfh	IL-6, IL-21	*Bcl-6*, Ascl2	CXCR5, PD-1, and IL-21	PP, ILF?	Induce IgA production by GC B cells to maintain a healthy microbiota
iTreg	TGFβ, IL-2	*Foxp3*, STAT5	IL-10, TGFβ	mLN, PP, CP, ILF, and LP	Suppressor capacity, keep homeostatic balance in gut

Table 2 | CD4$^+$ T cell plasticity in the gut.

Plasticity in the intestine	Capacity	Features of hybrid cell/ex-Th lineage cell	Origin	Developmental mechanism	Function in the gut	References
Th1/Th2	Th1/Th2 hybrid cells	Tbet$^+$ CXCR3$^+$ IFNg$^+$ GATA-3$^+$ IL-33R$^+$ IL-4$^+$ IL-13$^+$ IL-15$^+$	Naïve T cells	*H. polygyrus* infection → transcription factor balance	Gut function unknown; ↓ delayed-type hypersensitivity ↓ allergic airway inflammation	(13)
Th17/Th1	Th17/Th1 hybrid cells	RORγt$^+$ Tbet$^+$ IL-17$^+$ IFNγ^+ CD161$^+$ (only in humans) $\beta 7^+$ CCR6$^+$	Naive T cells	Cytokine-induced upregulation of Tbet	Associated with Crohn's disease	(14–21)
	ex-Th17^{Th1} cells	Tbet$^+$ RORγt$^-$ IL-17$^-$ IFNγ^+ $\beta 7^+$ CCR6$^+$	Committed Th17 cells			
Th17/Th2	Th17/Th2	RORγt$^+$ GATA-3$^+$ IL-4$^+$ GM-CSF$^+$ IL-17$^+$	Not investigated	CD4-dependent Bcl11b-knock down or IL-4 treatment of EAE mice	↓ EAE (by redirecting lymphocytes to the gut)	(22)
Th17-to-Treg	Co-expression of Treg and Th17 markers not shown		Committed Th17 cells	PPARγ activation that promotes iTreg induction	↓ T cell transferred colitis	(23)
Treg-to-Th17	Treg/Th17 hybrid cells	Foxp3$^+$ RORγt$^+$ IL-17$^+$ $\beta 7^+$ CD103$^+$ suppressive	Committed Treg cells	Micro-environmental cues in PPs of Crohn's disease patients	↓ Crohn's disease	(24, 25)
Th17/Tfh	ex-Th17^{Tfh}	RORγt$^-$ IL-17$^-$ Bcl-6$^+$ CXCR5$^+$ PD-1$^+$ IL-21$^+$	Committed Th17 cells	Not IL-23	Required for IgA-producing B cells	(26)
Treg/Tfh	ex-Treg^{Tfh} cells	Foxp3$^-$ Bcl-6$^+$, IL-21$^+$, CXCR5$^+$, CD40L$^+$, ICOS$^+$, PD-1$^+$, and CD28$^+$	Committed Treg cells	Micro-environment of PPs. Requirement for B cells and CD40:CD40L interaction. Involvement of IL-6 and autocrine IL-21	Induced GC formation in PPs and IgA-producing cells in the gut	(27, 28)
CD4$^+$/cytotoxic CD4$^+$ T cells	CD4$^+$ CTLs	CD4$^+$ CD8$\alpha\alpha^+$Runx3$^+$ ThPOK$^-$ granzyme B$^+$	CD4$^+$ T cells	Continuous antigenic stimulation, IL-15, non-pathogenic microorganisms, TGFβ, RA	↓ Colitis	(29, 30)

expression many months after systemic infection with LCMV. Earlier work from the same group has shown that the development of LCMV-specific Th1/Th2 hybrid cells originating from antigen-experienced Th2 cells required TCR engagement, not just a "Th1 milieu" provided by LCMV challenge and are stable *in vivo* for months (35).

Functionally, the Th1/Th2 hybrid cells have the capacity to elicit Th1 and Th2 cell responses but with a decreased Th-specific potency compared their single identity counterpart. Mice that received *in vitro* derived Th1/Th2 cells before the induction of type-1 inflammation showed signs for delayed-type hypersensitivity but not as strong as after a transfer of pure Th1 cells. Similarly, the transfer of Th1/Th2 cells reduced the signs for induced allergic airway inflammation compared to a Th2 cell transfer (13).

Th17/Th1 CELL PLASTICITY

In health, Th17 cells preferentially home to small intestinal LP (26) and are important for intestinal homeostasis [reviewed in Ref. (36)]. Th17 cells are characterized by the expression of IL-17A, IL-17F, and IL-22 and the lineage-defining transcription factor RORγt (37–39), which acts in co-operation with other transcription factors, including aryl hydrocarbon receptor (AhR) and RORα (40, 41). Shortly after the first descriptions of Th17 cells, cells making both IL-17 and IFNγ, so called double producers, were noted. In the intestine of patients with Crohn's disease (CD), IL-17A IFNγ-double positive $CD4^+$ T cells co-expressing RORγt and Tbet have been found (14), sometimes with frequencies above those of single positive T cells (15). Cosmi et al. characterized these double producers further and found that virtually all $IL\text{-}17^+IFN\gamma^+CD4^+$ T cells, as well as Th17 cells expressed the lectin-like surface molecule CD161 (15). This led them to conclude that human Th17 and Th17/Th1 cells exclusively originate from an NKT-like $CD161^+CD4^+$ T cell precursor. Furthermore, Kleinschek et al. showed that $CD161^+CD4^+$ T cells preferentially home to the gut due to their high expression levels of CCR6 and integrin β7. They confirmed that these cells can be induced to produce IFNγ in addition to IL-17 (16). In mice, colitis studies revealed not only the presence of Th1/Th17 hybrid cells (17–19) but also that Th17 cells, initially unable to produce IFNγ, abolish IL-17 production completely and switch on IFNγ (ex-$Th17^{Th1}$) (18, 20, 42).

Hirota et al. used an IL-17-fate reporter mouse that permanently marks IL-17-producing cells to show that these ex-$Th17^{Th1}$ cells undergo a near complete switch from Th17 cell to Th1 cell, except for the maintenance of IL-1R and AhR expression as remnants of their former identity (26). Since Th1 cells are not known for the expression of the IL-1R, ex-$Th17^{Th1}$ cells are unique within the Th1 lineage in the ability to respond to the acute phase reactant IL-1. AhR expression has been shown to increase Th17 cell activity and particularly drive the expression of IL-22 (40). It is currently not known what the role of AhR is in ex-$Th17^{Th1}$ cells, however, it is tempting to speculate that there is a role in coordinating IL-22 production at barrier sites such as the intestine, where IL-22R is expressed by epithelial cells (43). IL-22 deficiency worsens the colitis induced by either dextran sodium sulfate or by T cell transfer (44), and results in reduced secretion of antimicrobial agents important for maintaining epithelial health (45, 46). Interestingly, AhR has been shown essential for the long-term maintenance of lymphoid cells, such as innate lymphoid cells (ILC) type 3, intraepithelial lymphocytes (IELs), and tissue resident cells, at epithelial barrier sites (47–49). This suggests that ex-$Th17^{Th1}$ cells may be maintained in the intestine providing long-term protection or upholding aberrant immunity, in part through IL-22 signaling, with the help of AhR ligands.

Because the frequency and number of IL-17/IFNγ double producers are increased in the gut of CD patients (14), they have been implicated in disease pathogenesis. However, it is unknown if the presence of Th17/Th1 hybrid cells in CD patients are a cause or a consequence of the disease. These hybrid cells could develop as a bystander product of inflammation, or might drive the initial inflammatory response. In colitis models, the pathogenicity of Th1/Th17 hybrid cells and ex-Th17 cells is linked with Tbet. However, the role for Tbet in the pathogenicity of Th17 cells remains controversial (50–53) and switching to Th17/Th1 or $IFN\gamma^+$ex-Th17 might involve Runx family members in co-operation with Tbet (54).

Th17/Th2 CELL PLASTICITY

Naïve T cell activation *in vitro* in the presence of IL-4 inhibits RORγt expression and IL-17 production (55), which makes the existence of T cells with a hybrid phenotype of Th17/Th2 cells seem unlikely. However, *in vivo* studies identified $CD4^+$ T cells simultaneously expressing IL-4 and IL-17 (22). These Th17/Th2 hybrid cells were reported to be present in draining LNs and mLNs of mice with experimental autoimmune encephalomyelitis (EAE) that either had a CD4-specific Bcl11b-deficency or were treated with IL-4. In EAE, Th17 cells are pathogenic when they gain access to the central nervous system (CNS), contributing to CNS inflammation. EAE-induced Bcl11b-deficient mice showed a delayed onset and reduced disease severity, attributed to a redirection of T helper cells away from a draining LN/CNS route to the intestine. Even though an accumulation of Th17 cells in the intestine has been reported to cause colitis these mice were asymptomatic.

Th17-TO-Treg CELL PLASTICITY

A different approach was chosen to address Th17 cell plasticity by Carbo et al. (23). Computational modeling predicated a role of the nuclear receptor peroxisome proliferator-activated receptor gamma (PPARγ) in a phenotype switch from Th17-to-Treg cell in the murine gut. *In silico*, PPARγ activation of fully differentiated Th17 cells reduced IL-17 and RORγt, while initiating Foxp3 expression. *In vitro*, analysis confirmed these *in silico* predictions. Polarized Th17 cells treated with pioglitazone, a synthetic PPARγ agonist, induced Foxp3 and inhibited RORγt and IL-17A expression. This effect was not observed in PPARγ-deficient Th17 cells. Mice that received pioglitazone orally to activate PPARγ recovered from transferred colitis, with a phenotypic switch in transferred T cells, from a predominantly Th17 phenotype to an iTreg cell phenotype characterized by decreased IL-17 and RORγt and increased expression of Foxp3.

In humans, $IL\text{-}17^+$ $FOXP3^+$ T cells were identified in inflamed intestinal mucosa of patients with CD, but not in patients with ulcerative colitis or healthy controls (24). These Treg/Th17 cells shared characteristics of Th17 and Treg cells, expressing *RORC* (encoding RORγt) and CD161 and showing Treg-typical suppressor activity *in vitro*. In addition, the majority these FOXP3$^+$IL-17$^+$ T cells expressed CCR6, a receptor that mediates homing to skin and mucosal tissues (56) and high levels of integrin α4β7 and CD103, markers for gut-homing potential. Analysis of the TCR repertoire suggested that FOXP3$^+$IL-17$^+$ cells develop from FOXP3$^+$ Tregs when exposed to inflammatory signals in the gut (24) and *in vitro* stimulation of FOXP3$^+$ circulating cells can result in IL-17 expression (57). In human tonsils obtained after routine tonsillectomy, up to 25% of the FOXP3$^+$CD4$^+$ T cell population can produce IL-17 upon activation (25). These FOXP3$^+$IL-17 producers are CCR6$^+$, co-express *RORC* and *FOXP3* and display cell-contact dependent suppressive properties (25). Whilst FOXP3$^+$IL-17$^+$ cells in the LP appear unique to areas of intestinal inflammation in CD (24), in tonsil they are much more readily identifiable (25). Together these observations suggest that heterogeneity in the GALT micro-environment can influence Th17–Treg plasticity. Intriguingly, the FOXP3$^+$IL-17$^+$ T cells from CD patients also express IFNγ, IL-22, and IL-21 (24), suggesting plasticity not just between Th17 and Treg, but with other CD4$^+$ effector states.

Th17/Tfh CELL PLASTICITY

In addition to a Th17-to-Th1 conversion, Th17 cells can acquire a Tfh cell phenotype (26), including expression of Bcl-6, the transcription factor that is both necessary and sufficient for the formation of Tfh (58–60). Tfh provide antigen-specific help to germinal center (GC) B cells via CD40L, IL-4, and IL-21 (61). The only GALT to contain GCs are the PP and mLNs, and within these structures Tfh act to select high-affinity GC B cells to exit the PP GC as long-lived IgA secreting plasma cells and memory B cells (62). An IL-17-fate reporter mouse was used to show that transfer of Th17 cells into a T cell deficient recipient could support high-affinity IgA production in the GCs of PPs by converting into Tfh cells (26). Interestingly, this conversion resulted in the loss of IL-17 expression and other Th17 associated features to enable these cells to effectively switch into Tfh cells in the PP. The physiological relevance of these ex-Th17^{Tfh} cells in host defense or in microbial homeostasis remains to be elucidated. But, the essential role for Th17 cells in the production of high-affinity IgA (26) suggests that this Th17 to Tfh cell switch is critical for IgA-dependent immune responses.

IgA production in the gut can occur outside the GC but the IgA species are low-affinity, with little somatic hypermutation (63). The production of GC-derived IgA is essential for the maintenance of bacterial communities in the gut. Mice that express a mutated form of activation-induced cytidine deaminase (AIDG23S) that allows class switch to IgA but not somatic hypermutation have alterations of the gut microbiota, suggesting that IgA derived from the PP GC response is essential for maintaining homeostasis of the gut microbiota (64). This demonstrates that high-affinity IgA promotes healthy microbiota, rather than target it for elimination like IgG derived from the LN and spleen (62). The production of immunoglobulin that nourishes commensal microbiota is one of the features that discriminates the function of GALT GCs from peripheral GCs, and may be one of the reasons that GALT GC T cells exhibit plasticity that is not observed in the GCs of lymph nodes and spleen. Selective IgA deficiency (OMIM 137100) is a common incidental finding amongst blood donors (with numerous reports since the 1970s), without any particular symptomatology originally appreciated [reviewed in Ref. (65)]. However, it has recently been reported that IgA-deficient persons have increased frequency of gastrointestinal and respiratory infections, and of allergy and autoimmunity (66).

Treg-TO-Tfh CELL PLASTICITY

In mice, Th17 cells are not unique in their ability to switch to a Tfh cell phenotype, also Foxp3$^+$ cells have been reported to be able to do this in the PP GCs (27, 28). The first study used adoptive transfer of CD4$^+$EGFP$^+$ cells from spleen or LNs of Foxp3–EGFP reporter mice into T cell deficient mice (27). Whilst 80% of Foxp3$^+$ T cells switched off Foxp3 expression in the PPs, about half of the transferred cells kept their Foxp3$^+$ profile in the LP of the small intestine as well as in the spleen. The ex-Treg^{Tfh} cells that form in the PP expressed Bcl-6 and also IL-21, CXCR5, CD40L, ICOS, PD-1, and CD28, all associated with Tfh cell function (61). Functionally, it has been shown that these ex-Treg^{Tfh} cells induce GC formation in PPs and facilitate IgA-producing cells in the gut (27). These findings appear in contrast with the work of Hirota et al. that identified ex-Th17^{Tfh} cells (26). In the study by Hirota et al., mucosal Foxp3$^+$ T cells transferred into TCRα$^{-/-}$ hosts did not differentiate into Tfh cells, induce GC B cells or IgA production. It remains unclear whether differences in the models (Tsuji: CD3ε$^{-/-}$ recipients; Hirota: TCRα$^{-/-}$ recipients) or source of cells transferred (Tsuji: spleen and LN, Hirota: mucosal origin) or intestinal environment of the transfer recipients explain the discrepancies. In a separate study, Takahashi et al. transferred iTreg cells into TCRα$^{-/-}$ mice and showed that these cells can lose Foxp3 expression and become Tfh in the PP (67). Intriguingly, transferred iTreg cells were more likely to lose Foxp3 expression in the PP than in the spleen, suggesting that the micro-environment of the gut affects the plasticity of Tregs. The conversion of Treg-to-Tfh in the gut is controlled, in part, by expression of microRNA-10a that suppresses Bcl-6 and Ncor2, thereby repressing of Treg-to-Tfh conversion in the gut (67).

Not all Tregs within the PP convert into Tfh, however, there is a regulatory population of CD4$^+$ T cells in GCs; T follicular regulatory cells (Tfr) (68–70). Tfr are the progeny of Foxp3$^+$CD4$^+$ cells that share phenotypic characteristics of Tfh cells, including CXCR5, PD-1, and Bcl-6 expression. In peripheral secondary lymphoid organs, Tfr control the size and output of the GC response (68–70). In PP GCs, Tfr control the quality of IgA produced, which in turn promotes diversity within the microbial community of the gut (28). Taken together, conversion of Treg-to-Tfh in the gut is finely balanced to ensure the ratio of Tfh to Tfr within the PP supports high-affinity IgA production and homeostasis of commensal bacteria.

Th2-TO-Tfh CELL PLASTICITY

The gastrointestinal helminth parasite *H. polygyrus* has been shown to give raise to Th1/Th2 hybrid cells but also been suggested give rise to Th2/Tfh hybrid cells (71). These hybrids were described as IL-4 producing CD4$^+$ cells expressing CXCR5, ICOS and PD-1, Bcl-6 and IL-21 and that localized in B cell follicles of mLNs after *H. polygyrus* infection. Zaretsky et al. found similar IL-4^+CXCR5^+PD-1^+ Th cells after immunization with schistosomiasis soluble egg antigen (72). A later study using dual reporters for IL-4 and IL-13 and *N. brasiliensis* infection demonstrated that Tfh phenotype cells express IL-4 but not IL-13, whereas Th2 cells express both prototypic Th2 cytokines. Importantly, IL-4^+ Tfh cells are Bcl-6^+ and do not express high levels of GATA-3, suggesting that these cells are Tfh cells that produce IL-4 rather than *bona fide* Th2/Tfh hybrids (73).

CD4$^+$ T CELL INTO CYTOTOXIC CD4$^+$ T CELL CONVERSION

Among the CD4$^+$ IELs a population of cells has been described that lost its CD4-lineage transcription factor ThPOK and acquired the CD8-lineage transcription factor Runx3 (29, 30). The induction of Runx3 expression by CD4$^+$ T cells was associated with expression of CD8αα, the natural killer cell – and CTL-related molecule 2B4 (CD244) and Tbet (29). In addition, these cells expressed granzyme and the activation-induced degranulation marker CD107a (LAMP-1) (30). As well as closely resembling mature CD8$^+$ CTLs, these cells showed high cytolytic activity. At the same time, these cells lose their ability to produce IL-17 and to express RORγt (29, 30). Fate-mapping and adoptive transfer experiments by Mucida et al. showed that CD4$^+$ CTLs originate from ThPOK$^+$ naive CD4$^+$ T cells (30).

The loss of ThPOK together with the inability to produce IL-17 in the intestine had physiological implications on the development of colitis. Conditional deletion of ThPOK in CD4$^+$ T cells prior to their transfer into lymphopenic Rag$^{-/-}$ deficient mice enhanced the differentiation of CD4$^+$CD8α$^+$ CTLs in the gut of the recipients, which, as a consequence, saw a reduction in intestinal inflammation compared with controls (29). By contrast, the transfer of Runx3-deficient CD4$^+$ T cells resulted in an exacerbated intestinal inflammation, but provided recipient mice with increased protection against infection with the enteropathogenic bacterium *Citrobacter rodentium* (29). A role of CD4$^+$ CTL cells in celiac disease is suggested by their restriction to MHC class II, their induction by dietary antigen, responsiveness to IL-15, and cytotoxic potential (30).

MECHANISMS OF CD4$^+$ T CELL PLASTICITY

Very little is known about the underlying mechanisms determining CD4$^+$ T cell plasticity. It is likely that the same factors that are involved in T cell differentiation are implicated in a phenotype switch, but this remains largely untested.

The development of some CD4$^+$ T hybrid cells or ex-Th lineage cells seem to predominantly take place in the intestine, indicating that the micro-environment has a major influence on CD4$^+$ T cell plasticity and identity. For example, the micro-environmental cues contributing to a phenotype switch between Th17 and Tfh seem to be unique to the PP, as the plasticity of Th17 cells toward a Tfh cell fate was restricted to the micro-environment of PPs and did not occur in peripheral LNs (26). Likewise, transferred Foxp3$^+$ T cells lost Foxp3 expression and acquired Tfh features preferentially in the PPs (27, 65). Further evidence of the unique nature of the PP comes from *in vitro* stimulation assays in which APCs from PP and spleen generate different CD4$^+$ effectors (74, 75).

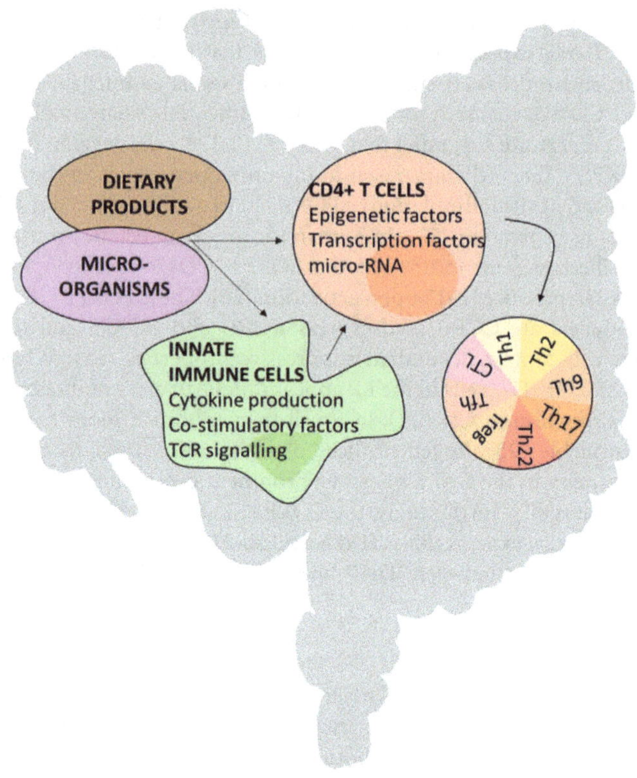

FIGURE 2 | Possible mechanisms of CD4$^+$ T cell plasticity in the gut.

Factors enabling CD4$^+$ T cell plasticity could, in part, originate from the microbiota or dietary products that effect CD4$^+$ T cells either directly or indirectly via innate immune cells. These extrinsic cues can alter transcription factor and microRNA expression and epigenetic markers such as histone modifications (**Figure 2**). For example, microRNA-10a dampens the conversion of Treg cells to both Th17 and Tfh cell fates (67). In addition, the cellular composition of the GALT, enriched in non-conventional lymphocytes such as ILCs, IEL populations of TCRγδ$^+$, and CD8αα$^+$TCRαβ$^+$ T cells and mucosal associated innate NKT cells, is substantially different compared with other secondary lymphoid organs and will contribute to a different environment in which T cells encounter antigen and are maintained.

MICROBIOTA

The nature of antigen or metabolic products provided by the gut microbiota plays a role in T cell plasticity. There are a number of examples where CD4$^+$ T cell subsets are expanded in response to particular microbial species and their products. Using germ-free mice, a mixture of 17 *Clostridia* species were selected from human gut flora for their ability to induce mucosal Tregs (76). Introduction of these 17 strains mitigated colitis and allergic diarrhea models (76). This protective effect is mediated by short chain fatty acids, products of these 17 bacteria (and of *Bacteroides fragilis*, also shown to induce Tregs) (77). The microbiome is shaped, in part by induced Tregs, and mice lacking induced

Tregs are more susceptible to colitis and asthma (78). Thus the gut microbiome is implicated in the protection of autoimmunity and autoinflammation both in the gut and at distant sites. Recent work provides evidence for a symbiosis between $CD4^+$ T cell subsets and the microbiome (28). Lack of Tfr resulted in poor quality IgA production and a limited biodiversity of the microbiome. The presence of Tfr permitted a more diverse microbiome including a larger representation of non-pathogenic *Clostridia* (28), which establishes a positive feedback loop between $CD4^+$ cells and the microbiome mediated through SCFA, Foxp3 expression, and IgA production. This narrowing of the microbiome and subsequently SCFA deplete environment might explain the association between IgA deficiency and allergy and autoimmunity (66). Taken together, these studies provide evidence that the gut microbiota and $CD4^+$ T cell fate within the gut are inter-dependent, with each affecting the composition of the other.

$CD4^+CD8\alpha^+$ CTLs are absent from the intestines of germ-free mice and of mice mono-colonized with segmented filamentous bacteria (SFB), but appear in the intestines following reconstitution with specific non-pathogenic microorganisms (30). Little is known about the mechanisms how antigens originating from microbiota induce a phenotype switch. However, data on Th17 cell differentiation indicate that SFB colonization promotes Th17 cell commitment by the expression of inflammation-associated genes, such as the gene for serum amyloid A (SAA) (79). Some Th17 cells from murine gut have TCR specific for SFB-derived antigen (80). In addition, it has been shown that ATP derived from commensal bacteria activates $CD70^{high}$ $CD11c^{low}$ cells in the LP, leading to enhanced differentiation of Th17 cells (81). Therefore, changes in the concentration of SAA or ATP could either induce a switch toward Th17 phenotype or destabilize Th17 cell commitment toward another phenotype.

DIETARY PRODUCTS

Dietary products, mainly after being processed by microorganisms, can induce phenotype switch. PPARγ has been identified to induce a Th17-to-Treg cell switch (23). This nuclear receptor regulates fatty acid storage and glucose metabolism. Therefore, consumption of food containing certain fatty acids may promote a phenotype switch from Th17-to-Treg cells. Several dietary products have been reported to promote or inhibit lineage commitment [reviewed in Ref. (2)]. It is likely that these factors are also candidates to induce a phenotype switch of $CD4^+$ T cells. In addition, dietary products could influence a phenotype switch by affecting metabolic and signaling pathways and epigenetic status.

INNATE IMMUNE CELLS: PROVIDERS OF COSTIMULATION AND CYTOKINES

Innate immune cells are abundant in the GALT. They have the potential to influence $CD4^+$ T cell plasticity via their determination of the micro-environment via the secretion of soluble mediators, expression of co-stimulatory molecules, and via their potential to act as APCs. Mucida et al. demonstrated that continuous activation of $CD4^+$ T cells by oral administration of an antigen is necessary for a phenotype switch to $CD4^+$ CTLs (30). It has been reported previously that antigen dose and peptide/TCR affinity can influence Th commitment (82).

Co-stimulatory factors have been shown to play a role in Treg-to-Tfh plasticity. Blocking the interaction of CD40, expressed on APCs such as B cells and DCs, with CD40L, found on T cells, is able to prevent a phenotype switch from Treg cell to Tfh cell (27).

The role of cytokines in Th17 cell plasticity has been studied by several investigators but has not yet been fully elucidated. However, it is clear that IL-23-dependent pathway does play an important role. In *Helicobacter hepaticus*-induced typhlocolitis, mRNA levels for IL-23p19 were elevated after bacterial inoculation and *ex vivo* $IL\text{-}17A^+$ cells isolated from the colitic intestine expressed both subunits of the IL-23R, indicating that IL-23 acts on Th17 cells to induce a program resulting in IFNγ production (18). T cell transfer studies also showed that IL-23 is required for the appearance of $IL\text{-}17A^+IFN\gamma^+$ double-producing T cells in the intestine. Transferred naive $CD4^+$ T cells developed to Th1/Th17 hybrid cells in $Rag^{-/-}$ mice, but not in $p19^{-/-}$ $RAG^{-/-}$ mice [lacking IL-23; (21)]. These studies were extended by Ahern et al. demonstrating that in the intestine the emergence of $IL\text{-}17A^+IFN\gamma^+$ double-producing Th cells, but not IL-17A single producing Th cells, requires T cell-intrinsic IL-23 signaling by transferring $IL\text{-}23R^{-/-}CD45RB^{high}$ $CD4^+$ T cells into full hosts (17). In humans, $CD161^+CD4^+$ T cells from CD patients readily produce IL-17 and IFNγ upon stimulation with IL-23, whereas, in healthy subjects, IL-1β was required alongside IL-23 (16).

The role of IL-12, the primary cytokine inducing Th1 cell differentiation, in mediating Th17-to-Th1 cell conversion remains controversial. *In vitro*, obtained results differ from those data being observed in *in vivo* models. Upon transfer of naive $CD4^+$ T cells, Th17/Th1 cells were detected in the mLNs of IL12p35-Rag-double deficient mice (lacking IL-12), demonstrating that IL-12 is negligible in Th1/Th17 induction in the intestine (21). In contrast, Lee et al. showed *in vitro* that in both IL-23 and IL-12 are able to switch off IL-17 and enhance IFNγ production in a STAT4- and Tbet-dependent manner. It has also been shown that *ex vivo* Th17 cells can be converted into a Th1-like phenotype following IFNγ-induced expression of Tbet and acquisition of IL-12Rβ2 surface expression (83, 84). Lee et al. investigated the effect of additional cytokines on Th17 cell plasticity and found that Th17 cells require TGFβ for sustained expression of IL-17F and IL-17A (20).

Although the precise role of IL-23 in the Th17-to-Th1 cell conversion requires further investigation, it does not seem to play an essential role in a phenotype switch from Th17 to Tfh cell. Th17 cells can give rise to Tfh cells in IL-23-competent and -deficient mice (26). For a phenotype switch from Tregs to Tfh cells it has been shown that the cytokine IL-6 can to down-regulate Foxp3, and this may be relevant to Treg plasticity in the IL-6 rich PPs (85).

TRANSCRIPTION FACTORS

Transcription factors maintain and instruct lineage programs by complex mechanisms, often involving several cooperating transcription factors, and their binding and access to specific DNA sequences. The expression of lineage determining transcription factors is induced by multiple factors in the micro-environment, including cytokines. Their regulation falls outside the scope of this review, but their interactions are of importance in maintaining Th identity and are likely to play a prominent role in ultimately generating hybrid Th cells and Th identity conversions. Co-expression of IFNγ and Th2-associated cytokines in the same T cell seems to be enabled by signals that keep both Tbet and GATA-3 expression in balance, which is in contrast to studies examining chromatin modification at *Tbx21* and *Gata3* (86, 87).

The loss of a single transcription factor can tip the balance in favor of an alternative lineage. In Bcl11b-deficient mice, GATA-3 expression in Th17 cells is unrestrained, resulting in GATA-3-mediated IL-4 production (22). This change in cell phenotype feeds back to the micro-environment, and has further implications for T cell biology. For example, the cytokine mix produced by Th2/Th17 hybrid cells triggers gut-imprinting properties in DCs. IL-4 together with GM-CSF enhance the expression of the enzyme RALDH2 in DCs (88, 89), leading to elevated levels of RA (90) that imprint gut-homing properties on T cells, such as α4β7 and CCR9 (91). Similarly, the termination of ThPOK in mature $CD4^+$ T cells enables the de-repression of the CTL program (30), resulting in MHC class II restricted $CD4^+$ T cells with a cytotoxic effector function. This process can be further promoted by Runx3 (29).

The factors responsible for carefully balancing two transcriptional programs within a single T cell may be present together from the moment of T cell differentiation or may be induced later. *In vitro*, data have shown that expression of one differentiation program is often found to be mutually exclusive with factors from another (55). Yet, differentiation of some programs are characterized by co-expression of two pathways from the start, such as seen with iTreg differentiation in which T cells co-express Foxp3 and RORγt from the start (25). These *in vitro* observations are often not recapitulated *in vivo* and vice versa. This highlights missing links in our understanding of which factors are required to determine full Th effector cell differentiation, which factors enable T cells to postpone the identity decision, as well as those that can still interfere at later stages.

EPIGENETICS

The observed stability or plasticity of Th subsets is governed by the epigenetic regulation of the key transcription factors and cytokines and their access to downstream genes (92). Whether a particular gene is poised for expression is controlled by the chromatin structure and histone or DNA modification state. Wei et al. evaluated the histone H3 methylation status over the entire genome in a variety of defined Th subsets (87). Promoter regions for *Tbx21* (encoding Tbet) in Th1 cells and *Rorc* (encoding RORγt) in Th17 cells displayed a permissive methylation state (H3K4me3) associated with full expression of these master regulators in each lineage. However, the promoter region for *Tbx21* in Th17 cells had a bivalent status characterized by H3K4me3/H3K27me3, reflecting the relative instability of these cells and their potential to acquire another Th cell phenotype. In addition, it has been shown that treatment of naïve T cells under Treg polarizing conditions with the fatty acid, butyrate, enhances permissive acetylation in the promoter region of the *Foxp3* locus. Butyrate, being a large bowel fermentation product, provides a link between microbial products and Treg cells by epigenetic mechanisms. Beyond histone modifications, miRNAs offer a further tuning of gene expression and $CD4^+$ phenotype, as illustrated earlier.

FUNCTION

$CD4^+$ T cell plasticity is important in the resolution of infections but can contribute to immunopathogenesis. The ability to switch or combine effector phenotypes can generally be seen as a very useful feature in the arsenal of the adaptive immune system. It is an additional tool providing flexibility to adequately control rapidly changing microorganisms. It allows the retention of TCRs with a useful track record while displaying a high degree of flexibility and adaptation depending on local environmental cues. Therefore, a phenotype switch may facilitate the ability to respond more quickly to changing immunological challenges and to successfully terminate immune responses after pathogen clearance. This flexibility may be especially important and useful at epithelial interfaces, where luminal content is constantly changing and the largest population of microorganism is encountered.

The ability to switch from one phenotype to another or obtain features from two effector programs increases the efficiency of a response. Combining effector mechanisms would enable the control of complex organisms that have evolved ways to deal with one predominant effector subset. This implies that effector programs can co-exists within one T cell, while the co-existences of different effector subset within the same micro-environment may be harder to achieve and maintain. It is worth noting that reports on Th cells displaying a hybrid phenotype highlight that such cells are less effective in dealing with situations where one part of their identity is required compared with the single identity T cells. This indicates that each identity is weakened by the presence of the transcriptional program of the other, a feature that could be abused by microorganisms. Conversely, producing these "weakened" T cells may be method of peripheral tolerance – in an inflamed milieu, T cells are stimulated under polarizing conditions and develop a single identity, whereas non-inflamed milieu offers conditions less favorable to any single identity and the "weakened" T cells are tolerized.

An additional physiological role for $CD4^+$ T cell plasticity is the gaining of specific functional features that require aspects of the previous full identity combined with a very specific trade. This is the case for Tfh cells that can develop from committed Th17 or Treg cells. In case of ex-$Th17^{Tfh}$ cells, they represent a subset of Tfh cells that are specialized to promote high-affinity IgA production in the GCs of PPs. A similar specialized role in GC B cell support is likely the case for ex-$Treg^{Tfh}$. These Tfh adopters have only been found in the PP and only support IgA production, demonstrating that this plasticity is unique to the gut environment.

Lastly, the transcriptional programs of each T cell effector subset may not be compatible with long-term survival. Effector cells that switch to a Th1 cell phenotype, may be maintained better as memory cells due to the activity mediated by Tbet. Recent reports describe a role of Tbet expression gradient as a regulator of $CD4^+$ T cell memory formation, with highly Th1-polarized $Tbet^+$ cells displaying end-effector features and a short lifespan, whereas Th cells with a lower expression of Tbet are able to enter the long-lived memory T cell pool (93, 94). This is to some degree mimicked by the finding that long-lived ex-Th17 cells acquired Tbet expression, albeit at levels lower than their Th1 counterparts.

From a therapeutic viewpoint, contemplating a deliberately induced phenotype switch could be used to up- or down-regulate the different effector arms of the adaptive immune response. Dampening $CD4^+$ T cell function would be useful for autoimmune disorders including CD and multiple sclerosis. In a colitis model, oral pioglitazone induces a switch from Th17 to an iTreg phenotype, improving disease and in EAE (a model of MS) pathogenic Th17 cells can be redirected to gut, again improving disease. Enhanced $CD4^+$ T cell responses could improve cancer surveillance and clearance. Whilst phenotypic switching appears to occur in very specific circumstances, some of these conditions are encountered spontaneously in healthy animals. Thus strategies to induce phenotype switching, with minimal side effects or co-morbidities, might be identifiable.

CONCLUSION

The nuanced view of Th differentiation suggested that within any $CD4^+$ effector population there are varying ratios of lineage determining transcription factors in each cell, with correspondingly graded cellular phenotypes. In GALT these ratios integrate a number of different signals – microbial products, dietary influences, costimulation, cytokines, and epigenetic modifications. Variation in these signals and their interpretation is the substrate for heterogeneity of $CD4^+$ T cells. As these microbial and dietary cues are unique to GALT, perhaps even unique to the most luminal GALT, such as PP, they could together provide a micro-environment permissive for plasticity, in contrast to other secondary lymphoid organs, where plasticity is less frequently reported and where much of the rigid *in vivo* definitions of the $CD4^+$ subsets were derived. Whether the phenotypic switches described herein are unique to an *in entero* environment is unknown. It is possible that similar blurring of $CD4^+$ subsets occurs at other mucosal sites, balancing tolerance, protection, and immunopathology with the need to maintain a diverse microbiome. To understand the precise factors underlying plasticity is relevant for our understanding of host (and microbiomial) health, host defense, pathogenesis of various gastrointestinal diseases and also for development and optimization of vaccines, where an enforced Tfh phenotype is desired.

ACKNOWLEDGMENTS

Verena Brucklacher-Waldert is supported by the Deutsche Forschungsgemeinschaft (DFG BR 4253/1-1 Forschungsstipendium). Edward J. Carr is an academic clinical trainee, funded by the NIHR. Michelle A. Linterman is supported by the BBSRC. Marc Veldhoen is supported by a BBSRC ISPG grant and the ERC (No. 280307 – Epithelial_Immunol).

REFERENCES

1. Mestecky J, Lamm ME, Strober W, Bienenstock J, McGhee JR, Mayer L. *Mucosal Immunology*. 3rd ed. London: Elsevier Academic Press (2005).
2. Veldhoen M, Brucklacher-Waldert V. Dietary influences on intestinal immunity. *Nat Rev Immunol* (2012) **12**(10):696–708. doi:10.1038/nri3299
3. Bentley R, Meganathan R. Biosynthesis of vitamin K (menaquinone) in bacteria. *Microbiol Rev* (1982) **46**(3):241–80.
4. Randall TD, Mebius RE. The development and function of mucosal lym- phoid tissues: a balancing act with micro-organisms. *Mucosal Immunol* (2014) 7(3):455–66. doi:10.1038/mi.2014.11
5. Mowat AM. Anatomical basis of tolerance and immunity to intestinal antigens. *Nat Rev Immunol* (2003) **3**(4):331–41. doi:10.1038/nri1057
6. Zygmunt B, Veldhoen M. T helper cell differentiation more than just cytokines. *Adv Immunol* (2011) **109**:159–96. doi:10.1016/B978-0-12-387664-5.00005-4
7. Zhu J, Yamane H, Paul WE. Differentiation of effector CD4 T cell populations. *Annu Rev Immunol* (2010) **28**(1):445–89. doi:10.1146/annurev-immunol- 030409-101212
8. Curotto de Lafaille MA, Lafaille JJ. Natural and adaptive foxp3+ regulatory T cells: more of the same or a division of labor? *Immunity* (2009) **30**(5):626–35. doi:10.1016/j.immuni.2009.05.002
9. Bluestone JA, Mackay CR, O'Shea JJ, Stockinger B. The functional plasticity of T cell subsets. *Nat Rev Immunol* (2009) **9**(11):811–6. doi:10.1038/nri2654
10. Kamada N, Seo S-U, Chen GY, Nunez G. Role of the gut microbiota in immunity and inflammatory disease. *Nat Rev Immunol* (2013) **13**(5):321–35. doi:10.1038/nri3430
11. Veldhoen M. The role of T helper subsets in autoimmunity and allergy. *Curr Opin Immunol* (2009) **21**(6):606–11. doi:10.1016/j.coi.2009.07.009
12. O'Shea JJ, Paul WE. Mechanisms underlying lineage commitment and plastic- ity of helper CD4+ T cells. *Science* (2010) **327**(5969):1098–102. doi:10.1126/ science.1178334
13. Peine M, Rausch S, Helmstetter C, Fröhlich A, Hegazy AN, Kühl AA, et al. Stable T-bet+ GATA-3+ Th1/Th2 hybrid cells arise in vivo, can develop directly from naive precursors, and limit immunopathologic inflammation. *PLoS Biol* (2013) **11**(8):e1001633. doi:10.1371/journal.pbio.1001633
14. Annunziato F, Cosmi L, Santarlasci V, Maggi L, Liotta F, Mazzinghi B, et al. Phenotypic and functional features of human Th17 cells. *J Exp Med* (2007) **204**(8):1849–61. doi:10.1084/jem.20070663
15. Cosmi L, De Palma R, Santarlasci V, Maggi L, Capone M, Frosali F, et al. Human interleukin 17-producing cells originate from a CD161+CD4+ T cell precursor. *J Exp Med* (2008) **205**(8):1903–16. doi:10.1084/jem.20080397
16. Kleinschek MA, Boniface K, Sadekova S, Grein J, Murphy EE, Turner SP, et al. Cir- culating and gut-resident human Th17 cells express CD161 and promote intesti- nal inflammation. *J Exp Med* (2009) **206**(3):525–34. doi:10.1084/jem.20081712
17. Ahern PP, Schiering C, Buonocore S, McGeachy MJ, Cua DJ, Maloy KJ, et al. Interleukin-23 drives intestinal inflammation through direct activity on T cells. *Immunity* (2010) **33**(2):279–88. doi:10.1016/j.immuni.2010.08.010
18. Morrison PJ, Bending D, Fouser LA, Wright JF, Stockinger B, Cooke A, et al. Th17-cell plasticity in *Helicobacter hepaticus*-induced intestinal inflammation. *Mucosal Immunol* (2013) **6**(6):1143–56. doi:10.1038/mi.2013.11
19. Kullberg MC, Jankovic D, Feng CG, Hue S, Gorelick PL, McKenzie BS, et al. IL-23 plays a key role in *Helicobacter hepaticus*-induced T cell-dependent colitis. *J Exp Med* (2006) **203**(11):2485–94. doi:10.1084/jem.20061082
20. Lee YK, Turner H, Maynard CL, Oliver JR, Chen D, Elson CO, et al. Late devel- opmental plasticity in the T helper 17 lineage. *Immunity* (2009) **30**(1):92–107. doi:10.1016/j.immuni.2008.11.005
21. Hue S, Ahern P, Buonocore S, Kullberg MC, Cua DJ, McKenzie BS, et al. Interleukin-23 drives innate and T cell-mediated intestinal inflammation. *J Exp Med* (2006) **203**(11):2473–83. doi:10.1084/jem.20061099
22. Califano D, Sweeney KJ, Le H, VanValkenburgh J, Yager E, O'Connor WJr, et al. Diverting T helper cell trafficking through increased plasticity atten- uates autoimmune encephalomyelitis. *J Clin Invest* (2014) **124**(1):174–87. doi:10.1172/jci70103
23. Carbo A, Hontecillas R, Kronsteiner B, Viladomiu M, Pedragosa M, Lu P, et al. Systems modeling of molecular mechanisms controlling cytokine-driven CD4+ T cell differentiation and phenotype plasticity. *PLoS Comput Biol* (2013) **9**(4):e1003027. doi:10.1371/journal.pcbi.1003027
24. Hovhannisyan Z, Treatman J, Littman DR, Mayer L. Characterization of interleukin-17-producing regulatory T cells in inflamed intestinal mucosa from patients with inflammatory bowel diseases. *Gastroenterology* (2011) **140**(3):957–65. doi:10.1053/j.gastro.2010.12.002
25. Voo KS, Wang YH, Santori FR, Boggiano C, Arima K, Bover L, et al. Identifica- tion of IL-17-producing FOXP3+ regulatory T cells in humans. *Proc Natl Acad Sci U S A* (2009) **106**(12):4793–8. doi:10.1073/pnas.0900408106
26. Hirota K, Turner JE, Villa M, Duarte JH, Demengeot J, Steinmetz OM, et al. Plasticity of Th17 cells in Peyer's patches is responsible for the induc- tion of T cell-dependent IgA responses. *Nat Immunol* (2013) **14**(4):372–9. doi:10.1038/ni.2552
27. Tsuji M, Komatsu N, Kawamoto S, Suzuki K, Kanagawa O, Honjo T, et al. Preferential generation of follicular B helper T cells from Foxp3+ T cells in gut Peyer's patches. *Science* (2009) **323**(5920):1488–92. doi:10.1126/science. 1169152
28. Kawamoto S, Maruya M, Kato LM, Suda W, Atarashi K, Doi Y, et al. Foxp3+ T cells regulate immunoglobulin a selection and facilitate diversification of bacterial species responsible for immune homeostasis. *Immunity* (2014) **41**(1):152–65. doi:10.1016/j.immuni.2014.05.016
29. Reis BS, Rogoz A, Costa-Pinto FA, Taniuchi I, Mucida D. Mutual

expression of the transcription factors Runx3 and ThPOK regulates intestinal CD4+ T cell immunity. *Nat Immunol* (2013) **14**(3):271–80. doi:10.1038/ni.2518

30. Mucida D, Husain MM, Muroi S, van Wijk F, Shinnakasu R, Naoe Y, et al. Transcriptional reprogramming of mature CD4(+) helper T cells generates dis- tinct MHC class II-restricted cytotoxic T lymphocytes. *Nat Immunol* (2013) **14**(3):281–9. doi:10.1038/ni.2523
31. Maynard CL, Weaver CT. Intestinal effector T cells in health and disease. *Immu- nity* (2009) **31**(3):389–400. doi:10.1016/j.immuni.2009.08.012
32. Arumugam M, Raes J, Pelletier E, Le Paslier D, Yamada T, Mende DR, et al. Enterotypes of the human gut microbiome. *Nature* (2011) **473**(7346):174–80. doi:10.1038/nature09944
33. Mosmann TR, Cherwinski H, Bond MW, Giedlin MA, Coffman RL. Two types of murine helper T cell clone. I. Definition according to profiles of lymphokine activities and secreted proteins. *J Immunol* (1986) **136**(7):2348–57.
34. Antebi YE, Reich-Zeliger S, Hart Y, Mayo A, Eizenberg I, Rimer J, et al. Mapping differentiation under mixed culture conditions reveals a tunable continuum of T cell fates. *PLoS Biol* (2013) **11**(7):e1001616. doi:10.1371/journal.pbio.1001616
35. Hegazy AN, Peine M, Helmstetter C, Panse I, Frohlich A, Bergthaler A, et al. Interferons direct Th2 cell reprogramming to generate a stable GATA-3(+)T- bet(+) cell subset with combined Th2 and Th1 cell functions. *Immunity* (2010) **32**(1):116–28. doi:10.1016/j.immuni.2009.12.004
36. Maloy KJ, Kullberg MC. IL-23 and Th17 cytokines in intestinal homeostasis. *Mucosal Immunol* (2008) **1**(5):339–49. doi:10.1038/mi.2008.28
37. Veldhoen M, Hocking RJ, Atkins CJ, Locksley RM, Stockinger B. TGFbeta in the context of an inflammatory cytokine milieu supports de novo differentiation of IL-17-producing T cells. *Immunity* (2006) **24**(2):179–89. doi:10.1016/j.immuni. 2006.01.001
38. Weaver CT, Hatton RD, Mangan PR, Harrington LE. IL-17 family cytokines and the expanding diversity of effector T cell lineages. *Annu Rev Immunol* (2007) **25**:821–52. doi:10.1146/annurev.immunol.25.022106.141557
39. Ivanov II, McKenzie BS, Zhou L, Tadokoro CE, Lepelley A, Lafaille JJ, et al. The orphan nuclear receptor RORgammat directs the differentiation pro- gram of proinflammatory IL-17+ T helper cells. *Cell* (2006) **126**(6):1121–33. doi:10.1016/j.cell.2006.07.035
40. Veldhoen M, Hirota K, Westendorf AM, Buer J, Dumoutier L, Renauld JC, et al. The aryl hydrocarbon receptor links TH17-cell-mediated autoimmunity to envi- ronmental toxins. *Nature* (2008) **453**(7191):106–9. doi:10.1038/nature06881
41. Yang XO, Pappu BP, Nurieva R, Akimzhanov A, Kang HS, Chung Y, et al. Thelper 17 lineage differentiation is programmed by orphan nuclear receptors ROR alpha and ROR gamma. *Immunity* (2008) **28**(1):29–39. doi:10.1016/j.immuni. 2007.11.016
42. Bending D, De laPeñaH, Veldhoen M, Phillips JM, Uyttenhove C, Stockinger B, et al. Highly purified Th17 cells from BDC2.5NOD mice convert into Th1- like cells in NOD/SCID recipient mice. *J Clin Invest* (2009) **119**(3):565–72. doi:10.1172/jci37865
43. Wolk K, Kunz S, Witte E, Friedrich M, Asadullah K, Sabat R. IL-22 increases the innate immunity of tissues. *Immunity* (2004) **21**(2):241–54. doi:10.1016/j. immuni.2004.07.007
44. Zenewicz LA, Yancopoulos GD, Valenzuela DM, Murphy AJ, Stevens S, Flavell RA. Innate and adaptive interleukin-22 protects mice from inflammatory bowel disease. *Immunity* (2008) **29**(6):947–57. doi:10.1016/j.immuni.2008.11.003
45. Zheng Y, Valdez PA, Danilenko DM, Hu Y, Sa SM, Gong Q, et al. Interleukin-22 mediates early host defense against attaching and effacing bacterial pathogens. *Nat Med* (2008) **14**(3):282–9. doi:10.1038/nm1720
46. Aujla SJ, Chan YR, Zheng M, Fei M, Askew DJ, Pociask DA, et al. IL-22 medi- ates mucosal host defense against Gram-negative bacterial pneumonia. *Nat Med* (2008) **14**(3):275–81. doi:10.1038/nm1710
47. Kiss EA, Vonarbourg C, Kopfmann S, Hobeika E, Finke D, Esser C, et al. Natural aryl hydrocarbon receptor ligands control organogenesis of intestinal lymphoid follicles. *Science* (2011) **334**(6062):1561–5. doi:10.1126/science.1214914
48. Li Y, Innocentin S, Withers DR, Roberts NA, Gallagher AR, Grigorieva EF, et al. Exogenous stimuli maintain intraepithelial lymphocytes via aryl hydrocarbon receptor activation. *Cell* (2011) **147**(3):629–40. doi:10.1016/j.cell.2011.09.025
49. Zaid A, Mackay LK, Rahimpour A, Braun A, Veldhoen M, Carbone FR, et al. Persistence of skin-resident memory T cells within an epidermal niche. *Proc Natl Acad Sci U S A* (2014) **111**(14):5307–12. doi:10.1073/pnas.1322292111
50. Yang Y, Weiner J, Liu Y, Smith AJ, Huss DJ, Winger R, et al. T-bet is essen- tial for encephalitogenicity of both Th1 and Th17 cells. *J Exp Med* (2009) **206**(7):1549–64. doi:10.1084/jem.20082584
51. Duhen R, Glatigny S, Arbelaez CA, Blair TC, Oukka M, Bettelli E. Cutting edge: the pathogenicity of IFN-gamma-producing Th17 cells is independent of T-bet. *J Immunol* (2013) **190**(9):4478–82. doi:10.4049/jimmunol.1203172
52. O'Connor RA, Cambrook H, Huettner K, Anderton SM. T-bet is essential for Th1-mediated, but not Th17-mediated, CNS autoimmune disease. *Eur J Immunol* (2013) **43**(11):2818–23. doi:10.1002/eji.201343689
53. Grifka-Walk HM, Lalor SJ, Segal BM. Highly polarized Th17 cells induce EAE via a T-bet independent mechanism. *Eur J Immunol* (2013) **43**(11):2824–31. doi:10.1002/eji.201343723
54. Wang Y, Godec J, Ben-Aissa K, Cui K, Zhao K, Pucsek AB, et al. The tran- scription factors T-bet and Runx are required for the ontogeny of pathogenic interferon-gamma-producing T helper 17 cells. *Immunity* (2014) **40**(3):355–66. doi:10.1016/j.immuni.2014.01.002
55. Harrington LE, Hatton RD, Mangan PR, Turner H, Murphy TL, Murphy KM, et al. Interleukin 17-producing CD4+ effector T cells develop via a lin- eage distinct from the T helper type 1 and 2 lineages. *Nat Immunol* (2005) **6**(11):1123–32. doi:10.1038/ni1254
56. Liao F, Rabin RL, Smith CS, Sharma G, Nutman TB, Farber JM. CC-chemokine receptor 6 is expressed on diverse memory subsets of T cells and determines responsiveness to macrophage inflammatory protein 3 alpha. *J Immunol* (1999) **162**(1):186–94.
57. Koenen HJ, Smeets RL, Vink PM, van Rijssen E, Boots AM, Joosten I. Human CD25highFoxp3pos regulatory T cells differentiate into IL-17-producing cells. *Blood* (2008) **112**(6):2340–52. doi:10.1182/blood-2008-01-133967
58. Yu D, Rao S, Tsai LM, Lee SK, He Y, Sutcliffe EL, et al. The transcriptional repres- sor Bcl-6 directs T follicular helper cell lineage commitment. *Immunity* (2009) **31**(3):457–68. doi:10.1016/j.immuni.2009.07.002
59. Johnston RJ, Poholek AC, DiToro D, Yusuf I, Eto D, Barnett B, et al. Bcl6 and Blimp-1 are reciprocal and antagonistic regulators of T follicular helper cell dif- ferentiation. *Science* (2009) **325**(5943):1006–10. doi:10.1126/science.1175870
60. Nurieva RI, Chung Y, Martinez GJ, Yang XO, Tanaka S, Matskevitch TD, et al. Bcl6 mediates the development of T follicular helper cells. *Science* (2009) **325**(5943):1001–5. doi:10.1126/science.1176676
61. Linterman MA, Liston A, Vinuesa CG. T-follicular helper cell differentiation and the co-option of this pathway by non-helper cells. *Immunol Rev* (2012) **247**(1):143–59. doi:10.1111/j.1600-065X.2012.01121.x
62. Kato LM, Kawamoto S, Maruya M, Fagarasan S. Gut TFH and IgA: key players for regulation of bacterial communities and immune homeostasis. *Immunol Cell Biol* (2014) **92**(1):49–56. doi:10.1038/icb.2013.54
63. Bergqvist P, Stensson A, Lycke NY, Bemark M. T cell-independent IgA class switch recombination is restricted to the GALT and occurs prior to manifest germinal center formation. *J Immunol* (2010) **184**(7):3545–53. doi:10.4049/jimmunol.0901895
64. Shinkura R, Ito S, Begum NA, Nagaoka H, Muramatsu M, Kinoshita K, et al. Sep- arate domains of AID are required for somatic hypermutation and class-switch recombination. *Nat Immunol* (2004) **5**(7):707–12. doi:10.1038/ni1086
65. Yel L. Selective IgA deficiency. *Clin Immunol* (2010) **30**(1):10–6. doi:10.1007/ s10875-009-9357-x
66. Aytekin C, Tuygun N, Gokce S, Dogu F, Ikinciogullari A. Selective IgA deficiency: clinical and laboratory features of 118 children in Turkey. *Clin Immunol* (2012) **32**(5):961–6. doi:10.1007/s10875-012-9702-3
67. Takahashi H, Kanno T, Nakayamada S, Hirahara K, Sciume G, Muljo SA, et al. TGF-beta and retinoic acid induce the microRNA miR-10a, which targets Bcl-6 and constrains the plasticity of helper T cells. *Nat Immunol* (2012) **13**(6):587–95. doi:10.1038/ni.2286
68. Linterman MA, Pierson W, Lee SK, Kallies A, Kawamoto S, Rayner TF, et al. Foxp3+ follicular regulatory T cells control the germinal center response. *Nat Med* (2011) **17**(8):975–82. doi:10.1038/nm.2425
69. Chung Y, Tanaka S, Chu F, Nurieva RI, Martinez GJ, Rawal S, et al. Follicular reg- ulatory T cells expressing Foxp3 and Bcl-6 suppress germinal center reactions. *Nat Med* (2011) **17**(8):983–8. doi:10.1038/nm.2426
70. Wollenberg I, Agua-Doce A, Hernandez A, Almeida C, Oliveira VG, Faro J, et al. Regulation of the germinal center reaction by Foxp3+ follicular regulatory T cells. *Immunol* (2011) **187**(9):4553–60. doi:10.4049/jimmunol.1101328
71. King IL, Kroenke MA, Segal BM. GM-CSF-dependent, CD103+ dermal dendritic cells play a critical role in Th effector cell differentiation after subcutaneous immunization. *J Exp Med* (2010) **207**(5):953–61. doi:10.1084/jem.20091844
72. Glatman Zaretsky A, Taylor JJ, King IL, Marshall FA, Mohrs M, Pearce EJ. T fol- licular helper cells differentiate from Th2 cells in response to helminth antigens. *J Exp Med* (2009) **206**(5):991–9. doi:10.1084/jem.20090303
73. Liang HE, Reinhardt RL, Bando JK, Sullivan BM, Ho IC, Locksley RM. Diver- gent expression patterns

of IL-4 and IL-13 define unique functions in allergic immunity. *Nat Immunol* (2012) **13**(1):58–66. doi:10.1038/ni.2182

74. Harper HM, Cochrane L, Williams NA. The role of small intestinal antigen- presenting cells in the induction of T-cell reactivity to soluble protein antigens: association between aberrant presentation in the lamina propria and oral tol- erance. *Immunology* (1996) **89**(3):449–56. doi:10.1046/j.1365-2567.1996.d01-760.x

75. Iwasaki A, Kelsall BL. Freshly isolated Peyer's patch, but not spleen, dendritic cells produce interleukin 10 and induce the differentiation of T helper type 2 cells. *J Exp Med* (1999) **190**(2):229–39. doi:10.1084/jem.190.2.229

76. Atarashi K, Tanoue T, Oshima K, Suda W, Nagano Y, Nishikawa H, et al. Treg induction by a rationally selected mixture of *Clostridia* strains from the human microbiota. *Nature* (2013) **500**(7461):232–6. doi:10.1038/nature12331

77. Smith PM, Howitt MR, Panikov N, Michaud M, Gallini CA, Bohlooly YM, et al. The microbial metabolites, short-chain fatty acids, regulate colonic Treg cell homeostasis. *Science* (2013) **341**(6145):569–73. doi:10.1126/science.1241165

78. Josefowicz SZ, Niec RE, Kim HY, Treuting P, Chinen T, Zheng Y, et al. Extrathymi- cally generated regulatory T cells control mucosal TH2 inflammation. *Nature* (2012) **482**(7385):395–9. doi:10.1038/nature10772

79. Ivanov II, Atarashi K, Manel N, Brodie EL, Shima T, Karaoz U, et al. Induc- tion of intestinal Th17 cells by segmented filamentous bacteria. *Cell* (2009) **139**(3):485–98. doi:10.1016/j.cell.2009.09.033

80. Yang Y, Torchinsky MB, Gobert M, Xiong H, Xu M, Linehan JL, et al. Focused specificity of intestinal T17 cells towards commensal bacterial antigens. *Nature* (2014) **510**(7503):152–6. doi:10.1038/nature13279

81. Atarashi K, Nishimura J, Shima T, Umesaki Y, Yamamoto M, Onoue M, et al. ATP drives lamina propria TH17 cell differentiation. *Nature* (2008) **455**(7214):808–12. doi:10.1038/nature07240

82. Tao X, Grant C, Constant S, Bottomly K. Induction of IL-4-producing CD4+ T cells by antigenic peptides altered for TCR binding. *J Immunol* (1997) **158**(9):4237–44.

83. Bending D, Newland S, Krejci A, Phillips JM, Bray S, Cooke A. Epigenetic changes at Il12rb2 and Tbx21 in relation to plasticity behavior of Th17 cells. *J Immunol* (2011) **186**(6):3373–82. doi:10.4049/jimmunol.1003216

84. Lexberg MH, Taubner A, Albrecht I, Lepenies I, Richter A, Kamradt T, et al. IFN- gamma and IL-12 synergize to convert in vivo generated Th17 into Th1/Th17 cells. *Eur J Immunol* (2010) **40**(11):3017–27. doi:10.1002/eji.201040539

85. Yang XO, Nurieva R, Martinez GJ, Kang HS, Chung Y, Pappu BP, et al. Molecular antagonism and plasticity of regulatory and inflammatory T cell programs. *Immunity* (2008) **29**(1):44–56. doi:10.1016/j.immuni.2008.05.007

86. Usui T, Preiss JC, Kanno Y, Yao ZJ, Bream JH, O'Shea JJ, et al. T-bet regulates Th1 responses through essential effects on GATA-3 function rather than on IFNG gene acetylation and transcription. *J Exp Med* (2006) **203**(3):755–66. doi:10.1084/jem.20052165

87. Wei G, Abraham BJ, Yagi R, Jothi R, Cui K, Sharma S, et al. Genome-wideanaly- ses of transcription factor GATA3-mediated gene regulation in distinct T cell types. *Immunity* (2011) **35**(2):299–311. doi:10.1016/j.immuni.2011.08.007

88. Iwata M, Hirakiyama A, Eshima Y, Kagechika H, Kato C, Song SY. Retinoic acidimprintsgut-homing specificity on T cells. *Immunity* (2004) **21**(4):527–38. doi:10.1016/j.immuni.2004.08.011

89. Manicassamy S, Pulendran B. Retinoic acid-dependent regulation of immune responses by dendritic cells and macrophages. *Semin Immunol* (2009) **21**(1):22–7. doi:10.1016/j.smim.2008.07.007

90. Yokota Y, Mansouri A, Mori S, Sugawara S, Adachi S, Nishikawa S, et al. Develop- ment of peripheral lymphoid organs and natural killer cells depends on the helix- loop-helix inhibitor Id2. *Nature* (1999) **397**(6721):702–6. doi:10.1038/17812

91. Kunkel EJ, Campbell JJ, Haraldsen G, Pan J, Boisvert J, Roberts AI, et al. Lym- phocyte CC chemokine receptor 9 and epithelial thymus-expressed chemokine (TECK) expression distinguish the small intestinal immune compartment: epithelial expression of tissue-specific chemokines as an organizing principle in regional immunity. *J Exp Med* (2000) **192**(5):761–8. doi:10.1084/jem.192.5.761

92. O'Shea JJ, Lahesmaa R, Vahedi G, Laurence A, Kanno Y. Genomic views of STAT function in CD4+ T helper cell differentiation. *Nat Rev Immunol* (2011) **11**(4):239–50. doi:10.1038/nri2958

93. Pepper M, Pagan AJ, Igyarto BZ, Taylor JJ, Jenkins MK. Opposing signals from the Bcl6 transcription factor and the interleukin-2 receptor generate T helper 1 central and effector memory cells. *Immunity* (2011) **35**(4):583–95. doi:10.1016/j.immuni.2011.09.009

94. Marshall HD, Chandele A, Jung YW, Meng H, Poholek AC, Parish IA, et al. Dif- ferential expression of Ly6C and T-bet distinguish effector and memory Th1 CD4(+) cell properties during viral infection. *Immunity* (2011) **35**(4):633–46. doi:10.1016/j.immuni.2011.08.016

13

Role of T cell receptor affinity in the efficacy and specificity of adoptive T cell therapies

Jennifer D. Stone* and David M. Kranz*

Department of Biochemistry, University of Illinois, Urbana, IL, USA

Edited by:
Bruno Laugel, Cardiff University, UK

Reviewed by:
Christopher E. Rudd, University of Cambridge, UK
Yuri Sykulev, Thomas Jefferson University, USA
John Stephen Bridgeman, Cardiff University, UK

***Correspondence:**
Jennifer D. Stone and David M. Kranz, Department of Biochemistry, University of Illinois, 600 South Mathews Avenue, Urbana, IL 61801, USA
e-mail: jstone@illinois.edu; d-kranz@illinois.edu

Over the last several years, there has been considerable progress in the treatment of cancer using gene modified adoptive T cell therapies. Two approaches have been used, one involving the introduction of a conventional αβ T cell receptor (TCR) against a pepMHC cancer antigen, and the second involving introduction of a chimeric antigen receptor (CAR) consisting of a single-chain antibody as an Fv fragment linked to transmembrane and signaling domains. In this review, we focus on one aspect of TCR-mediated adoptive T cell therapies, the impact of the affinity of the αβ TCR for the pepMHC cancer antigen on both efficacy and specificity. We discuss the advantages of higher-affinity TCRs in mediating potent activity of CD4 T cells. This is balanced with the potential disadvantage of higher-affinity TCRs in mediating greater self-reactivity against a wider range of structurally similar antigenic peptides, especially in synergy with the CD8 co-receptor. Both TCR affinity and target selection will influence potential safety issues. We suggest pre-clinical strategies that might be used to examine each TCR for possible on-target and off-target side effects due to self-reactivities, and to adjust TCR affinities accordingly.

Keywords: adoptive T cell therapy, TCR affinity, T cell sensitivity, T cell cross-reactivity, tumor-associated epitopes

INTRODUCTION

Immunotherapies of cancer use either passive or active approaches to recruit immune cells against tumor cells. Although most passive strategies to date have involved monoclonal antibodies, a growing body of work shows that T cells may provide more immediate and potent anti-tumor cell activity. In the most common adoptive T cell approaches under investigation, genes that encode a T cell receptor (TCR) or a chimeric antibody-based receptor (chimeric antigen receptor, CAR) are introduced into *ex vivo* activated T cells from a patient. Both receptors have shown significant promise, but the properties of these receptors that yield the most effective responses continue to be explored. In addition, because of their potency and sensitivity, adoptive T cells can present safety issues that have not generally been seen with antibodies. Aspects of TCR-mediated adoptive T cell approaches are reviewed here.

TCR-MEDIATED ADOPTIVE T CELL THERAPIES

It has been a reasonable tenet that the potency of TCR-mediated adoptive T cell therapies could be improved by using class I-restricted TCRs that are able to function both in their normal context, CD8 T cells, and in CD4 T cells. While CD8 T cell activities against cancer are important, recruitment of CD4 T cells to the site of a tumor can result in direct tumor control (1) and provide a cytokine milieu that promotes the function and survival of CTLs and NK cells (2–9), and CTL proliferation within tumors (10). CD4 T cells can also take on a cytotoxic phenotype, killing tumor cells directly (11, 12). Finally, CD4 T cells contribute to IFNγ-dependent mechanisms of angiogenesis inhibition (13, 14) and enhanced innate and adaptive responses (15, 16).

The recruitment of CD4 T cells with class I MHC-restricted TCRs is, however, confounded by the fact that most TCRs with class I specificity require co-expression of CD8 for full activity. Nevertheless, some TCRs have been shown to mediate activity without CD8 suggesting that they have higher "functional avidity" (7, 17–23). Experimental studies using CD8 binding-impaired MHCs (24) or T cells that do or do not express co-receptor (25, 26) have defined affinity thresholds above which TCRs can respond to class I MHC without a requirement for CD8. There are now many approaches available to isolate or engineer TCRs that exhibit higher affinities and thus, act independent of CD8 (27–32).

ROLE OF CD8 IN ENHANCING T CELL SENSITIVITY

The dual roles of the CD8 co-receptor in binding to the class I MHC ligand and in signaling have been the topic of many investigations. The synergy between the TCR and CD8 allows just a few class I complexes on a target cell to stimulate cytolysis (33, 34). This exquisite sensitivity has evolved to allow our immune system to identify a potential target cell as "foreign" under conditions where the processed antigen levels are extremely low.

It has been argued that CD8 functions primarily by bringing the intracellular kinase Lck together with the TCR/CD3 complex (35). It should also be noted that CD8 binding to non-cognate pepMHC has a profound impact on increasing T cell sensitivity, and that the overall surface density of pepMHC is important in the contribution of CD8 (36, 37). Accordingly, MHC density on tumor cells can play a role in the function of both CD8 and the antigen-specific TCR.

Regardless of the exact mechanism, CD8 synergy with the TCR is so effective that cytolytic activity of CTLs can be induced even with very low TCR affinities [e.g., 300 μM (38, 39)]. This might be particularly important in the case of CD8 T cell responses against self-cancer antigens, where the TCR affinities appear to be lower than TCR affinities against foreign antigens (40, 41), most likely due to negative selection in the thymus. The TCR affinity threshold in the thymus that promotes negative selection is thought to be set very low in order to reduce the risk of peripheral autoimmune reactions (42–46). However, the well-known ability of CD8 to synergize with very low affinity TCRs also presents issues of undesirable autoreactivities against structurally similar self-peptides, when the affinity of the TCR against the cognate tumor antigen is increased (see below).

TCR:pepMHC AFFINITIES

Given the central role of TCR affinity in both driving T cell activity and in conferring the specificity of the reaction, we summarize concepts of affinity and its measurement here. More thorough reviews have been published elsewhere [e.g., (40, 47, 48)]. One straightforward way to describe TCR binding to pepMHC is as a simple, one-to-one interaction involving a bimolecular binding reaction:

$$\text{TCR} + \text{pepMHC} \underset{k_{off}}{\overset{k_{on}}{\rightleftharpoons}} \text{TCR:pepMHC}$$

where k_{on} indicates the association rate of the interaction, and k_{off} describes the dissociation rate of the interaction. Additional parameters describing the binding can be determined from these association and dissociation rates, including the half-life $[t_{1/2} = \ln(2)/k_{off}]$ and the equilibrium binding constant $(K_d = 1/K_a = [\text{TCR}][\text{pepMHC}]/[\text{TCR:pepMHC}] = k_{off}/k_{on})$. The equilibrium binding constant may also be measured with equilibrium (or estimated from quasi-equilibrium) binding experiments, using techniques such as Scatchard plots or other fitting of the bound vs. free equation for K_d. In this review, we do not describe the key role of peptide affinity for the MHC product, but this parameter is also critical in the assessment of which peptide(s) to target (49–52).

The bimolecular binding equation above is used to describe the interaction between two free molecules in solution, with 3D mobility. Using soluble versions of pepMHC and/or TCR and measurement techniques such as binding to cell surfaces or surface plasmon resonance, a variety of models relating TCR binding parameters to T cell triggering have been developed (40). These included models based on the dissociation rate (k_d) such as "kinetic proofreading" (53), which suggested that a critical $t_{1/2}$ threshold must be exceeded for T cell activation to occur. An extension of this model proposed an "optimal dwell time" (54), incorporating the concept that exceptionally long $t_{1/2}$ values would result in reduced activity at low antigen density as a consequence of reduced serial triggering of multiple TCRs by each cognate pepMHC molecule (55). This model, which predicts reduced sensitivity of TCRs with long half-lives seems to be contradicted by very high-affinity TCRs engineered via directed evolution that can mediate sensitive T cell responses to low amounts of antigen (56).

Because the TCR, CD8, and pepMHC all exist as integral cell surface proteins on opposing cells, each present in various numbers, the corresponding multivalent interactions have been difficult to deconvolute from cell-free affinity measurements. Initial exceptions to the correlation between k_{off} and activity among TCR:pepMHC pairs led to consideration of the value of k_{on} in the overall interaction (57–59). In the 2C system, which benefits from a large repertoire of reagents, measurements of pepMHC affinities by competition with a TCR clonotypic antibody on the live T cell surface gave good correlation with sensitivity and activity of 2C T cells against those targets (38). This approach allows direct measurement of the cell surface affinities, but unfortunately due to the lack of appropriate antibody reagents, most TCRs can not be probed in this manner. More recently, using careful statistical analyses and experimentation, a confinement time model of TCR triggering highlighted the contribution of k_{on} and potential re-binding of the same TCR:pepMHC (60). *In situ* measurements of TCR:pepMHC binding to opposing 2D surfaces were also performed, using single-molecule fluorescence resonance energy transfer (61) or mechanical force and contact surface area measurements (62). These studies revealed that binding parameters were altered/accelerated under the more physiological geometries, showing high correlation between faster on-rates, lower 2D-K_d values, and more potent agonist activity.

Regardless of the type of K_d measurement, 2D or 3D, or the involvement of kinetics, it is reasonable to conclude that TCR:pepMHC systems exhibit a: (1) minimum affinity threshold required to be stimulated by cognate pepMHC, (2) a maximum affinity threshold above which there is no longer improvement in sensitivity (or even a reduction in sensitivity), and (3) that these affinity-minima and -maxima will have different ranges, depending on whether the cognate co-receptors (CD8 for a class I pepMHC and CD4 for a class II pepMHC) are present.

ROLE OF TCR AFFINITY IN MEDIATING ACTIVITY OF CD4 AND CD8 T CELLS AGAINST A CLASS I MHC ANTIGEN

Class I MHC is engaged by the CD8 co-receptor with relatively low affinity ($K_d \sim$ 10–200 μM), that varies by allele (35, 63–67). Nevertheless, CD8 participation can increase sensitivity of a T cell to its cognate class I pepMHC complex by one-million fold (56), reviewed in (67). Accordingly, in the targeting of class I pepMHC, normal wild-type affinity TCRs in the range of 10–300 μM [reviewed in (40)] are sufficient to provide very sensitive responses (**Figure 1**). Indeed, normal CD8 T cells have been shown to respond to as few as one to three agonist pepMHC complexes on the surface of a cell (33, 34) due to the synergy with CD8. The ability of CD8 to synergize with even very low affinity TCRs [$K_d >$ 300 μM (25, 67, 68)] can be advantageous in the normal anti-tumor setting, as most anti-self (and, hence, anti-tumor) pepMHC reactive T cells would have been deleted in the thymus if they exhibited even modest affinities. Based on studies with various TCRs against class I pepMHC, the minimal affinity required for CD8 T cell activity appears to be in the range of 300 μM, whereas the optimal affinity above which there is no additional *in vitro* or *in vivo* improvement is about 10 μM (24, 26, 69, 70). However, there has been some evidence that higher-affinity TCRs yield faster T cell reactions, but reduced sensitivity at lower pepMHC densities (71, 72).

As indicated, it has been shown that CD4 T cell responses against tumors are very beneficial, a process that can be achieved by transducing CD4 T cells with TCRs that have higher affinities

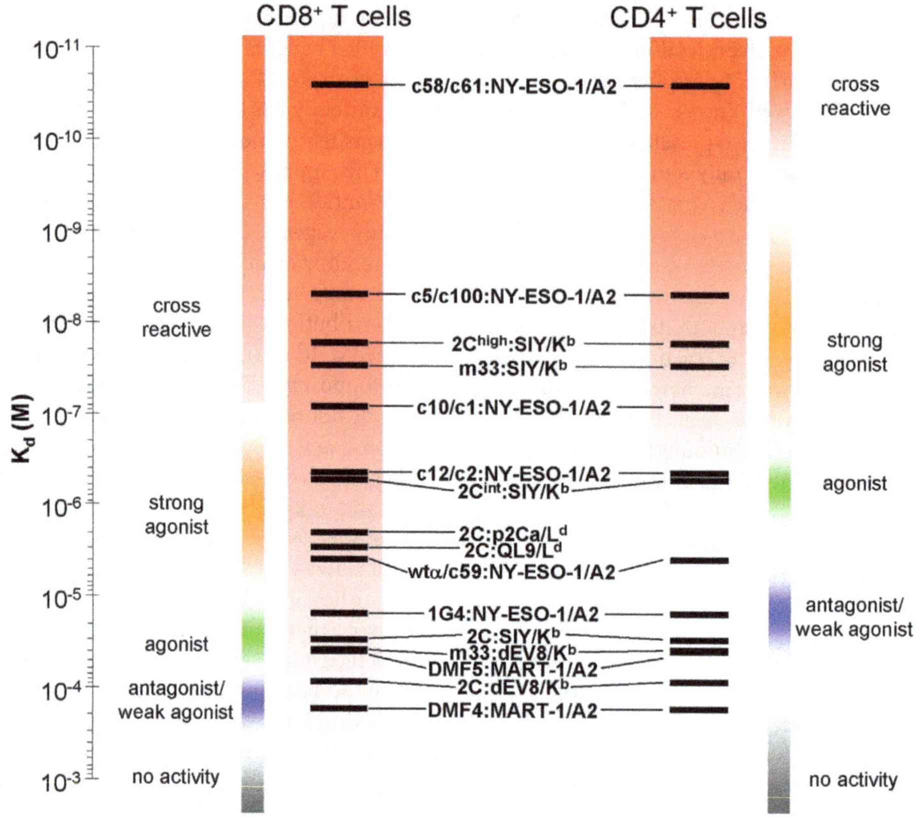

FIGURE 1 | Relationship between T cell activities and TCR affinities for a class I pepMHC antigen, in either CD8 or CD4 T cells. Various TCRs whose affinity for their target class I pepMHC complexes have been measured are depicted on an affinity scale (K_d). The relative activity ranges for those receptors are listed for those TCRs expressed in CD8 (left) and CD4 (right) T cells. The activity boundaries are approximated from the best-known systems. Sensitivity at low TCR affinities is achieved due to TCR synergy with the CD8 co-receptor. This same principle can yield CD8-dependent, undesirable cross reactivities with structurally similar self-peptides.

($K_d < 10\ \mu M$) against a class I MHC tumor antigen (25, 29, 73) (**Figure 1**). Even for CD4 T cells, however, there seems to exist an affinity threshold for class I pepMHC above which T cell activation occurs in the absence of the cognate peptide, as was seen for a picomolar-affinity TCR against HLA-A2/NY-ESO-1 (157–165) (73). This CD4 T cell activation appears to be due to the interaction of the affinity-engineered TCR with one or more self-pepMHC complexes with affinities above the CD8-independent threshold (i.e., $K_d < 10\ \mu M$).

Raising the affinity of a TCR in order to achieve optimal CD4 T cell activity (i.e., CD8 independence) also increases the risk that the same TCR, in a CD8 T cell, will mediate activity against structurally related self-peptides. In this scenario, TCR affinities for such a self-peptide-MHC that were below the threshold (e.g., $K_d > 300\ \mu M$, in the presence of CD8) for the wild-type TCR may now be elevated to $<300\ \mu M$ with the affinity-enhanced TCR. In summary, in CD4 T cells a high-affinity TCR against a cognate pepMHC would need to cross-react with a structurally related self pepMHC at an affinity of at least $10\ \mu M$ to stimulate autoreactivity, whereas in CD8 T cells a high-affinity TCR against a cognate pepMHC would need to cross-react with a structurally related self pepMHC at an affinity of only $300\ \mu M$ to stimulate autoreactivity, due to the synergy of CD8.

The consequences of these self-peptide cross-reactions can be varied. In one case (see 2C system below), a higher-affinity TCR introduced into CD8 T cells resulted in self-peptide reactivity and rapid deletion of the transduced CD8 T cells. While increased cross-reactivity by the mouse high-affinity TCR m33 in CD8 T cells resulted in deletion (74–76), several clinical trials in humans resulted in dangerous pathologies caused by the introduced T cells. The reasons for the difference in outcome are not entirely clear. One possibility is that the expression pattern of the cross-reactive epitope influences the outcome; for example, one cross-reactive epitope with the high-affinity m33 TCR, dEV8, is expressed ubiquitously, possibly overwhelming the introduced CD8 T cells and leading to AICD or even fratricide. By contrast, for cross-reactive epitopes that are tissue restricted (see below), the T cells may be able to persist and ultimately to mediate localized tissue destruction. Using appropriate animal models with tissue-restricted antigens, and adoptively transferred T cell with higher-affinity TCRs, it should be possible to investigate systematically the cause for different outcomes.

AFFINITY OF THE TCR CORRELATES WITH REACTIVITY FOR STRUCTURALLY RELATED PEPTIDES

Given the central role of the TCR:pepMHC interaction in activity and specificity it is not surprising that significant efforts have gone into dissecting the interface, often residue by residue. Of particular relevance is the role that TCR affinity plays in the recognition of structurally similar peptides, as such peptides could represent potential off-target safety issues. In order to consider this issue, we provide below a non-exhaustive review of several systems: the mouse class I pepMHC-specific TCR (2C), a mouse class II pepMHC-specific TCR (3.L2), and human TCRs against the cancer antigens MART-1, NY-ESO, MAGE-A3, and WT1. We focus on the activities mediated against the cognate peptides and, where available, structurally related peptides.

MOUSE 2C TCR AGAINST CLASS I ANTIGENS

The murine 2C T cell system (77, 78) has been studied extensively, from the level of central tolerance (79), to the level of structure/function (80–82), to its use in many tumor models (76, 83, 84). The CD8 T cell clone 2C was induced in a BALB.B mouse ($H\text{-}2^b$) by an alloresponse to the $H\text{-}2^d$ tumor P815 (85). The 2C TCR was shown to mediate positive-selection by K^b (79), and a potential self-peptide, called dEV8, involved in this selection has been identified (86, 87). A synthetic peptide, called SIY, that acts as a strong agonist in the context of K^b was also identified (88).

The known reactions of 2C with a variety of ligands (K^b, L^d, and K^{bm3}) have provided a model system to study TCR degeneracy (89). Affinities for the allogeneic ligands [p2Ca/L^d and QL9/L^d $K_d \sim 1\ \mu M$ (90, 91)], the putative positive-selection ligand [dEV8/K^b, $K_d \sim 80\ \mu M$ (90)], and the strong agonist ligand [SIY/K^b, $K_d \sim 30\ \mu M$ (26, 90, 91)] have been measured by various methods. The structure of this receptor in complex with dEV8/K^b was the first mouse TCR:pepMHC to be determined (80). Since then, the structures of the 2C TCR in complex with L^d ligands (81, 82) and K^b ligands (80, 92) have been solved, showing how the complementarity determining regions (CDR) accommodate the various ligands. CD8 2C T cells, have also been used to probe the exquisite sensitivity of T cells, suggesting that only a few agonist pepMHC molecules (or even one) on a target cell can mediate activity (33, 34). Finally, the 2C system and the strong agonist peptide SIY was used by Schreiber and colleagues to reveal the process of tumor antigen cross-presentation on stroma (83, 93, 94), and more recently the system has been exploited by Jacks and colleagues to reveal aspects of peripheral tumor tolerance (84) and the importance of mutated peptide antigens in immunoediting (95).

In the context of the present review, the 2C TCR ($K_d = 1\ \mu M$ for QL9/L^d, and $30\ \mu M$ for SIY/K^b) was also the first to be engineered for higher affinity by directed evolution, first against QL9/L^d (96) and then against SIY/K^b (71). A yeast display library of CDR3α mutants in the 2C single-chain TCR (scTCR) were selected with QL9/L^d to yield various mutants, including m6 with a K_d value of 10 nM (91, 96, 97). The same 2C scTCR library, selected with SIY/K^b, yielded various mutants including m33 with a K_d value of 30 nM (26, 71, 91). Stimulation of a T cell hybridoma expressing the higher-affinity TCR variants showed that they exhibited increased sensitivity to agonist peptide presentation (71, 97). In addition to sensitive agonist responses, binding of high-affinity TCR variants to structurally related pepMHC complexes were also increased (**Figure 2A**) (39, 71, 96, 97).

In addition to a broader range of reactivity with single-amino acid substitutions in the agonist peptide, the higher-affinity TCR m33 (isolated against the ligand SIY, with 1000-fold higher affinity) also showed CD8-dependent activity against the structurally similar self-peptide dEV8 (71). Although the m33 TCR only exhibited about a twofold increase in affinity for the self-pepMHC dEV8/K^b, this increase was sufficient for CD8 T cells expressing m33 to be stimulated by both exogenous dEV8 and endogenous peptides presented by $H\text{-}2^b$ cells such as C57BL/6 splenocytes (71). While the sequence of dEV8 only contains two amino acids in common with the strong agonist SIY (SIY: SIYRYYGL; dEV8: EQYKFYSV), they are very similar structurally (**Figure 2B**), and can be considered to be analogous to single-amino acid substitutions of agonist peptides. This notion forms the basis of the more detailed discussion below concerning the examination of structurally similar self-peptides.

It is important to point out that in contrast to an increase in affinity for structurally similar pepMHC complexes (i.e., m6 TCR with QL9 and its variants, or m33 TCR with SIY and dEV8), the affinities of engineered 2C variant TCRs were not increased toward structurally dissimilar ligands. For example, the high-affinity TCRs m6 and m13 selected against the allogeneic ligand QL9/L^d, had reduced affinities for the syngeneic ligand SIY/K^b (91).

MOUSE TCR 3L2 AND ITS LIGANDS

Similar effects of increased affinity were observed for the class II-restricted TCR system called 3.L2 (98, 99). The 3.L2 TCR was derived from a CD4 T cell clone against a peptide from the minor d allele of the b chain of mouse hemoglobin, presented in complex with $I\text{-}E^k$. The 3.L2 TCR was engineered by yeast surface display for increased affinity to the Hb/class II pepMHC complex. A panel of TCRs with an affinity range from the wild-type 3.L2 [K_d 20 μM (99, 100)] to the highest affinity variant, m15 (K_d 25 nM) were isolated (99). In the case of these higher-affinity TCR variants, there were no apparent increases in CD4 T cell activity for the agonist pepMHC. This may be a result of a wild-type affinity already above the optimal activation threshold for this complex. However, the ability to respond to single-amino acid substitutions of the Hb peptide was much broader for the TCRs with increased affinity (99, 101). A recent study showed that even a TCR (m2) with a modest improvement in affinity (twofold) for Hb/$I\text{-}E^k$ mediated broader peptide reactivity, and enhanced thymic negative selection (102). Thus, like the 2C system, the 3.L2 system also showed that structurally similar peptides have a higher probability of stimulating T cells that express affinity-enhanced TCRs.

HUMAN TCRs

A prioritized list of cancer-associated peptide antigens has been compiled, setting quantitative values on various properties, including antigenicity, relationship to oncogenicity, and specificity (103). Among the panel of peptides, some have been the antigenic peptides targeted by TCRs in adoptive T cell therapies. These include, most prominently, MART-1 (29), NY-ESO-1 (104, 105), MAGE-A3 (106), and WT1 (107, 108). Various strategies to improve the affinity, and it is hoped thus the efficacy, of TCRs for the adoptive

A

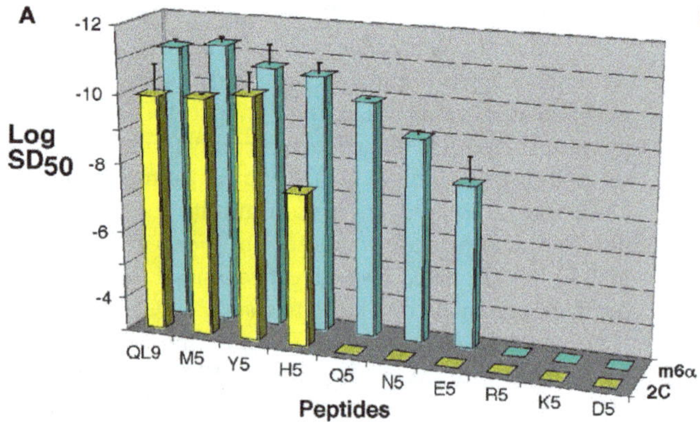

B

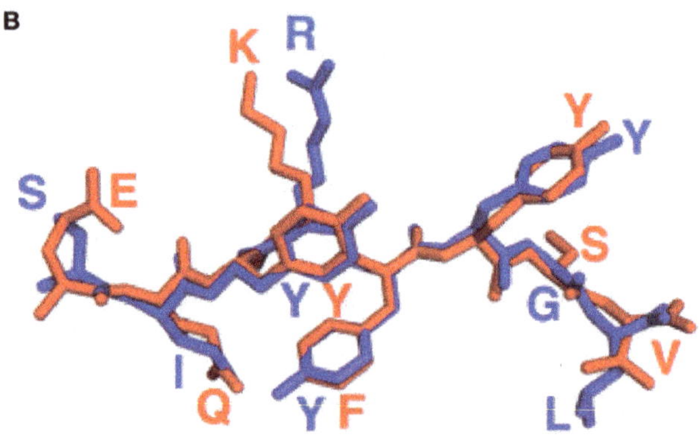

C

Protein	Peptide Sequence
SIY	SIYRYYGL
BLAST SEARCH	
serine protease 29 precursor	RIYRYYWA
ferrochelatase, mitochondrial	AIYRYYNE

D

Protein	Peptide Sequence
SIY	SIYRYYGL
PROTEOME SCANNING ***"XX[YFW][RKH][YFW][YFW][GSAT][LIVM]"***	
Cornichon homolog 3 (Drosophila), isoform CRA_a	LFYHFWSM
G-protein coupled receptor 84	LGYRYFAV
Integral membrane protein 2B	YLYKYFAL
Interferon-inducible protein AIM2	KRFKYFAL
Isoform 2 AND 4 of Transcription Factor RFX4	EWYHYYGI
Likely orthologue of H. sapiens chromosome 9 ORF 84	PAFKYYAI
MCG147124	ARFRYFSL
MCG15234, isoform CRA_a AND CRA_b	IGFKFFAM
Membrane-associated phosphatidylinositol transfer protein 1 AND 2	VEFRYWGM
MHC class II regulatory factor RFX1	SKYHYYGL
Myosin regulatory light chain 2, ventricular/cardiac muscle isoform	NVWRFWGI
NADH dehydrogenase [ubiquinone] complex I, assembly factor 7	ERFHFFAL
NADH dehydrogenase 1 [ubiquinone] 1 alpha subcomplex subunit 4	EQYKFYSV
NmrA-like family domain-containing protein 1	NMFRFYTL
Protein 1700010H22Rik	NFFKFFTL
Protein Fam47e	RCWRYWTL
Protein Gm9956	SCFKFFTV
Protein Omt2a (Fragment)	IGFKFFAM
Protein sel-1 homolog 2	TAFKYFSM
Protein Vmn1r68	RDFKYYSI
Ryanodine receptor 3	STFKFYTM
Sodium leak channel non-selective protein	IVFRFFSI
Spectrin beta chain	DKFRFFSM
Tail-anchored protein insertion receptor WRB	LIWKYYSV
Terminal uridylyltransferase 7	TTYKYFAL
Transcription factor RFX3 AND DNA-binding protein RFX2, RFX6	SKYHYYGI
Transmembrane 9 superfamily member 3	ETYKYFSL
Tumor necrosis factor ligand superfamily member 11	SEFHFYSI
Uncharacterized protein KIAA0825 homolog	QMWHYFSL
WD repeat domain phosphoinositide-interacting protein 2	SGYKFFSL
XK-related protein 2	LVFKYFGV
XK-related protein 4	FCWHFFTI

FIGURE 2 | T cell receptor affinity, specificity, and cross-reactivity in the 2C TCR system. **(A)** The m6α TCR engineered from the 2C TCR for increased affinity for QL9/L^d exhibited more sensitive reactivity with structurally related peptides with single-amino acid substitutions. Sensitization doses of various QL9 position 5 variant peptides for IL-2 production by CD8-negative TCR transfectants are shown. The log of the SD_{50} value was plotted for each of the peptides used to stimulate 2C TCR (yellow bars) and m6α TCR (blue bars) transfectants [*Reproduced with permission from Ref. (56)]. **(B)** The 2C TCR reacts with the agonist SIY peptide/K^b complex and the putative positive-selecting peptide dEV8/K^b complex with K_d values of 30 and 80 μM, respectively. While the sequences share only two amino acids in common, they are structurally very similar [shown here aligned from their H2-K^b-bound structures, SIY in blue and dEV8 in red; PDB IDs 1G6R (92) and 2CKB (173)]. **(C)** Performing a protein BLAST search of the mouse proteome with the SIY peptide sequence string and an Expect value cut off of 5.0 yielded only two sequence-similar peptides. **(D)** Performing a proteome scan to find sequences similar to SIY, based in part on alanine scan data of the peptide epitope, and the tolerance for mutations at each position yielded 43 peptides considered to be similar (only 33 sequences predicted to bind with SYFPEITHI scores >16 are shown). Using this technique, the putative positive-selecting peptide, and the self-peptide that reacts with the higher affinity TCR m33 (71), called dEV8 was identified (shown in bold, highlighted in yellow).

T cell therapy trials have been taken. While anti-tumor responses have been observed, there have been serious adverse events with MART-1 TCRs due to on-target/off-tumor activity (109), and lethal events with MAGE-3 TCRs due apparently to off-target cross-reactivity with structurally similar epitopes (110, 111). For these reasons, we summarize below various aspects of reactivities mediated by TCRs against four of the candidates for adoptive T cell therapies (MART-1, MAGE-A3, NY-ESO-1, and WT1).

MART-1

MART-1, a differentiation antigen upregulated on the surface of melanoma cells, contains the well-studied HLA-A2-restricted peptide epitope AAGIGILTV [27–35] (112) and its N-terminal extended variant EAAGIGILTV [26–35] (113). CD8 T cell clone M1F12 (now called DMF4) against this peptide was isolated from a patient with an anti-tumor response (114). The DMF4 TCR has a relatively low affinity (K_d 170 μM) for the predicted endogenous epitope, AAGIGILTV/HLA-A2 (115). The DMF4 TCR was used in one of the first trials of gene modified adoptive T cell transfer in humans (116). While relatively low overall response rates were reported [4/31, or 13%, with 17 patients reported in the original publication (109, 116)], the study represented an important step toward proof of concept for TCR gene therapies.

In an attempt to improve the efficacy of MART-1-directed TCR gene therapy, a second generation T cell clone called DMF5, with higher functional avidity and detectable activity in CD4 T cells, was isolated (117). The affinity of DMF5 (K_d 40 μM) (115) was higher than DMF4, but interestingly still lower than the murine wild-type receptor 2C (K_d 30 μM) [Note: like DMF5, the 2C TCR exhibited some activity in CD4 T cells *in vitro*, although *in vivo* anti-tumor activity of CD4 T cells with the 2C TCR was less effective than the higher-affinity TCR m33, with a K_d of 30 nM (76)]. Similarly, because DMF5 showed greater *in vitro* activity than DMF4 in CD4 T cells, it was hypothesized that DMF5-transduced T cells might mediate improved anti-melanoma responses (109). Indeed, objective response rates were higher in the DMF5 trial (30 vs. 13%). However, unlike patients treated with DMF4, patients treated with DMF5 experienced a marked cytokine (IFN-γ) spike and serious skin rashes 3–5 days after T cell transfer. The cytokine spike induced was ~9-fold higher for patients treated with the affinity-enhanced DMF5 TCR when compared with previous patients who received cells with the DMF4 TCR, suggesting that the TCR reactivity was related to these results. Furthermore, since IFN-γ is produced by activated T cells, and patients were lymphodepleted prior to transduced T cell infusion (and still showed signs of lymphodepletion at the 3- to 5-day time point), it is likely that the cytokines were derived from the transferred cells. Importantly, DMF5 also mediated high rates of anterior uveitis, hearing loss, and dizziness, presumably due to reactions to MART-1 expressed in the normal eye and ear (109). Accordingly, these responses were characterized as on target/off tumor, and were only revealed by the potency of T cells transduced with the higher-affinity DMF5 TCR.

MAGE-A3

MAGE-A3 is a cancer-testis antigen and a member of a larger MAGE family. A related family member, MAGE-A1, was the first immunogenic gene found to elicit a natural CTL response in a melanoma patient (118). MAGE-A3 was identified several years later (119) and is one of the most commonly expressed MAGE family genes in cancers of different epithelial origins [reviewed in (120)]. Several peptide epitopes from MAGE-A3 have been identified, restricted by various MHC alleles. Here, we focus on the HLA-A2-restricted epitope, MAGE-A3 [112–120]: KVAELVHFL, which was the epitope targeted in a recent trial that resulted in the deaths of two patients (111), although a recent clinical trial with a MAGE-A3 epitope (EVDPIGHLY [161–169]) restricted by HLA-A1 also showed cross-reactivity, cardiovascular toxicity, and lethality in a clinical trial (110).

A high-avidity TCR was generated by vaccinating an HLA-A2 transgenic mouse with the MAGE-A3 [112–120] peptide (106). As murine CD8 does not bind efficiently to HLA-A2, T cells generated against peptide/HLA-A2 complexes in these mice presumably have affinities above the CD8 independence threshold, and would be sufficient to recruit CD4 as well as CD8 T cells. Human CD8, but not CD4, T cells expressing the MAGE-A3 [112–120]-specific TCR stained with soluble pepMHC tetramers, and were activated *in vitro* by MAGE-expressing tumor cells. To identify a TCR with even higher avidity, various point mutations in the CDR3α were examined for improved T cell activity (29), revealing an A118T variant that raised the functional avidity of the TCR, and mediated improved CD4 T cell activity (106). T cells transduced with these MAGE-A3/HLA-A2 TCRs were also screened against structurally similar peptides from other MAGE family members. An epitope from MAGE-A12 (differing only by a Val to Met substitution at position 2) was recognized indistinguishably from MAGE-A3, and detectable responses were seen with similar peptides from MAGE-A2 and MAGE-A6.

The MAGE-A3 A118T TCR was recently used in adoptive T cell therapy in nine melanoma patients (111). Five patients experienced objective regression of their tumors, including one complete response and one durable partial response that persisted for over 12 months. However, unexpected neurological toxicity was observed in three MAGE-A3 patients, resulting in two patient deaths. High levels of CD4 T cells with the murine TCR were detected in the cerebrospinal fluid of the patients that experienced toxicity, although brain infiltrating T cells were predominantly CD8 (CD4 T cells were rare). Cells expanded from the cerebrospinal fluid of one of the patients who succumbed showed specific IFN-γ release when stimulated with MAGE-A3$^+$/HLA-A2$^+$ tumor cells.

To identify potential cross-reactive epitopes that might have accounted for these toxicities, a BLAST search of the MAGE-A3 peptide, KVAELVHFL, was conducted with the human genome, revealing various candidates (111). The peptides were synthesized and tested for their ability to stimulate CD8 T cells transduced with the MAGE-A3 A118T TCR. One peptide (SAAELVHFL from EPS8L2, for epidermal growth factor receptor kinase substrate 8-like protein 2) was reactive, but transfection of the full EPS8L2 gene into HLA-A2-positive cells did not stimulate activity. However, staining of brain sections with anti-MAGE family antibodies, as well as testing with Q-RT-PCR, revealed a subset of neurons that expressed MAGE genes, including MAGE-A12 (111). Thus, it was suggested that T cell recognition of the structurally similar peptide from MAGE-A12 likely accounted for the neuronal toxicity.

NY-ESO-1

NY-ESO-1 (or LAGE-1) is also a cancer-testis antigen that is expressed on a variety of tumors from different origins [reviewed in (121)]. An NY-ESO-1 peptide (NY-ESO-1 [157–165], SLLMWITQC) restricted by HLA-A2 was identified using CTL lines from a melanoma patient (122). A CD8-dependent TCR called 1G4 that is specific for this epitope was shown to have K_d value of 15 μM for the NY-ESO/A2 complex (104, 105).

As the native NY-ESO peptide bound poorly to HLA-A2, and was less active in solution due to reactions of the C-terminal cysteine (123), there have been efforts to design improved peptide analogs. Toward this effort, a positional alanine scan (124) indicated that P3-Leu, P4-Met, P5-Trp, P7-Thr, and P8-Gln were important for T cell recognition, while a crystal structure of the HLA-A2-bound peptide (125) showed that P2-Leu, P3-Leu, P6-Ile, and P9-Cys were unlikely to contact the TCR directly. To eliminate the problems with the cysteine at P9, and to improve HLA-A2 binding, various P9 substitutions have been tested (104, 123, 125). A peptide with a valine substitution (SLLMWITQV) bound better to A2, was more stable in solution (123), and stimulated 1G4 T cells more effectively than the wild-type peptide *in vitro* (104). However, vaccination strategies with the C165V peptide did not lead to efficient cross-reactivity with the wild-type peptide (126), likely due to a repositioning of the peptide main chain with the different anchor residue at P9 (127).

While vaccination for NY-ESO-1 remains challenging, adoptive T cell therapy for this epitope has been shown to be effective and safe, even with a higher-affinity TCR variant of 1G4. Several single-site CDR mutants of the 1G4 TCR increased affinity and mediated improved activity of CD4 T cells (29). The 1G4-α95LY TCR has been tested clinically in melanoma and synovial cell sarcoma with a significant benefit (overall response rate of 45 and 67%, respectively), and a good safety profile has been reported for the 17 treated patients (128).

In a separate strategy, the 1G4 TCR has been modified for higher affinity by phage display yielding affinities as high as 26 pM (129, 130). The highest affinity TCRs yielded self-reactivity in both CD8 and CD4 T cells (73) (**Figure 1**). A high-affinity (50 pM) variant generated by phage display has also been produced as a soluble, bispecific fusion with anti-CD3 to redirect T cells to NY-ESO *in vitro* and in a human xenograft model in mice (131, 132).

WT1

Wilms' tumor antigen (WT1) is a zinc-finger transcription factor that plays a significant role in embryogenesis but is minimally expressed in normal adult tissues. It is overexpressed in most leukemias, and in several other tumor types [reviewed in (133, 134)]. The recent prioritization of tumor-associated peptides (103) ranked WT1 as the top target due to its immunogenicity, restricted expression in normal tissues, and a strong correlation with tumorigenesis. An immunogenic HLA-A2-restricted epitope, WT1 [126–134]: RMFPNAPYL has been characterized (107, 135). Interestingly, the identical peptide sequence is present in the mouse WT1 homolog, and has been shown to be an immunogenic epitope in the context of H2-D^b (136, 137). [Note: a TCR targeting WT1 [235–243], restricted by HLA-A*2402 (138), is also being explored for adoptive immunotherapy, with reported efficacy and safety in pre-clinical systems (139); this peptide and TCR are not discussed further here.]

To date, several WT1 vaccination trials in mice and humans have been undertaken, showing excellent safety profiles but low response rates [reviewed in (140)]. A recent study (141) showed that only clones of low functional avidity for HLA-A2:WT1 [126–134] could be isolated from HLA-A2-positive individuals, while clones of higher functional avidity could be obtained from HLA-A2-negative individuals through allogeneic stimulation *in vitro*. However, the allogeneic clones showed promiscuous reactivity to different HLA-A2-bound peptides (141), highlighting that caution should be taken when taking advantage of allogeneic stimulation to isolate tumor-specific TCRs of improved affinity. A limited trial where anti-WT1 CTL clones were elicited *ex vivo* from patients, in the presence of IL-21, and re-introduced showed substantial persistence of the WT1-specific T cells (108). The results also suggested an improved response over WT1 vaccines, while maintaining favorable safety. Looking toward adoptive T cell therapy, a WT1 [126–134]/A2-specific TCR isolated from peptide-specific, allo-induced CTLs (107, 142), exhibited good anti-tumor responses in a mouse xenograft model with TCR-transduced T cells (143, 144). A more recent study targeting WT1 for adoptive T cell therapies described a novel strategy to reduce endogenous TCR levels by using a targeted zinc-finger nuclease, followed by introduction of their WT1-specific TCR. This approach resulted in enhancement of overall functional avidity due to the higher T cell surface levels of the exogenous WT1-specific TCR (145).

With the possibility for improvement of anti-WT1 CD4 T cell responses with higher-affinity TCRs, our lab, working with Greenberg and colleagues has previously engineered an enhanced affinity (CD8-independent) TCR against the murine WT1/D^b complex (137, 146), and we have recently engineered a higher-affinity human TCR against WT1/HLA-A2 (unpublished). The mouse and human TCRs are being tested in mouse models with analysis of potential on-target/off-tumor responses, or cross-reactivity with structurally related pepMHCs (see below). Adoptive transfer studies with CD8 T cells and the mouse TCR against WT1/D^b have shown no signs of toxicity in the mouse models (146).

DOES THE ADVANTAGE OF HIGHER-AFFINITY TCRs IN CD4 T CELLS OUTWEIGH THE POTENTIAL DISADVANTAGE WITH SELF-REACTIVITY?

Given the connection between sensitivity and cross-reactivity with TCRs in CD8 T cells, it is reasonable to ask if the recruitment of CD4 T cells with higher-affinity TCRs is worth the risk of self-reactivity (by transducing all peripheral T cells including CD8 T cells). As described above, redirected CD4 T cells provide an opportunity for direct destruction of the tumor by the effector CD4 T cells. Our recent findings (76) and results from others (75) suggest that nanomolar affinity TCRs are more potent in CD4 T cells than wild-type TCRs. In fact, the only treatment which resulted in long-term control of established tumors, with no outgrowth, was CD4 T cells transduced with the 30-nM affinity TCR m33 (76).

We suggest that the major importance of CD4 T cell recruitment will be that they provide a cytokine milieu that facilitates the generation of endogenous responses against multiple class I MHC-restricted cancer antigens. These antigens might include individual unique peptides with tumor-specific, patient-specific mutations. Such mutated peptides have recently been shown to represent the dominant epitopes of an effective immune response that drives immunoediting (95, 147). Accordingly, it will be important to identify strategies that allow TCRs to mediate CD4 T cell activity, ultimately enabling a broad anti-cancer immune response. Since adoptive T cell therapies currently are configured to introduce the same TCR into both CD4 and CD8, an important issue is whether it is possible to improve current pre-clinical approaches to assess potential self-reactivity and consequent toxicity.

One possible strategy to take advantage of high-affinity TCRs in immunotherapy would be to separate CD4 and CD8 T cells *ex vivo* for transduction with separate TCR variants, as has been done in mouse studies (74–76). The CD4 T cells could be transduced with nanomolar affinity TCRs, while the CD8 T cells could be transduced with a reduced affinity version of the receptor. The method for creating a lowered affinity version of a TCR is fairly straightforward, as conserved residues in the CDR2 loops may be substituted, reducing the overall binding affinity of the TCR while maintaining the peptide specificity. Using a library of receptors with different residues at a single CDR2β position in the m33 and 2C TCRs, we recently showed that a range of binding affinities were achieved by the resulting receptor variants, and certain variants were sufficiently lowered in affinity to minimize cross-reactivity in CD8 T cells, but retain CD4 T cell activity (74). Several conserved positions in TCRs have been characterized [reviewed in (148)] which could be mutated to achieve lower-affinity variants of an anti-tumor TCR.

It is of course possible that adoptive T cell therapy could be combined with checkpoint blockade treatment to interfere with negative signals transmitted to T cells, for example from interactions of molecules such as CTLA-4 or PD-1 and their ligands, B7 and PD-L1 or PD-L2, respectively [reviewed in (149)]. With the advent of checkpoint blockade treatments, including antibodies that inhibit CTLA-4 (FDA-approved Ipilimumab) and PD-1 (or its ligand PD-L1), it is possible that lower-affinity TCRs will have improved efficacy in adoptive T cell therapies. Clinically, checkpoint blockade [reviewed in (150)] has been used to enhance endogenous T cell responses against a tumor. In melanoma patients, ipilimumab treatment showed a survival benefit, either alone or with a gp100 peptide-based vaccine, over the peptide vaccine alone (151). Patients treated with ipilimumab often exhibited tissue restricted, immune-related adverse autoimmune effects. Recently, there has been considerable excitement about blocking PD-1 signaling. As the PD-1 ligands, PD-L1 and PD-L2, are specifically upregulated at sites of inflammation and on many tumors (149), PD-1 blockade may more directly target immunosuppression in the tumor with fewer side effects than with CTLA-4. PD-1 blockade, currently in clinical trials in the form of several different antibodies (152–155), has shown promising response rates [up to 52% objective response rate in advanced melanoma patients treated with the MK-3475 (lambrolizumab) PD-1 blocking antibody (155)], but these treatments were also associated with immune-related adverse effects, although at lower rates than CTLA-4 blockade. In combination with checkpoint blockade, it is possible that a lower-affinity TCR could act with higher potency in an adoptive T cell therapy setting, as has been seen in a mouse model (156). It remains to be seen if this may have similar safety concerns as with higher-affinity TCRs, in terms of cross-reactivity, or on-target/off-tumor responses.

POTENTIAL STRATEGIES TO EVALUATE SELF-REACTIVITY RISKS ASSOCIATED WITH HIGHER-AFFINITY TCRs

Along with the promise of adoptive therapy with engineered TCR-transduced T cells has come the very real dangers of on-target/off-tumor toxicity (as seen in the MART-1 trial) and cross-reactivity with similar epitopes in normal tissues (as seen in the MAGE-A3 trial). Several important techniques are already in use to check for cross-reactivity, including *in vitro* screening of CD4 and CD8 T cells transduced with tumor-specific TCRs, using as antigen-presenting cells various lines derived from normal tissues. However, to safely take advantage of this therapeutic strategy and avoid serious adverse effects, it will be imperative to develop expanded strategies to screen candidate TCRs for safety and potential cross-reactivity prior to delivery into human patients. We propose below a combination of *in silico*, *in vitro*, and *in vivo* (murine) strategies to enhance current screens prior to clinical trials. In each case, we argue that having an engineered, high-affinity TCR would be of significant value in revealing potential safety concerns, even if a lower-affinity TCR may be desirable in a clinical setting, especially in CD8 T cells (75, 76). It is relatively easy to introduce mutations at one of several, well-characterized locations in the TCR [reviewed in (148)] that can reliably reduce affinity while maintaining specificity and anti-tumor activity (74).

One way to attempt to detect possible cross reactivities for a given TCR will be to take advantage of the vast amount of information available through genomic and proteomic databases. A standard protein BLAST (Basic Logical Alignment Search Tool, blastp algorithm)[1] search can be conveniently performed using the NCBI web interface, revealing similar sequences to a given peptide ranked with an Expect (E) value. The E value is a measure of the statistical significance of a particular match compared to random chance in the entire proteome, with lower E values being more significantly similar to the search string. As a model, the mouse proteome was searched by BLAST for sequences similar to the SIY peptide, which acts as an $H2\text{-}K^b$-restricted agonist for the 2C TCR, but is not actually contained within the mouse proteome. This search revealed two peptides with Expect values <5.0 (**Figure 2C**). However, the previously identified positive-selecting antigen, dEV8, was not identified in the BLAST search, even extending the accepted E value up to 10,000. Thus, BLAST searches alone do not capture the criteria that would be best used to search for MHC-binding peptides with potentially similar TCR-contact residues.

All peptides identified through *in silico* screens were tested in MHC-binding prediction algorithms with arbitrary cut-off values used previously for distinguishing qualitative binders vs. non-binders. Algorithms examined here included SYFPEITHI with a cutoff of >16 for binders (157)[2]; BIMAS with a cutoff of estimated $t^{1/2} > 30\,s$[3]; Artificial Neural Network [ANN; (158)], and Stabilized Matrix Method [SMM (159)]. ANN and SMM were both applied with a cut-off value of $IC_{50} < 500$ nM, and both were accessed through the Immune Epitope Database (IEDB) Analysis Resource[4]. A plot of predicted MHC-binding values for epitopes discussed in this review are shown in **Figure 3A**. It has been estimated that an IC_{50} cutoff of 500 nM by ANN or SMM yields 80% or higher (up to 97%) accuracy in predicting MHC binders, depending on allele (160). However, it is important to keep in mind that some MHC-binding peptides may be missed using a threshold such as this; for example, using 500 nM as a binding threshold for netMHCpan $H2\text{-}K^b$ binding predictions would omit p2Ca, a peptide which is known to form a complex with $H2\text{-}K^b$ and stimulate 2C T cells (161).

[1] http://blast.ncbi.nlm.nih.gov/
[2] http://www.syfpeithi.de/Scripts/MHCServer.dll/EpitopePrediction.htm
[3] http://bimas.dcrt.nih.gov/molbio/hla_bind
[4] http://tools.iedb.org/analyze/html/mhc_binding.html#

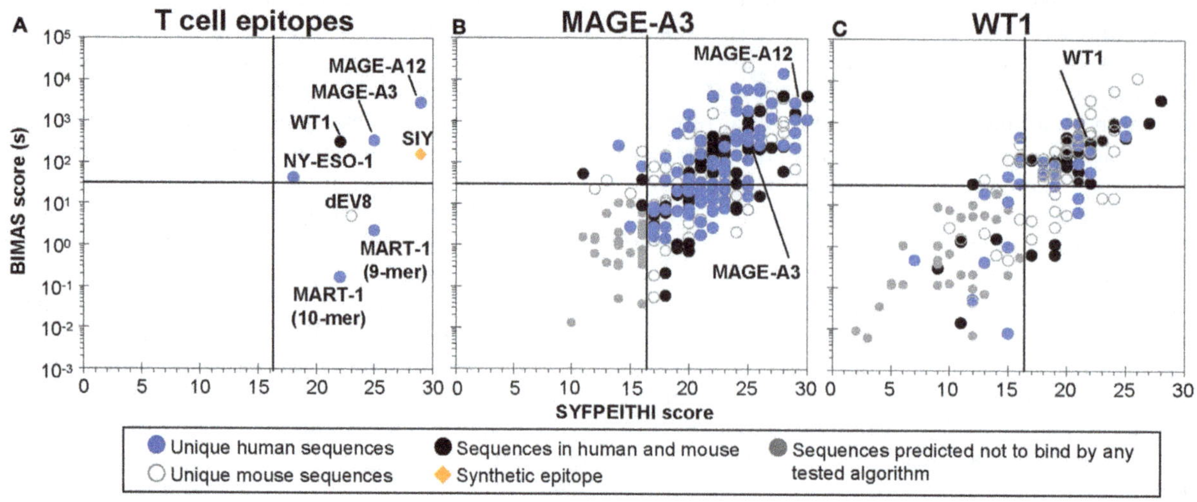

D

A2-restricted epitope	MAGE-A3[112-120]		WT1[126-134]	
Sequence	KVAELVHFL		RMFPNAPYL	
Search String	[KRHSG][VMILA][AVILMED] [EDK][LIVMA]**X**[HSTAQN][FYW][LVIM]		[RKH][MILV][FYW][PASTG]**X** [GAST][PAST][FYW][YFVILM]	
Search Type*	Without gaps	With gaps	Without gaps	With gaps
Theoretical maximum number peptides yielded#	3,780,000	532,980,000	1,036,800	146,188,800
Total human peptide sequences matching	134	830	13	78
Total matching peptides predicted to bind HLA-A2§	98	448	11	56
% predicted binders identically covered by the mouse genome	41	42	64	54

* Without gaps indicates that the search was conducted for the string as stated only; With gaps indicates that the search also allowed a single, 1 residue gap (any amino acid) in the sequence at any position

\# if search were applied to a set containing every possible combination of amino acids

§ Using a 500nM IC_{50} cut-off value for binding predictions to HLA-A2 with the ANN and SMM prediction algorithms

FIGURE 3 | Analysis of selected tumor epitopes for homologous sequences in the human and mouse proteomes. **(A)** MHC-binding prediction scores for a set of characterized T cell epitopes, including six HLA-A2-restricted human tumor-associated epitopes. **(B)** MHC-binding predictions for peptides identified in a MAGE-A3 [112–120] homology scan (no gaps) of the human and mouse proteomes. **(C)** MHC-binding predictions for peptides identified in a WT1 [126–134] homology scan of the human and mouse proteomes (including an allowed, single-amino acid gap). For **(B,C)**, peptides were subjected to ANN and SMM prediction algorithms along with SYFPEITHI and BIMAS, and prediction to bind above the arbitrary thresholds described in the text in any of the algorithms was taken to indicate a potential binder. **(D)** A comparison of MAGE-A3 and WT1 proteome scan results. The total number of predicted binders identified in the human proteome and the percent of the binders identically found in the mouse proteome for both epitopes (searched without gaps) are highlighted in yellow.

Using the MHC-binding principles, an alternative strategy to BLAST is to scan the full proteome for sequence motifs that: (1) preserve critical residues (or conservative mutations) ideally identified by positional single-site substitutions of the peptide epitope, and (2) allow other residues to vary more widely. A similar strategy was used to identify potential positive-selecting ligands for the OT-1 TCR, scanning for MHC-binding motifs, and then scoring for similarity among the predicted TCR contacts to the H2-K^b-restricted ovalbumin peptide, OVA (87). For our current efforts, using previous alanine scan information for the SIY peptide (SIYRYYGL) that stimulates the 2C TCR (39), a search motif was designed as "*XX[YFW][RKH][YFW][YFW][GSAT][LIVM]*," where "X" indicates that any residue would be acceptable at that position, and bracketed residues indicate that one of those limited set of residues would be acceptable. If every possible sequence were available in the proteome, the 2C homology search, as designed, would yield 518,400 sequences (20 × 20 × 3 × 3 × 3 × 3 × 4 × 4). Scanning the mouse proteome [the complete *Mus musculus* proteome from The Universal Protein Knowledgebase (UniProtKB), 73,947 entries] with this motif identified 43 peptides, of which 33 were predicted to bind well to H2-K^b (in this case, defining binders using a SYFPEITHI cutoff of 17 or higher, see **Figure 2D**). Importantly, this strategy identified, among the 33 peptides, dEV8 from the NADH dehydrogenase, which as described above is known to react with 2C TCR and the higher-affinity m33 TCR.

We propose that the yield of identified, predicted MHC-binding peptides when searching the proteome in this manner provides a reasonable estimate of the possible number of self-reactive peptides, and a tractable number of candidates that could be tested for reactivity with a higher-affinity TCR (like m33) in CD8 T cells. Of course, the identified peptides are influenced by the design of the search string, as well as the accuracy of binding predictions. To improve the ability of searches like this to comprehensively identify all potentially cross-reactive peptides, an epitope of interest should be evaluated for the ability of substituted peptides to activate its specific TCR. Value can be obtained from simple, single-point alanine substitutions, as can be seen from the ability of the murine proteome scan to identify the dEV8 peptide (with only two amino acids in common with the agonist peptide, **Figure 2D**) when guided by alanine substitutions of SIY for binding and stimulation of the 2C TCR (39).

While the search strategies for structurally similar peptides may identify potential problematic cross-reactive epitopes, this strategy alone can not identify structurally dissimilar peptides which act as agonists. It is possible that such peptides could be identified using combinatorial peptide library techniques, where individual positions/residues are held constant in each peptide pool, and stimulation is evaluated (162, 163).

To evaluate *in silico* strategies for human tumor targeting, BLAST searches of the HLA-A2-restricted epitopes for MART-1, NY-ESO-1, MAGE-A3, and WT1 were performed in the human proteome; similarity was defined with an Expect value cut off of 5.0. Within this range of similarity, the MART-1 (27–35) and WT1 (126–134) described above were identified as unique within the proteome. NY-ESO-1 (157–165) yielded two additional peptides rated similar within these criteria; however, neither was predicted to bind to HLA-A2. By contrast, MAGE-A3 (112–120) yielded fourteen sequences that were similar within this range of Expect values, of which 10 were other members of the MAGE family. All of the MAGE-similar peptides were predicted to have some binding to HLA-A2 (SYFPEITHI score greater than 16 or BIMAS off-rate >30 s).

Two of the epitopes, MAGE-A3 and WT1, were used further as the basis for a scan for structurally similar peptide sequences, as done with SIY. The contribution of each peptide position to T cell recognition has not been systematically studied for these epitopes; however, some data on substitutions is available (106, 111, 164–166). Using these data, and striving to maintain structural homology/conservative mutations, proteome search strings were generated, and applied to both the human and murine proteomes. This strategy thus further aimed to determine what fraction of potentially cross-reactive, structurally similar epitopes would be represented in both the human and murine proteomes. This information could be useful in examining what fraction of potential cross-reactive epitopes might reveal toxicities in a mouse model (see below).

If every possible sequence were available in the proteome, the MAGE-A3, and WT1 searches would yield ~3,800,000 and ~1,040,000 sequences, respectively. Applying the searches to the human proteome (the complete *Homo sapiens* proteome downloaded from UniProtKB, 134,787 entries) yielded 134 sequences similar to the MAGE-A3 epitope and 13 sequences similar to the WT1 peptide. Thus, consistent with the BLAST search, WT1-like sequences were about 10-fold more rare in the human proteome than MAGE-A3-like sequences. We also allowed the search string to include a single random amino acid gap anywhere in the peptide sequence for WT1, yielding larger theoretical search maxima (e.g., 146,000,000 for WT1, almost 40-fold larger than the theoretical search size without gaps for MAGE-A3, 3,800,000). When even that search string for WT1 was applied to the human proteome, only 78 peptides were identified, still half as many as identified with the MAGE-A3 search string without gaps (134 peptides). It should be noted that for most TCRs, insertion of a single residue (i.e., "gap") in the peptide may significantly alter the bound conformation of the peptide, resulting in a loss of recognition of the epitope. Using a combinatorial library scanning approach where peptide pools of different length were tested for the ability to stimulate different TCRs, it has been shown that TCRs have restricted length preferences in the peptide epitopes that they recognize (163). Thus, it remains to be seen whether the addition of "gaps" in a search string are of any value. This can be readily determined by activity analysis of cognate peptides that have the various single-amino acid insertions.

The MAGE-A3 and WT1-related peptides were further screened using the binding prediction algorithms listed above, and peptides predicted to bind by the ANN or SMM algorithms ($IC_{50} < 500$ nM) were designated as potential binders, resulting in 98 and 11 peptides for MAGE-A3 and WT1, respectively. Interestingly, of these epitopes, 41 and 64%, respectively, were identically represented in the mouse proteome, with many others having highly homologous sequences. The distribution of homologous sequences identified through these screens, and their presence uniquely in the human proteome, the mouse proteome, or identically in both is shown in **Figures 3B,C** (where the WT1-like peptides in **Figure 3C** also include those with single-amino acid gaps). A summary of the search results for these two epitopes can be seen in **Figure 3D**. The number of peptides identified by this type of search in all three cases (SIY, MAGE-A3, and WT1) is readily amenable to small-scale synthesis and *in vitro* testing for T cell stimulation by peptide-loaded, HLA-A2-positive APCs. We propose this straightforward screen to evaluate cross reactivities with structurally similar epitopes. Peptides with reactivities would be followed with more detailed analysis of gene transcript levels in different tissues, and studies of the ability of the gene-product to be processed and presented.

Proteome searches using a particular motif can not assess all potential cross-reactive peptide epitopes, especially those without structural similarity. Hence, we propose that an additional *in vitro* screening strategy may be useful. For example, an open reading frame (ORF) library (167, 168) covering genes from the human proteome would be transfected into HLA-A2-positive APCs. ORF libraries have been used in yeast two-hybrid systems toward mapping the protein "interactome," (169) and recently the human ORFome is being developed in a lentiviral vector system, which would allow for convenient application to mammalian cell transduction (168, 170). This would provide another opportunity to identify unpredicted cross reactivities, and such libraries would provide a resource available for screening virtually any TCR, restricted by the appropriate HLA alleles.

Finally, we propose expanded use of HLA transgenic mice to screen for safety. As mentioned above, 40–65% of peptides identified in MAGE-A3 and WT1 homology screens were identical in mouse and human, providing a rationale for using a mouse screen to identify at least some of the potentially adverse cross reactivities. The system would ideally involve the use of mouse T cells transduced with human TCRs (human V regions linked to mouse C regions), as these would provide syngeneic cell:cell adhesion systems for optimal activities. TCR-transduced mouse CD4 and CD8 T cells could be transferred to the transgenic HLA-A2/D^d hybrid MHCs (AAD, available from Jackson Labs) which allows cells to present HLA-A2 peptide epitopes while still engaging mouse CD8. This system could be tested with various affinity TCRs in order to push the limits of safety and efficacy.

A significant advantage of the mouse system would be the opportunity to also generate additional transgenic mice on the AAD background, where the tumor gene of interest (e.g., MART-1, MAGE-A3, or NY-ESO-1) is expressed under the relevant mouse promoter. Such models could reveal on-target/off-tumor activities due to uncharacterized expression of the target gene in normal tissue, either at low levels or by a low-frequency cell subset. As the WT1 [126–134] epitope is identical in the mouse and human proteins, this provides an opportunity to assess safety without the generation of the human WT1 transgene.

CONCLUDING REMARKS

While there will always remain a risk of unpredicted reactivities in patients receiving adoptive T cell therapies, we believe that the use of TCRs with different affinities and specificities in an expanded set of pre-clinical approaches, as described here, will identify some of the possible problems. Proteome search approaches provide a measure of the number of related self-peptides that could pose safety concerns with adoptive T cell therapies. In addition, the number of peptides represented in the proteome predicted to be similar to a given epitope should correlate with the extent of central tolerance that might exist against a cancer peptide. In this regard, this type of analysis might be considered for peptide vaccines (e.g., lower numbers of homologous peptides may correlate with higher frequencies of peripheral T cells that have escaped negative selection). Further safeguards at the initial clinical stage, such as reduction in the number of T cells delivered, may be considered. Significant progress has also been made in the development of suicide genes or alternative approaches that could allow rapid deletion of T cells before a dangerous reaction reaches the critical stage (171, 172). Finally, transfer of only CD4 T cells may be desirable as they can mediate strong anti-tumor effects and potential for helping endogenous immune responses, but CD4 T cells may not exhibit the CD8-dependent cross reactivities that the same TCRs mediate in CD8 T cells.

ACKNOWLEDGMENTS

We thank members of the lab, past and present, for valuable contributions to the development of these concepts. We also thank Hans Schreiber and Phil Greenberg for discussions and long-standing collaborative work with our lab. Research in the lab has been funded by grants from the National Institutes of Health (R01 GM55767 and P01 CA97296, to David M. Kranz) and the Melanoma Research Alliance (to David M. Kranz), and a Samuel and Ruth Engelberg/Irvington Institute Postdoctoral Fellowship of the Cancer Research Institute to Jennifer D. Stone.

REFERENCES

1. Perez-Diez A, Joncker NT, Choi K, Chan WF, Anderson CC, Lantz O, et al. CD4 cells can be more efficient at tumor rejection than CD8 cells. *Blood* (2007) **109**:5346–54. doi:10.1182/blood-2006-10-051318
2. Surman DR, Dudley ME, Overwijk WW, Restifo NP. Cutting edge: CD4+ T cell control of CD8+ T cell reactivity to a model tumor antigen. *J Immunol* (2000) **164**:562–5.
3. Novy P, Quigley M, Huang X, Yang Y. CD4 T cells are required for CD8 T cell survival during both primary and memory recall responses. *J Immunol* (2007) **179**:8243–51.
4. Oh S, Perera LP, Terabe M, Ni L, Waldmann TA, Berzofsky JA. IL-15 as a mediator of CD4+ help for CD8+ T cell longevity and avoidance of TRAIL-mediated apoptosis. *Proc Natl Acad Sci U S A* (2008) **105**:5201–6. doi:10.1073/pnas.0801003105
5. Nakanishi Y, Lu B, Gerard C, Iwasaki A. CD8(+) T lymphocyte mobilization to virus-infected tissue requires CD4(+) T-cell help. *Nature* (2009) **462**:510–3. doi:10.1038/nature08511
6. Bos R, Sherman LA. CD4+ T-cell help in the tumor milieu is required for recruitment and cytolytic function of CD8+ T lymphocytes. *Cancer Res* (2010) **70**:8368–77. doi:10.1158/0008-5472.CAN-10-1322
7. Ray S, Chhabra A, Chakraborty NG, Hegde U, Dorsky DI, Chodon T, et al. MHC-I-restricted melanoma antigen specific TCR-engineered human CD4+ T cells exhibit multifunctional effector and helper responses, in vitro. *Clin Immunol* (2010) **136**:338–47. doi:10.1016/j.clim.2010.04.013
8. Restifo NP, Dudley ME, Rosenberg SA. Adoptive immunotherapy for cancer: harnessing the T cell response. *Nat Rev Immunol* (2012) **12**:269–81. doi:10.1038/nri3191
9. Stroncek DF, Berger C, Cheever MA, Childs RW, Dudley ME, Flynn P, et al. New directions in cellular therapy of cancer: a summary of the summit on cellular therapy for cancer. *J Transl Med* (2012) **10**:48. doi:10.1186/1479-5876-10-48
10. Wang LX, Shu S, Disis ML, Plautz GE. Adoptive transfer of tumor-primed, in vitro-activated, CD4+ T effector cells (TEs) combined with CD8+ TEs provides intratumoral TE proliferation and synergistic antitumor response. *Blood* (2007) **109**:4865–76. doi:10.1182/blood-2006-09-045245
11. Quezada SA, Simpson TR, Peggs KS, Merghoub T, Vider J, Fan X, et al. Tumor-reactive CD4(+) T cells develop cytotoxic activity and eradicate large established melanoma after transfer into lymphopenic hosts. *J Exp Med* (2010) **207**:637–50. doi:10.1084/jem.20091918
12. Xie Y, Akpinarli A, Maris C, Hipkiss EL, Lane M, Kwon EK, et al. Naive tumor-specific CD4(+) T cells differentiated in vivo eradicate established melanoma. *J Exp Med* (2010) **207**:651–67. doi:10.1084/jem.20091921
13. Qin Z, Blankenstein T. CD4+ T cell – mediated tumor rejection involves inhibition of angiogenesis that is dependent on IFN gamma receptor expression by nonhematopoietic cells. *Immunity* (2000) **12**:677–86. doi:10.1016/S1074-7613(00)80218-6
14. Ibe S, Qin Z, Schuler T, Preiss S, Blankenstein T. Tumor rejection by disturbing tumor stroma cell interactions. *J Exp Med* (2001) **194**:1549–59. doi:10.1084/jem.194.11.1549
15. Hunder NN, Wallen H, Cao J, Hendricks DW, Reilly JZ, Rodmyre R, et al. Treatment of metastatic melanoma with autologous CD4+ T cells against NY-ESO-1. *N Engl J Med* (2008) **358**:2698–703. doi:10.1056/NEJMoa0800251

16. Liu Z, Noh HS, Chen J, Kim JH, Falo LD Jr, You Z. Potent tumor-specific protection ignited by adoptively transferred CD4+ T cells. *J Immunol* (2008) **181**:4363–70.
17. Kuball J, Schmitz FW, Voss RH, Ferreira EA, Engel R, Guillaume P, et al. Cooperation of human tumor-reactive CD4+ and CD8+ T cells after redirection of their specificity by a high-affinity p53A2.1-specific TCR. *Immunity* (2005) **22**:117–29. doi:10.1016/j.immuni.2004.12.005
18. Morris EC, Tsallios A, Bendle GM, Xue SA, Stauss HJ. A critical role of T cell antigen receptor-transduced MHC class I-restricted helper T cells in tumor protection. *Proc Natl Acad Sci U S A* (2005) **102**:7934–9. doi:10.1073/pnas.0500357102
19. Roszkowski JJ, Lyons GE, Kast WM, Yee C, Van Besien K, Nishimura MI. Simultaneous generation of CD8+ and CD4+ melanoma-reactive T cells by retroviral-mediated transfer of a single T-cell receptor. *Cancer Res* (2005) **65**:1570–6. doi:10.1158/0008-5472.CAN-04-2076
20. Tsuji T, Yasukawa M, Matsuzaki J, Ohkuri T, Chamoto K, Wakita D, et al. Generation of tumor-specific, HLA class I-restricted human Th1 and Tc1 cells by cell engineering with tumor peptide-specific T-cell receptor genes. *Blood* (2005) **106**:470–6. doi:10.1182/blood-2004-09-3663
21. Willemsen R, Ronteltap C, Heuveling M, Debets R, Bolhuis R. Redirecting human CD4+ T lymphocytes to the MHC class I-restricted melanoma antigen MAGE-A1 by TCR alphabeta gene transfer requires CD8alpha. *Gene Ther* (2005) **12**:140–6. doi:10.1038/sj.gt.3302388
22. Kessels HW, Schepers K, van den Boom MD, Topham DJ, Schumacher TN. Generation of T cell help through a MHC class I-restricted TCR. *J Immunol* (2006) **177**:976–82.
23. Chhabra A, Yang L, Wang P, Comin-Anduix B, Das R, Chakraborty NG, et al. CD4+CD25- T cells transduced to express MHC class I-restricted epitope-specific TCR synthesize Th1 cytokines and exhibit MHC class I-restricted cytolytic effector function in a human melanoma model. *J Immunol* (2008) **181**:1063–70.
24. Laugel B, van den Berg HA, Gostick E, Cole DK, Wooldridge L, Boulter J, et al. Different T cell receptor affinity thresholds and CD8 coreceptor dependence govern cytotoxic T lymphocyte activation and tetramer binding properties. *J Biol Chem* (2007) **282**:23799–810. doi:10.1074/jbc.M700976200
25. Chervin AS, Stone JD, Bowerman NA, Kranz DM. Cutting edge: inhibitory effects of CD4 and CD8 on T cell activation induced by high-affinity noncognate ligands. *J Immunol* (2009) **183**:7639–43. doi:10.4049/jimmunol.0901664
26. Chervin AS, Stone JD, Holler PD, Bai A, Chen J, Eisen HN, et al. The impact of TCR-binding properties and antigen presentation format on T cell responsiveness. *J Immunol* (2009) **183**:1166–78. doi:10.4049/jimmunol.0900054
27. Molloy PE, Sewell AK, Jakobsen BK. Soluble T cell receptors: novel immunotherapies. *Curr Opin Pharmacol* (2005) **5**:438–43. doi:10.1016/j.coph.2005.02.004
28. Richman SA, Kranz DM. Display, engineering, and applications of antigen-specific T cell receptors. *Biomol Eng* (2007) **24**:361–73. doi:10.1016/j.bioeng.2007.02.009
29. Robbins PF, Li YF, El-Gamil M, Zhao Y, Wargo JA, Zheng Z, et al. Single and dual amino acid substitutions in TCR CDRs can enhance antigen-specific T cell functions. *J Immunol* (2008) **180**:6116–31.
30. Haidar JN, Pierce B, Yu Y, Tong W, Li M, Weng Z. Structure-based design of a T-cell receptor leads to nearly 100-fold improvement in binding affinity for pepMHC. *Proteins* (2009) **74**:948–60. doi:10.1002/prot.22203
31. Zoete V, Irving MB, Michielin O. MM-GBSA binding free energy decomposition and T cell receptor engineering. *J Mol Recognit* (2010) **23**:142–52. doi:10.1002/jmr.1005
32. Stone JD, Chervin AS, Aggen DH, Kranz DM. T cell receptor engineering. *Methods Enzymol* (2012) **503**:189–222. doi:10.1016/B978-0-12-396962-0.00008-2
33. Sykulev Y, Joo M, Vturina I, Tsomides TJ, Eisen HN. Evidence that a single peptide-MHC complex on a target cell can elicit a cytolytic T cell response. *Immunity* (1996) **4**:565–71. doi:10.1016/S1074-7613(00)80483-5
34. Purbhoo MA, Irvine DJ, Huppa JB, Davis MM. T cell killing does not require the formation of a stable mature immunological synapse. *Nat Immunol* (2004) **5**:524–30. doi:10.1038/ni0604-658a
35. Artyomov MN, Lis M, Devadas S, Davis MM, Chakraborty AK. CD4 and CD8 binding to MHC molecules primarily acts to enhance Lck delivery. *Proc Natl Acad Sci U S A* (2010) **107**:16916–21. doi:10.1073/pnas.1010568107
36. Anikeeva N, Lebedeva T, Clapp AR, Goldman ER, Dustin ML, Mattoussi H, et al. Quantum dot/peptide-MHC biosensors reveal strong CD8-dependent cooperation between self and viral antigens that augment the T cell response. *Proc Natl Acad Sci U S A* (2006) **103**:16846–51. doi:10.1073/pnas.0607771103
37. Anikeeva N, Gakamsky D, Scholler J, Sykulev Y. Evidence that the density of self peptide-MHC ligands regulates T-cell receptor signaling. *PLoS ONE* (2012) **7**:e41466. doi:10.1371/journal.pone.0041466
38. Sykulev Y, Brunmark A, Jackson M, Cohen RJ, Peterson PA, Eisen HN. Kinetics and affinity of reactions between an antigen-specific T cell receptor and peptide-MHC complexes. *Immunity* (1994) **1**:15–22. doi:10.1016/1074-7613(94)90005-1
39. Bowerman NA, Colf LA, Garcia KC, Kranz DM. Different strategies adopted by K(b) and L(d) to generate T cell specificity directed against their respective bound peptides. *J Biol Chem* (2009) **284**:32551–61. doi:10.1074/jbc.M109.040501
40. Stone JD, Chervin AS, Kranz DM. T-cell receptor binding affinities and kinetics: impact on T-cell activity and specificity. *Immunology* (2009) **126**:165–76. doi:10.1111/j.1365-2567.2008.03015.x
41. Aleksic M, Liddy N, Molloy PE, Pumphrey N, Vuidepot A, Chang KM, et al. Different affinity windows for virus and cancer-specific T-cell receptors: implications for therapeutic strategies. *Eur J Immunol* (2012) **42**:3174–9. doi:10.1002/eji.201242606
42. Palmer E. Negative selection – clearing out the bad apples from the T-cell repertoire. *Nat Rev Immunol* (2003) **3**:383–91. doi:10.1038/nri1085
43. Hogquist KA, Baldwin TA, Jameson SC. Central tolerance: learning self-control in the thymus. *Nat Rev Immunol* (2005) **5**:772–82. doi:10.1038/nri1707
44. Naeher D, Daniels MA, Hausmann B, Guillaume P, Luescher I, Palmer E. A constant affinity threshold for T cell tolerance. *J Exp Med* (2007) **204**:2553–9. doi:10.1084/jem.20070254
45. Mathis D, Benoist C. Aire. *Annu Rev Immunol* (2009) **27**:287–312. doi:10.1146/annurev.immunol.25.022106.141532
46. Dissanayake D, Gronski MA, Lin A, Elford AR, Ohashi PS. Immunological perspective of self versus tumor antigens: insights from the RIP-gp model. *Immunol Rev* (2011) **241**:164–79. doi:10.1111/j.1600-065X.2011.01014.x
47. Bridgeman JS, Sewell AK, Miles JJ, Price DA, Cole DK. Structural and biophysical determinants of alphabeta T-cell antigen recognition. *Immunology* (2012) **135**:9–18. doi:10.1111/j.1365-2567.2011.03515.x
48. Huang J, Meyer C, Zhu C. T cell antigen recognition at the cell membrane. *Mol Immunol* (2012) **52**:155–64. doi:10.1016/j.molimm.2012.05.004
49. Yewdell JW, Bennink JR. Immunodominance in major histocompatibility complex class I-restricted T lymphocyte responses. *Annu Rev Immunol* (1999) **17**:51–88. doi:10.1146/annurev.immunol.17.1.51
50. Ohno S, Moriya O, Yoshimoto T, Hayashi H, Akatsuka T, Matsui M. Immunogenic variation between multiple HLA-A*0201-restricted, hepatitis C virus-derived epitopes for cytotoxic T lymphocytes. *Viral Immunol* (2006) **19**:458–67. doi:10.1089/vim.2006.19.458
51. Moutaftsi M, Salek-Ardakani S, Croft M, Peters B, Sidney J, Grey H, et al. Correlates of protection efficacy induced by vaccinia virus-specific CD8+ T-cell epitopes in the murine intranasal challenge model. *Eur J Immunol* (2009) **39**:717–22. doi:10.1002/eji.200838815
52. Engels B, Engelhard VH, Sidney J, Sette A, Binder DC, Liu RB, et al. Relapse or eradication of cancer is predicted by peptide-major histocompatibility complex affinity. *Cancer Cell* (2013) **23**:516–26. doi:10.1016/j.ccr
53. McKeithan TW. Kinetic proofreading in T-cell receptor signal transduction. *Proc Natl Acad Sci U S A* (1995) **92**:5042–6. doi:10.1073/pnas.92.11.5042
54. Kalergis AM, Boucheron N, Doucey MA, Palmieri E, Goyarts EC, Vegh Z, et al. Efficient T cell activation requires an optimal dwell-time of interaction between the TCR and the pMHC complex. *Nat Immunol* (2001) **2**:229–34. doi:10.1038/85286

55. Valitutti S, Muller S, Cella M, Padovan E, Lanzavecchia A. Serial triggering of many T-cell receptors by a few peptide-MHC complexes. *Nature* (1995) **375**:148–51. doi:10.1038/375148a0
56. Holler PD, Kranz DM. Quantitative analysis of the contribution of TCR/pepMHC affinity and CD8 to T cell activation. *Immunity* (2003) **18**:255–64. doi:10.1016/S1074-7613(03)00019-0
57. Rosette C, Werlen G, Daniels MA, Holman PO, Alam SM, Travers PJ, et al. The impact of duration versus extent of TCR occupancy on T cell activation: a revision of the kinetic proofreading model. *Immunity* (2001) **15**:59–70. doi:10.1016/S1074-7613(01)00173-X
58. Ely LK, Green KJ, Beddoe T, Clements CS, Miles JJ, Bottomley SP, et al. Antagonism of antiviral and allogeneic activity of a human public CTL clonotype by a single altered peptide ligand: implications for allograft rejection. *J Immunol* (2005) **174**:5593–601.
59. Tian S, Maile R, Collins EJ, Frelinger JA. CD8+ T cell activation is governed by TCR-peptide/MHC affinity, not dissociation rate. *J Immunol* (2007) **179**:2952–60.
60. Aleksic M, Dushek O, Zhang H, Shenderov E, Chen JL, Cerundolo V, et al. Dependence of T cell antigen recognition on T cell receptor-peptide MHC confinement time. *Immunity* (2010) **32**:163–74. doi:10.1016/j.immuni.2009.11.013
61. Huppa JB, Axmann M, Mortelmaier MA, Lillemeier BF, Newell EW, Brameshuber M, et al. TCR-peptide-MHC interactions in situ show accelerated kinetics and increased affinity. *Nature* (2010) **463**:963–7. doi:10.1038/nature08746
62. Huang J, Zarnitsyna VI, Liu B, Edwards LJ, Jiang N, Evavold BD, et al. The kinetics of two-dimensional TCR and pMHC interactions determine T-cell responsiveness. *Nature* (2010) **464**:932–6. doi:10.1038/nature08944
63. Garcia KC, Scott CA, Brunmark A, Carbone FR, Peterson PA, Wilson IA, et al. CD8 enhances formation of stable T-cell receptor/MHC class I molecule complexes. *Nature* (1996) **384**:577–81. doi:10.1038/384577a0
64. Wyer JR, Willcox BE, Gao GF, Gerth UC, Davis SJ, Bell JI, et al. T cell receptor and coreceptor CD8 alphaalpha bind peptide-MHC independently and with distinct kinetics. *Immunity* (1999) **10**:219–25. doi:10.1016/S1074-7613(00)80022-9
65. Gao GF, Rao Z, Bell JI. Molecular coordination of alphabeta T-cell receptors and coreceptors CD8 and CD4 in their recognition of peptide-MHC ligands. *Trends Immunol* (2002) **23**:408–13. doi:10.1016/S1471-4906(02)02282-2
66. Cole DK, Dunn SM, Sami M, Boulter JM, Jakobsen BK, Sewell AK. T cell receptor engagement of peptide-major histocompatibility complex class I does not modify CD8 binding. *Mol Immunol* (2008) **45**:2700–9. doi:10.1016/j.molimm.2007.12.009
67. Cole DK, Laugel B, Clement M, Price DA, Wooldridge L, Sewell AK. The molecular determinants of CD8 co-receptor function. *Immunology* (2012) **137**:139–48. doi:10.1111/j.1365-2567.2012.03625.x
68. Bowerman NA, Crofts TS, Chlewicki L, Do P, Baker BM, Christopher Garcia K, et al. Engineering the binding properties of the T cell receptor:peptide:MHC ternary complex that governs T cell activity. *Mol Immunol* (2009) **46**:3000–8. doi:10.1016/j.molimm.2009.06.012
69. Schmid DA, Irving MB, Posevitz V, Hebeisen M, Posevitz-Fejfar A, Sarria JC, et al. Evidence for a TCR affinity threshold delimiting maximal CD8 T cell function. *J Immunol* (2010) **184**:4936–46. doi:10.4049/jimmunol.1000173
70. Zhong S, Malecek K, Johnson LA, Yu Z, Vega-Saenz de Miera E, Darvishian F, et al. T-cell receptor affinity and avidity defines antitumor response and autoimmunity in T-cell immunotherapy. *Proc Natl Acad Sci U S A* (2013) **110**:6973–8. doi:10.1073/pnas.1221609110
71. Holler PD, Chlewicki LK, Kranz DM. TCRs with high affinity for foreign pMHC show self-reactivity. *Nat Immunol* (2003) **4**:55–62. doi:10.1038/ni863
72. Thomas S, Xue SA, Bangham CR, Jakobsen BK, Morris EC, Stauss HJ. Human T cells expressing affinity-matured TCR display accelerated responses but fail to recognize low density of MHC-peptide antigen. *Blood* (2011) **118**:319–29. doi:10.1182/blood-2010-12-326736
73. Zhao Y, Bennett AD, Zheng Z, Wang QJ, Robbins PF, Yu LY, et al. High-affinity TCRs generated by phage display provide CD4+ T cells with the ability to recognize and kill tumor cell lines. *J Immunol* (2007) **179**:5845–54.
74. Chervin AS, Stone JD, Soto CM, Engels B, Schreiber H, Roy EJ, et al. Design of T-cell receptor libraries with diverse binding properties to examine adoptive T-cell responses. *Gene Ther* (2012) **20**(6):634–44.
75. Engels B, Chervin AS, Sant AJ, Kranz DM, Schreiber H. Long-term persistence of CD4(+) but rapid disappearance of CD8(+) T cells expressing an MHC class I-restricted TCR of nanomolar affinity. *Mol Ther* (2012) **20**:652–60. doi:10.1038/mt.2011.286
76. Soto CM, Stone JD, Chervin AS, Engels B, Schreiber H, Roy EJ, et al. MHC-class I-restricted CD4 T cells: a nanomolar affinity TCR has improved anti-tumor efficacy in vivo compared to the micromolar wild-type TCR. *Cancer Immunol Immunother* (2012) **62**:359–69. doi:10.1007/s00262-012-1336-z
77. Eisen HN. Specificity and degeneracy in antigen recognition: yin and yang in the immune system. *Annu Rev Immunol* (2001) **19**:1–21. doi:10.1146/annurev.immunol.19.1.1
78. Chen J, Eisen HN, Kranz DM. A model T-cell receptor system for studying memory T-cell development. *Microbes Infect* (2003) **5**:233–40. doi:10.1016/S1286-4579(03)00016-9
79. Sha WC, Nelson CA, Newberry RD, Kranz DM, Russell JH, Loh DY. Positive and negative selection of an antigen receptor on T cells in transgenic mice. *Nature* (1988) **336**:73–6. doi:10.1038/336073a0
80. Garcia KC, Degano M, Stanfield RL, Brunmark A, Jackson MR, Peterson PA, et al. An alphabeta T cell receptor structure at 2.5 A and its orientation in the TCR-MHC complex. *Science* (1996) **274**:209–19. doi:10.1126/science.274.5285.209
81. Speir JA, Garcia KC, Brunmark A, Degano M, Peterson PA, Teyton L, et al. Structural basis of 2C TCR allorecognition of H-2Ld peptide complexes. *Immunity* (1998) **8**:553–62. doi:10.1016/S1074-7613(00)80560-9
82. Colf LA, Bankovich AJ, Hanick NA, Bowerman NA, Jones LL, Kranz DM, et al. How a single T cell receptor recognizes both self and foreign MHC. *Cell* (2007) **129**:135–46. doi:10.1016/j.cell.2007.01.048
83. Spiotto MT, Rowley DA, Schreiber H. Bystander elimination of antigen loss variants in established tumors. *Nat Med* (2004) **10**:294–8. doi:10.1038/nm999
84. DuPage M, Cheung AF, Mazumdar C, Winslow MM, Bronson R, Schmidt LM, et al. Endogenous T cell responses to antigens expressed in lung adenocarcinomas delay malignant tumor progression. *Cancer Cell* (2011) **19**:72–85. doi:10.1016/j.ccr.2010.11.011
85. Kranz DM, Sherman DH, Sitkovsky MV, Pasternack MS, Eisen HN. Immunoprecipitation of cell surface structures of cloned cytotoxic T lymphocytes by clone-specific antisera. *Proc Natl Acad Sci U S A* (1984) **81**:573–7. doi:10.1073/pnas.81.2.573
86. Tallquist MD, Yun TJ, Pease LR. A single T cell receptor recognizes structurally distinct MHC/peptide complexes with high specificity. *J Exp Med* (1996) **184**:1017–26. doi:10.1084/jem.184.3.1017
87. Santori FR, Kieper WC, Brown SM, Lu Y, Neubert TA, Johnson KL, et al. Rare, structurally homologous self-peptides promote thymocyte positive selection. *Immunity* (2002) **17**:131–42. doi:10.1016/S1074-7613(02)00361-8
88. Udaka K, Wiesmuller KH, Kienle S, Jung G, Walden P. Decrypting the structure of major histocompatibility complex class I-restricted cytotoxic T lymphocyte epitopes with complex peptide libraries. *J Exp Med* (1995) **181**:2097–108. doi:10.1084/jem.181.6.2097
89. Tallquist MD, Weaver AJ, Pease LR. Degenerate recognition of alloantigenic peptides on a positive-selecting class I molecule. *J Immunol* (1998) **160**:802–9.
90. Garcia KC, Tallquist MD, Pease LR, Brunmark A, Scott CA, Degano M, et al. Alphabeta T cell receptor interactions with syngeneic and allogeneic ligands: affinity measurements and crystallization. *Proc Natl Acad Sci U S A* (1997) **94**:13838–43. doi:10.1073/pnas.94.25.13838
91. Jones LL, Colf LA, Stone JD, Garcia KC, Kranz DM. Distinct CDR3 conformations in TCRs determine the level of cross-reactivity for diverse antigens, but not the docking orientation. *J Immunol* (2008) **181**:6255–64.
92. Degano M, Garcia KC, Apostolopoulos V, Rudolph MG, Teyton L, Wilson IA. A functional hot spot for antigen recognition in a superagonist TCR/MHC complex.

Immunity (2000) **12**:251–61. doi:10.1016/S1074-7613(00)80178-8
93. Spiotto MT, Yu P, Rowley DA, Nishimura MI, Meredith SC, Gajewski TF, et al. Increasing tumor antigen expression overcomes "ignorance" to solid tumors via crosspresentation by bone marrow-derived stromal cells. *Immunity* (2002) **17**:737–47. doi:10.1016/S1074-7613(02)00480-6
94. Spiotto MT, Schreiber H. Rapid destruction of the tumor microenvironment by CTLs recognizing cancer-specific antigens cross-presented by stromal cells. *Cancer Immun* (2005) **5**:8.
95. DuPage M, Mazumdar C, Schmidt LM, Cheung AF, Jacks T. Expression of tumour-specific antigens underlies cancer immunoediting. *Nature* (2012) **482**:405–9. doi:10.1038/nature10803
96. Holler PD, Holman PO, Shusta EV, O'Herrin S, Wittrup KD, Kranz DM. In vitro evolution of a T cell receptor with high affinity for peptide/MHC. *Proc Natl Acad Sci U S A* (2000) **97**:5387–92. doi:10.1073/pnas.080078297
97. Holler PD, Lim AR, Cho BK, Rund LA, Kranz DM. CD8(-) T cell transfectants that express a high affinity T cell receptor exhibit enhanced peptide-dependent activation. *J Exp Med* (2001) **194**:1043–52. doi:10.1084/jem.194.8.1043
98. Evavold BD, Allen PM. Separation of IL-4 production from Th cell proliferation by an altered T cell receptor ligand. *Science* (1991) **252**:1308–10. doi:10.1126/science.1833816
99. Weber KS, Donermeyer DL, Allen PM, Kranz DM. Class II-restricted T cell receptor engineered in vitro for higher affinity retains peptide specificity and function. *Proc Natl Acad Sci U S A* (2005) **102**:19033–8. doi:10.1073/pnas.0507554102
100. Kersh GJ, Kersh EN, Fremont DH, Allen PM. High- and low-potency ligands with similar affinities for the TCR: the importance of kinetics in TCR signaling. *Immunity* (1998) **9**:817–26. doi:10.1016/S1074-7613(00)80647-0
101. Donermeyer DL, Weber KS, Kranz DM, Allen PM. The study of high-affinity TCRs reveals duality in T cell recognition of antigen: specificity and degeneracy. *J Immunol* (2006) **177**:6911–9.
102. Lynch JN, Donermeyer DL, Weber KS, Kranz DM, Allen PM. Subtle changes in TCRalpha CDR1 profoundly increase the sensitivity of CD4 T cells. *Mol Immunol* (2013) **53**:283–94. doi:10.1016/j.molimm.2012.08.020
103. Cheever MA, Allison JP, Ferris AS, Finn OJ, Hastings BM, Hecht TT, et al. The prioritization of cancer antigens: a national cancer institute pilot project for the acceleration of translational research. *Clin Cancer Res* (2009) **15**:5323–37. doi:10.1158/1078-0432.CCR-09-0737
104. Chen JL, Dunbar PR, Gileadi U, Jager E, Gnjatic S, Nagata Y, et al. Identification of NY-ESO-1 peptide analogues capable of improved stimulation of tumor-reactive CTL. *J Immunol* (2000) **165**:948–55.
105. Boulter JM, Glick M, Todorov PT, Baston E, Sami M, Rizkallah P, et al. Stable, soluble T-cell receptor molecules for crystallization and therapeutics. *Protein Eng* (2003) **16**:707–11. doi:10.1093/protein/gzg087
106. Chinnasamy N, Wargo JA, Yu Z, Rao M, Frankel TL, Riley JP, et al. A TCR targeting the HLA-A*0201-restricted epitope of MAGE-A3 recognizes multiple epitopes of the MAGE-A antigen superfamily in several types of cancer. *J Immunol* (2011) **186**:685–96. doi:10.4049/jimmunol.1001775
107. Gao L, Bellantuono I, Elsasser A, Marley SB, Gordon MY, Goldman JM, et al. Selective elimination of leukemic CD34(+) progenitor cells by cytotoxic T lymphocytes specific for WT1. *Blood* (2000) **95**:2198–203.
108. Chapuis AG, Ragnarsson GB, Nguyen HN, Chaney CN, Pufnock JS, Schmitt TM, et al. Transferred WT1-reactive CD8+ T cells can mediate antileukemic activity and persist in post-transplant patients. *Sci Transl Med* (2013) **5**:174ra127. doi:10.1126/scitranslmed.3004916
109. Johnson LA, Morgan RA, Dudley ME, Cassard L, Yang JC, Hughes MS, et al. Gene therapy with human and mouse T-cell receptors mediates cancer regression and targets normal tissues expressing cognate antigen. *Blood* (2009) **114**:535–46. doi:10.1182/blood-2009-03-211714
110. Linette GP, Stadtmauer EA, Maus MV, Rapoport AP, Levine BL, Emery L, et al. Cardiovascular toxicity and titin cross-reactivity of affinity enhanced T cells in myeloma and melanoma. *Blood* (2013) **122**:863–71. doi:10.1182/blood-2013-03-490565
111. Morgan RA, Chinnasamy N, Abate-Daga D, Gros A, Robbins PF, Zheng Z, et al. Cancer regression and neurological toxicity following anti-MAGE-A3 TCR gene therapy. *J Immunother* (2013) **36**:133–51. doi:10.1097/CJI.0b013e3182829903
112. Kawakami Y, Eliyahu S, Sakaguchi K, Robbins PF, Rivoltini L, Yannelli JR, et al. Identification of the immunodominant peptides of the MART-1 human melanoma antigen recognized by the majority of HLA-A2-restricted tumor infiltrating lymphocytes. *J Exp Med* (1994) **180**:347–52. doi:10.1084/jem.180.1.347
113. Castelli C, Storkus WJ, Maeurer MJ, Martin DM, Huang EC, Pramanik BN, et al. Mass spectrometric identification of a naturally processed melanoma peptide recognized by CD8+ cytotoxic T lymphocytes. *J Exp Med* (1995) **181**:363–8. doi:10.1084/jem.181.1.363
114. Hughes MS, Yu YY, Dudley ME, Zheng Z, Robbins PF, Li Y, et al. Transfer of a TCR gene derived from a patient with a marked antitumor response conveys highly active T-cell effector functions. *Hum Gene Ther* (2005) **16**:457–72. doi:10.1089/hum.2005.16.457
115. Borbulevych OY, Santhanagopolan SM, Hossain M, Baker BM. TCRs used in cancer gene therapy cross-react with MART-1/Melan-A tumor antigens via distinct mechanisms. *J Immunol* (2011) **187**:2453–63. doi:10.4049/jimmunol.1101268
116. Morgan RA, Dudley ME, Wunderlich JR, Hughes MS, Yang JC, Sherry RM, et al. Cancer regression in patients after transfer of genetically engineered lymphocytes. *Science* (2006) **314**:126–9. doi:10.1126/science.1129003
117. Johnson LA, Heemskerk B, Powell DJ Jr, Cohen CJ, Morgan RA, Dudley ME, et al. Gene transfer of tumor-reactive TCR confers both high avidity and tumor reactivity to nonreactive peripheral blood mononuclear cells and tumor-infiltrating lymphocytes. *J Immunol* (2006) **177**:6548–59.
118. van der Bruggen P, Traversari C, Chomez P, Lurquin C, De Plaen E, van den Eynde B, et al. A gene encoding an antigen recognized by cytolytic T lymphocytes on a human melanoma. *Science* (1991) **254**:1643–7. doi:10.1126/science.1840703
119. Gaugler B, van den Eynde B, van der Bruggen P, Romero P, Gaforio JJ, De Plaen E, et al. Human gene MAGE-3 codes for an antigen recognized on a melanoma by autologous cytolytic T lymphocytes. *J Exp Med* (1994) **179**:921–30. doi:10.1084/jem.179.3.921
120. Caballero OL, Chen YT. Cancer/testis (CT) antigens: potential targets for immunotherapy. *Cancer Sci* (2009) **100**:2014–21. doi:10.1111/j.1349-7006.2009.01303.x
121. Gnjatic S, Nishikawa H, Jungbluth AA, Gure AO, Ritter G, Jager E, et al. NY-ESO-1: review of an immunogenic tumor antigen. *Adv Cancer Res* (2006) **95**:1–30. doi:10.1016/S0065-230X(06)95001-5
122. Jager E, Chen YT, Drijfhout JW, Karbach J, Ringhoffer M, Jager D, et al. Simultaneous humoral and cellular immune response against cancer-testis antigen NY-ESO-1: definition of human histocompatibility leukocyte antigen (HLA)-A2-binding peptide epitopes. *J Exp Med* (1998) **187**:265–70. doi:10.1084/jem.187.2.265
123. Bownds S, Tong-On P, Rosenberg SA, Parkhurst M. Induction of tumor-reactive cytotoxic T-lymphocytes using a peptide from NY-ESO-1 modified at the carboxy-terminus to enhance HLA-A2.1 binding affinity and stability in solution. *J Immunother* (2001) **24**:1–9. doi:10.1097/00002371-200101000-00001
124. Romero P, Dutoit V, Rubio-Godoy V, Lienard D, Speiser D, Guillaume P, et al. CD8+ T-cell response to NY-ESO-1: relative antigenicity and in vitro immunogenicity of natural and analogue sequences. *Clin Cancer Res* (2001) **7**:766s–72.
125. Webb AI, Dunstone MA, Chen W, Aguilar MI, Chen Q, Jackson H, et al. Functional and structural characteristics of NY-ESO-1-related HLA A2-restricted epitopes and the design of a novel immunogenic analogue. *J Biol Chem* (2004) **279**:23438–46. doi:10.1074/jbc.M314066200
126. Khong HT, Yang JC, Topalian SL, Sherry RM, Mavroukakis SA, White DE, et al. Immunization of HLA-A*0201 and/or HLA-DPbeta1*04 patients with metastatic melanoma using epitopes from the NY-ESO-1 antigen. *J Immunother* (2004) **27**:472–7. doi:10.1097/00002371-200411000-00007
127. Chen JL, Stewart-Jones G, Bossi G, Lissin NM, Wooldridge L, Choi EM, et al. Structural and kinetic basis for heightened immunogenicity of T cell vaccines. *J Exp*

Med (2005) **201**:1243–55. doi:10.1084/jem.20042323

128. Robbins PF, Morgan RA, Feldman SA, Yang JC, Sherry RM, Dudley ME, et al. Tumor regression in patients with metastatic synovial cell sarcoma and melanoma using genetically engineered lymphocytes reactive with NY-ESO-1. *J Clin Oncol* (2011) **29**:917–24. doi:10.1200/JCO.2010.32.2537
129. Li Y, Moysey R, Molloy PE, Vuidepot AL, Mahon T, Baston E, et al. Directed evolution of human T-cell receptors with picomolar affinities by phage display. *Nat Biotechnol* (2005) **23**:349–54. doi:10.1038/nbt1070
130. Dunn SM, Rizkallah PJ, Baston E, Mahon T, Cameron B, Moysey R, et al. Directed evolution of human T cell receptor CDR2 residues by phage display dramatically enhances affinity for cognate peptide-MHC without increasing apparent cross-reactivity. *Protein Sci* (2006) **15**:710–21. doi:10.1110/ps.051936406
131. Liddy N, Bossi G, Adams KJ, Lissina A, Mahon TM, Hassan NJ, et al. Monoclonal TCR-redirected tumor cell killing. *Nat Med* (2012) **18**:980–7. doi:10.1038/nm.2764
132. McCormack E, Adams KJ, Hassan NJ, Kotian A, Lissin NM, Sami M, et al. Bi-specific TCR-anti CD3 redirected T-cell targeting of NY-ESO-1- and LAGE-1-positive tumors. *Cancer Immunol Immunother* (2013) **62**:773–85. doi:10.1007/s00262-012-1384-4
133. Scharnhorst V, van der Eb AJ, Jochemsen AG. WT1 proteins: functions in growth and differentiation. *Gene* (2001) **273**:141–61. doi:10.1016/S0378-1119(01)00593-5
134. Rosenfeld C, Cheever MA, Gaiger A. WT1 in acute leukemia, chronic myelogenous leukemia and myelodysplastic syndrome: therapeutic potential of WT1 targeted therapies. *Leukemia* (2003) **17**:1301–12. doi:10.1038/sj.leu.2402988
135. Oka Y, Elisseeva OA, Tsuboi A, Ogawa H, Tamaki H, Li H, et al. Human cytotoxic T-lymphocyte responses specific for peptides of the wild-type Wilms' tumor gene (WT1) product. *Immunogenetics* (2000) **51**:99–107. doi:10.1007/s002510050018
136. Gaiger A, Reese V, Disis ML, Cheever MA. Immunity to WT1 in the animal model and in patients with acute myeloid leukemia. *Blood* (2000) **96**:1480–9.
137. Stone JD, Aggen DH, Chervin AS, Narayanan S, Schmitt TM, Greenberg PD, et al. Opposite effects of endogenous peptide-MHC class I on T cell activity in the presence and absence of CD8. *J Immunol* (2011) **186**:5193–200. doi:10.4049/jimmunol.1003755
138. Ohminami H, Yasukawa M, Fujita S. HLA class I-restricted lysis of leukemia cells by a CD8(+) cytotoxic T-lymphocyte clone specific for WT1 peptide. *Blood* (2000) **95**:286–93.
139. Ochi T, Fujiwara H, Okamoto S, An J, Nagai K, Shirakata T, et al. Novel adoptive T-cell immunotherapy using a WT1-specific TCR vector encoding silencers for endogenous TCRs shows marked antileukemia reactivity and safety. *Blood* (2011) **118**:1495–503. doi:10.1182/blood-2011-02-337089
140. Van Driessche A, Berneman ZN, Van Tendeloo VF. Active specific immunotherapy targeting the Wilms' tumor protein 1 (WT1) for patients with hematological malignancies and solid tumors: lessons from early clinical trials. *Oncologist* (2012) **17**:250–9. doi:10.1634/theoncologist.2011-0240
141. Falkenburg WJ, Melenhorst JJ, van de Meent M, Kester MG, Hombrink P, Heemskerk MH, et al. Allogeneic HLA-A*02-restricted WT1-specific T cells from mismatched donors are highly reactive but show off-target promiscuity. *J Immunol* (2011) **187**:2824–33. doi:10.4049/jimmunol.1100852
142. Gao L, Xue SA, Hasserjian R, Cotter F, Kaeda J, Goldman JM, et al. Human cytotoxic T lymphocytes specific for Wilms' tumor antigen-1 inhibit engraftment of leukemia-initiating stem cells in non-obese diabetic-severe combined immunodeficient recipients. *Transplantation* (2003) **75**:1429–36. doi:10.1097/01.TP.0000061516.57346.E8
143. Xue SA, Gao L, Hart D, Gillmore R, Qasim W, Thrasher A, et al. Elimination of human leukemia cells in NOD/SCID mice by WT1-TCR gene-transduced human T cells. *Blood* (2005) **106**:3062–7. doi:10.1182/blood-2005-01-0146
144. Xue SA, Gao L, Thomas S, Hart DP, Xue JZ, Gillmore R, et al. Development of a Wilms' tumor antigen-specific T-cell receptor for clinical trials: engineered patient's T cells can eliminate autologous leukemia blasts in NOD/SCID mice. *Haematologica* (2010) **95**:126–34. doi:10.3324/haematol.2009.006486
145. Provasi E, Genovese P, Lombardo A, Magnani Z, Liu PQ, Reik A, et al. Editing T cell specificity towards leukemia by zinc finger nucleases and lentiviral gene transfer. *Nat Med* (2012) **18**:807–15. doi:10.1038/nm.2700
146. Schmitt TM, Aggen DH, Stromnes IM, Dossett ML, Richman SA, Kranz DM, et al. Enhanced-affinity murine T-cell receptors for tumor/self-antigens can be safe in gene therapy despite surpassing the threshold for thymic selection. *Blood* (2013) **122**:348–56. doi:10.1182/blood-2013-01-478164
147. Matsushita H, Vesely MD, Koboldt DC, Rickert CG, Uppaluri R, Magrini VJ, et al. Cancer exome analysis reveals a T-cell-dependent mechanism of cancer immunoediting. *Nature* (2012) **482**:400–4. doi:10.1038/nature10755
148. Marrack P, Scott-Browne JP, Dai S, Gapin L, Kappler JW. Evolutionarily conserved amino acids that control TCR-MHC interaction. *Annu Rev Immunol* (2008) **26**:171–203. doi:10.1146/annurev.immunol.26.021607.090421
149. Pardoll DM. The blockade of immune checkpoints in cancer immunotherapy. *Nat Rev Cancer* (2012) **12**:252–64. doi:10.1038/nrc3239
150. Callahan MK, Wolchok JD. At the bedside: CTLA-4- and PD-1-blocking antibodies in cancer immunotherapy. *J Leukoc Biol* (2013) **94**:41–53. doi:10.1189/jlb.1212631
151. Hodi FS, O'Day SJ, McDermott DF, Weber RW, Sosman JA, Haanen JB, et al. Improved survival with ipilimumab in patients with metastatic melanoma. *N Engl J Med* (2010) **363**:711–23. doi:10.1056/NEJMoa1003466
152. Berger R, Rotem-Yehudar R, Slama G, Landes S, Kneller A, Leiba M, et al. Phase I safety and pharmacokinetic study of CT-011, a humanized antibody interacting with PD-1, in patients with advanced hematologic malignancies. *Clin Cancer Res* (2008) **14**:3044–51. doi:10.1158/1078-0432.CCR-07-4079
153. Brahmer JR, Tykodi SS, Chow LQ, Hwu WJ, Topalian SL, Hwu P, et al. Safety and activity of anti-PD-L1 antibody in patients with advanced cancer. *N Engl J Med* (2012) **366**:2455–65. doi:10.1056/NEJMoa1200694
154. Topalian SL, Hodi FS, Brahmer JR, Gettinger SN, Smith DC, McDermott DF, et al. Safety, activity, and immune correlates of anti-PD-1 antibody in cancer. *N Engl J Med* (2012) **366**:2443–54. doi:10.1056/NEJMoa1200690
155. Hamid O, Robert C, Daud A, Hodi FS, Hwu WJ, Kefford R, et al. Safety and tumor responses with lambrolizumab (anti-PD-1) in melanoma. *N Engl J Med* (2013) **369**:134–44. doi:10.1056/NEJMoa1305133
156. Peng W, Liu C, Xu C, Lou Y, Chen J, Yang Y, et al. PD-1 blockade enhances T-cell migration to tumors by elevating IFN-gamma inducible chemokines. *Cancer Res* (2012) **72**:5209–18. doi:10.1158/0008-5472.CAN-12-1187
157. Rammensee H, Bachmann J, Emmerich NP, Bachor OA, Stevanovic S. SYFPEITHI: database for MHC ligands and peptide motifs. *Immunogenetics* (1999) **50**:213–9. doi:10.1007/s002510050595
158. Nielsen M, Lundegaard C, Worning P, Lauemoller SL, Lamberth K, Buus S, et al. Reliable prediction of T-cell epitopes using neural networks with novel sequence representations. *Protein Sci* (2003) **12**:1007–17. doi:10.1110/ps.0239403
159. Peters B, Sette A. Generating quantitative models describing the sequence specificity of biological processes with the stabilized matrix method. *BMC Bioinformatics* (2005) **6**:132. doi:10.1186/1471-2105-6-132
160. Kosmrlj A, Read EL, Qi Y, Allen TM, Altfeld M, Deeks SG, et al. Effects of thymic selection of the T-cell repertoire on HLA class I-associated control of HIV infection. *Nature* (2010) **465**:350–4. doi:10.1038/nature08997
161. Eisen HN, Hou XH, Shen C, Wang K, Tanguturi VK, Smith C, et al. Promiscuous binding of extracellular peptides to cell surface class I MHC protein. *Proc Natl Acad Sci U S A* (2012) **109**:4580–5. doi:10.1073/pnas.1201586109
162. Wooldridge L, Ekeruche-Makinde J, van den Berg HA, Skowera A, Miles JJ, Tan MP, et al. A single autoimmune T cell receptor recognizes more than a million different peptides. *J Biol Chem* (2012) **287**:1168–77. doi:10.1074/jbc.M111.289488
163. Ekeruche-Makinde J, Miles JJ, van den Berg HA, Skowera A, Cole DK, Dolton G, et al. Peptide length determines the outcome of TCR/peptide-MHCI engagement. *Blood* (2013) **121**:1112–23. doi:10.1182/blood-2012-06-437202

164. Pinilla-Ibarz J, May RJ, Korontsvit T, Gomez M, Kappel B, Zakhaleva V, et al. Improved human T-cell responses against synthetic HLA-0201 analog peptides derived from the WT1 oncoprotein. *Leukemia* (2006) **20**:2025–33. doi:10.1038/sj.leu.2404380
165. Al Qudaihi G, Lehe C, Negash M, Al-Alwan M, Ghebeh H, Mohamed SY, et al. Enhancement of lytic activity of leukemic cells by CD8+ cytotoxic T lymphocytes generated against a WT1 peptide analogue. *Leuk Lymphoma* (2009) **50**:260–9. doi:10.1080/10428190802578478
166. Borbulevych OY, Do P, Baker BM. Structures of native and affinity-enhanced WT1 epitopes bound to HLA-A*0201: implications for WT1-based cancer therapeutics. *Mol Immunol* (2010) **47**:2519–24. doi:10.1016/j.molimm.2010.06.005
167. Rual JF, Hirozane-Kishikawa T, Hao T, Bertin N, Li S, Dricot A, et al. Human ORFeome version 1.1: a platform for reverse proteomics. *Genome Res* (2004) **14**:2128–35. doi:10.1101/gr.2973604
168. Yang X, Boehm JS, Yang X, Salehi-Ashtiani K, Hao T, Shen Y, et al. A public genome-scale lentiviral expression library of human ORFs. *Nat Methods* (2011) **8**:659–61. doi:10.1038/nmeth.1638
169. Rual JF, Venkatesan K, Hao T, Hirozane-Kishikawa T, Dricot A, Li N, et al. Towards a proteome-scale map of the human protein-protein interaction network. *Nature* (2005) **437**:1173–8. doi:10.1038/nature04209
170. Skalamera D, Ranall MV, Wilson BM, Leo P, Purdon AS, Hyde C, et al. A high-throughput platform for lentiviral overexpression screening of the human ORFeome. *PLoS ONE* (2011) **6**:e20057. doi:10.1371/journal.pone.0020057
171. Kieback E, Charo J, Sommermeyer D, Blankenstein T, Uckert W. A safeguard eliminates T cell receptor gene-modified autoreactive T cells after adoptive transfer. *Proc Natl Acad Sci U S A* (2008) **105**:623–8. doi:10.1073/pnas.0710198105
172. Marin V, Cribioli E, Philip B, Tettamanti S, Pizzitola I, Biondi A, et al. Comparison of different suicide-gene strategies for the safety improvement of genetically manipulated T cells. *Hum Gene Ther Methods* (2012) **23**:376–86. doi:10.1089/hgtb.2012.050
173. Garcia KC, Degano M, Pease LR, Huang M, Peterson PA, Teyton L, et al. Structural basis of plasticity in T cell receptor recognition of a self peptide-MHC antigen. *Science* (1998) **279**:1166–72. doi:10.1126/science.279.5354.1166

14

Young T cells age during a redirected anti-tumor attack: chimeric antigen receptor-provided dual costimulation is half the battle

***Andreas A. Hombach*[1,2] *and Hinrich Abken*[1,2] ***

[1] *Center for Molecular Medicine Cologne, University of Cologne, Cologne, Germany*
[2] *Department I Internal Medicine, University Hospital Cologne, Cologne, Germany*

Edited by:
Bruno Laugel, Cardiff University School of Medicine, UK

Reviewed by:
Per Thor Straten, University Hospital Herlev Denmark, Denmark
Christoph Renner, University Hospital Basel, Switzerland

****Correspondence:***
Hinrich Abken, Center for Molecular Medicine Cologne, University Hospital Cologne, Robert-Koch-Str. 21, D-50931 Köln, Germany
e-mail: hinrich.abken@uk-koeln.de

Adoptive therapy with chimeric antigen receptor (CAR)-redirected T cells showed spectacular efficacy in the treatment of leukemia in recent early phase trials. Patient's T cells were *ex vivo* genetically engineered with a CAR, amplified and re-administered to the patient. While T cells mediating the primary response were predominantly of young effector and central memory phenotype, repetitive antigen engagement irreversible triggers T cell maturation leaving late memory cells with the KLRG1$^+$ CD57$^+$ CD7$^-$ CCR7$^-$ phenotype in the long-term. These cells preferentially accumulate in the periphery, are hypo-responsive upon TCR engagement and prone to activation-induced cell death. A recent report indicates that those T cells can be rescued by CAR provided CD28 and OX40 (CD134) stimulation. We discuss the strategy with respect to prolong the anti-tumor response and to improve the over-all efficacy of adoptive cell therapy.

Keywords: adoptive cell therapy, chimeric antigen receptor, memory T cells, CD28, OX40

ADOPTIVE THERAPY WITH CAR ENGINEERED T CELLS SHOWED SPECTACULAR EFFICACY IN EARLY PHASE TRIALS

Recent success in the immune therapy of malignant diseases has sustained the promise that the immune system can control cancer in the long-term. On the other hand, tumor-specific T cells are rare in cancer patients making their isolation and *ex vivo* amplification to therapeutic numbers necessary. To overcome the situation strategies were developed to engraft T cells with defined specificity by genetic engineering; the so-called "T-body" strategy equips patient's T cells with a recombinant trans-membrane receptor molecule which is composed in the extracellular part of an antibody-type recognition domain for MHC-independent binding and in the intracellular part of T cell activating domains, mostly the TCR CD3ζ endodomain linked to a costimulatory domain like CD28, OX40, or 4-1BB (Gross and Eshhar, 1992; Eshhar, 2008). Such a chimeric antigen receptor (CAR) redirects T cells in an antigen-specific fashion producing specific T cell activation toward defined targets.

Second generation CAR's providing CD28 costimulation along with the primary CD3ζ signal more effectively activate T cells than CAR's with CD3ζ signaling only. This is basically due to the CD28 mediated improvement of T cell effector functions and the protection from activation-induced cell death resulting in prolonged persistence *in vivo* (Savoldo et al., 2011). Other costimulatory domains of the CD28 family, like 4-1BB (CD137), also improves T cell persistence (Milone et al., 2009; Song et al., 2011). Each individual costimulatory signal, however, differentially orchestrates the effector functions including cytokine secretion, amplification, and cytolytic activity (Hombach and Abken, 2011) which allows to modulate the anti-tumor response in a fine-tuned fashion.

Current clinical trials are utilizing second generation CARs to ensure prolonged persistence of engineered T cells *in vivo*. T cells engineered with a 4-1BB-ζ CAR targeting CD19 recently produced spectacular efficacy toward refractory leukemia in patients with high tumor burden (Kalos et al., 2011; Grupp et al., 2013). Further studies in other centers are also reporting encouraging clinical responses using CD28-ζ CAR T cells (Brentjens et al., 2011; Kochenderfer et al., 2012). The general success of these studies is likely due to repetitive tumor cell killing by CAR T cells; additionally, the targeted CD19 is also expressed by healthy B cells which re-stimulate the CAR T cells independently of the targeted tumor cells. The situation in targeting solid tumors, however, is more complex, in particular with respect to immune repression, and may require supporting strategies as discussed in a recent review (Gilham et al., 2012). We here address an additional aspect which is attracting increasing attention and which is of equal relevance for the success in adoptive cell therapy: the progression of CAR redirected T cells into terminal maturation upon repetitive antigen encounter.

REPETITIVE CAR ENGAGEMENT PRODUCES LATE EFFECTOR MEMORY CELLS WITH ALTERED FUNCTIONAL CAPACITIES

Chimeric antigen receptor engineered young T cells, the majority of them with central memory phenotype, are adoptively transferred to the patient since these cells showed superior in mediating an anti-tumor response in pre-clinical models (Klebanoff et al., 2005). Repetitive binding to cognate antigen, however, induces CAR T cells to amplify, as T cells physiologically do upon TCR/CD28 engagement or TCR stimulation in presence of IL-2. Extensive amplification, however, substantially impacts the anti-tumor efficacy of CAR T cells in the long-term. After

<2 weeks of cell divisions *in vitro*, T cells progress in maturation and alter their functional properties, associated by a change in phenotype (**Figure 1**). Repetitive antigen engagement converts naïve and central memory T cells to cells with a CCR7$^-$ CD62L^{low} CD57$^+$ KLRG1$^+$ effector memory phenotype with CD45RO^{high} CD45RA^{low} and CD27^{low} CD28^{low} expression. CAR mediated maturation occurs in both CD8$^+$ and CD4$^+$ T cells and does not happen when cell division is blocked. The process is observed in a mouse tumor model in which after adoptive transfer of young CCR7$^+$ CAR T cells the majority of tumor infiltrating CAR T cells are of CCR7^{low} phenotype (Hombach et al., 2013). One consequence is that the capacity of those cells to re-enter the lymph and to re-circulate is diminished since CCR7 is required for T cell homing into secondary lymphoid organs (Sallusto et al., 1999; Müller and Lipp, 2003; Bromley et al., 2005; Klebanoff et al., 2005; Moschovakis and Förster, 2012). Inability of CCR7$^-$ T cells to re-circulate, on the other hand, may be of advantage since most solid cancer lesions occur in the periphery. The assumption is sustained by the observation that CCR7$^-$ CAR T cells persist in higher numbers in the tumor lesion although both the CCR7$^+$ and CCR7$^-$ subset T cells equally efficiently target to the tumor (Hombach et al., 2013). Paradoxically, the anti-tumor response of CCR7$^-$ CAR T cells is less efficient than that of CCR7$^+$ T cells when redirected by a CD28-ζ CAR. This is moreover unexpected since CCR7$^-$ T cells secrete higher amounts of pro-inflammatory cytokines like IFN-γ and harbor higher levels of cytolytic effector molecules like perforin and granzymes compared to CCR7$^+$ T cells. Detailed analyses revealed that CCR7$^-$ T cells are prone to spontaneous and activation-induced cell death which is insufficiently prevented by CAR mediated CD28 costimulation (Hombach et al., 2013). Similar observations were reported for CD57$^+$ T cells (Chattopadhyay et al., 2009) and which is in contrast to CCR7$^+$ T cells.

Simultaneous CD28 and OX40 costimulation reduces the high propensity of CCR7$^-$ T cells to undergo apoptosis (Hombach et al., 2013). OX40 promotes Bcl-xL and Bcl-2 expression, enhances the survival of antigen-experienced effector T cells and improves the generation of antigen-specific T cell memory (Rogers

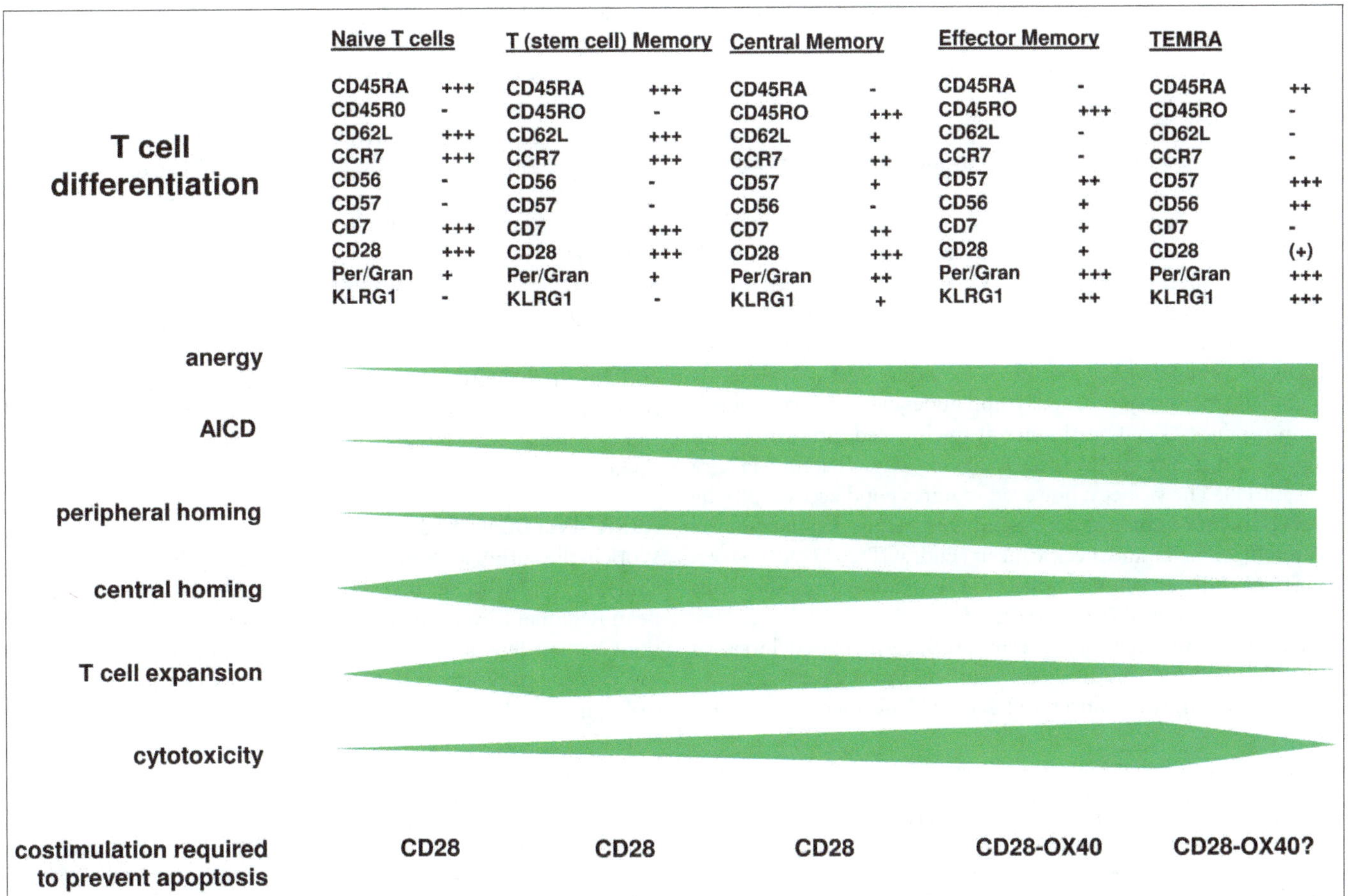

FIGURE 1 | T cell maturation is accompanied by altered functional properties. CAR engineered T cells progress in maturation when the CAR repetitively engages cognate antigen as physiologically occurs upon TCR/CD28 signaling. While CAR engineered "young" memory T cells are transferred to the patient, the cells expand and undergo further differentiation leaving effector memory T cells at the tumor lesion which require additional signals for being protected from anergy and activation-induced cell death. On the other hand, those more matured cells have increased cytolytic potential making them highly effective in the anti-tumor attack. Engineering T cells with a combined CD28-OX40 CAR which prevents apoptosis of matured CCR7$^-$ T cells is one of the upcoming strategies to solve the situation and to improve the anti-tumor efficacy in the long-term.

et al., 2001). In combination with CD28 in a so-called "third generation" CD28-OX40 CAR, combined costimulation improved survival and cytolytic activities of CCR7$^-$ T cells toward targeted cancer cells (Hombach et al., 2013). Similar results were obtained with CD62L$^-$ T cells which mature from CCR7$^-$ CD62L$^+$ T cells upon stimulation (Hombach and Abken, 2011). The combination of costimulatory signals achieves the effect since OX40 alone does not provide benefit in this context whereas CD28 costimulation alone, which prevents CCR7$^+$ T cell apoptosis, does not reduce the number of apoptotic CCR7$^-$ cells. Taken together adoptive cell therapy will benefit from redirecting T cells by a CD28-OX40 CAR to provide protection from apoptosis when young cells progress in maturation.

PERSPECTIVES: HOW TO MAINTAIN AN ANTI-TUMOR RESPONSE IN THE LONG-TERM?

Several factors together are required to rescue matured CAR T cells for the anti-tumor response in the long-term.

First, any T cell subset converts to effector memory cells upon repetitive antigen engagement and amplification and in each stage of maturation requires appropriate costimulation to escape cell death; consequently, harnessing young T cells with a CD28-OX40 CAR will be beneficial and will rescue CCR7$^-$ cells when produced during an anti-tumor attack.

Second, CCR7$^-$ T cells persist in peripheral lesions due to their inability to re-enter the lymph, thereby increasing the probability for successful cancer cell killing. To improve their accumulation at the tumor site T cells were additionally engineered with the CCR2 receptor (Moon et al., 2011). Alternatively, CAR engineered T cells are injected into the tumor lesion taking advantage of the plethora of different effector T cell subsets in fighting cancer while circumventing the limitations in T cell trafficking. In contrast, i.v. injected T cells become stuck in the lungs for hours and subsequently accumulate in liver, spleen, and lymph nodes, while regional application produces T cell persistence at the injected tumor site with only local diffusion within the following days (Parente-Pereira et al., 2011). The strategy, however, requires good accessibility by direct puncture or by endoscopy and is currently evaluated in the treatment of head and neck cancer (EudraCT 2012-001654-25, NCT01722149) or will be applied to the treatment of cutaneous lymphoma (EudraCT 2011-003125-10).

Third, effector memory T cells produce increased levels of pro-inflammatory cytokines and cytolytic molecules, both contributing to improve cancer cell killing. Late memory T cells, however, are TCR hypo-responsive which is due to an inefficient formation of the TCR synapse as a result of galectin-3 anchoring of TCR components. Interestingly, formation of a transgenic CAR synapse in those cells is not affected making them fully responsive to CAR targets (Rappl et al., 2012).

Since T cell expansion is mandatory to establish adoptively transferred T cells in the long-term, sufficient space is provided to transferred T cells by non-myeloablative lympho-depleting preconditioning followed by IL-2 administration to sustain expansion; other cytokines like IL-7 and IL-15 are also explored (Weber et al., 2011). Extensive T cell amplification, on the other hand, produces effector memory T cells which then need to be protected from activation-induced cell death. Other costimulation than by CD28 and OX40 may also provide benefit to those cells, for instance 4-1BB (Song et al., 2011). Co-signaling by 4-1BB and CD28 may also provide an advantage to matured T cells, however, needs to be evaluated in detail. The effect of each combination of costimulatory signals, however, cannot be predicted since the CAR with its linked endodomains provides simultaneous signaling while in the physiological situation the signals occur individually in a well-defined temporal and spatial order. An elegant solution of the dilemma is the use of virus-specific T cells which are further matured by the immune system and have some significant properties needed for effective anti-cancer therapy. These cells obtain survival and costimulatory signals when engaging virus-infected cells by their TCR. Current trials use EBV or CMV specific, autologous T cells engineered with a first or second generation CAR, for instance directed against ErbB2 (NCT01109095), CD30 (NCT01192464), CD19 (NCT00709033; NCT01475058; NCT01430390; NCT00840853; NCT01195480), or GD-2 (NCT00085930). Virus-specific T cells are long-lived in pre-clinical models *in vivo*, have a great capacity to amplify and are particularly applied in the context of allogeneic stem cell transplantation where they protect from virus re-activation and tumor relapse while having low risk of inducing graft versus host disease.

ACKNOWLEDGMENTS

Work in the author's laboratory is supported by the Deutsche Krebshilfe, the Wilhelm Sander-Stiftung, the European Union (European Regional Development Fund – Investing in your future) and the German federal state North Rhine-Westphalia (NRW), and the Fortune program of the Medical Faculty of the University of Cologne.

REFERENCES

Brentjens, R. J., Rivière, I., Park, J. H., Davila, M. L., Wang, X., Stefanski, J., et al. (2011). Safety and persistence of adoptively transferred autologous CD19-targeted T cells in patients with relapsed or chemotherapy refractory B-cell leukemias. *Blood* 118, 4817–4828. doi:10.1182/blood-2011-04-348540

Bromley, S. K., Thomas, S. Y., and Luster, A. D. (2005). Chemokine receptor CCR7 guides T cell exit from peripheral tissues and entry into afferent lymphatics. *Nat. Immunol.* 6, 895–901. doi:10.1038/ni1240

Chattopadhyay, P. K., Betts, M. R., Price, D. A., Gostick, E., Horton, H., Roederer, M., et al. (2009). The cytolytic enzymes granyzme A, granzyme B, and perforin: expression patterns, cell distribution, and their relationship to cell maturity and bright CD57 expression. *J. Leukoc. Biol.* 85, 88–97. doi:10.1189/jlb.0208107

Eshhar, Z. (2008). The T-body approach: redirecting T cells with antibody specificity. *Handb. Exp. Pharmacol.* 181, 329–342. doi:10.1007/978-3-540-73259-4_14

Gilham, D. E., Debets, R., Pule, M., Hawkins, R. E., and Abken, H. (2012). CAR-T cells and solid tumors: tuning T cells to challenge an inveterate foe. *Trends Mol. Med.* 18, 377–384. doi:10.1016/j.molmed.2012.04.009

Gross, G., and Eshhar, Z. (1992). Endowing T cells with antibody specificity using chimeric T cell receptors. *FASEB J.* 6, 3370–3378.

Grupp, S. A., Kalos, M., Barrett, D., Aplenc, R., Porter, D. L., Rheingold, S. R., et al. (2013). Chimeric antigen receptor-modified T cells for acute lymphoid leukemia. *N. Engl. J. Med.* 368, 1509–1518. doi:10.1056/NEJMoa1215134

Hombach, A. A., and Abken, H. (2011). Costimulation by chimeric antigen receptors revisited the T cell antitumor response benefits from combined CD28-OX40 signalling. *Int. J. Cancer* 129, 2935–2944. doi:10.1002/ijc.25960

Hombach, A. A., Chmielewski, M., Rappl, G., and Abken, H. (2013). Adoptive immunotherapy with redirected T cells produces CCR7(-) cells that are trapped in the periphery and benefit from combined CD28-OX40 costimulation. *Hum. Gene Ther.* 24, 259–269. doi:10.1089/hum.2012.247

Kalos, M., Levine, B. L., Porter, D. L., Katz, S., Grupp, S. A., Bagg, A., et al. (2011). T cells with chimeric antigen receptors have potent antitumor effects and can establish memory in patients with advanced leukemia. *Sci. Transl. Med.* 3, 95ra73. doi:10.1126/scitranslmed.3002842

Klebanoff, C. A., Gattinoni, L., Torabi-Parizi, P., Kerstann, K., Cardones, A. R., Finkelstein, S. E., et al. (2005). Central memory self/tumor-reactive CD8+ T cells confer superior antitumor immunity compared with effector memory T cells. *Proc. Natl. Acad. Sci. U.S.A.* 102, 9571–9576. doi:10.1073/pnas.0503726102

Kochenderfer, J. N., Dudley, M. E., Feldman, S. A., Wilson, W. H., Spaner, D. E., Maric, I., et al. (2012). B-cell depletion and remissions of malignancy along with cytokine-associated toxicity in a clinical trial of anti-CD19 chimeric-antigen-receptor-transduced T cells. *Blood* 119, 2709–2720. doi:10.1182/blood-2011-10-384388

Milone, M. C., Fish, J. D., Carpenito, C., Carroll, R. G., Binder, G. K., Teachey, D., et al. (2009). Chimeric receptors containing CD137 signal transduction domains mediate enhanced survival of T cells and increased antileukemic efficacy in vivo. *Mol. Ther.* 17, 1453–1464. doi:10.1038/mt.2009.83

Moon, E. K., Carpenito, C., Sun, J., Wang, L.-C. S., Kapoor, V., Predina, J., et al. (2011). Expression of a functional CCR2 receptor enhances tumor localization and tumor eradication by retargeted human t cells expressing a mesothelin-specific chimeric antibody receptor. *Clin. Cancer Res.* 17, 4719–4730. doi:10.1158/1078-0432.CCR-11-0351

Moschovakis, G. L., and Förster, R. (2012). Multifaceted activities of CCR7 regulate T-cell homeostasis in health and disease. *Eur. J. Immunol.* 42, 1949–1955. doi:10.1002/eji.201242614

Müller, G., and Lipp, M. (2003). Shaping up adaptive immunity: the impact of CCR7 and CXCR5 on lymphocyte trafficking. *Microcirculation* 10, 325–334. doi:10.1080/mic.10.3-4.325.334

Parente-Pereira, A. C., Burnet, J., Ellison, D., Foster, J., Davies, D. M., van der Stegen, S., et al. (2011). Trafficking of CAR-engineered human T cells following regional or systemic adoptive transfer in SCID beige mice. *J. Clin. Immunol.* 31, 710–718. doi:10.1007/s10875-011-9532-8

Rappl, G., Riet, T., Awerkiew, S., Schmidt, A., Hombach, A. A., Pfister, H., et al. (2012). The CD3-zeta chimeric antigen receptor overcomes TCR Hypo-responsiveness of human terminal late-stage T cells. *PLoS ONE* 7:e30713. doi:10.1371/journal.pone.0030713

Rogers, P. R., Song, J., Gramaglia, I., Killeen, N., and Croft, M. (2001). OX40 promotes Bcl-xL and Bcl-2 expression and is essential for long-term survival of CD4 T cells. *Immunity* 15, 445–455. doi:10.1016/S1074-7613(01)00191-1

Sallusto, F., Lenig, D., Förster, R., Lipp, M., and Lanzavecchia, A. (1999). Two subsets of memory T lymphocytes with distinct homing potentials and effector functions. *Nature* 401, 708–712. doi:10.1038/44385

Savoldo, B., Ramos, C. A., Liu, E., Mims, M. P., Keating, M. J., Carrum, G., et al. (2011). CD28 costimulation improves expansion and persistence of chimeric antigen receptor-modified T cells in lymphoma patients. *J. Clin. Invest.* 121, 1822–1826. doi:10.1172/JCI46110

Song, D.-G., Ye, Q., Carpenito, C., Poussin, M., Wang, L.-P., Ji, C., et al. (2011). In vivo persistence, tumor localization, and antitumor activity of CAR-engineered T cells is enhanced by costimulatory signaling through CD137 (4-1BB). *Cancer Res.* 71, 4617–4627. doi:10.1158/0008-5472.CAN-11-0422

Weber, J., Atkins, M., Hwu, P., Radvanyi, L., Sznol, M., and Yee, C. (2011). White paper on adoptive cell therapy for cancer with tumor-infiltrating lymphocytes: a report of the CTEP subcommittee on adoptive cell therapy. *Clin. Cancer Res.* 17, 1664–1673. doi:10.1158/1078-0432.CCR-10-2272

15

Structure-based, rational design of T cell receptors

V. Zoete[1], M. Irving[1,2], M. Ferber[1], M. A. Cuendet[1,3] and O. Michielin[1,2,4,5]*

[1] Molecular Modeling Group, Swiss Institute of Bioinformatics, Lausanne, Switzerland
[2] Lausanne Cancer Center, Lausanne, Switzerland
[3] Department of Chemistry, New York University, New York, USA
[4] Department of Research, University Hospital Center and University of Lausanne, Lausanne, Switzerland
[5] Ludwig Center for Cancer Research of the University of Lausanne, Lausanne, Switzerland

Edited by:
Bruno Laugel, Cardiff University School of Medicine, UK

Reviewed by:
Salvatore Valitutti, Institut National de la Santé et de la Recherche Médicale, France
Roland Hugo Stote, Centre National de la Recherche Scientifique, France
Pierre J. Rizkallah, Institute of Infection and Immunity, School of Medicine, Cardiff University, UK

***Correspondence:**
O. Michielin, Molecular Modeling Group, Swiss Institute of Bioinformatics, Quartier UNIL-Sorge – Batiment Genopode, CH-1015 Lausanne, Switzerland
e-mail: olivier.michielin@unil.ch

Adoptive cell transfer using engineered T cells is emerging as a promising treatment for metastatic melanoma. Such an approach allows one to introduce T cell receptor (TCR) modifications that, while maintaining the specificity for the targeted antigen, can enhance the binding and kinetic parameters for the interaction with peptides (p) bound to major histocompatibility complexes (MHC). Using the well-characterized 2C TCR/SIYR/H-2K(b) structure as a model system, we demonstrated that a binding free energy decomposition based on the MM-GBSA approach provides a detailed and reliable description of the TCR/pMHC interactions at the structural and thermodynamic levels. Starting from this result, we developed a new structure-based approach, to rationally design new TCR sequences, and applied it to the BC1 TCR targeting the HLA-A2 restricted NY-ESO-$1_{157-165}$ cancer-testis epitope. Fifty-four percent of the designed sequence replacements exhibited improved pMHC binding as compared to the native TCR, with up to 150-fold increase in affinity, while preserving specificity. Genetically engineered $CD8^+$ T cells expressing these modified TCRs showed an improved functional activity compared to those expressing BC1 TCR. We measured maximum levels of activities for TCRs within the upper limit of natural affinity, $K_D = \sim 1 - 5\,\mu M$. Beyond the affinity threshold at $K_D < 1\,\mu M$ we observed an attenuation in cellular function, in line with the "half-life" model of T cell activation. Our computer-aided protein-engineering approach requires the 3D-structure of the TCR-pMHC complex of interest, which can be obtained from X-ray crystallography. We have also developed a homology modeling-based approach, TCRep 3D, to obtain accurate structural models of any TCR-pMHC complexes when experimental data is not available. Since the accuracy of the models depends on the prediction of the TCR orientation over pMHC, we have complemented the approach with a simplified rigid method to predict this orientation and successfully assessed it using all non-redundant TCR-pMHC crystal structures available. These methods potentially extend the use of our TCR engineering method to entire TCR repertoires for which no X-ray structure is available. We have also performed a steered molecular dynamics study of the unbinding of the TCR-pMHC complex to get a better understanding of how TCRs interact with pMHCs. This entire rational TCR design pipeline is now being used to produce rationally optimized TCRs for adoptive cell therapies of stage IV melanoma.

Keywords: molecular modeling, protein-engineering, TCR, TCR-pMHC, immunotherapy, adoptive transfer, cancer

INTRODUCTION

Recognition by the $CD8^+$ T cell receptor (TCR) of immunogenic peptide (p) presented by class I major histocompatibility complexes (MHC) is a key event in the specific immune response against virus-infected cells or tumor cells. Binding of the TCR to the pMHC complex leads to T cell activation and killing of the target cell (1). The TCR is composed of two chains, α and β, that pair on the surface of the T cell to form a heterodimeric receptor on the surface of the T cell. Each chain is composed of a constant domain that anchors the protein in the cell membrane and of a variable domain that confers antigen recognition (**Figure 1**). The TCR contacts pMHC molecules via the 6 complementarity-determining regions (CDR), three each from the α and β chains (**Figure 2**). These CDRs constitute the hypervariable regions of the two V domains, called Vα and Vβ (2–4). They are generated by somatic gene rearrangement and negatively selected in the thymus against reactivity with endogenic pMHCs. CDR3α and CDR3β are the most diverse regions of the TCR and thus play a major role in antigen specificity. The CDR1 and CDR2 loops of the α and β chains predominantly make contact with the MHC molecule. The strength of the interaction between TCR and pMHC has been shown to play an important role in the T cell activation (5–9). However, the kinetics of the TCR/pMHC interaction is also determinant in T cell activation (10, 11). Consequently, understanding the biophysical properties of the TCR/pMHC interaction is of great interest for the prediction of the T cell activation, and for

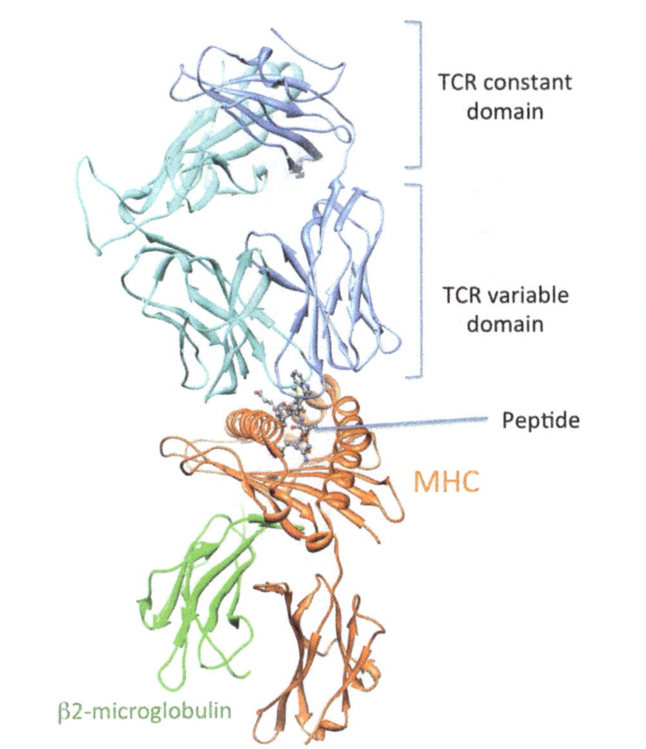

FIGURE 1 | 3D-structure of the TCR-pMHC complex. (1G4 TCR bound to NY-ESO-1/HLA-A201, entry 2BNR (124) of the PDB). TCRα, TCRβ, MHC, and b2-microglobulin are colored in blue, cyan, orange, and green, respectively. The NY-ESO-1 peptide is displayed in ball and stick.

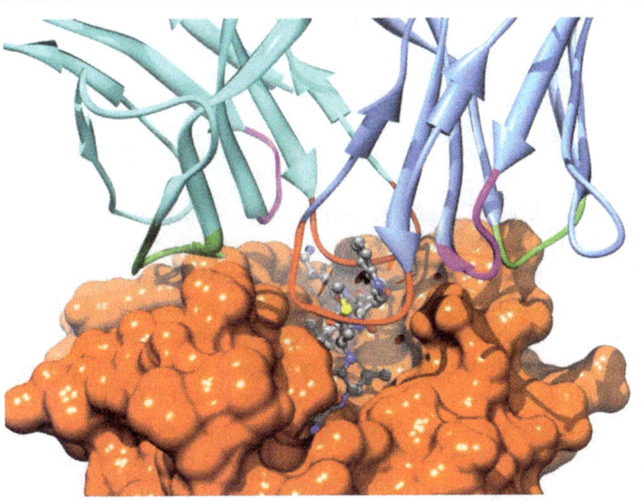

FIGURE 2 | Position of the TCR CDRs over the pMHC surface. CDR1s, CDR2s, and CDR3s are colored in magenta, green, and red, respectively.

the rational TCR optimization toward improved adoptive transfer cancer therapy (12, 13).

This review will focus on the different computer-aided techniques we developed and used to study the TCR-pMHC complex from a structural and thermodynamic point of view. First we present the results obtained by steered molecular dynamics (SMD) simulations of molecular recognition events occurring during the TCR-pMHC complex formation. Second, we describe the different approaches we developed to derive structural models of TCR-pMHC complexes for a large TCR repertoire. Third, we summarize our approaches to estimate the binding free energy for the TCR association to pMHC. Finally, we present our *in silico* structure-based protein-engineering approach that enables the fine-tuning of TCR-pMHC binding parameters.

INVESTIGATING TCR-pMHC INTERACTIONS USING STEERED MD SIMULATIONS

The structure of ~66 TCR-pMHC complexes are known to date (14) among which ~25 are unique complexes. The compared features of these structures were the object of extensive reviews (1, 15, 16). In addition, binding kinetics and thermodynamics of many complexes have been measured (17). The general picture that emerges is that T cell activation requires TCR-pMHC binding to fall within a certain range of affinity and kinetics. However, clear structural determinants of TCR specificity have remained elusive. A single mutation can change a peptide from agonist to antagonist, but the same TCR can recognize various peptides with different binding modes. Thus TCRs can be exquisitely specific while displaying a high degree of cross-reactivity. In addition, TCRs use extremely varied thermodynamic strategies to bind to pMHCs, ranging from entropy-favored to entropy-opposed.

A system that exemplifies both the sensitivity of TCR recognition and its potential for cross-reactivity with different binding strategies is the Tax nonapeptide (LLFGYPVYV) from the HTLV-1 virus presented by the HLA-A0201 MHC. This pMHC is a strong agonist for the A6 TCR but the P6A peptide mutant (Pro replaced by Ala at position 6, see **Figure 3A**) dramatically reduces the binding affinity and abrogates T cell activation (18). On the other hand, the B7 TCR, which has the same α chain as A6 but a different β chain, is also activated by the Tax peptide presented by the same MHC. B7 binds with an affinity similar to A6, but the binding is entropically opposed, whereas A6 binding is entropically favored, outlining a completely different binding mechanism (19) (see **Figure 3B**).

Detailed aspects of protein–protein interactions can be characterized by SMD simulations, in which the dissociation is actuated by an external force acting on the protein. A typical reaction coordinate for protein–protein dissociation is the distance between the centers of mass of each protein. In the following, we call this reaction coordinate ξ. In the case of the TCR-pMHC, we assumed that the dissociation happens in the direction perpendicular to the cellular membranes (see **Figure 3C**). We also assumed that there is no substantial conformational rearrangement upon dissociation (except possibly in the CDRs and in the peptide), which is supported by the similarity of X-ray structures of bound and unbound TCRs or pMHCs. To enforce these assumptions during the SMD, we devised the individual pulling scheme (20) in which each non-H atom (except CDRs and peptide) is subjected to an individual harmonic potential. As shown on **Figure 3D**, the center of mass distance ξ is increased by collectively shifting the reference positions of the individual potentials. For each TCR-pMHC complex,

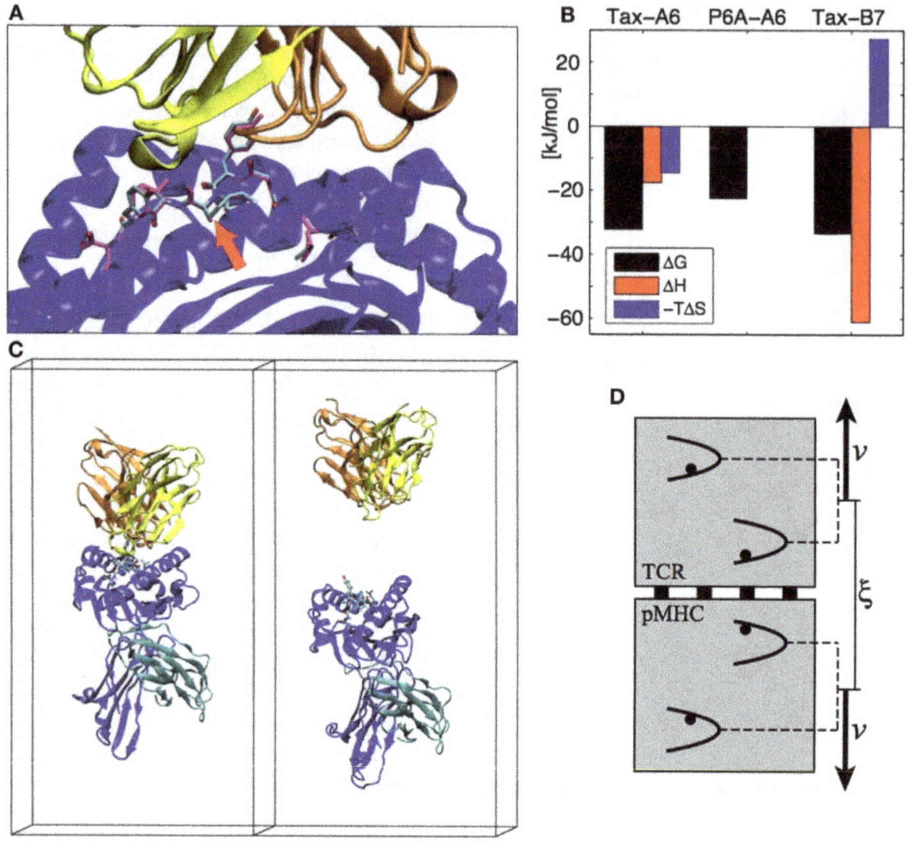

FIGURE 3 | (A) The A6 TCR (yellow and orange) bound to the HLA-A2 MHC (blue) presenting the Tax peptide (cyan). The P6A peptide mutant is overlaid in magenta (PDB entry 1AO7). The site of the P6A mutation is indicated by a red arrow. **(B)** Experimental TCR binding thermodynamics. For P6A-A6, no entropy/enthalpy measurements are available. References are given in the text. **(C)** TCR-pMHC complex in its simulation box before and after the SMD simulation (water molecules not shown). **(D)** The individual pulling scheme used to dissociate the proteins. The distance ξ between the centers of mass is increased at rate 2ν. Each backbone heavy atom is subjected to an individual harmonic potential. All individual potentials move in concert, with their relative positions fixed to their values in the crystal structure.

we performed about 150 unbinding trajectories of 4 ns each during which ξ is gradually increased by 2 nm from the bound state distance to reach a final conformation as shown on the right panel of **Figure 3C**. The simulations were performed with the Gromacs software (21) using the Gromos 45a3 force field (22) with explicit water molecules.

With about 150 trajectories we were able to obtain converged ensemble averages of many observables at any given protein–protein separation, including for highly fluctuating quantities involving solvent molecules. In particular, we established maps of H-bonds or of non-polar contacts for all residues of the TCR and pMHC as a function of ξ. As an example, **Figure 4B** shows an H-bond occurrence map for the OH group on the Tyr5 side-chain of the Tax peptide in the Tax-A6 system. We see that α-S31 is the main TCR H-bonding partner in the bound state, but that new H-bonds are formed with α-S100 in the transition state. Overall, our simulations have shown that the number and diversity of H-bonds occurring in a protein complex largely exceeds what is apparent from the crystal structures. Using this methodology, detailed maps such as **Figure 4B** can be established for any interaction to any atom in the system, depending on the biological question of interest.

For all three TCR-pMHC complexes, we monitored energy variations in different parts of the system upon dissociation. **Figure 4C** shows that there are differences in TCR-pMHC interaction energies between the complexes. But these are largely compensated by effects in the internal protein reorganization energy (**Figure 4D**), solvent-protein interaction energy (**Figure 4E**), and solvent internal energy (**Figure 4F**). As a general lesson for protein–protein interactions, we retain that the solvent plays a key role in two different ways. First, variations of solvation energies exceed contributions from the proteins themselves upon binding. Second, specific water molecules trapped at the interface can influence the binding mechanism and thermodynamics (data not shown). In the present case, these two aspects happen to be also the two major factors differentiating A6 and B7 binding.

Focusing on the bound state of the TCR-pMHC complexes, the decomposition of the average interaction energy among CDRs brings valuable insights. **Figure 4A** illustrates the differences between the A6 and B7 binding modes, with a much less prominent

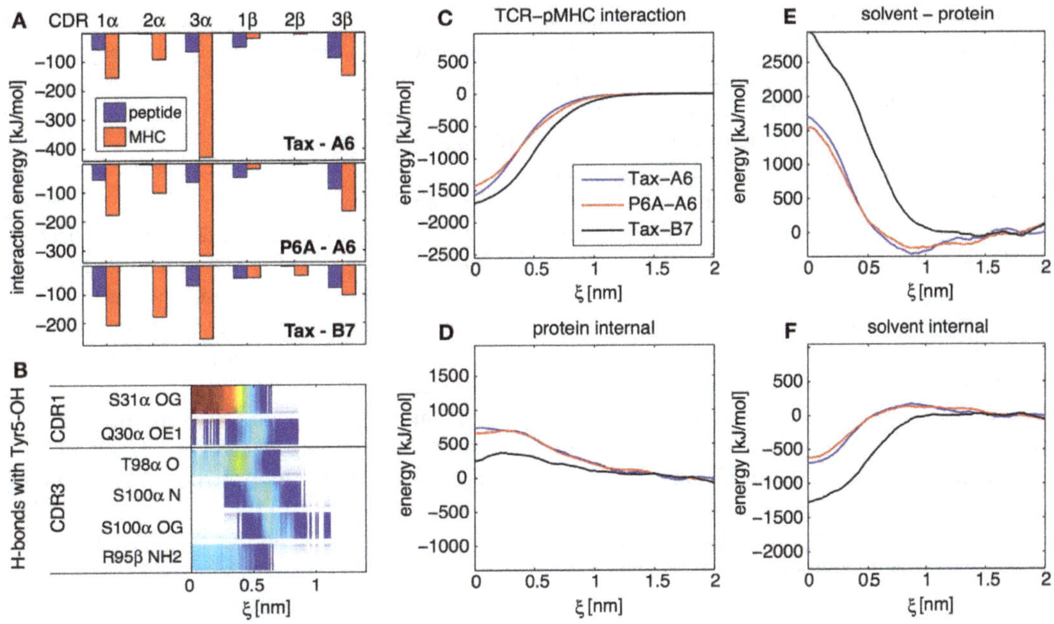

FIGURE 4 | Results from the SMD dissociation of three TCR-pMHC complexes. **(A)** Average interaction energy in the bound complexes, partitioned in CDR and peptide/MHC contributions. **(B)** Focus on the OH group on the side-chain of the peptide Tyr 5 residue. The color bars indicate the average occurrence of H-bonds with TCR atoms as a function of center of mass separation ξ. Red means that the H-bond is formed almost all the time, blue indicate a rare interaction. **(C)** Interaction energy between the TCR and the pMHC for all three complexes, as a function of ξ. **(D)** Total internal energy (bonded and non-bonded) of TCR and pMHC. **(E)** Solvent-protein interaction energy. **(F)** Solvent internal energy. The contributions from **(C–F)** add up to the total system energy.

contribution of CDR3α for B7. Generally for all complexes, **Figure 4A** shows that, while CDR2 interacts mostly with MHC, both CDR1 and CDR3 interact equally with peptide and MHC, even at large distance, as confirmed by our H-bond occurrence maps (not shown). Therefore, our simulations do not support the two-step model (23) for TCR engagement, in which the CDR1 and CDR2 preferentially contact the MHC at large distance, while the CDR3 establishes final contacts to "read" the peptide mainly at short distances.

Overall, although the P6A-A6 complex has a very different affinity compared to the wild-type Tax-A6, both complexes share very similar features in terms of specific H-bonds or energy contributions. On the other hand, the Tax-B7 complex has a binding affinity similar to that of Tax-A6, but uses a completely different binding mechanism. The B7 TCR creates a very different set of H-bonds and hydrophobic contacts to the pMHC and makes a very different usage of the solvent, which reflects in a different partition of the binding energy. In retrospect, as noted previously by Baker and coworkers (24), it is not so surprising to observe active TCRs with very different binding mechanisms. Indeed, if TCRs are issued from random sequence variation and selection upon pMHC binding affinity and kinetics only, each TCR is likely to adopt its own unique pMHC binding strategy as long as it matches these criteria.

TCR-pMHC HOMOLOGY MODELING

PIONEERING STUDY OF TCR-pMHC HOMOLOGY MODELING

The recent development and use of experimental techniques to determine sequences of TCRs that bind to a pMHC complex (25), led to the collection of large repertoires of TCR sequences with given pMHC specificities (26, 27). Understanding the selection mechanism that causes this gene usage can be facilitated by the introduction of structural information regarding the underlying TCR-pMHC complexes. This information can be used to identify conserved 3D binding motifs that are not obvious from repertoire sequences alone (28), to suggest explanations regarding the impact of TCR mutation on its affinity for given pMHCs (29) and ultimately to support the rational engineering of TCRs with particular binding properties (7, 30). Experimental structural techniques such as X-ray crystallography or NMR provide direct and valuable information regarding the 3D-structures of macromolecules. Unfortunately, they require the production of the protein, can be time consuming, and are thus hardly applicable to the analysis of large repertoires of tens to hundreds of TCRs. According to the 3D-structure database of the international ImMunoGenetics information system [IMGT/3D-structure-DB (31, 32)] the 3D-structure of 66 TCR-pMHC complexes have been determined experimentally so far. This number is negligible compared to the vast TCR diversity created by genetic rearrangements of the TCR V, D, and J genes. Indeed, the number of unique TCRβ chains in blood has been estimated to be of the order of 10^6 (33, 34). There is thus a need for tools able to predict the 3D-structure of TCR-pMHC complexes from the amino acid sequences of their components.

The pioneering work of Michielin et al. (29) provided a remarkable demonstration of the feasibility and the predictive ability of TCR-pMHC 3D-structure modeling. The authors used a murine

T1 TCR, specific for a photoreactive derivative of the Plasmodium berghei circumsporozoite (PbCS) 253–260 nonapeptide presented by the K_D class I MHC (35). Fifty mutants involving the TCR's CDR, the MHC's α1 and α2 helices and the peptide were prepared and the association constants between the TCR and the pMHC were measured (35). A first homology model was built for the wild-type TCR-pMHC complex with the MODELLER program (36–38), using the four TCR structures available at that time (39–42) and the structure of H-2Kb MHC (43) as templates. These structures provided good templates for the β-sheet framework of the TCR, and of the α helices/β-sheet of the MHC grooves. The high secondary structure content of these regions imposed strong restrictions on their backbone conformation according to the MODELLER algorithm, which facilitates the modeling of those parts. In contrast, the CDR loops of TCRs have a very low level of sequence identity and no specific secondary structure, which obviously limits the efficiency of modeling by homology. The CDR loops conformation obtained in the first homology model were thus refined using a simulated annealing technique (44), followed by clustering the generated conformations based on their relative Cartesian coordinate root mean square deviation (RMSD). A final conformation was chosen from a well-populated, low-energy cluster, whose structure was compatible with the experimental mutational data. All but three of the 50 mutations found qualitative explanation in the model in terms of breaking of a significant TCR/pMHC interaction. In addition, the model suggested that a TCR pocket could form upon binding to accommodate the peptide hapten, explaining the high level of affinity of the T1 TCR for this pMHC ($K_D \sim 10$ nM), and demonstrating predictive capabilities for the modeling approach that go beyond reproducing only the structural features present in the templates. Since more X-ray structures of TCR-ligand complexes are continuously determined, it could be expected that the range of applicability and the accuracy of such a modeling approach would improve, since there is no limitation to the number of simultaneous templates that can be used.

TCRep 3D

The first study described above (29) led to the development of TCRep 3D, as a generalization of the TCR-pMHC modeling approach (28). TCRep 3D is an approach dedicated to the prediction of high-quality 3D-structures that can provide a functional insight on the interaction between a TCR and a pMHC. It includes by design minimal input and optimal automation, to analyze wide sets of sequences of TCRs belonging to a common TCR repertoire.

The modeling pipeline is composed of two modules (see **Figure 5**): (i) homology modeling of the TCR-pMHC complex and (ii) *ab initio* CDR loops structure optimization. First, the user provides the sequence of the target complex and a list of preferred templates. By default, all the TCR-pMHC templates of the Protein Data Bank are used. The global structure of the complex is modeled by homology. It could be possible to couple this step to computer-aided approaches for the docking of peptide antigens into MHC molecules (45), in case the peptide binding mode could not be correctly predicted by homology modeling. Each CDR loop is then subsequently refined while the rest of the complex remains rigid. The MODELLER (38) software is used for the two modules.

The originality of TCRep 3D resides in the specific bias that we impose to the system during the structural sampling. Canonical restraints available from the literature (46) are added to the backbone dihedral angles of CDR1 and 2 to limit the conformational space accessible to the loops. We developed an iterative sampling

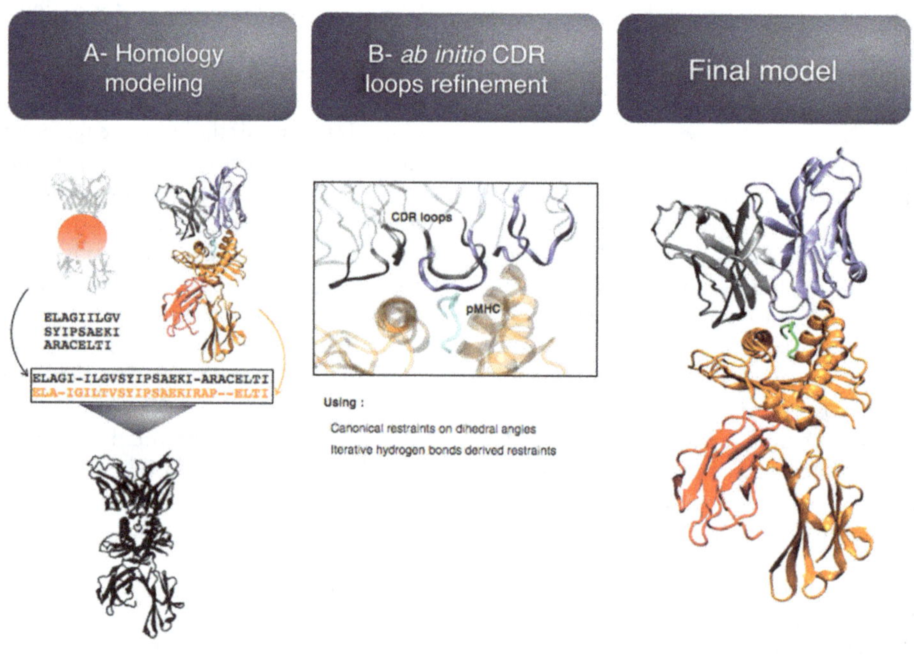

FIGURE 5 | Key steps of the TCRep 3D modeling procedure.

method that identifies potential hydrogen bonds between TCR and pMHC, and converts them into modeling restraints. The scoring function was adapted accordingly, to favor structures that satisfy most of the canonical restraints, and display potential hydrogen bonds. We demonstrated that TCRep 3D is significantly more efficient than common loop modeling approaches in predicting CDR loops conformations.

At the time of the study, TCRep 3D produced one TCR-pMHC structure in 7 days on a single CPU. However, the modeling can be parallelized on a computing grid, and the computation time scales efficiently with the number of CPUs used, allowing the user to quickly model a large number of sequences.

TCRep 3D has been successfully applied to experimentally determined sets of sequences of TCRs that recognize given cancer epitopes.

(a) In a study on HLA-A*0201/Melan-A-specific CD8 T cells (47), the modeling of the TCR-pMHC 3D-structure revealed the structural feature that explained how two distinct sets of TCR performed differently in recognizing a naturally occurring decamer variant of the Melan-A peptide. One of the TCR subsets could not make proper interactions with the glutamic acid at position 1 of the peptide because of the location and structural properties of the CDR1α (see **Figures 6A,B**).

(b) The analysis of HLA-A*0201/NY-ESO-$1_{157-165}$ specific $CD8^+$ T cells from five melanoma patients showed a preferential usage of three Vβ genes. Additionally, experimental evidence on the importance of the Met4-Trp5 pair of the NY-ESO-$1_{157-165}$ antigen were found, suggesting that those two contact residues make critical interactions with the TCR, regardless of the gene segment usage (26). The modeling of the corresponding TCR-pMHC structures revealed a striking mechanism of selection through the presence of a single conserved glycine residue situated in the center of all CDR3β. An *in vitro* experimental functional study of mutations of this amino acid combined with *in silico* modeling of several mutants was performed. All mutations resulted in dramatic structural changes associated with complete experimental loss of affinity of the TCR to NY-ESO-1/HLA-A*0201 (28).

LONG-RANGE DRIVING FORCE FOR TCR ORIENTATION

Over the years, successive releases of TCR-pMHC crystal structures have revealed the variety of native binding orientations that the TCR can adopt. Recent studies reported a range of more than 45° in the TCR binding angles relative to the MHC (48), depending on the peptide, the MHC, and the α/β pairing of the TCR. Although the challenge of TCR binding mode prediction has been recurrently discussed, only a few studies have focused on predicting the actual binding mode of given TCR-pMHC (49, 50). Therefore, all methods and applications relied on the existence of at least one TCR-pMHC crystal structure.

In order to understand the molecular basis that governs TCR orientation upon binding, we tested a simplified rigid approach on all published TCR-pMHC crystal structures (48), which allowed scanning quickly multiple orientations of the TCR relative to the pMHC. In this approach, the TCR was moved 6–12 Å away from the pMHC molecule along the TCR principal axis (see **Figure 7A**). Subsequently, the TCR was rotated around that same axis until a complete revolution was obtained (see **Figure 7B**). The effective energy of the system was computed every 5°, as the sum of the intermolecular energy and the solvation free energy, using the CHARMM22 force field (51, 52) in combination with the FACTS implicit solvation model (53).

We demonstrated that the sum of the Coulomb interaction and the electrostatic solvation energies is sufficient to identify the native TCR orientation as the energetic minimum upon rotation (see **Figure 7C**). Importantly, despite the rigid-body simplification, the results were robust upon small structural variations of the TCR such as changes induced by MD simulations. We also tested our approach on crystal structures of unbound TCRs, which were confronted to pMHCs. Accurate energy minima were also identified, suggesting that perfect shape complementarity is not required to obtain a reliable signal. The long-distance interactions during the TCR approach appear to be independent of the binding process itself, since the binding orientation is reliably identified without considering either short-range energy terms or CDR induced fit upon binding.

Furthermore, we decomposed the effective energy into per-residue contributions, in an approach that is similar to the

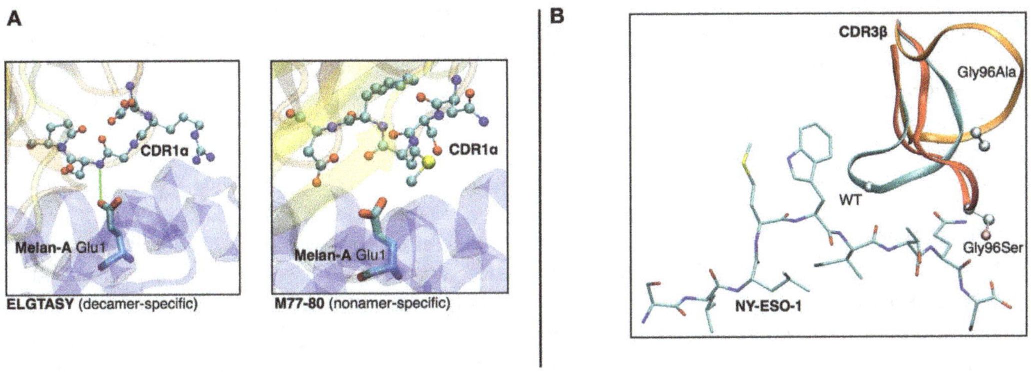

FIGURE 6 | (A) Structural differences between nona- vs. decamer-specific TCR bound to Melan-A(ELA)/HLA– A*0201. The green line identifies the hydrogen bond that is formed between CDR1α and Glu1 of the peptide. No favorable interactions were identified between M77-80 and the decamer variant of Melan-A. **(B)** *In silico* mutation results in NY-ESO-1 repertoire. The dramatic structural rearrangement of the mutated CDR3β confirms the importance of the central Gly.

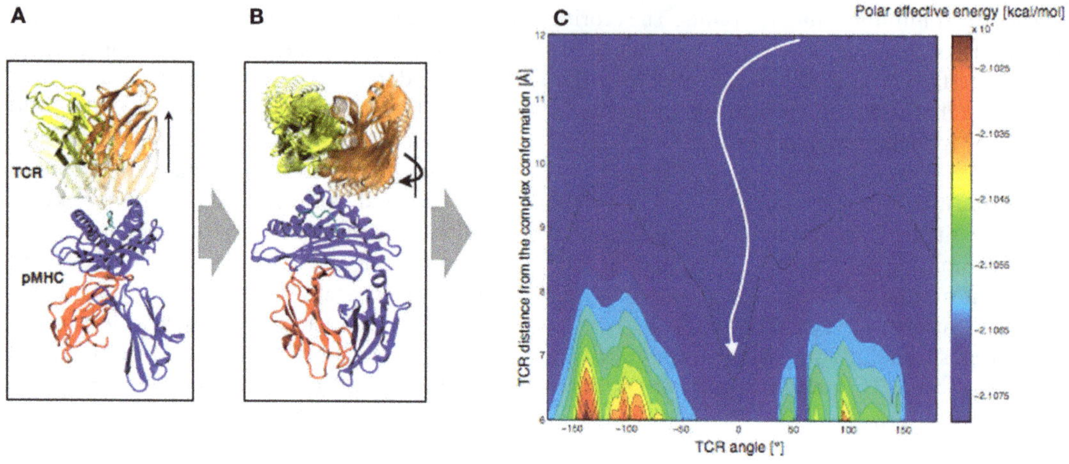

FIGURE 7 | Rigid displacement protocol. **(A)** Rigid TCR translation along the principal axis. **(B)** Rigid TCR rotation around the principal axis. **(C)** Landscape representation of the TCR-pMHC polar energy as a function of the TCR/pMHC distance and the TCR angle. 0° corresponds to the native orientation of the bound conformation.

Molecular Mechanics – Generalized Born Surface Area (MM-GBSA) energy decompositions (54). The contributions of structural sub-groups to the profile of the TCR/pMHC interaction energy during rotation were calculated, to estimate their role in the overall orientation. Results showed that most of the driving force (>90%) leading to the orientation of the TCR is defined by CDR1,2/MHC interactions. This is in agreement with previous observations, revealing a ring of charged residues at the pMHC interface, which interacts with CDR1,2 with complementary charges (48). We reported that the role of the CDR3/peptide interaction is of lesser importance at long-distance.

In turn, such knowledge of the structure may be used as a preliminary approach in the process of modeling protein/protein interactions. More specifically, the rigid search for an energetic minimum upon TCR rotation may become a complementary module of TCRep 3D, to search for the correct binding mode, after modeling the TCR and the pMHC independently. We attempted to predict the binding mode of the A6 TCR with tax/HLA-A*0201, after modeling the TCR by homology. The effective energy minimum upon rotation was computed for 500 homology models, and we obtained an average shift of 12.2° from the orientation of the crystal structure. This demonstrated the potential of the approach as a component of a TCR-pMHC structural prediction pipeline (55). The approach is also easily applicable to other types of protein complexes, provided that the association is also driven by long-range electrostatic interactions.

FREE ENERGY CALCULATIONS

APPLICATION OF THE THERMODYNAMIC INTEGRATION METHOD FOR TCR-pMHC BINDING FREE ENERGY DIFFERENCES

T cell receptor recognition can exhibit exquisite specificity upon single peptide mutation. In the A6/Tax/HLA-A0201 complex described above (Tax-A6), mutating the Ala at position 6 to a Pro (P6A) turns the Tax peptide from a strong agonist into a weak antagonist. These systems were extensively studied experimentally (18, 56) and the binding free energy difference between the Tax-A6 and the P6A-A6 complexes was found to be $\Delta\Delta G = 2.90 \pm 0.20$ kcal/mol. (see **Figure 3B**). These results are difficult to rationalize from the structure alone, as there is almost no difference between the conformations of the Tax-A6 and P6A-A6 complexes (see **Figure 3A**, red arrow). To gain a better understanding of the effect of the mutation on TCR recognition, we used free energy simulation to analyze in detail the origin of the binding free energy difference (57).

As we will see below, calculating the binding free energy by simulating the entire TCR-pMHC unbinding process itself is difficult. Instead, the present method uses the thermodynamic cycle shown in **Figure 8A** to reformulate the problem,

$$\Delta\Delta G^{\text{Binding}}_{\text{P6A}} = \Delta G^{\text{Binding}}_{\text{P6}} - \Delta G^{\text{Binding}}_{\text{A6}} = \Delta G^{\text{P6}\rightarrow\text{A6}}_{\text{Bound}} - \Delta G^{\text{P6}\rightarrow\text{A6}}_{\text{Unbound}}. \quad (1)$$

This means that we can obtain $\Delta\Delta G^{\text{Binding}}_{\text{P6A}}$ by computing the P6 → A6 mutation free energy in both the unbound and the bound states. Among the different methods available to calculate mutation free energy differences (58, 59), we chose thermodynamic integration (60, 61). We define an interpolated potential energy function $U(r, \lambda)$ that is equivalent to the potential energy function of the wild-type for $\lambda = 0$ (Pro) and to that of the P6A mutant for $\lambda = 1$ (Ala). The free energy difference can be obtained through

$$\Delta G^{\text{P6}\rightarrow\text{A6}}_{\text{Bound}} = \int_0^1 \left\langle \frac{\partial U(r,\lambda)}{\partial \lambda} \right\rangle_\lambda d\lambda.$$

Here, $\langle\cdot\rangle_\lambda$ represents an ensemble average at fixed λ. In practice, we perform a set of simulations at discrete λ-values and evaluate the integral above numerically. The number and position of λ-values required for accurate integration depends on the smoothness of the $\langle \frac{\partial U}{\partial \lambda} \rangle_\lambda$ function. To construct an appropriate interpolating potential energy function, a dual topology scheme was used, as shown on **Figure 8B**. For vanishing atoms, only the non-bonded interactions are scaled, while the bonded interactions are left unchanged (62). As we did not use soft-core potentials

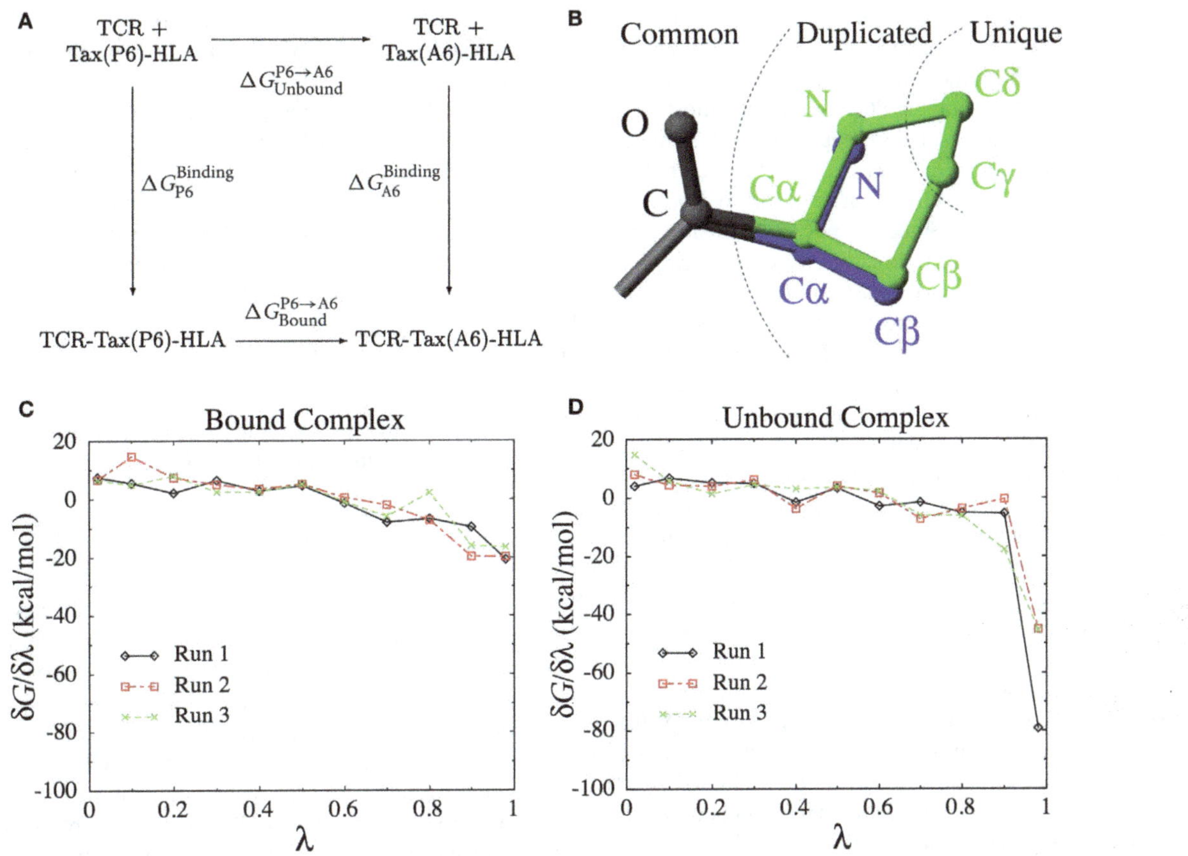

FIGURE 8 | (A) The thermodynamic cycle underlying Eq. 1. **(B)** The dual topology scheme used to interpolate the potential energy function between the Pro side-chain (green) and the Ala side-chain (blue). Common atoms are unaffected, Duplicated atoms change type and non-bonded parameters. Unique atoms vanish, with their non-bonded interactions switched to zero and their bonded interactions unchanged. **(C)** Derivatives of the free energy obtained for each λ-value in three independent runs for the bound complex. **(D)** Idem for the unbound complex.

(63) for vanishing atoms, special care was taken in the limit of $\lambda \rightarrow 0$ and $\lambda \rightarrow 1$ to deal with the singularities of the Coulomb and Lennard-Jones potentials.

Starting from the crystal structures for both the unbound (64) and the bound complex (18), MD simulations were performed in the CHARMM program (51) with the CHARMM22 force field (52). The proteins were locally solvated in a sphere of 16 Å surrounding the peptide using the stochastic boundary method (65). The set of λ-values used were $\lambda = 0.02$, 0.1, 0.2, 0.3, 0.4, 0.5, 0.6, 0.7, 0.8, 0.9, 0.98. After 100 ps of initial equilibration, data was collected for 30 ps at each λ-value, separated by 10 ps equilibration time after each λ update. Three simulations with independent initial velocities were produced.

The simulations were structurally stable with average RMSD of non-H atoms no greater than 0.8 Å with respect to the crystal structures. The average free energy derivatives obtained in the three different runs are shown on **Figures 8C,D** for the bound and unbound states, respectively. In the unbound state (**Figure 8D**), the derivative takes very large values close to $\lambda = 1$, due to the interaction of the vanishing Pro atoms with the solvent molecules. This does not happen in the bound state, because the vanishing atoms are concealed from the solvent in the void created by the protein pocket.

Three different schemes were tested for the extrapolation to $\lambda = 0$ and $\lambda = 1$, using linear, quadratic or $\lambda^{-3/4}$ functions. The integration over all λ-values was performed using the trapezoidal rule. The final result is $\Delta\Delta G^{Binding}_{P6A} = 2.9 \pm 1.1$ kcal/mol, which compares very favorably with the experimental value of 2.9 ± 0.2 kcal/mol.

One of the major strengths of the method lies in the linearity of Eq. 1, which allows decomposing as a sum of contributions form different types of interactions and/or of different parts of the system. Given that the total free energy difference is in good agreement with experiment, there is a good chance that the decomposition provides meaningful insights on the mechanisms leading to TCR specificity.

A notable contribution to $\Delta\Delta G$ (+0.64 kcal/mol) arises from the difference in solvation free energy of the mutated residue: in the unbound structure, the Tax P6 residue is solvent-exposed with around 35% of its surface accessible to water molecules. The A6 mutant has fewer exposed hydrophobic groups, which entails a more modest solvation penalty in the unbound state.

This stabilizes the unbound state of the P6A mutant relative to the wild-type, which in turn makes P6A-A6 binding less favorable The rest of the peptide contributes a modest 0.38 kcal/mol to $\Delta\Delta G$.

The total contribution of the TCR in the bound state is around +0.8 kcal/mol destabilizing the P6A mutant, the most significant part of which is due to the CDR3α loop. Most of this energy arises from the van der Waals term, in accord with the fact that the TCR provides good surface complementarity for the hydrophobic side-chain of the Pro residue. Since the pocket is already present in the Tax-A6 complex, there is no large free energy cost needed to induce it, in contrast to what is found in the solvent. The TCR residues that contribute the most to the TCR specificity for the wild-type peptide are N30 from the CDR1α, D99, and S100 from the CDR3α, and G97, L98, A99, G100, G101 from the CDR3β.

The most important contribution to $\Delta\Delta G$ (1.26 kcal/mol) arises from the difference in interactions with the MHC. This is due to a conformational change that takes place in the Tax P6 region upon TCR engagement. In the Tax system, the cost of this conformational change is balanced by a very favorable interaction of the Pro ring with hydrophobic residues of the MHC groove, which does not take place with the shorter Ala side-chain. This is an example of how a conformational change taking place along the physical binding pathways translates into a free energy contribution along the alchemical pathways.

Overall, it emerges that the total binding free energy difference between the wild-type and the mutant peptide consists of four contributions that are similar in magnitude. The self-interaction of the peptide and the change in the interaction between the peptide and the three portions of its environment (TCR, HLA-A2, and solvent) all contribute between 0.5 and 1.2 kcal/mol to stabilizing the wild-type complex. This important result was not evident from the X-ray structures or the experimental data. Interestingly, these calculations show that accurate free energy differences could be obtained although most of the complexity of this system was ignored in our relatively short simulations including only the mutated side-chain and its local environment.

ASSESSING THE APPLICABILITY OF THE JARZYNSKI IDENTITY TO CALCULATE TCR-pMHC BINDING FREE ENERGY PROFILES

In classical thermodynamics, the dissipative work $W_{A\rightarrow B}$ needed to bring a system from state A to state B is greater than the free energy difference ΔG_{AB} between the two states, with equality only in adiabatic conditions. Conversely, a recent result in non-equilibrium statistical mechanics, the Jarzynski identity (JI) states that (66, 67)

$$e^{-\beta\Delta G_{AB}} = \left\langle e^{-\beta W_{A\rightarrow B}} \right\rangle_0 .$$

Here, $\beta = (k_B T)^{-1}$, with T the temperature and k_B the Boltzmann constant. The average $\langle\cdot\rangle_0$ is taken over canonically distributed initial conditions in state A. The JI was proven to hold in the case of thermostated molecular dynamics (66–69). The JI was applied with some success to simulations of small molecular systems (68–71). Given the biological importance of the TCR-pMHC system, we were compelled to determine if the JI could be employed to calculate protein–protein binding free energy profiles from SMD trajectories of large protein–protein complexes (72). The free energy profile, or potential of mean force (PMF), is very relevant because in addition to the total binding free energy it provides estimates of k_{on} and k_{off} from the free energy barrier height.

In SMD, an external potential of the form $u(\xi(r), t)$ is used to steer the system from position A at time 0 to B at time t along the reaction coordinate ξ. This potential can be a simple harmonic potential or take a more complex form such as in the individual pulling scheme (72) presented in Section "Investigating TCR-pMHC Interactions Using Steered MD Simulations." If we are interested in the PMF along ξ, the JI can be written as (73),

$$e^{-\beta G(\xi)} \alpha \left\langle \delta[\xi(r) - \xi] e^{-\beta W(t)} \right\rangle_0 .$$

Importantly, $W(t)$ is the work accumulated by the perturbed system (including u), defined as (74),

$$W(t) = \int_0^t dt \frac{\partial u}{\partial t} (\xi(r), t) .$$

For each of the Tax-A6 and P6A-A6 complexes, we performed 150 trajectories starting from independent conformation of the bound complex. The TCR and pMHC centers of mass separation was increased by 2 nm over 4 ns. The resulting work profiles are shown on **Figure 9A** and the distribution of final work values is shown on **Figure 9B**. As expected if the system is not too far from equilibrium (71, 75), the distribution (in its central part) close to a Gaussian. To obtain the PMF, the work profiles $W(t)$ collected from multiple SMD simulations have to be postprocessed with three distinct operations:

1. Reduce from the biased system to the physical system (unbias);
2. Average over all $\xi(r)$ visited during the evolution to recover $G(\xi)$;
3. Estimate the exponential average $\left\langle e^{-\beta W} \right\rangle_0$.

Operations 1 and 2 are performed within a modified weighted histogram scheme (73) adapted to the case of the individual potentials (72). Operation 3 can be more problematic. If we apply direct exponential averaging, the estimated PMF is very close to the lowest measured work profile at a given ξ. In the case where the true free energy value lies in the unsampled lower tail of the work distribution, direct averaging will result in a large overestimation. Indeed, for the Tax-A6 complex, the work profiles of **Figure 9A** would result in a dissociation free energy around 250 kJ/mol, compared to the experimental value of 32.2 kJ/mol (18).

Instead of direct averaging, if we assume that the work distribution is Gaussian, we can estimate $G(\xi)$ with a second-order cumulant expansion (71, 75),

$$G(\xi) = \bar{W}(\xi) - \frac{\beta}{2}\sigma^2(\xi) .$$

Here, $\bar{W}(\xi)$ is the mean and σ the standard deviation of the work values at ξ obtained by applying operations 1 and 2 above to each trajectory independently. The resulting PMFs are shown on **Figure 9C**. The final dissociation free energies are −110 and

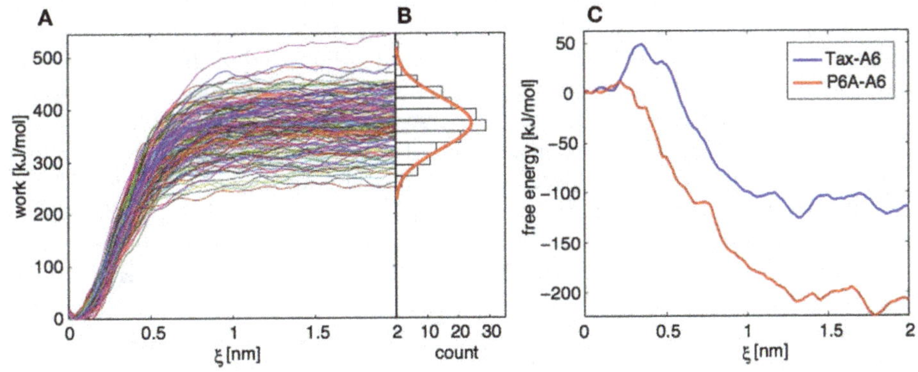

FIGURE 9 | Application of the Jarzynski identity to TCR-pMHC dissociation. **(A)** Work profiles collected in 152 independent trajectories for the Tax-P6A complex. **(B)** Histogram of the work distribution at $\xi = 2$ nm, with a fitted Gaussian distribution. **(C)** Free energy profiles calculated using the Jarzynski identity and the cumulant expansion method.

−210 kJ/mol for Tax-A6 and P6A-A6, respectively, which is a severe underestimation of the experimental values of 32.5 and 22.5 kJ/mol. We note that the calculated values should be corrected for translational and rotational entropic contributions to be compared to standard state free energy measurements, but this does not improve the results.

Our results show that direct averaging produces a strong overestimation of $G(\xi)$, which could be fixed only by sampling an extremely large number of trajectories to get enough low work values. Conversely, the cumulant expansion produces a strong underestimation of $G(\xi)$, which shows that the real work distribution has a shorter lower tail than the Gaussian distribution. Repeating the calculations with datasets of similar sizes and slightly different conditions showed the reproducibility of these findings.

Overall, this example illustrates the severe sampling difficulties that hamper the application of the JI to systems with sizeable dissipation. These difficulties have been evidenced by other researchers in systematic convergence studies of the JI method (76–79).

ESTIMATION OF RESIDUE CONTRIBUTION TO THE BINDING FREE ENERGY OF THE TCR/pMHC ASSOCIATION USING MM-PB(GB)SA

In the Molecular Mechanics – Poisson Boltzman Surface Area (MM-PBSA), or its variant the MM-GBSA, the binding free energy, ΔG_{bind}, is written as the sum of the gas phase contribution, $\Delta H_{\text{bind}}^{\text{gas}}$, the desolvation free energy of the system upon binding, ΔG_{desolv}, and an entropic contribution, $-T\Delta S$ (80):

$$\Delta G_{\text{bind}} = \Delta H_{\text{bind}}^{\text{gas}} + \Delta G_{\text{desolv}} - T\Delta S.$$

The term $\Delta H_{\text{bind}}^{\text{gas}}$ is constituted by the van der Waals (ΔH_{vdw}) and electrostatic (ΔH_{elec}) interaction energies between the two partners in the complex, and their conformational energy change upon binding, ΔH_{intra}:

$$\Delta H_{\text{bind}}^{\text{gas}} = \Delta H_{\text{elec}} + \Delta G_{\text{vdW}} + \Delta H_{\text{intra}}.$$

ΔG_{desolv} is the difference between the solvation free energy, ΔG_{solv}, of the complex and that of the isolated parts. ΔG_{solv} is divided into the electrostatic, $\Delta G_{\text{elec, solv}}$, and the non-polar, $\Delta G_{\text{np, solv}}$, contributions,

$$\Delta G_{\text{solv}} = \Delta G_{\text{elec,solv}} + \Delta G_{\text{np,solv}}.$$

$\Delta G_{\text{elec, solv}}$ is calculated by solving the exact Poisson or the Poisson–Boltzmann (PB) equation (81, 82) in MM-PBSA, and the much faster but approximate Generalized Born (GB) model (83) in MM-GBSA (84). The term $\Delta G_{\text{np,solv}}$, which can be considered as the sum of a cavity term and a solute–solvent van der Waals term, is assumed to be proportional to the solvent accessible surface area (SASA) (85),

$$\Delta G_{\text{np,solv}} = \gamma SASA + b.$$

The entropy term can be decomposed into translational, S_{trans}, rotational, S_{rot}, and vibrational S_{vib}, contributions. These terms are calculated using standard equations of statistical mechanics (54, 86).

In the standard MM-PB(GB)SA protocol, all these energy terms are typically averaged over several hundreds of frames extracted from multi-nanosecond MD simulation trajectories, generally performed in explicit solvent. Those explicit water molecules are removed prior to energy calculations. In principle, three trajectories should be performed, one for the complex and one for each of the isolated partners, and the energy terms calculated using the corresponding simulation. However, a frequent, less computationally demanding, approximation consists in performing only one MD simulation for the complex (54). The terms relative to one isolated partner are then calculated after removing the atoms of the other partner in the frames extracted from the MD simulation of the complex. In this variant, the conformational energy change upon association is therefore neglected ($\Delta H_{\text{intra}} = 0$), and the influence of conformational changes on the other energy terms are not captured.

MM-PB(GB)SA has been used successfully to identify the hot-spots of protein–protein association and to determine the effect of mutations on association processes (84, 87–90). Two approaches can be considered. The computational alanine scanning (CAS) approach (91) is directly comparable to its experimental counterpart. In this approach, ΔG_{bind} values are calculated for the wild-type system, as well as for several mutants in which one residue has been replaced by an alanine. The difference in ΔG_{bind} between the wild-type system and the mutants can be used to estimate the role played by each residue in the association process. Alternatively, it is possible to perform a binding free energy decomposition (BFED) for the wild-type system (84). In this approach, the contributions to ΔG_{bind} arising from groups of atoms, typically single residues, or even backbone or side-chain, are estimated from the wild-type system by performing a pairwise decomposition of the MM-PB(GB)SA terms (88, 90). BFED, which requires only one binding free energy calculation, is faster than CAS. In addition, BFED provides the possibility to study contributions from non-mutable groups of atoms, such as the backbone. However, contrarily to CAS, BFED results cannot be compared directly to an experimental alanine scanning.

To assess the ability of the MM-GBSA approach to identify quantitatively the hot-spots residues for the TCR/pMHC association, we performed a study of the 2C TCR/SIYR/H-2Kb system using both the CAS and BFED methods (90). This system was chosen because both the experimental 3D-structure and the results of an experimental alanine scanning were available at that time (92). A very good correlation was found between the residue contributions to ΔG_{bind} from both methods, with a correlation coefficient of 0.94, highlighting the interest in the faster BFED approach. A correlation coefficient of $R = 0.67$ was found between experimentally determined activity differences for alanine mutants and the calculated binding free energy changes upon mutation.

Our results also showed that BFED provided a more detailed and reliable description of the interactions between the TCR and pMHC molecules when including entropic terms. When the entropy was taken into account, the correlation coefficient was increased to 0.72. It was noticeable that the correlation obtained when neglecting the entropy term, which is very computationally expensive to calculate, was sufficient to quantify and rank the importance of the residues for TCR/pMHC association. Altogether, these pioneering results suggested that the BFED for the TCR-pMHC system provides a detailed and reliable enough description of the interactions between the molecules to be used as an *in silico* investigation tool in TCR protein-engineering.

COMPUTER-AIDED PROTEIN ENGINEERING

BACKGROUND

Patients with diverse types of cancer develop tumor-specific $CD4^+$ and $CD8^+$ T cell responses. Although these responses are typically unable to contain solid tumor growth or hematological malignancies, clinical studies have revealed the adoptive transfer of *ex vivo* expanded autologous tumor-specific T cells to be a promising immunotherapeutic approach to cancer treatment (13). A limitation, however, is that TCRs which bind tumor associated/self antigen are often of relatively low affinity. TCRs generally bind pMHC in the range of $K_D = 1\text{–}100\,\mu\text{M}$ (93). However, as a result of the thymic negative selection whereby T cells with high-affinity TCRs for "self" antigens are eliminated to prevent autoimmunity, TCRs specific for "self" tumor associated antigens tend to be weaker-binders compared to TCRs specific for "non-self" peptides (94). Thus, the development of tumor-targeting TCRs to endow them with optimal binding properties, both in terms of fine-specificity against the targeted pMHC, and kinetic/affinity parameters that confer maximum cellular responsiveness, is a field of intense research toward cancer immunotherapy development (95).

The relative importance of the roles played by the TCR/pMHC binding affinity (K_D), and individual kinetic parameters (k_{on} and k_{off}), on T cell activation, has been intensively studied recently (11). The emerging consensus hypothesizes the existence of a TCR/pMHC "dwell-time"(96) enabling the sequential interaction of TCRs with a rare antigenic pMHC complex – a process known as "serial triggering" – and conferring an optimal T cell activation (97). It has also been demonstrated that both k_{on} and k_{off} define the "effective half-life" of a TCR/pMHC interaction (98). Thus, K_D, k_{on}, and k_{off} do all contribute to T cell activation and their optimizations should be addressed concomitantly by TCR engineering techniques for cancer immunotherapy.

As introduced earlier, TCRs contact pMHC antigens via the six CDRs (**Figure 2**), with CDR3α and CDR3β mainly bound over the peptide, and CDR1 and CDR2, α and β, making more contacts with MHC. It could thus be expected that mutations of CDR3s would be more likely to maintain peptide specificity than mutants of CDR1s and CDR2s. Indeed, several mutagenesis studies produced high-affinity TCRs bearing mutations on CDR3α and CDR3β that were found to be peptide-specific (99–102). However, other studies also discovered high-affinity mutants in CDR1 and CDR2 retaining peptide specificity despite the close proximity of the mutated region to MHC residues (99, 103). This indicates that all six CDRs can serve as a focus for mutagenesis to generate higher-affinity TCRs, while still potentially retaining substantial peptide specificity (2, 93).

Several efforts have been performed to optimize TCRs (93), which mainly consist in experimental yeast (100, 101, 104–106), phage (18, 102, 103, 107), and mammalian cell (108, 109) display techniques. These approaches were able to increase the affinity of the TCR by a factor of 100–10^6, leading to K_D as low as 26 pM (102). Although very efficient to increase the K_D, these techniques lead to TCRs bearing multiple mutations, without providing a straightforward control of the effect of each one. Such TCRs are prone to alloreactivity due to peptide-independent binding of MHCs (95, 110).

Detailed control of the effect of each mutation at the atomic level can be provided by *in silico* rational protein-engineering techniques (111–115). Recently, Haidar et al. (116) engineered the human A6 TCR for enhanced affinity toward the Tax peptide/HLA-A2 MHC complex. Rapidly, the authors created a set of 219 fitted scoring functions, aiming to reproduce the binding affinity change upon 648 mutations of the ovomucoid turkey inhibitor molecule, using energy and statistically derived potential terms. Each function was then tested against the affinity changes of a first set of 11 A6 TCR mutants, and evaluated by correlation. The function reproducing the best the affinity changes on A6 TCR (named ZAFFI score) was retained to suggest new mutations. Due to the significant number of non-binding mutations generated using only the ZAFFI score, the authors further developed the ZAFFI filter function. The latter, trained by a Monte Carlo method on the 36 first A6 TCR point mutations, was employed to filter out mutations with potentially bad electrostatic contacts. In total 59 mutants were tested. Twelve were found to be better binders than the wild-type TCR, as measured experimentally by Surface Plasmon resonance (SPR). It must be noted that some non-binders were generated on purpose to help training the ZAFFI score and filter. All mutations found in this study to increase the binding were hydrophobic substitutions that enhanced the interface complementarity. No mutation introducing new significant electrostatic contacts, and thus potentially increasing the selectivity of the TCR/pMHC binding, was found positive. Despite the use of fitted scoring function and filter that hampers its straightforward translation to non-TCR systems, this interesting study illustrated the feasibility of a rational *in silico* approach to design TCR with higher affinities. It opened the road to new approaches, with physically sound and non-fitted universal free energy estimates, straightforward transferability, and high success rates.

METHODOLOGY AND RESULTS ON BC1 TCR

Encouraged by the results of our BFED method in reproducing the outcome of a alanine scanning experiment on the TCR/SIYR/H-2Kb system (90), we decided to develop a new structure-based approach, based on MM-GBSA free energy calculations, to rationally design new TCR sequences. Our approach can be divided into several steps. First, the importance of each wild-type TCR residue for the TCR/pMHC association is estimated using a MM-GBSA BFED. Then, based on the TCR-pMHC structure and the residue contributions to the binding, mutations are designed for the residues showing the most promising opportunities of enhancement for the interaction with the pMHC. These putative sequence modifications are finally selected for experimental testing based on the estimated binding free energy gain, $\Delta\Delta G_{\text{bind}}$. The latter was obtained by calculating the contribution of each residue to the binding free energy change upon a given mutation, $\Delta\Delta G^{\text{res}}_{\text{bind}}$, as the difference between the residue contribution for the mutated complex, $\Delta G^{\text{res,mut}}_{\text{bind}}$, and that for the wild-type complex, $\Delta G^{\text{res}}_{\text{bind}}$:

$$\Delta\Delta G^{\text{res}}_{\text{bind}} = \Delta G^{\text{res,mut}}_{\text{bind}} - \Delta G^{\text{res}}_{\text{bind}}.$$

$\Delta G^{\text{res}}_{\text{bind}}$ and $\Delta G^{\text{res,mut}}_{\text{bind}}$ values were calculated from MD simulations of the wild-type and the corresponding mutated TCR-pMHC, respectively. The binding free energy difference upon a given mutation, $\Delta\Delta G_{\text{bind}}$, was finally obtained by summing the $\Delta\Delta G^{\text{res}}_{\text{bind}}$ values over the mutated residue and all the residues in contact with it. This local summation was preferred to a summation over all residues of the TCR-pMHC complex since it suppresses the errors arising from residues far from the site of the sequence modification, and making no contribution to the mutation effect.

We have applied our computer-aided protein-engineering approach to the BC1 TCR (26, 117). This TCR was discovered from a long-surviving melanoma patient (LAU #155) with a naturally occurring CD8$^+$ T cell response against the immunodominant cancer-testis epitope NY-ESO-1$_{157\text{–}165}$ (SLLMWITQC), presented by the commonly expressed MHC class I allele HLA-A*0201. The expression profile of NY-ESO-1 makes it an attractive target for cancer immunotherapy. It is indeed expressed by several solid tumors, including melanoma, as well as hematological malignancies (myelomas, lymphomas, and leukemias), while in normal tissue its expression is limited to the testis cells (118–122). Interestingly, recent studies have shown that an immune response against NY-ESO-1 can convey an important clinical benefit for the patient. Seventy-seven percent of patients treated with the CTLA-4 blocking antibody ipilimumab showed favorable clinical outcome if they had a detectable CD8$^+$ T cell responses against NY-ESO-1, compared to only 14% otherwise (123). Our *in silico* approach was facilitated by the existence of the crystal structure of the 1G4 TCR bound to NY-ESO-1/HLA-A*201 (124), PDB ID 2BNR, available in the protein databank (125). The sequence of the latter differs only from that of the BC1 TCR by four residues: Thr95α, Ser96α, Asn97β, and Thr98β of the 1G4 TCR, are replaced by Gln95α, Thr96 α, Ala97β, and Ala98β in BC1 TCR, respectively. These sequence modifications were introduced in the 1G4 X-ray structure before applying our approach. Noticeably, three crystal structures of free and bound 1G4 TCR were solved after we performed our simulations (126). These affinity-enhanced TCRs contain mutations in the CDR3 loops or in both the CDR2 and CDR3 loops, which were obtained by *in vitro* directed evolution (102). They revealed that the binding mode for the high-affinity TCRs was identical to that of the wild-type TCR, with only limited changes in the mutated CDRs. A previous assessment by Zhao et al., of six phage library-derived 1G4 TCR variants demonstrated three categories of TCR specificity related to affinity; (i) super-high-affinity TCR (26 pM) which completely lacked specificity, (ii), mid-range affinity TCR (5 and 85 nM) that were specific only in the absence of CD8 co-engagement, and, (iii), intermediate-range affinity TCR (0.4 and 4 μM) that maintained specificity (107). By taking a rational computer-aided approach to TCR engineering, we were able to design a new original set of TCR variants. We enhanced the TCR/pMHC binding interactions in a "step-by-step" manner, targeting change to specific kinetic parameters, and limiting overall gain in affinity as well as potential for cross-reactivity.

Twenty four of the most promising mutations identified using this approach, spanning 11 different residues of the CDRs (see **Figure 10**), were introduced into the BC1 TCR sequence. The engineered proteins were produced using a mammalian cell expression system, purified and tested by titration ELISA. We found a qualitative agreement between the calculated $\Delta\Delta G_{\text{bind}}$ values and the experimental results. Thirteen (54%) of the mutations proposed by our approach showed improved affinity for the pMHC, compared to the wild-type TCR (Zoete et al., in preparation). We obtained an excellent correlation of $R = 0.85$ between the calculated $\Delta\Delta G_{\text{bind}}$ and the measured co-logarithm of the optical density measured by ELISA titration. Only three outliers were found: Vβ A51V, Y94N, and A51D. Their presence might be explained by conformational rearrangements upon mutation, minimally accessible during the MD simulations. This correlation illustrates the efficiency with which the $\Delta\Delta G_{\text{bind}}$ calculated with our method allows for the rational selection of TCR sequence modifications potentially increasing its affinity for pMHC.

For quantitative TCR/pMHC binding measurements some of the TCRs were refolded from bacterial inclusion bodies and analyzed by SPR. We began by producing TCR

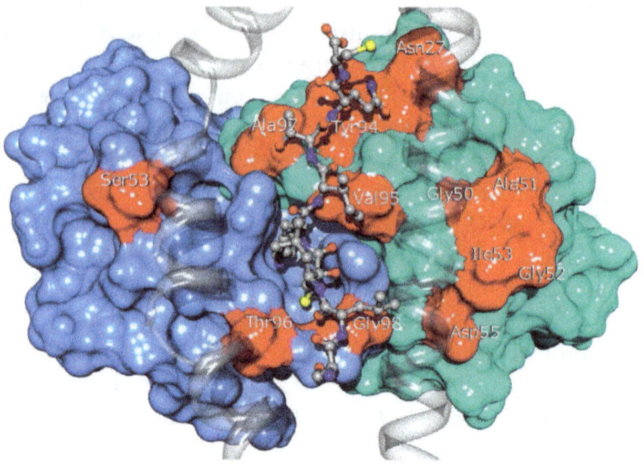

FIGURE 10 | Location of the BC1 TCR residues for which sequence modifications were designed. TCRα and β are shown as blue and cyan surfaces. Modified residues are colored in red. The NY-ESO-1 peptide is shown in ball and stick and the MHC as a transparent ribbon. Only the α1 and α2 helices of MHC are displayed, for the clarity of the figure.

Table 1 | Binding affinity of rationally designed BC1 TCR variants [from Ref. (7)] measured by SPR.

TCR mutations	K_D (μM)
β-V49I	Near non-binding
Wild-type	21.4
β-G50A	4.62
β-A97L	2.69
β-G50A + A51E	1.91
β-G50A + A51E + A97L	0.91
α-S53W + β-G50A + A51E	0.4
α-S53W + β-G50A + A51E + A97L	0.14
β-G50A + A51I + G52Q + I53T	0.015

having one amino acid change. The best single replacement TCR had 52-fold improvement in K_D (Zoete et al., in preparation). Then, we gradually increased affinity by step-wise combination of rationally selected replacements in both the β-chain and the α-chain. As predicted by modeling and assessed by SPR binding assays, we found the following progression in K_D (**Table 1**): WT (21.4 μM) > β-G50A (4.6 μM) > β- G50A + A51E (1.9 μM) > β-G50A + A51E + A97L (0.91 μM) > β-G50A + βA51E-βA97L + α-S53W (0.14 μM) (Zoete et al., in preparation) (7). Our method thus allows for the design of TCRs with fine tuned K_D values, potentially leading to T cells with optimal activity (7). This is in contrast with experimental display approaches which tend to select the tightest-binding TCRs that can potentially surpass an "affinity threshold of specificity," as has been reported for the 1G4 TCR (107). We found a very satisfying correlation between the calculated energies and the pK_D and k_{off} values measured by SPR (Zoete et al., in preparation).

Importantly, we found that our approach was able to predict successfully mutations toward both non-polar and polar residues, contrary to previous studies where only designed mutations toward non-polar residues were successful in increasing the experimental affinity (116). To take place, polar interactions, such as hydrogen bond or ionic interaction, require an appropriate match of chemical functionalities and precise geometrical constrains between interacting partners. Therefore, they provide an essential contribution to the directionality and the specificity of molecular recognition (127). This point is critical to the development of TCRs for immunotherapies. It is indeed essential that TCRs maintain their specificity, and do not acquire novel antigen specificities that might cause off-target toxicity upon the adoptive transfer of genetically engineered T cells to patients. Two rationally designed sequence modifications provide interesting examples regarding the detailed control provided by our approach on the binding process. Mutation β-A51E introduces an ionic interaction between the new glutamate side-chain and MHC Arg75 (**Figure 11A**), translating into a calculated favorable $\Delta\Delta G_{bind}$. This replacement produced a fourfold experimental improvement in K_D as measured by SPR (8). This mutation thus increases the affinity for the pMHC through better interactions with the MHC molecule, and therefore cannot be expected to increase the selectivity for the peptide antigen. Interestingly, we also designed the β-A97D variant, which introduces a new hydrogen bond between TCR and the peptide Thr7 side-chain (**Figure 11B**). The overall effect of this modification was somewhat unfavorable to the binding, as shown by the experimental titration ELISA and calculated $\Delta\Delta G_{bind}$ values (Zoete et al., in preparation). However, despite the decreased activity, this mutation is interesting for the putative gain in selectivity for the NY-ESO-1 system thanks to the new polar interaction taking place between the TCR and the peptide.

An experimental alanine scanning of the peptide supported this idea. The affinity of several TCR mutants (β-G50A/A51E, A97L, A97D, I53W, V95L, and Y94N) for the different mutated pMHC were measured by titration ELISA and compared to the results for the wild-type TCR. All mutated TCR showed affinities similar to the wild-type TCR for all the peptide mutants. The only exception was the β-A97D TCR mutant, which did not bind to the peptide T7A mutant contrary to the wild-type TCR. This experimental result is in good agreement with the *in silico* data showing that all those TCR mutations modified the interactions with the MHC rather than with the peptide with the exception of β-A97D which exchanges a hydrogen bond with the peptide Thr7 side-chain. The β-A97L TCR mutant, which makes non-polar contact with the side-chain of peptide Thr7 but no hydrogen bond, is less affected by the Thr7 mutation to Ala than the β-A97D TCR variant. Thus, although the β-A97D modification is somewhat unfavorable to the binding, it could be useful to introduce it in engineered TCRs targeting NY-ESO-1, in addition to other variations increasing the affinity, in order to obtain more selective TCRs.

The selectivity of TCRs designed by our approach was tested experimentally. We observed no interaction of our TCRs with any non-cognate pMHC complexes. In addition, tetramer binding studies with an extensive panel of non-cognate pMHC revealed that the TCR variants expressed at the cell-surface were also HLA-A*0201/NY-ESO-$1_{157-165}$ –specific (7).

The binding free energy calculations used in our approach are physics-based and not reliant on *ad hoc* model fitting. We

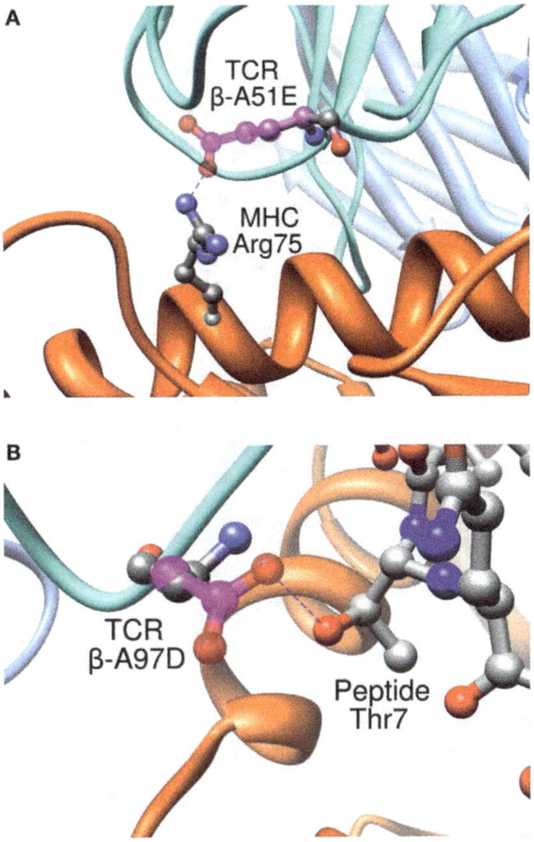

FIGURE 11 | Interaction between pMHC and the modified residues of the β-A51E (A) and β-A97D TCR variants (B). TCR wild-type residues are shown in ball and stick, colored according to the atom types. Modified residues are colored in magenta. New hydrogen bonds are shown as dotted blue lines.

can thus expect that our design strategy is highly transferable to any protein/protein interaction of known structure and biological interest.

INTERMEDIATE TCR/pMHC BINDING PARAMETERS CONFER MAXIMUM BIOLOGICAL RESPONSES

In order to efficiently screen our extensive panel of modeled BC1 TCR variants we began by establishing a mammalian cell expression system for TCR production. HEK-293 cells were PEI co-transfected with pHYK8 plasmids encoding the α- and β-chains, each under control of the CMV promoter. Following the strategy of Chang et al. an acidic-basic zipper was incorporated to facilitate heterodimeric chain pairing (128). Following 5–7 days culture in serum-free medium, the TCR variants were HIS-tag purified from the supernatants (yields were up to ~3 mg/L) and compared to the wild-type TCR by titration ELISA for binding plate-captured pMHC. Single and multiple amino acid replacements were assessed in the α- and β-chains. Over 60% showed enhanced pMHC binding as compared to the wild-type TCR. Further, binding of the TCR variants against an Ala replacement scan of the NY-ESO-$1_{157–165}$ peptide (SLLMWITQC) revealed near identical patterns of recognition, suggesting a conserved mechanism of binding. For all TCR variants, M160, W161, I162, and Q164 were critical contact residues as their replacement with Ala abolished TCR/pMHC binding (7, 8).

The TCR chains were subcloned into pGMT7 for their expression as inclusion bodies in BL21(DE3)pLys bacterial cells and subsequent TCR refolding by dialysis (129). The binding affinity and kinetics for a panel of TCRs having various combinations of amino acid replacements in CDR2-β, CDR3-β, and CDR2-α, were measured by SPR using the BIACore 3000. Most natural TCRs bind pMHC with weak affinity, in the range of 1–100 μM, as a result of slow association (10^3–10^4 $M^{-1}s^{-1}$), and fast rates of dissociation (typically a half-life of seconds at 37°C) (1, 10, 130), reflecting the need for T lymphocytes to detect a virtually limitless repertoire of foreign epitopes while avoiding autoreactivity, and the fact that they do not undergo somatic hypermutation as do antibodies. The eight TCRs chosen amongst our panel incrementally increased in affinity from 21.4 μM for the wild-type one, to extreme physiologic affinity at 15 nM (summarized in **Table 1**).

Lentiviral constructs were built to assess the activity of the rationally designed TCRs in transduced primary human $CD8^+$ T cells and identify those able to confer maximum activity levels. A range of functions were assessed for the transduced $CD8^+$ T cells including Ca^{2+} flux, intracellular signaling, cell-surface TCR clustering, target-cell killing, and cytokine/chemokine release. All activity levels for affinity-enhanced TCRs uniformly increased from that of the wild-type TCR, reaching a peak for TCRs within the upper range of natural affinity, 1–5 μM. Beyond this affinity, in the supraphysiological range, however, activity levels began to drop, both in the presence and absence of CD8 co-receptor engagement, usually reaching a minimum for the extreme supraphysiological affinity TCR (1, 7, 8, 10, 130). However, under experimental conditions in which the T cells were exposed to target-cells pulsed with high concentration of NY-ESO-$1_{157–165}$ peptide this attenuation in activity for the supraphysiological affinity TCR was no longer observed. This phenomenon is illustrated in **Figure 12**. Importantly, no non-specific reactivity was observed for any of the rationally designed TCRs (7, 8).

Over the years two main models of T cell activation have emerged [reviewed in Stone et al. (11)]. For the "affinity model" (101, 131) the total number of TCRs bound to pMHCs at equilibrium is thought to regulate T cell activity levels. The "half-life model" proposes that the TCR must stay bound with sufficiently strength/duration for productive signaling and also enable the serial engagement of the "rare" antigenic pMHC complex by adjacent TCR for the amplification of signal (i.e., the TCRs must have an optimal dwell-time) (96, 97, 132–134). Although the half-life of a TCR/pMHC interaction has traditionally been calculated from k_{off} values ($t_{1/2} = \ln 2/k_{off}$), recent work by Aleksic et al. has elegantly demonstrated that for TCRs having faster association rates there can be rapid TCR/pMHC re-engagement rather than a lateral diffusion of TCRs in the cell membrane to prolong the effective half-life of the TCR/pMHC interaction. Thus, both k_{off} and k_{on} can contribute to TCR/pMHC dwell or confinement time (135). Overall our findings correspond to the "half-life" model of T cell activation. Presumably the supraphysiological affinity TCRs are limiting the serial engagement but at high peptide concentrations this is not an issue as the TCR can find more pMHC molecules

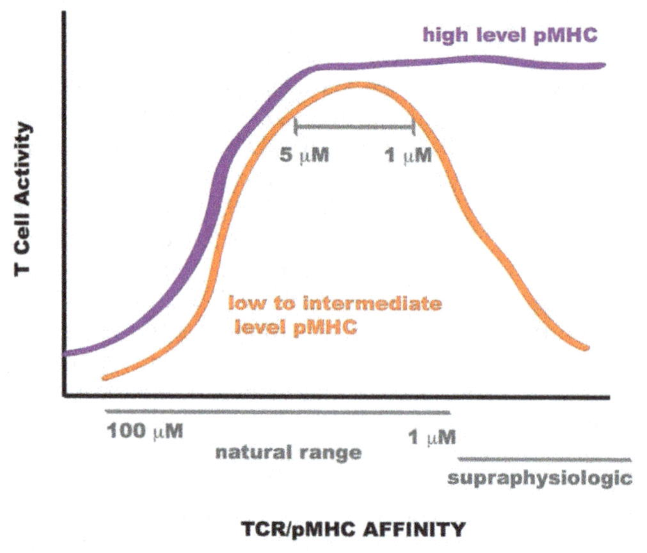

FIGURE 12 | Sketch of T cell activity as a function of TCR-pMHC affinity. At low to intermediate levels of pMHC, T-cell activity is optimal for TCR within K_D range 1–5 μM (orange curve). At high levels of pMHC T-cell activity is not attenuated for supraphysiologic affinity TCR (purple curve).

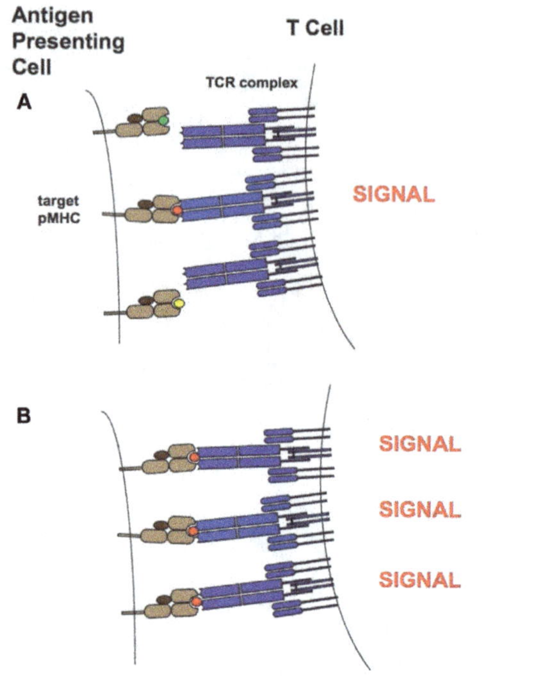

FIGURE 13 | T-cell activation in the presence of limiting (A) or saturating levels (B) of target pMHC complex. In the case where target pMHC concentration is limiting, TCRs of too high-affinity may inhibit serial engagement and thereby attenuate T-cell activity levels. MHCs are colored in light brown, β2-microglobulins in dark brown, TCRs in blue and peptide antigens are shown as small green, red, and yellow circles. The peptide colored in red corresponds to the specific antigen.

on the target-cell-surface. This is demonstrated in **Figure 13**. Our work also demonstrated the value of a modeling approach because TCRs with particular binding parameters, i.e., falling within an optimal affinity range, either through faster on-rates or slower off-rates, can be developed to enable maximum T cell activity levels.

CONCLUSION

We found that the synergy between *in silico* design, and *in vitro* testing using both soluble molecules and transfected cells is key to the design of improved TCRs to be used in adoptive cell transfer therapies. Using an innovative structural approach based on recent *in silico* techniques, we have developed a method to rationally optimize the surface of the TCR to increase its affinity for pMHC. As opposed to library screening, we propose a step-wise, incremental optimization of the TCR. This allows the preservation of the favorable initial properties of the TCR through the various cycles. Our optimization method can selectively target contacts involving the MHC or the peptide, thus maintaining a good balance between overall affinity and specificity. In addition, modifying only a few amino acids reduces the risk of obtaining undesired cross-recognition or raising anti-TCR antibodies *in vivo*. This rational optimization approach is therefore very promising to the design of TCRs for adoptive T cell immunotherapy clinical trials.

The application of our TCR engineering approach to the tumor-targeting BC1 TCR targeted to the A2/NY-ESO-$1_{157-165}$ antigen identified several original single mutations of the CDR loops conferring increased experimental affinity for pMHC compared to the wild-type TCR. T cells expressing some of the affinity-enhanced TCR showed better overall functionality, including improved killing of both peptide-loaded T2 cells and melanoma tumor cell lines, higher proliferative capacity, and increased levels of cytokine/chemokine secretion, as compared to wild-type TCR expressing T cells. For all functional assays, we observed a gain in $CD8^+$ T cell activity level with increase in affinity, with a peak at an affinity of ~1–5 μM. Beyond this affinity we observed a progressive decrease in activity levels. We are currently testing the relative activity of the different TCRs *in vivo* in a mouse model. The successful candidates are planned to enter a phase I clinical trial program for stage IV melanoma. As the methods presented here are general and transferable to any TCR-pMHC complex, other cancer types will follow shortly.

In parallel to direct applications of the existing approach, we will take advantage of the methodological work presented above to improve our *in silico* TCR optimization method. The development of homology-based approaches to model the 3D-structure of TCR-pMHC complexes potentially extends the use of our method to TCR repertoires for which no X-ray structure is available. The detailed picture of the TCR/pMHC interaction emerging from the MD simulations showed the presence of single water molecules trapped at the interface (20). Including these interfacial waters in the BFED scheme would improve accuracy in some cases. Close residues at protein–protein interfaces can display collaborative effects that result in the non-additivity of their contributions to the binding free energy, which will have to be taken into account in the next generation of TCR optimization methods. Noticeably, because the binding free energy decomposition method used is physics-based, without any *ad hoc* parameters, our *in silico* techniques are straightforwardly transferable to other types of macromolecular protein complexes.

ACKNOWLEDGMENTS

This work was supported by the Swiss National Center of Competence in Research and the Swiss National Science Foundation grants 3200B0-103173 (to O. Michielin) and by OncoSuisse grants OCS 01381-08-2003 (to O. Michielin) and 02555-02-2010 (to O. Michielin and V. Zoete). Molecular graphics images were produced using VMD and the UCSF Chimera package from the resources for Biocomputing, Visualization, and Informatics at the University of California, San Francisco, CA, USA. We thank the Vital-IT group from the Swiss Institute of Bioinformatics for providing the computational resources.

REFERENCES

1. Rudolph MG, Stanfield RL, Wilson IA. How TCRs bind MHCs, peptides, and coreceptors. *Annu Rev Immunol* (2006) **24**:419–66. doi:10.1146/annurev.immunol.23.021704.115658
2. Burrows SR, Chen Z, Archbold JK, Tynan FE, Beddoe T, Kjer-Nielsen L, et al. Hard wiring of T cell receptor specificity for the major histocompatibility complex is underpinned by TCR adaptability. *Proc Natl Acad Sci U S A* (2010) **107**:10608–13. doi:10.1073/pnas.1004926107
3. Garcia KC, Adams EJ. How the T cell receptor sees antigen-a structural view. *Cell* (2005) **122**:333–6. doi:10.1016/j.cell.2005.07.015
4. Godfrey DI, Rossjohn J, McCluskey J. The fidelity, occasional promiscuity, and versatility of T cell receptor recognition. *Immunity* (2008) **28**:304–14. doi:10.1016/j.immuni.2008.02.004
5. Davis MM, Boniface JJ, Reich Z, Lyons D, Hampl J, Arden B, et al. Ligand recognition by alpha beta T cell receptors. *Annu Rev Immunol* (1998) **16**:523–44. doi:10.1146/annurev.immunol.16.1.523
6. Dietrich P-Y, Le Gal F-A, Dutoit V, Pittet MJ, Trautman L, Zippelius A, et al. Prevalent role of TCR alpha-chain in the selection of the preimmune repertoire specific for a human tumor-associated self-antigen. *J Immunol* (2003) **170**:5103–9.
7. Irving M, Zoete V, Hebeisen M, Schmid D, Baumgartner P, Guillaume P, et al. Interplay between T cell receptor binding kinetics and the level of cognate peptide presented by major histocompatibility complexes governs $CD8^+$ T cell responsiveness. *J Biol Chem* (2012) **287**:23068–78. doi:10.1074/jbc.M112.357673
8. Schmid DA, Irving MB, Posevitz V, Hebeisen M, Posevitz-Fejfar A, Sarria J-CF, et al. Evidence for a TCR affinity threshold delimiting maximal CD8 T cell function. *J Immunol* (2010) **184**:4936–46. doi:10.4049/jimmunol.1000173
9. Valmori D, Dutoit V, Schnuriger V, Quiquerez A-L, Pittet MJ, Guillaume P, et al. Vaccination with a Melan-A peptide selects an oligoclonal T cell population with increased functional avidity and tumor reactivity. *J Immunol* (2002) **168**:4231–40.
10. Krogsgaard M, Davis MM. How T cells "see" antigen. *Nat Immunol* (2005) **6**:239–45. doi:10.1038/ni1173
11. Stone JD, Chervin AS, Kranz DM. T-cell receptor binding affinities and kinetics: impact on T-cell activity and specificity. *Immunology* (2009) **126**:165–76. doi:10.1111/j.1365-2567.2008.03015.x
12. Restifo NP, Dudley ME, Rosenberg SA. Adoptive immunotherapy for cancer: harnessing the T cell response. *Nat Rev Immunol* (2012) **12**:269–81. doi:10.1038/nri3191
13. Rosenberg SA, Restifo NP, Yang JC, Morgan RA, Dudley ME. Adoptive cell transfer: a clinical path to effective cancer immunotherapy. *Nat Rev Cancer* (2008) **8**:299–308. doi:10.1038/nrc2355
14. Khan JM, Cheruku HR, Tong JC, Ranganathan S. MPID-T2: a database for sequence-structure-function analyses of pMHC and TR/pMHC structures. *Bioinformatics* (2011) **27**:1192–3. doi:10.1093/bioinformatics/btr104
15. Gras S, Burrows SR, Turner SJ, Sewell AK, McCluskey J, Rossjohn J. A structural voyage toward an understanding of the MHC-I-restricted immune response: lessons learned and much to be learned. *Immunol Rev* (2012) **250**:61–81. doi:10.1111/j.1600-065X.2012.01159.x
16. Wang J-H, Reinherz EL. The structural basis of αβ T-lineage immune recognition: TCR docking topologies, mechanotransduction, and co-receptor function. *Immunol Rev* (2012) **250**:102–19. doi:10.1111/j.1600-065X.2012.01161.x
17. Armstrong KM, Insaidoo FK, Baker BM. Thermodynamics of T-cell receptor-peptide/MHC interactions: progress and opportunities. *J Mol Recognit* (2008) **21**:275–87. doi:10.1002/jmr.896
18. Ding YH, Baker BM, Garboczi DN, Biddison WE. Four A6-TCR/peptide/HLA-A2 structures that generate very different T cell signals are nearly identical. *Immunity* (1999) **11**:45. doi:10.1016/S1074-7613(00)80080-1
19. Davis-Harrison RL, Armstrong KM, Baker BM. Two different T cell receptors use different thermodynamic strategies to recognize the same peptide/MHC ligand. *J Mol Biol* (2005) **346**:533–50. doi:10.1016/j.jmb.2004.11.063
20. Cuendet MA, Zoete V, Michielin O. How T cell receptors interact with peptide-MHCs: a multiple steered molecular dynamics study. *Proteins* (2011) **79**:3007–24. doi:10.1002/prot.23104
21. Lindahl E, Hess B, van der Spoel D. GROMACS 3.0: a package for molecular simulation and trajectory analysis. *J Mol Mod* (2001) **7**:306.
22. Daura X, Mark AE, van Gunsteren WF. Parametrization of aliphatic CHn united atoms of GROMOS96 force field. *J Comput Chem* (1998) **19**:535–47. doi:10.1002/(SICI)1096-987X(19980415)19:5<535::AID-JCC6>3.0.CO;2-N
23. Wu LC, Tuot DS, Lyons DS, Garcia KC, Davis MM. Two-step binding mechanism for T-cell receptor recognition of peptide MHC. *Nature* (2002) **418**:552–6. doi:10.1038/nature00920
24. Gagnon SJ, Borbulevych OY, Davis-Harrison RL, Baxter TK, Clemens JR, Armstrong KM, et al. Unraveling a hotspot for TCR recognition on HLA-A2: evidence against the existence of peptide-independent TCR binding determinants. *J Mol Biol* (2005) **353**:556–73. doi:10.1016/j.jmb.2005.08.024
25. Boudinot P, Marriotti-Ferrandiz ME, Pasquier LD, Benmansour A, Cazenave P-A, Six A. New perspectives for large-scale repertoire analysis of immune receptors. *Mol Immunol* (2008) **45**:2437–45. doi:10.1016/j.molimm.2007.12.018
26. Derré L, Bruyninx M, Baumgaertner P, Ferber M, Schmid D, Leimgruber A, et al. Distinct sets of alphabeta TCRs confer similar recognition of tumor antigen NY-ESO-$1_{157-165}$ by interacting with its central Met/Trp residues. *Proc Natl Acad Sci U S A* (2008) **105**:15010–5. doi:10.1073/pnas.0807954105
27. Romero P, Dunbar PR, Valmori D, Pittet M, Ogg GS, Rimoldi D, et al. *Ex vivo* staining of metastatic lymph nodes by class I major histocompatibility complex tetramers reveals high numbers of antigen-experienced tumor-specific cytolytic T lymphocytes. *J Exp Med* (1998) **188**:1641–50. doi:10.1084/jem.188.9.1641
28. Leimgruber A, Ferber M, Irving M, Hussain-Kahn H, Wieckowski S, Derré L, et al. TCRep 3D: an automated *in silico* approach to study the structural properties of TCR repertoires. *PLoS ONE* (2011) **6**:e26301. doi:10.1371/journal.pone.0026301
29. Michielin O, Luescher I, Karplus M. Modeling of the TCR-MHC-peptide complex. *J Mol Biol* (2000) **300**:1205–35. doi:10.1006/jmbi.2000.3788
30. Zoete V, Irving MB, Michielin O. MM-GBSA binding free energy decomposition and T cell receptor engineering. *J Mol Recognit* (2010) **23**:142–52. doi:10.1002/jmr.1005
31. Ehrenmann F, Lefranc M-P. IMGT/3D structure-DB: querying the IMGT database for 3D structures in immunology and immunoinformatics (IG or antibodies, TR, MH, RPI, and FPIA). *Cold Spring Harb Protoc* (2011) **2011**:750–61. doi:10.1101/pdb.prot5637
32. Ehrenmann F, Kaas Q, Lefranc M-P. IMGT/3D structure-DB and IMGT/DomainGapAlign: a database and a tool for immunoglobulins or antibodies, T cell receptors, MHC, IgSF and MhcSF. *Nucleic Acids Res* (2010) **38**:D301–7. doi:10.1093/nar/gkp946
33. Arstila TP, Casrouge A, Baron V, Even J, Kanellopoulos J, Kourilsky P. A direct estimate of the human alphabeta T cell receptor diversity. *Science* (1999) **286**:958–61. doi:10.1126/science.286.5441.958

34. Robins HS, Campregher PV, Srivastava SK, Wacher A, Turtle CJ, Kahsai O, et al. Comprehensive assessment of T-cell receptor beta-chain diversity in alphabeta T cells. *Blood* (2009) **114**:4099–107. doi: 10.1182/blood-2009-04-217604
35. Kessler B, Michielin O, Blanchard CL, Apostolou I, Delarbre C, Gachelin G, et al. T cell recognition of hapten. Anatomy of T cell receptor binding of a H-2kd-associated photoreactive peptide derivative. *J Biol Chem* (1999) **274**:3622–31. doi:10.1074/jbc.274.6.3622
36. Eswar N, Webb B, Marti-Renom MA, Madhusudhan MS, Eramian D, Shen M-Y, et al. Comparative protein structure modeling using Modeller. *Curr Protoc Bioinformatics* (2006) **5**:Unit5.6.
37. Martí-Renom MA, Stuart AC, Fiser A, Sánchez R, Melo F, Sali A. Comparative protein structure modeling of genes and genomes. *Annu Rev Biophys Biomol Struct* (2000) **29**:291–325. doi:10.1146/annurev.biophys.29.1.291
38. Sali A, Blundell TL. Comparative protein modelling by satisfaction of spatial restraints. *J Mol Biol* (1993) **234**:779–815. doi:10.1006/jmbi.1993.1626
39. Bentley GA, Boulot G, Karjalainen K, Mariuzza RA. Crystal structure of the beta chain of a T cell antigen receptor. *Science* (1995) **267**:1984–7. doi:10.1126/science.7701320
40. Fields BA, Ober B, Malchiodi EL, Lebedeva MI, Braden BC, Ysern X, et al. Crystal structure of the V alpha domain of a T cell antigen receptor. *Science* (1995) **270**:1821–4. doi:10.1126/science.270.5243.1821
41. Garboczi DN, Ghosh P, Utz U, Fan QR, Biddison WE, Wiley DC. Structure of the complex between human T-cell receptor, viral peptide and HLA-A2. *Nature* (1996) **384**:134–41. doi:10.1038/384134a0
42. Garcia KC, Degano M, Pease LR, Huang M, Peterson PA, Teyton L, et al. Structural basis of plasticity in T cell receptor recognition of a self peptide-MHC antigen. *Science* (1998) **279**:1166–72. doi:10.1126/science.279.5354.1166
43. Fremont DH, Stura EA, Matsumura M, Peterson PA, Wilson IA. Crystal structure of an H-2Kb-ovalbumin peptide complex reveals the interplay of primary and secondary anchor positions in the major histocompatibility complex binding groove. *Proc Natl Acad Sci U S A* (1995) **92**:2479–83. doi:10.1073/pnas.92.7.2479
44. Fiser A, Do RK, Sali A. Modeling of loops in protein structures. *Protein Sci* (2000) **9**:1753–73. doi:10.1110/ps.9.9.1753
45. Fagerberg T, Cerottini J-C, Michielin O. Structural prediction of peptides bound to MHC class I. *J Mol Biol* (2006) **356**:521–46. doi:10.1016/j.jmb.2005.11.059
46. Al-Lazikani B, Lesk AM, Chothia C. Canonical structures for the hypervariable regions of T cell alphabeta receptors. *J Mol Biol* (2000) **295**:979–95. doi:10.1006/jmbi.1999.3358
47. Derré L, Ferber M, Touvrey C, Devevre E, Zoete V, Leimgruber A, et al. A novel population of human melanoma-specific CD8 T cells recognizes Melan-AMART-1 immunodominant nonapeptide but not the corresponding decapeptide. *J Immunol* (2007) **179**:7635–45.
48. Khan JM, Ranganathan S. Understanding TR binding to pMHC complexes: how does a TR scan many pMHC complexes yet preferentially bind to one. *PLoS ONE* (2011) **6**:e17194. doi:10.1371/journal.pone.0017194
49. Roomp K, Domingues FS. Predicting interactions between T cell receptors and MHC-peptide complexes. *Mol Immunol* (2011) **48**:553–62. doi:10.1016/j.molimm.2010.10.014
50. Varani L, Bankovich AJ, Liu CW, Colf LA, Jones LL, Kranz DM, et al. Solution mapping of T cell receptor docking footprints on peptide-MHC. *Proc Natl Acad Sci U S A* (2007) **104**:13080–5. doi:10.1073/pnas.0703702104
51. Brooks BR, Brooks CL, Mackerell AD, Nilsson L, Petrella RJ, Roux B, et al. CHARMM: the biomolecular simulation program. *J Comput Chem* (2009) **30**:1545–614. doi:10.1002/jcc.21287
52. Mackerell AD, Bashford D, Bellott M, Dunbrack RL, Evanseck JD, Field MJ, et al. All-atom empirical potential for molecular modeling and dynamics studies of proteins. *J Phys Chem B* (1998) **102**:3586–616. doi:10.1021/jp973084f
53. Haberthür U, Caflisch A. FACTS: fast analytical continuum treatment of solvation. *J Comput Chem* (2008) **29**:701–15. doi:10.1002/jcc.20832
54. Zoete V, Meuwly M, Karplus M. Study of the insulin dimerization: binding free energy calculations and per-residue free energy decomposition. *Proteins* (2005) **61**:79–93. doi:10.1002/prot.20528
55. Ferber M, Zoete V, Michielin O. T-cell receptors binding orientation over peptide/MHC class I is driven by long-range interactions. *PLoS ONE* (2012) **7**:e51943. doi:10.1371/journal.pone.0051943
56. Baker BM, Gagnon SJ, Biddison WE, Wiley DC. Conversion of a T cell antagonist into an agonist by repairing a defect in the TCR/peptide/MHC interface: implications for TCR signaling. *Immunity* (2000) **13**:475–84. doi:10.1016/S1074-7613(00)00047-9
57. Michielin O, Karplus M. Binding free energy differences in a TCR-peptide-MHC complex induced by a peptide mutation: a simulation analysis. *J Mol Biol* (2002) **324**:547–69. doi:10.1016/S0022-2836(02)00880-X
58. Christ CD, Mark AE, van Gunsteren WF. Basic ingredients of free energy calculations: a review. *J Comput Chem* (2010) **31**:1569–82. doi:10.1002/jcc.21450
59. Cuendet MA, Zoete V, Michielin O. Molecular Dynamics-based Free Energy Simulations. In: Schwede T, Peitsch M editors. *Computational Structural Biology*. Singapore: World Scientific Publishing (2008). p. 513–48.
60. Gao J, Kuczera K, Tidor B, Karplus M. Hidden thermodynamics of mutant proteins: a molecular dynamics analysis. *Science* (1989) **244**:1069–72. doi:10.1126/science.2727695
61. Kirkwood JG. Statistical mechanics of fluid mixture. *J Chem Phys* (1935) **3**:300–13. doi:10.1063/1.1749657
62. Boresch S, Karplus M. The role of bonded terms in free energy simulations: 1. Theoretical analysis. *J Phys Chem A* (2013) **103**:103–18. doi:10.1021/jp981628n
63. Beutler TC, Mark AE, van Schaik RC, Gerber PB, van Gunsteren WF. Avoiding singularities and numerical instabilities in free energy calculations based on molecular simulations. *Chem Phys Lett* (1994) **222**:529–39. doi:10.1016/0009-2614(94)00397-1
64. Madden DR, Garboczi DN, Wiley DC. The antigenic identity of peptide-MHC complexes: a comparison of the conformations of five viral peptides presented by HLA-A2. *Cell* (1993) **75**:693–708. doi:10.1016/0092-8674(93)90490-H
65. Brooks CL, Brünger A, Karplus M. Active site dynamics in protein molecules: a stochastic boundary molecular-dynamics approach. *Biopolymers* (1985) **24**:843–65. doi:10.1002/bip.360240509
66. Jarzynski C. A non-equilibrium equality for free energy differences. *Phys Rev Lett* (1997) **78**:2690–3. doi:10.1103/PhysRevLett.78.2690
67. Jarzynski C. Equilibrium free energy differences from nonequilibrium measurements: a master equation approach. *Phys Rev E* (1997) **56**:5018–35. doi:10.1103/PhysRevE.56.5018
68. Cuendet MA. Statistical mechanical derivation of Jarzynski's identity for thermostated non-Hamiltonian dynamics. *Phys Rev Lett* (2006) **96**:120602. doi:10.1103/PhysRevLett.96.120602
69. Cuendet MA. The Jarzynski identity derived from general Hamiltonian or non-Hamiltonian dynamics reproducing NVT or NPT ensembles. *J Chem Phys* (2006) **125**:144109–144109–12. doi:10.1063/1.2338535
70. Isralewitz B, Davis-Harrison RL, Baudry J, Armstrong KM, Gullingsrud J, Baker BM, et al. Steered molecular dynamics investigations of protein function. *J Mol Graphics Modell* (2001) **19**:13. doi:10.1016/S1093-3263(00)00133-9
71. Park S, Schulten K. Calculating potentials of mean force from steered molecular dynamics information. *J Chem Phys* (2004) **120**:5946–61. doi:10.1063/1.1651473
72. Cuendet MA, Michielin O. Protein-protein interaction investigated by steered molecular dynamics: the TCR-pMHC complex. *Biophys J* (2008) **95**:3575–90. doi:10.1529/biophysj.108.131383
73. Hummer G, Szabo A. Free energy reconstruction from non-equilibrium single-molecule pulling experiments. *Proc Natl Acad Sci U S A* (2001) **98**:3658–61. doi:10.1073/pnas.071034098
74. Schurr JM, Fujimoto BS. Equalities for the non-equilibrium work transferred from an external potential to a molecular system. analysis of single-molecule extension experiments. *J Phys Chem B* (2003) **107**:14007–19. doi:10.1021/jp0306803
75. Hendrix DA, Jarzynski C. A "fast growth" method of computing free energy differences. *J Chem Phys* (2001) **114**:5974. doi:10.1063/1.1353552

76. Oberhofer H, Dellago C, Geissler PL. Biased sampling of non-equilibrium trajectories: can fast switching simulations outperform conventional free energy calculation methods? *J Phys Chem B* (2005) **109**:6902–15. doi:10.1021/jp044556a
77. Rudolph MG, Zuckerman DM, Stanfield RL, Woolf TB, Wilson IA. Systematic finite-sampling inaccuracy in free energy differences and other non-linear quantities. *J Stat Phys* (2004) **114**:1303. doi:10.1023/B:JOSS.0000013961.84860.5b
78. Shirts MR, Pande VS. Comparison of efficiency and bias of free energies computed by exponential averaging, the Bennett acceptance ratio, and thermodynamic integration. *J Chem Phys* (2005) **122**:144107. doi:10.1063/1.1873592
79. Ytreberg FM, Swendsen RH, Zuckerman DM. Comparison of free energy methods for molecular systems. *J Chem Phys* (2006) **125**:184114. doi:10.1063/1.2378907
80. Kollman PA, Massova I, Reyes C, Kuhn B, Huo S, Chong L, et al. Calculating structures and free energies of complex molecules: combining molecular mechanics and continuum models. *Acc Chem Res* (2000) **33**:889–97. doi:10.1021/ar000033j
81. Gilson MK, Honig B. Calculation of the total electrostatic energy of a macromolecular system: solvation energies, binding energies, and conformational analysis. *Proteins* (1988) **4**:7–18. doi:10.1002/prot.340040104
82. Gilson MK, Honig BH. Energetics of charge-charge interactions in proteins. *Proteins* (1988) **3**:32–52. doi:10.1002/prot.340030104
83. Still WC, Tempczyk A, Hawley RC, Hendrickson T. Semianalytical treatment of solvation for molecular mechanics and dynamics. *J Am Chem Soc* (1990) **112**:6127–9. doi:10.1021/ja00172a038
84. Gohlke H, Kiel C, Case DA. Insights into protein-protein binding by binding free energy calculation and free energy decomposition for the Ras-Raf and Ras-RalGDS complexes. *J Mol Biol* (2003) **330**:891–913. doi:10.1016/S0022-2836(03)00610-7
85. Amidon GL, Yalkowsky SH, Anik ST, Valvani SC. Solubility of non-electrolytes in polar solvents. V. Estimation of the solubility of aliphatic monofunctional compounds in water using a molecular surface area approach. *J Phys Chem* (2013) **79**:2239–46. doi:10.1021/j100588a008
86. Tidor B, Karplus M. The contribution of vibrational entropy to molecular association. The dimerization of insulin. *J Mol Biol* (1994) **238**:405–14. doi:10.1006/jmbi.1994.1300
87. Guo J, Wang X, Sun H, Liu H, Yao X. The molecular basis of IGF-II/IGF2R recognition: a combined molecular dynamics simulation, free-energy calculation and computational alanine scanning study. *J Mol Model* (2012) **18**:1421–30. doi:10.1007/s00894-011-1159-4
88. Lafont V, Schaefer M, Stote RH, Altschuh D, Dejaegere A. Protein-protein recognition and interaction hot spots in an antigen-antibody complex: free energy decomposition identifies "efficient amino acids." *Proteins* (2007) **67**:418–34. doi:10.1002/prot.21259
89. Oberlin M, Kroemer R, Mikol V, Minoux H, Tastan E, Baurin N. Engineering protein therapeutics: predictive performances of a structure-based virtual affinity maturation protocol. *J Chem Inf Model* (2012) **52**:2204–14. doi:10.1021/ci3001474
90. Zoete V, Michielin O. Comparison between computational alanine scanning and per-residue binding free energy decomposition for protein-protein association using MM-GBSA: application to the TCR-p-MHC complex. *Proteins* (2007) **67**:1026–47. doi:10.1002/prot.21395
91. Massova I, Kollman PA. Computational alanine scanning to probe protein-protein interactions: a novel approach to evaluate binding free energies. *J Am Chem Soc* (1999) **121**:8133–43. doi:10.1021/ja990935j
92. Degano M, Garcia KC, Apostolopoulos V, Rudolph MG, Teyton L, Wilson IA. A functional hot spot for antigen recognition in a superagonist TCR/MHC complex. *Immunity* (2000) **12**:251–61. doi:10.1016/S1074-7613(00)80178-8
93. Richman SA, Kranz DM. Display, engineering, and applications of antigen-specific T cell receptors. *Biomol Eng* (2007) **24**:361–73. doi:10.1016/j.bioeng.2007.02.009
94. Cole DK, Pumphrey NJ, Boulter JM, Sami M, Bell JI, Gostick E, et al. Human TCR-binding affinity is governed by MHC class restriction. *J Immunol* (2007) **178**:5727–34.
95. Johnson LA, Morgan RA, Dudley ME, Cassard L, Yang JC, Hughes MS, et al. Gene therapy with human and mouse T-cell receptors mediates cancer regression and targets normal tissues expressing cognate antigen. *Blood* (2009) **114**:535–46. doi:10.1182/blood-2009-03-211714
96. Kalergis AM, Boucheron N, Doucey MA, Palmieri E, Goyarts EC, Vegh Z, et al. Efficient T cell activation requires an optimal dwell-time of interaction between the TCR and the pMHC complex. *Nat Immunol* (2001) **2**:229–34. doi:10.1038/85286
97. Valitutti S. The serial engagement model 17-years after: from tcr triggering to immunotherapy. *Front Immunol* (2012) **3**:272. doi:10.3389/fimmu.2012.00272
98. Aleksic M, Dushek O, Zhang H, Shenderov E, Chen J-L, Cerundolo V, et al. Dependence of T cell antigen recognition on T cell receptor-peptide MHC confinement time. *Immunity* (2010) **32**:163–74. doi:10.1016/j.immuni.2009.11.013
99. Chlewicki LK, Holler PD, Monti BC, Clutter MR, Kranz DM. High-affinity, peptide-specific T cell receptors can be generated by mutations in CDR1, CDR2 or CDR3. *J Mol Biol* (2005) **346**:223–39. doi:10.1016/j.jmb.2004.11.057
100. Holler PD, Holman PO, Shusta EV, O'Herrin S, Wittrup KD, Kranz DM. *In vitro* evolution of a T cell receptor with high affinity for peptide/MHC. *Proc Natl Acad Sci U S A* (2000) **97**:5387–92. doi:10.1073/pnas.080078297
101. Holler PD, Kranz DM. Quantitative analysis of the contribution of TCR/pepMHC affinity and CD8 to T cell activation. *Immunity* (2003) **18**:255–64. doi:10.1016/S1074-7613(03)00019-0
102. Li Y, Moysey R, Molloy PE, Vuidepot A-L, Mahon T, Baston E, et al. Directed evolution of human T-cell receptors with picomolar affinities by phage display. *Nat Biotechnol* (2005) **23**:349–54. doi:10.1038/nbt1070
103. Dunn SM, Rizkallah PJ, Baston E, Mahon T, Cameron B, Moysey R, et al. Directed evolution of human T cell receptor CDR2 residues by phage display dramatically enhances affinity for cognate peptide-MHC without increasing apparent cross-reactivity. *Protein Sci* (2006) **15**:710–21. doi:10.1110/ps.051936406
104. Bowerman NA, Crofts TS, Chlewicki L, Do P, Baker BM, Christopher Garcia K, et al. Engineering the binding properties of the T cell receptor:peptide:MHC ternary complex that governs T cell activity. *Mol Immunol* (2009) **46**:3000–8. doi:10.1016/j.molimm.2009.06.012
105. Buonpane RA, Moza B, Sundberg EJ, Kranz DM. Characterization of T cell receptors engineered for high affinity against toxic shock syndrome toxin-1. *J Mol Biol* (2005) **353**:308–21. doi:10.1016/j.jmb.2005.08.041
106. Kieke MC, Sundberg E, Shusta EV, Mariuzza RA, Wittrup KD, Kranz DM. High affinity T cell receptors from yeast display libraries block T cell activation by superantigens. *J Mol Biol* (2001) **307**:1305–15. doi:10.1006/jmbi.2001.4560
107. Zhao Y, Bennett AD, Zheng Z, Wang QJ, Robbins PF, Yu LYL, et al. High-affinity TCRs generated by phage display provide $CD4^+$ T cells with the ability to recognize and kill tumor cell lines. *J Immunol* (2007) **179**:5845–54.
108. Chervin AS, Aggen DH, Raseman JM, Kranz DM. Engineering higher affinity T cell receptors using a T cell display system. *J Immunol Methods* (2008) **339**:175–84. doi:10.1016/j.jim.2008.09.016
109. Kessels HW, van Den Boom MD, Spits H, Hooijberg E, Schumacher TN. Changing T cell specificity by retroviral T cell receptor display. *Proc Natl Acad Sci U S A* (2000) **97**:14578–83. doi:10.1073/pnas.97.26.14578
110. Hawkins RE, Gilham DE, Debets R, Eshhar Z, Taylor N, Abken H, et al. Development of adoptive cell therapy for cancer: a clinical perspective. *Hum Gene Ther* (2010) **21**:665–72. doi:10.1089/hum.2010.086
111. Barrozo A, Borstnar R, Marloie G, Kamerlin SCL. Computational protein engineering: bridging the gap between rational design and laboratory evolution. *Int J Mol Sci* (2012) **13**:12428–60. doi:10.3390/ijms131012428
112. Karanicolas J, Kuhlman B. Computational design of affinity and specificity at protein-protein interfaces. *Curr Opin Struct Biol* (2009) **19**:458–63. doi:10.1016/j.sbi.2009.07.005
113. Pantazes RJ, Maranas CD. OptCDR: a general computational method for the design of antibody complementarity determining regions for

targeted epitope binding. *Protein Eng Des Sel* (2010) **23**:849–58. doi:10.1093/protein/gzq061

114. Pantazes RJ, Grisewood MJ, Maranas CD. Recent advances in computational protein design. *Curr Opin Struct Biol* (2011) **21**:467–72. doi:10.1016/j.sbi.2011.04.005
115. Samish I, MacDermaid CM, Perez-Aguilar JM, Saven JG. Theoretical and computational protein design. *Annu Rev Phys Chem* (2011) **62**:129–49. doi:10.1146/annurev-physchem-032210-103509
116. Haidar JN, Pierce B, Yu Y, Tong W, Li M, Weng Z. Structure-based design of a T-cell receptor leads to nearly 100-fold improvement in binding affinity for pepMHC. *Proteins* (2009) **74**:948–60. doi:10.1002/prot.22203
117. Le Gal F-A, Ayyoub M, Dutoit V, Widmer V, Jäger E, Cerottini J-C, et al. Distinct structural TCR repertoires in naturally occurring versus vaccine-induced CD8^{+} T-cell responses to the tumor-specific antigen NY-ESO-1. *J Immunother* (2005) **28**:252–7. doi:10.1097/01.cji.0000161398.34701.26
118. Atanackovic D, Arfsten J, Cao Y, Gnjatic S, Schnieders F, Bartels K, et al. Cancer-testis antigens are commonly expressed in multiple myeloma and induce systemic immunity following allogeneic stem cell transplantation. *Blood* (2007) **109**:1103–12. doi:10.1182/blood-2006-04-014480
119. Chen YT, Scanlan MJ, Sahin U, Türeci O, Gure AO, Tsang S, et al. A testicular antigen aberrantly expressed in human cancers detected by autologous antibody screening. *Proc Natl Acad Sci U S A* (1997) **94**:1914–8. doi:10.1073/pnas.94.5.1914
120. Liggins AP, Lim SH, Soilleux EJ, Pulford K, Banham AH. A panel of cancer-testis genes exhibiting broad-spectrum expression in haematological malignancies. *Cancer Immun* (2010) **10**:8.
121. Lim SH, Austin S, Owen-Jones E, Robinson L. Expression of testicular genes in haematological malignancies. *Br J Cancer* (1999) **81**:1162–4. doi:10.1038/sj.bjc.6690824
122. Marsh S, Parham P, Barber LD. *The HLA Factsbook.* (1999).
123. Yuan J, Adamow M, Ginsberg BA, Rasalan TS, Ritter E, Gallardo HF, et al. Integrated NY-ESO-1 antibody and CD8^{+} T-cell responses correlate with clinical benefit in advanced melanoma patients treated with ipilimumab. *Proc Natl Acad Sci U S A* (2011) **108**:16723–8. doi:10.1073/pnas.1110814108
124. Chen J-L, Stewart-Jones G, Bossi G, Lissin NM, Wooldridge L, Choi EML, et al. Structural and kinetic basis for heightened immunogenicity of T cell vaccines. *J Exp Med* (2005) **201**:1243–55. doi:10.1084/jem.20042323
125. Rose PW, Bi C, Bluhm WF, Christie CH, Dimitropoulos D, Dutta S, et al. The RCSB Protein Data Bank: new resources for research and education. *Nucleic Acids Res* (2013) **41**:D475–82. doi:10.1093/nar/gks1200
126. Sami M, Rizkallah PJ, Dunn S, Molloy P, Moysey R, Vuidepot A, et al. Crystal structures of high affinity human T-cell receptors bound to peptide major histocompatibility complex reveal native diagonal binding geometry. *Protein Eng Des Sel* (2007) **20**:397–403. doi:10.1093/protein/gzm033
127. Hubbard RE, Haider MK. Hydrogen bonds in proteins: role and strength. *Encyclopedia of Life Science* (2001). 1–6.
128. Chang HC, Bao Z, Yao Y, Tse AG, Goyarts EC, Madsen M, et al. A general method for facilitating heterodimeric pairing between two proteins: application to expression of alpha and beta T-cell receptor extracellular segments. *Proc Natl Acad Sci U S A* (1994) **91**:11408–12. doi:10.1073/pnas.91.24.11408
129. Boulter JM, Glick M, Todorov PT, Baston E, Sami M, Rizkallah P, et al. Stable, soluble T-cell receptor molecules for crystallization and therapeutics. *Protein Eng* (2003) **16**:707–11. doi:10.1093/protein/gzg087
130. Janin J. The kinetics of protein-protein recognition. *Proteins* (1997) **28**:153–61. doi:10.1002/(SICI)1097-0134(199706)28:2<153::AID-PROT4>3.0.CO;2-G
131. Tian S, Maile R, Collins EJ, Frelinger JA. CD8^{+} T cell activation is governed by TCR-peptide/MHC affinity, not dissociation rate. *J Immunol* (2007) **179**:2952–60.
132. Kersh EN, Shaw AS, Allen PM. Fidelity of T cell activation through multistep T cell receptor zeta phosphorylation. *Science* (1998) **281**:572–5. doi:10.1126/science.281.5376.572
133. McKeithan TW. Kinetic proofreading in T-cell receptor signal transduction. *Proc Natl Acad Sci U S A* (1995) **92**:5042–6. doi:10.1073/pnas.92.11.5042
134. Valitutti S, Müller S, Cella M, Padovan E, Lanzavecchia A. Serial triggering of many T-cell receptors by a few peptide-MHC complexes. *Nature* (1995) **375**:148–51. doi:10.1038/375148a0
135. Dushek O, Aleksic M, Wheeler RJ, Zhang H, Cordoba S-P, Peng Y-C, et al. Antigen potency and maximal efficacy reveal a mechanism of efficient T cell activation. *Sci Signal* (2011) **4**:ra39. doi:10.1126/scisignal.2001430

16

Monitoring the dynamics of T cell clonal diversity using recombinant peptide: MHC technology

J. Lori Blanchfield, Shayla K. Shorter and Brian D. Evavold*

Department of Microbiology and Immunology, Emory University, Atlanta, GA, USA

Edited by:
Bruno Laugel, Cardiff University School of Medicine, UK

Reviewed by:
Nick Gascoigne, Scripps Research Institute, USA
Peter Sun, National Institutes of Health, USA
Johannes Huppa, Medical University of Vienna, Austria

***Correspondence:**
Brian D. Evavold, Department of Microbiology and Immunology, Emory University, 1510 Clifton Road, Atlanta, GA 30322, USA
e-mail: bevavol@emory.edu

The capacity to probe antigen specific T cells within the polyclonal repertoire has been revolutionized by the advent of recombinant peptide:MHC (pMHC) technology. Monomers and multimers of pMHC molecules can enrich for and identify antigen specific T cells to elucidate the contributions of T cell frequency, localization, and T cell receptor (TCR) affinity during immune responses. Two-dimensional (2D) measurements of TCR–pMHC interactions are at the forefront of this field because the biological topography is replicated such that TCR and pMHC are membrane anchored on opposing cells, allowing for biologically pertinent measures of TCR antigen specificity and diversity. 2D measurements of TCR-pMHC kinetics have also demonstrated increased fidelity compared to three-dimensional surface plasmon resonance data and are capable of detecting T cell affinities that are below the detection level of most pMHC multimers. Importantly, 2D techniques provide a platform to evaluate T cell affinity and antigen specificity against multiple protein epitopes within the polyclonal repertoire directly *ex vivo* from sites of ongoing immune responses. This review will discuss how antigen specific pMHC molecules, with a focus on 2D technologies, can be used as effective tools to evaluate the range of TCR affinities that comprise an immune response and more importantly how the breadth of affinities determine functional outcome against a given exposure to antigen.

Keywords: kinetics, 2D assays, T cell activation, recombinant pMHC, T cell affinity

DETECTION OF ANTIGEN SPECIFIC T CELLS

The ability to mount an effective immune response is essential to the survival of a living organism. Adaptive immunity in particular allows vertebrates a defense mechanism against countless pathogens. Antigen receptors on lymphocyte surfaces allow for recognition of a specific target, leading to activation and subsequent expansion of effector cells. This process is heavily dependent on affinity and on/off rate binding kinetics of the receptor for antigen. Though it is generally accepted that the highest affinity and thus most fit lymphocytes are selectively expanded (1, 2), the exact affinities of lymphocytes needed for an optimal immune response are still unknown.

During the course of a B cell response, somatic hypermutation in the germinal center allows for editing of the B cell receptor (BCR) to improve the affinity of the responding cells. This process involves the introduction of random mutations in the antigen binding site that can result in enhanced recognition of the target antigen. B cell affinity maturation allows higher affinity cells to outcompete less fit, lower affinity clones. While T cells also selectively expand responders based on specificity for antigen, T cells do not undergo receptor editing to improve the specificity of the response. Of interest, some reports have shown that mature T cells can re-express V(D)J recombination machinery and facilitate rearrangement of the T cell receptor (TCR) (3, 4). As the concept of TCR editing in the periphery may require further investigation, this review will assume that the TCR is fixed once the T cell has matured and entered the periphery. From the predetermined TCR repertoire, mature T cells are still able to generate diverse antigen specific polyclonal responses. This leads to the questions of what affinity range defines an optimal T cell response and what technology is best suited to evaluate this aspect of T cell diversity.

One way to detect diversity of the TCR repertoire is through the analysis of antigen driven changes in Vβ chain usage and complimentary determining region (CDR3) sequences during the course of an immune response. The αβ chains of the conventional TCR are encoded by V, D, J genes. Recombination of these gene segments concomitant with nucleotide insertions and imprecise joining events yields highly diverse T cell receptors. The CDR3 region, formed from the joining of the αβ TCR chains, directly contacts the antigen in the binding groove and thus reflects the antigen specificity of the clone (5). Studies show that during the course of an immune response, certain Vβ chains are preferentially expanded to create a unique signature of antigen specificity and clonal dominance of an immune response (6–8). Spectratyping or immunoscope analysis is a technique in which the sequence length of the CDR3 is derived from the DNA of bulk clonal populations typically identified by Vβ usage (9). CDR3 sequence length has been used to subset and characterize T cell clonal populations for specific antigens (10, 11). Tracking CDR3 lengths and Vβ profiles can also provide insight in monitoring disease progression and for diagnostic purposes (12–15). Though repertoire analyses via these methods have revealed useful information, they lack the fine resolution to assess the diversity of a T cell clonal response. For example, these methods are primarily done on bulk cellular populations resulting in conclusions based on a population average rather than on individual clones. More recent inquiries have shown this critical limitation fails to identify the paired TCRα and β chains responsible for the antigen recognition (16) and as a result, attempts to modify the techniques for single-clone analysis are being pursued (17). Future research combining single-cell analyses of TCRαβ chain usage along with functional readouts and kinetic measurements will greatly enhance our knowledge of the T cells that comprise the polyclonal repertoire.

The detection of antigen specific T cells concomitant with the characterization of their functional responsiveness has been key to providing insights into the factors that promote pathogenic specific and protective immunity. Historically, the tracking of antigen specific T cells in a polyclonal environment has been performed with functional assays assessing proliferation, production of cytokines, cytotoxic mediators, and protein markers of cell activation. These indirect markers are important for characterizing T cell phenotype but may poorly represent the entire polyclonal repertoire because detection depends on antigen dose utilized in the assay as well as the efficiency of the assay itself. Stimulation with high dose, cognate antigen may negatively bias T cell detection toward a low affinity profile by eliminating the higher affinity clones though activation induced cell death (18), while low dose cognate antigen may selectively detect cells with higher affinity TCR. Therefore, a direct means for quantifying antigen specific T cells utilizing recombinant cognate or variant peptide:MHC (pMHC) molecules could provide more sensitive analytical tools for assessing the complexity of the entire responding T cell population (19).

The development of recombinant pMHC molecules for detection of a myriad of MHC class I and II epitopes from both foreign (bacteria, viruses, and parasites) and self proteins (tumors and targets of autoimmune attack) provide a method for specific assessment or targeting of the T cell repertoire. Multimers of pMHC, especially the biotin:streptavidin-based pMHC tetramer technology, provide accessible tools to determine the frequency of antigen specific T cells via flow cytometry (19) and to deplete antigen specific T cells *in vivo* (20, 21). Importantly, tetramers are useful for enumerating and enriching antigen specific T cells. The fluorophore attached to tetramers can allow for the "pull down" or enrichment of antigen specific cells from a polyclonal population for downstream applications such as determining precursory frequency of tetramer positive cells (22, 23). The efficiency of detection by multimers is due to the aggregation of TCR:antigen interactions that increase avidity and circumvent the short half life of interactions between TCR and pMHC (19, 24). MHC class I and II tetramers are the most commonly utilized multimer largely because monomers and dimers exhibited insufficient binding kinetics for TCR to facilitate detection by flow cytometry and were less stimulatory than tetramers (25). Advancements on multimer technology have been focused on increasing avidity through creation of progressively higher order oligomers, most notably the commercially available 5-armed pentamers (26–28) or 10-armed dextramers (29, 30). Despite the increased avidity provided by these reagents, multimers of higher order magnitude beyond pentamers provide, at most, modest increases in sensitivity of T cell detection (29, 30), possibly due to the physical constraints needed for multiple simultaneous TCR–pMHC interactions (31). Even in the case of pMHC tetramers, it is unlikely that all four monomers bind simultaneously due to steric hindrances (25, 32).

The efficiency of pMHC molecules to detect antigen specific T cells is also dependent on peptide orientation within the MHC groove. Peptide-MHC anchor residues, which typically lie at positions 1, 4, 6, and 9 of the core peptide for MHC class II, are key to the stability of the peptide within the MHC. Variations in the amino acid residues that contact MHC, termed MHC variant peptides, can weaken or stabilize the interaction between TCR and pMHC (33–36). Though MHC variant peptides have been used to stabilize interactions with MHC to enhance T cell detection, these modifications could confound downstream analyses. For instance, these changes could modify the secondary structure, altering the TCR contact residues (37, 38) and may impact accurate kinetic and functional analysis. Furthermore the non-covalent interactions between peptide and MHC class II are of particular concern because the binding groove is open at both ends and can allow for the peptide to slide into different binding registers and influence TCR detection of the pMHC complex (39). For example, we and others identified three to four peptide registers in the well described $OVA_{323-339}$ 17-mer peptide (40, 41) that have made uniform recombinant pMHC monomer production and especially the creation of tetramers somewhat difficult (41). One method to improve the tetramer production is through the use of a limited set of linker amino acids used to covalently attach peptide to the N-terminus of the MHC class II molecule (42). In addition, multiple binding registers can be limited by creating a disulfide bond or "lock" engineered via a cysteine residue on the peptide and on the MHC as reported for insulin B_{9-23}, $OVA_{323-339}$, and $HA_{126-138}$ peptides (41, 43). Despite the effective use of recombinant pMHC and tetramers for the identification of antigen reactive T cells, their use as direct measures of TCR frequency and affinity during an immune response can be problematic.

MEASURING TCR AFFINITY FOR pMHC

A critical determinant for an antigenic response is the strength of signal derived through the TCR (44, 45). Although many factors contribute to the translation of signals into a biological response (i.e., costimulation (46), duration of signal (47, 48), etc.), affinity is a major parameter that establishes and controls the contribution of all additional factors in this response. Characterization of T cell response dynamics requires methods to obtain biophysical measures of affinity and kinetic on/off rates between TCR and recombinant pMHC. Many of the models describing T cell activation have been postulated based on kinetic-binding data from three-dimensional (3D) and two-dimensional (2D) binding assays.

Purified TCR and pMHC proteins can be used to study binding kinetics in 3D using techniques such as surface plasmon resonance (SPR). In this case, TCR and pMHC protein interactions occur in a fluid filled 3D space and affinity is measured in terms of the molar concentration needed to generate binding; TCR-pMHC affinity can range from 1 to 100 μM while the half life of the interaction can range from 10 to 100 s (49–52). SPR analysis provided the biophysical basis for models correlating TCR binding kinetics and T cell triggering in order to explain the functional differences seen between agonists, weak agonists, and antagonists (53–55). The most popular models are the kinetic proofreading and kinetic discrimination models, which ascribe optimal T cell responses to binding kinetics that allow sufficient time for TCR triggering (53, 54, 56, 57). Ligands that stimulate outside of this optimal time range, i.e., too long or too short, will not lead to a productive response according to these models. Despite the accuracy of these models in predicting agonist responses, several instances were identified where the biophysical measures did not relate to T cell activation state, particularly in response to weaker ligands (51, 57–62). These exceptions raised questions regarding the accuracy of 3D kinetic measurements derived from purified molecules to reflect the kinetics of proteins within the membrane environment. 3D assays are also limited in their ability to assess the full scope of a response due to the difficulty in purifying TCR from all participating antigen specific T cells. Therefore, alternative technologies are needed to probe the breadth of a polyclonal T cell response.

Analysis of receptor/ligand interactions using 2D technologies provides a physiologically relevant context in which to assay TCR affinity and the scope of polyclonal T cell responses because the TCR and pMHC are bound within cell membranes. Therefore these assays, namely the fluorescent based assays of FRAP and FRET, as well as the mechanical based micropipette techniques, biomembrane force probe and flow cell, can potentially better interrogate T cell kinetics with pMHC (63–69). The interactions between pMHC and TCR were found to occur more rapidly when analyzed in 2D rather than 3D, lending support to the serial triggering model where high affinity interactions generate fast off rates and rapid on-rates amenable for sampling multiple pMHC (69, 70). For the most part, one cannot readily convert the 2D area based measurements to 3D volume based affinities and on rates. A conversion of affinity from 2D FRET data to 3D measurements was suggested based on approximations of the contact area and intercellular volume between the T cell and surrogate APC bilayer (66). The approximations of contact area and intercellular volume are difficult to attain for T cells, which possibly explains why there is a discrepancy between the converted 3D K_d and SPR values for the MCC agonist and T102S weak agonist peptides. In contrast, the 2D and 3D half-life measurements are comparable because they are reported in units of time, yet in 2D, the time of interaction is more rapid than found in 3D analyses (66, 70).

We have focused on the mechanical 2D micropipette adhesion frequency assay as it provides a novel platform for evaluating T cell antigen specificity, frequency, and cross reactivity between epitopes within a polyclonal repertoire. Importantly, small numbers of T cells can be individually analyzed directly *ex vivo* from the blood and sites of ongoing immune responses. This assay allows for the visualization of TCR binding events with pMHC on opposing cells via a modified inverted microscope (**Figure 1**). The T cell and pMHC coated red blood cell are placed on opposing micropipettes and moved in and out of contact by means of a piezoelectric actuator for a defined contact and retraction cycle that will facilitate a binding event at equilibrium (71). A binding event is seen as distension of the RBC membrane on the video monitor as the cells are moved out of contact. The concentration of pMHC monomer coating on the RBC is optimized to yield an average binding frequency between 10 and 90% for several repeated

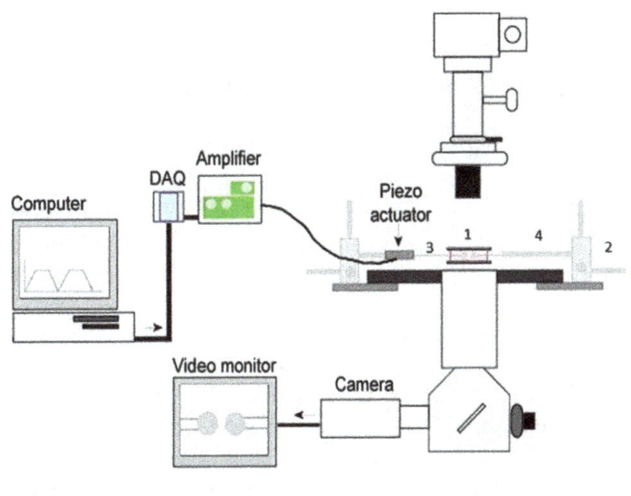

FIGURE 1 | The basic 2D micropipette adhesion frequency assay system. The foundation for this system is an inverted microscope. The stage has been modified with a metal adapter (1) to rest a media filled chamber containing the T cells and pMHC coated RBCs above the 100× oil immersion objective lens. The stage is also fitted with course micromanipulators (2) allowing for the movement of the micropipettes (3) within the chamber. The micropipettes are attached to a hydraulic pressure system (not shown) by means of a micropipette holder (4) allowing for individual cells to be aspirated and held within the chamber. A piezoelectric actuator is attached to one micropipette holder such that it can be moved in and out of contact with the opposing cell. The DAQ, digital acquisition board, converts the cyclical digital signal from a computer program to an analog voltage signal that drives the piezoelectric actuator. Cells can be visualized on the video monitor and adhesion events can be subsequently recorded.

contacts (usually 50 contacts). The micropipette assay is sufficiently sensitive to measure the binding of a single receptor-ligand bond, a feature that cannot be achieved with pMHC multimer technology. The higher sensitivity of the micropipette assay is not based on increased valency but likely due to the 2D orientation of the pMHC and TCR incorporated within the cell membranes. This closely replicates the interaction as it would occur between two cells and allows for measurement of TCR: pMHC kinetic parameters in a biologically relevant context. The effective 2D binding affinity, with a detection range from high to low, 10^{-2} to 10^{-7} μm^4, is a composite term that incorporates the affinity (K_a) and the contact area (A_c) between the T cell and surrogate APC. Derivation of the effective 2D binding affinity (A_cK_a) requires quantification of the receptor density (m_r), the ligand density (m_l), and the frequency of adhesion (P_a) between the cells as represented by $A_cK_a = -\ln(1 - P_a)/m_r m_l$ (71, 72). The adhesion frequency assay is the fundamental model of 2D mechanical assays where binding frequencies can be used to derive affinities and on/off rate kinetic readouts (73). The biomembrane force probe is a modified adhesion frequency assay that can allow for detection of individual bonds with increased sensitivity for detecting faster on/off rates and it can be modified to readout the effects of force on the bond between TCR and pMHC (73). Furthermore, the 2D micropipette system can be altered to permit visualization of functional fluorescent readouts such as calcium signaling, which has already been integrated into the FRET based 2D assays (66). The capacity of multiple readouts and increased sensitivity with the 2D mechanical tools is evidence for the power/significance of these techniques.

BREADTH OF AFFINITY IN THE POLYCLONAL REPERTOIRE

The affinity of TCRs for antigen can be discussed at both the single clone and population levels. A single TCR clone expands into multiple daughter cells that will possess a measurable but narrow range in affinity despite expressing an identical TCR. A polyclonal population of cells will possess a wider range or distribution of affinities comprised of all TCR clones activated to expand in response to any specific antigenic stimuli. Additionally, TCRs by their very nature are degenerate or crossreactive and can interact with many different peptide antigens. The estimated α:β TCR diversity is $\sim 10^{18}$, a seemingly large number that is significantly reduced to several hundred millions of T cells during thymocyte maturation (74, 75). Even with these reduced numbers, T cells still possess the ability to respond to most possible antigens. Therefore, the ability of a single TCR to recognize multiple antigens, albeit with varying degrees of affinity, is critical to increase the number of T cells that recognize each antigen.

The concept of TCR degeneracy is demonstrated by the capacity of monoclonal TCRs to recognize MHC variant peptides or altered peptide ligands, defined as epitopes with modified affinity for cognate TCR (76, 77). They also provide insight into the effective affinity range recognized by a single TCR. For instance, OT-I $CD8^+$ TCR transgenic T cells exhibit a Vα2/Vβ5 rearranged TCR that recognizes the cognate SIINFEKL (OVA) peptide on H2-K^b with a high 2D effective affinity ($\sim 10^{-3}\ \mu m^4$). Modifying this peptide sequence changes the affinity of OT-1 TCR for pMHC generating a breadth of affinities (70) that can alter downstream functional outcomes to yield agonist (A2, 2D affinity of $\sim 10^{-4}\ \mu m^4$), weak agonist (G4 and E1, 2D affinity of $\sim 10^{-5}\ \mu m^4$), or antagonist (V-OVA and R4, 2D affinity of $\sim 10^{-6}\ \mu m^4$) responses (70). Overall the OT-1 TCR exhibits an approximate, 1000-fold range in affinities depending on the peptide being presented by MHC class I. Additional T cells will have to be analyzed to determine whether this breadth of the 2D affinity range is characteristic of all $CD8^+$ or $CD4^+$ T cells.

The identification that a single TCR can exhibit a broad range of affinities to different peptide antigens led to the study of the array of affinities found within a polyclonal $CD4^+$ T cell response against one peptide antigen. The breadth of 2D effective affinities for a single antigen within a polyclonal population exhibited a Gaussian distribution possessing a defined mean and standard deviation. For example, $CD4^+$ T cells primed with the LCMV (lymphocytic choriomeningitis virus) GP_{61-80} peptide epitope, showed between a 100- and 1000-fold range of affinities by the 2D micropipette assay with a mean of $4.21 \pm 1.48 \times 10^{-4}\ \mu m^4$ (78). A similar distribution and range with a lower mean affinity $1.63 \pm 0.48 \times 10^{-5}\ \mu m^4$ was also observed for the polyclonal response against the myelin oligodendrocyte glycoprotein self antigen MOG_{35-55} (78). As one would expect, the analysis of a single TCR does not replicate the affinity range found within a polyclonal population. It is currently unclear how well conclusions made based on monoclonal models informs on the polyclonal response to the same antigen (79). This is affirmed by comparing the 2D affinities between the monoclonal $CD4^+$ SMARTA T cell clone and the polyclonal $CD4^+$ T cell population. Both populations are specific for the same GP_{66-77}: IA^b antigen, but the monoclonal SMARTA population only represents a fraction of the affinity breadth seen in the polyclonal response. In this case, the monoclonal cells have a mean affinity of $\sim 10^{-3}\ \mu m^4$ which is $\sim$10-fold higher than the mean polyclonal affinity of $\sim 10^{-4}\ \mu m^4$ [**Figure 2A** adapted from Ref. (48, 78)]. Although the SMARTA TCR is monoclonal, it is interesting that this TCR exhibits a range of affinities, albeit more narrow than the responding polyclonal T cells. An affinity range can even be detected

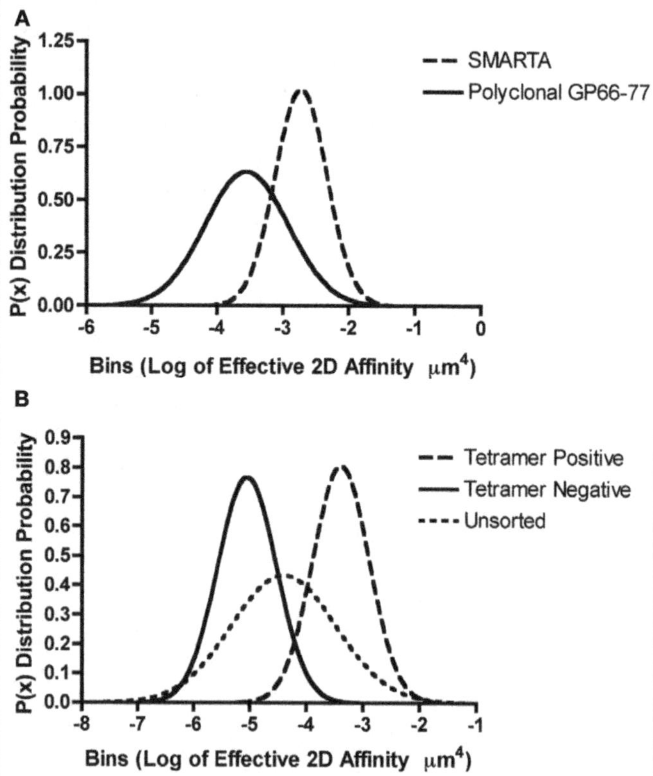

FIGURE 2 | Range of TCR affinities for an individual pMHC in a polyclonal repertoire. (A,B) Gaussian distributions were modeled for the described T cells by utilizing previously published effective 2D affinity means and standard deviations using the equation $P(x) = 1/[\sigma \times \mathrm{sqrt}(2\pi) \times e\hat{}(-(X-\mu)\hat{}2/(2s\hat{}2))]$ where $P(x)$ is the probability density function or distribution, σ is the standard deviation, X is the variate or bin interval, and μ is the mean log of the TCR affinities. **(A)** The monoclonal SMARTA T cells and the polyclonal GP_{61-80} population both recognize GP_{66-77}: IA^b. The 2D micropipette adhesion frequency assay was used to determine the mean effective 2D affinities and standard deviations as previously reported (48, 78). Gaussian distributions indicated that SMARTA T cells exhibit a higher log of affinity μm^4 ($-2.7 + 0.39$) $\sim$10-fold higher than the polyclonal T cell populations ($-3.5 + 0.63$), indicating that monoclonal population underrepresented the polyclonal affinity range. **(B)** The 2D micropipette adhesion frequency assay was used to ascertain the mean effective 2D affinities and standard deviations for the polyclonal GP_{61-80} repertoire (unsorted) and FACS sorted GP_{66-77}: IA^b tetramer positive and negative populations (78). Gaussian distributions indicated that both the tetramer positive ($\sim$peak at -3.0) and tetramer negative ($\sim$peak at -5.0) populations under represented the range of affinities exhibited by the polyclonal (unsorted) repertoire.

among TCRs expressed on a single T cell because FRET analyses with the 5C.C7 CD4$^+$ TCR have shown a 250-fold 2D affinity range for MCC between microclusters of the same cell (66). Furthermore, monoclonal models are often thought to represent the highest affinity TCRs within a polyclonal response, which is not necessarily the case. Clones are often selected *in vitro* for optimal growth, effector function, and reagent availability for tracking the TCR *in vivo*. For example, we have found that the transgenic 2D2 TCR, widely used for the study of demyelinating autoimmune disease, is of low affinity for its antigenic ligand yet shows measurable reactivity through proliferation and cytokine production assays (48, 80).

While the ability to track antigen specific T cells within a polyclonal repertoire has been revolutionized by the use of pMHC tetramers recent investigations call into question the fidelity of these reagents to sufficiently capture all participating effectors in an immune response. Our laboratory and others have shown a discrepancy in the use of tetramers to determine the breadth of CD4$^+$ T cell responses. Tetramers will not detect T cells where the affinity of the TCR for antigen is below the avidity threshold needed for binding. We have estimated this 2D effective affinity cutoff to be between 10^{-5} and 10^{-4} μm^4 for MHC class II restricted T cells; it is more difficult to define for MHC class I based tetramers as CD8 significantly contributes to the overall stability and binding while CD4 does not (48, 78, 81). Analysis of the tetramer positive subset of polyclonal GP_{66-77} reactive T cells showed enrichment for higher affinity T cells with a mean 2D affinity of $\sim 10^{-3}$ μm^4 as compared to the affinity of the intact polyclonal T cell population of $\sim 10^{-4}$ or the tetramer negative T cells $\sim 10^{-5}$ μm^4 (78). Of interest, the tetramer positive and negative cells are a subset of the overall polyclonal affinity repertoire [**Figure 2B**, adapted from Ref. (78)]. For both the self and pathogen specific CD4$^+$ T cell response, the percentage of tetramer reactivity was lower and did not correlate to the percentage of cytokine responders or the frequency of antigen specific T cells measured by the 2D micropipette adhesion frequency assay (78). Therefore, the sole use of tetramers to monitor the antigen specificity, frequency, magnitude, and affinity of a polyclonal repertoire in order to predict the overall composition of an immune response appears somewhat limited, missing the contribution of the lower affinity T cells.

Underestimating the contribution of low affinity T cells is a significant issue for models of autoimmune disease where negative selection likely enriches for a low affinity repertoire reactive against self antigen. Our studies with MOG_{35-55} specific CD4$^+$ T cells indicated that tetramer generally reacted with 7–10% of T cells within the target organ, while functional effector responses and 2D affinity analysis detected much higher levels of cells (78). In the 2D2 TCR transgenic model of EAE, the 2D2 T cells promoted spontaneous paralytic disease (4%) or spontaneous optic neuritis (35%) (80). This TCR has very low affinity for antigen (48) and does not interact with MOG-specific tetramers and therefore contrasts with data suggesting low affinity or low avidity T cells are less pathogenic. Furthermore, retrogenic derived monoclonal TCR models suggest that TCR of low avidity can support the development of spontaneous EAE in the absence of higher avidity T cells (82). The challenge in studying the contributions of low affinity T cells has been the lack of reagents to do so. The 2D adhesion frequency assays gives us one such tool to characterize lower affinity T cells alongside the higher affinity contributors within a polyclonal population.

BENEFITS OF AN INCLUSIVE RESPONSE

To date, current models of T cell clonal expansion suggest that high affinity T cell clones are preferentially enriched over low affinity clones (83–85). As a result, many current T cell therapeutic initiatives seek to elicit or artificially create high affinity T cells to enhance pathogen specific and anti-tumor responses (86). However, recent investigations have shown that T cells manipulated to have supraphysiological affinity were unexpectedly less potent effectors than lower affinity counterparts due to triggering of inhibitory mechanisms (87, 88). It would therefore be plausible that an effective immune response may benefit from a balance of high, intermediate, and low affinity T cell responders.

Polyclonal TCR affinity composition can be shaped by TCR activation thresholds. For example, CD27 costimulation has been shown to support the emergence of lower affinity CD8$^+$ T cells that mediate greater protection against reinfection with an influenza variant (89). Similarly, clones with low functional avidity have been shown to be important in the maintenance of an effective anti-tumor response (90). Although affinity was not the sole focus of this study, reduction of $p56^{Lck}$ expression significantly decreased T cell sensitivity to activation which mimics a lower affinity response. These low affinity effectors were less susceptible to an exhausted phenotype and mediated better protection in subsequent rechallenge. Such investigations provide evidence for why low affinity clones may exist within the repertoire and how therapeutics to limit them may be shortsighted.

The role for low affinity T cell populations can be obscured by the nature of the assay used to analyze the response. In a study examining the therapeutic efficacy of tumor vaccines, high affinity clones (as determined by SPR) responded optimally in *in vitro* assays, but intermediate affinity clones mediated the best anti-tumor responses *in vivo* (91). Similarly, a study evaluating optimal T cell responses to peptide in the 5C.C7 model (85, 92) showed that intermediate affinity clones mediated the most optimal *in vivo* responses while high affinity clones demonstrated the strongest response *in vitro*. Future studies may benefit from understanding the interplay of individual T cell affinity subsets in the overall efficacy of tumor and pathogen specific responses. These findings underscore the potential role for lower affinity effectors in an immune response and therefore they should be an important consideration in the design of therapeutic interventions.

Understanding how T cell affinity mediates protective immunity also has important implications for vaccine design because recent studies have shown the priming agent and the adjuvant can alter the CD4$^+$ TCR affinity composition. In one study, vaccinations using either cytochrome C peptide or whole protein were compared (93). Though both vaccination regimens generated diverse clonal responses, peptide vaccines elicited high affinity dominated responses while protein vaccines generated a repertoire inclusive of both low and high affinity responses. The maintenance of low affinity effectors was found, at least in part, to require CD27–CD70 signaling. Another study demonstrated the ability of vaccine adjuvants to affect the affinity composition of T cells generated in response to pigeon cytochrome C, PCC (94). All the adjuvants tested were effective in enhancing a PCC-specific T cell response, but alum, IFA, and CFA induced lower avidity responses while CpG and monophosphoryl lipid A generated higher avidity responses as determined by pMHC tetramer and CDR3 spectrotyping. This observation suggests that adjuvants could differentially influence recruitment into the polyclonal response. The effect was dependent on the dispersive ability of the adjuvant and activation of different TLRs that resulted in changes in $CD4^+$ T cell recruitment and/or migration. It is worth noting that even adjuvant choice can affect the balance of low and high affinity clonotypes (94, 95) and should be furthered explored with 2D assays. The application of 2D based pMHC technologies to these questions will allow us to uniquely explore the breadth of TCR affinities and redefine our understanding of the dynamic interplay between TCR affinity subsets within the polyclonal repertoire.

CONCLUSION

The use of pMHC technology is at the forefront of monitoring antigen specific immune responses. We promote 2D mechanical based assays with purified pMHC for several reasons. First, they display increased sensitivity for detecting antigen specific T cells when compared to functional responses or pMHC tetramer based assays. Secondly, the polyclonal repertoire can be monitored without purification of individual TCRs because the analysis is carried out using intact T cells. Lastly, 2D assays provide a more accurate representation of the relationship between T cell affinity and functional responsiveness. The findings to date have highlighted the presence of antigen specific $CD4^+$ T cells exhibiting a range of affinities from low to high in both autoimmune and pathogen specific models. Low affinity, tetramer negative populations elicit effector functions and expand in response to antigen suggesting their capacity to contribute to adaptive immune responses. The idea that lower affinity T cells effectively compete within and contribute to the effector T cell repertoire at the very least modifies our view that high affinity T cell clones would dominate the lower affinity counterparts. Future work is needed to examine how affinity of the initial TCR:pMHC interaction contributes functionally to the initiation, maintenance, and/or resolution of a polyclonal immune response. In addition, we need sensitive techniques that allow for analysis of TCR crossreactivity and in the case of autoimmunity, epitope spread to new antigens. At this point in time, 2D based assays together with recombinant pMHC molecules are useful tools available to characterize individual T cell affinity contributions to the breadth of an immune response. Potential clinical outcomes for this research include the use of TCR affinity as a biomarker to monitor disease progression and to provide information for the development of high efficacy antigen specific therapies.

ACKNOWLEDGMENTS

Special thanks to Jinsung Hong (Georgia Institute of Technology) for the design of **Figure 1** and to Jennifer D. Hood (Emory University) and Lindsay J. Edwards (Beth Israel Deaconess Medical Center) for assistance with the editing of this manuscript. Financial support was provided by NIH grants 1R01AI096879 and 5R01NS071518. J. Lori Blanchfield is also funded by the National Multiple Sclerosis Society FG 1963A1/1.

REFERENCES

1. Berek C, Milstein C. Mutation drift and repertoire shift in the maturation of the immune response. *Immunol Rev* (1987) **96**:23–41. doi:10.1111/j.1600-065X.1987.tb00507.x
2. Busch DH, Pamer EG. T cell affinity maturation by selective expansion during infection. *J Exp Med* (1999) **189**(4):701–10. doi:10.1084/jem.189.4.701
3. Serra P, Amrani A, Han B, Yamanouchi J, Thiessen SJ, Santamaria P. RAG-dependent peripheral T cell receptor diversification in CD8+ T lymphocytes. *Proc Natl Acad Sci U S A* (2002) **99**(24):15566–71. doi:10.1073/pnas.242321099
4. Hale JS, Wubeshet M, Fink PJ. TCR revision generates functional CD4+ T cells. *J Immunol* (2010) **185**(11):6528–34. doi:10.4049/jimmunol.1002696
5. Chien YH, Davis MM. How alpha beta T-cell receptors "see" peptide/MHC complexes. *Immunol Today* (1993) **14**(12):597–602. doi:10.1016/0167-5699(93)90199-U
6. Moss PA, Moots RJ, Rosenberg WM, Rowland-Jones SJ, Bodmer HC, McMichael AJ, et al. Extensive conservation of alpha and beta chains of the human T-cell antigen receptor recognizing HLA-A2 and influenza A matrix peptide. *Proc Natl Acad Sci U S A* (1991) **88**(20):8987–90. doi:10.1073/pnas.88.20.8987
7. Turner SJ, Diaz G, Cross R, Doherty PC. Analysis of clonotype distribution and persistence for an influenza virus-specific CD8+ T cell response. *Immunity* (2003) **18**(4):549–59. doi:10.1016/S1074-7613(03)00087-6
8. Turner SJ, Doherty PC, McCluskey J, Rossjohn J. Structural determinants of T-cell receptor bias in immunity. *Nat Rev Immunol* (2006) **6**(12):883–94. doi:10.1038/nri1977
9. Pannetier C, Even J, Kourilsky P. T-cell repertoire diversity and clonal expansions in normal and clinical samples. *Immunol Today* (1995) **16**(4):176–81. doi:10.1016/0167-5699(95)80117-0
10. Pannetier C, Cochet M, Darche S, Casrouge A, Zöller M, Kourilsky P. The sizes of the CDR3 hypervariable regions of the murine T-cell receptor beta chains vary as a function of the recombined germ-line segments. *Proc Natl Acad Sci U S A* (1993) **90**(9):4319–23. doi:10.1073/pnas.90.9.4319
11. Currier JR, Deulofeut H, Barron KS, Kehn PJ, Robinson MA. Mitogens, superantigens, and nominal antigens elicit distinctive patterns of TCRB CDR3 diversity. *Hum Immunol* (1996) **48**(1-2):39–51. doi:10.1016/0198-8859(96)00076-6
12. Kim G, Kohyama K, Tanuma N, Matsumoto Y. Diagnosis and assessment of preclinical and clinical autoimmune encephalomyelitis using peripheral blood lymphocyte TCR. *Eur J Immunol* (1998) **28**(9):2751–9. doi:10.1002/(SICI)1521-4141(199809)28:09<2751::AID-IMMU2751>3.0.CO;2-J
13. Ria F, van den Elzen P, Madakamutil LT, Miller JE, Maverakis E, Sercarz EE. Molecular characterization of the T cell repertoire using immunoscope analysis and its possible implementation in clinical practice. *Curr Mol Med* (2001) **1**(3):297–304. doi:10.2174/1566524013363690
14. Okajima M, Wada T, Nishida M, Yokoyama T, Nakayama Y, Hashida Y, et al. Analysis of T cell receptor Vbeta diversity in peripheral CD4 and CD8 T lymphocytes in patients with autoimmune thyroid diseases. *Clin Exp Immunol* (2009) **155**(2):166–72. doi:10.1111/j.1365-2249.2008.03842.x

15. Memon SA, Sportès C, Flomerfelt FA, Gress RE, Hakim FT. Quantitative analysis of T cell receptor diversity in clinical samples of human peripheral blood. *J Immunol Methods* (2012) **375**(1-2):84–92. doi:10.1016/j.jim.2011.09.012
16. Dash P, McClaren JL, Oguin TH III, Rothwell W, Todd B, Morris MY, et al. Paired analysis of TCRalpha and TCRbeta chains at the single-cell level in mice. *J Clin Invest* (2011) **121**(1):288–95. doi:10.1172/JCI44752
17. Bonarius HP, Baas F, Remmerswaal EB, van Lier RA, ten Berge IJ, Tak PP, et al. Monitoring the T-cell receptor repertoire at single-clone resolution. *PLoS ONE* (2006) **1**:e55. doi:10.1371/journal.pone.0000055
18. Critchfield JM, Racke MK, Zúñiga-Pflücker JC, Cannella B, Raine CS, Goverman J, et al. T cell deletion in high antigen dose therapy of autoimmune encephalomyelitis. *Science* (1994) **263**(5150):1139–43. doi:10.1126/science.7509084
19. Altman JD, Moss PA, Goulder PJ, Barouch DH, McHeyzer-Williams MG, Bell JI, et al. Phenotypic analysis of antigen-specific T lymphocytes. *Science* (1996) **274**(5284):94–6. doi:10.1126/science.274.5284.94
20. Kappel BJ, Pinilla-Ibarz J, Kochman AA, Eng JM, Hubbard VM, Leiner I, et al. Remodeling specific immunity by use of MHC tetramers: demonstration in a graft-versus-host disease model. *Blood* (2006) **107**(5):2045–51. doi:10.1182/blood-2005-07-2828
21. Vincent BG, Young EF, Buntzman AS, Stevens R, Kepler TB, Tisch RM, et al. Toxin-coupled MHC class I tetramers can specifically ablate autoreactive CD8+ T cells and delay diabetes in nonobese diabetic mice. *J Immunol* (2010) **184**(8):4196–204. doi:10.4049/jimmunol.0903931
22. Moon JJ, Chu HH, Pepper M, McSorley SJ, Jameson SC, Kedl RM, et al. Naive CD4(+) T cell frequency varies for different epitopes and predicts repertoire diversity and response magnitude. *Immunity* (2007) **27**(2):203–13. doi:10.1016/j.immuni.2007.07.007
23. Chu HH, Moon JJ, Takada K, Pepper M, Molitor JA, Schacker TW, et al. Positive selection optimizes the number and function of MHCII-restricted CD4+ T cell clones in the naive polyclonal repertoire. *Proc Natl Acad Sci U S A* (2009) **106**(27):11241–5. doi:10.1073/pnas.0902015106
24. Stone JD, Artyomov MN, Chervin AS, Chakraborty AK, Eisen HN, Kranz DM. Interaction of streptavidin-based peptide-MHC oligomers (tetramers) with cell-surface TCRs. *J Immunol* (2011) **187**(12):6281–90. doi:10.4049/jimmunol.1101734
25. Boniface JJ, Rabinowitz JD, Wülfing C, Hampl J, Reich Z, Altman JD, et al. Initiation of signal transduction through the T cell receptor requires the multivalent engagement of peptide/MHC ligands [corrected]. *Immunity* (1998) **9**(4):459–66. doi:10.1016/S1074-7613(00)80629-9
26. Duplan V, Suberbielle E, Napper CE, Joly E, Saoudi A, Gonzalez-Dunia D. Tracking antigen-specific CD8+ T cells in the rat using MHC class I multimers. *J Immunol Methods* (2007) **320**(1-2):30–9. doi:10.1016/j.jim.2006.11.008
27. Davis MM, Altman JD, Newell EW. Interrogating the repertoire: broadening the scope of peptide-MHC multimer analysis. *Nat Rev Immunol* (2011) **11**(8):551–8. doi:10.1038/nri3020
28. Fierabracci A. The potential of multimer technologies in type 1 diabetes prediction strategies. *Diabetes Metab Res Rev* (2011) **27**(3):216–29. doi:10.1002/dmrr.1165
29. Batard P, Peterson DA, Devêvre E, Guillaume P, Cerottini JC, Rimoldi D, et al. Dextramers: new generation of fluorescent MHC class I/peptide multimers for visualization of antigen-specific CD8+ T cells. *J Immunol Methods* (2006) **310**(1-2):136–48. doi:10.1016/j.jim.2006.01.006
30. Massilamany C, Upadhyaya B, Gangaplara A, Kuszynski C, Reddy J. Detection of autoreactive CD4 T cells using major histocompatibility complex class II dextramers. *BMC Immunol* (2011) **12**:40. doi:10.1186/1471-2172-12-40
31. Bakker AH, Schumacher TN. MHC multimer technology: current status and future prospects. *Curr Opin Immunol* (2005) **17**(4):428–33. doi:10.1016/j.coi.2005.06.008
32. McMichael AJ, O'Callaghan CA. A new look at T cells. *J Exp Med* (1998) **187**(9):1367–71. doi:10.1084/jem.187.9.1367
33. Parkhurst MR, Salgaller ML, Southwood S, Robbins PF, Sette A, Rosenberg SA, et al. Improved induction of melanoma-reactive CTL with peptides from the melanoma antigen gp100 modified at HLA-A*0201-binding residues. *J Immunol* (1996) **157**(6):2539–48.
34. Ford ML, Evavold BD. Regulation of polyclonal T cell responses by an MHC anchor-substituted variant of myelin oligodendrocyte glycoprotein 35-55. *J Immunol* (2003) **171**(3):1247–54.
35. Ryan KR, McNeil LK, Dao C, Jensen PE, Evavold BD. Modification of peptide interaction with MHC creates TCR partial agonists. *Cell Immunol* (2004) **227**(1):70–8. doi:10.1016/j.cellimm.2004.01.003
36. Chen JL, Stewart-Jones G, Bossi G, Lissin NM, Wooldridge L, Choi EM, et al. Structural and kinetic basis for heightened immunogenicity of T cell vaccines. *J Exp Med* (2005) **201**(8):1243–55. doi:10.1084/jem.20042323
37. Novak EJ, Liu AW, Gebe JA, Falk BA, Nepom GT, Koelle DM, et al. Tetramer-guided epitope mapping: rapid identification and characterization of immunodominant CD4+ T cell epitopes from complex antigens. *J Immunol* (2001) **166**(11):6665–70.
38. Raddassi K, Kent SC, Yang J, Bourcier K, Bradshaw EM, Seyfert-Margolis V, et al. Increased frequencies of myelin oligodendrocyte glycoprotein/MHC class II-binding CD4 cells in patients with multiple sclerosis. *J Immunol* (2011) **187**(2):1039–46. doi:10.4049/jimmunol.1001543
39. Stadinski BD, Zhang L, Crawford F, Marrack P, Eisenbarth GS, Kappler JW. Diabetogenic T cells recognize insulin bound to IAg7 in an unexpected, weakly binding register. *Proc Natl Acad Sci U S A* (2010) **107**(24):10978–83. doi:10.1073/pnas.1006545107
40. Robertson JM, Jensen PE, Evavold BD. DO11.10 and OT-II T cells recognize a C-terminal ovalbumin 323-339 epitope. *J Immunol* (2000) **164**(9):4706–12.
41. Landais E, Romagnoli PA, Corper AL, Shires J, Altman JD, Wilson IA, et al. New design of MHC class II tetramers to accommodate fundamental principles of antigen presentation. *J Immunol* (2009) **183**(12):7949–57. doi:10.4049/jimmunol.0902493
42. Kozono H, White J, Clements J, Marrack P, Kappler J. Production of soluble MHC class II proteins with covalently bound single peptides. *Nature* (1994) **369**(6476):151–4. doi:10.1038/369151a0
43. Crawford F, Stadinski B, Jin N, Michels A, Nakayama M, Pratt P, et al. Specificity and detection of insulin-reactive CD4+ T cells in type 1 diabetes in the nonobese diabetic (NOD) mouse. *Proc Natl Acad Sci U S A* (2011) **108**(40):16729–34. doi:10.1073/pnas.1113954108
44. Gett AV, Sallusto F, Lanzavecchia A, Geginat J. T cell fitness determined by signal strength. *Nat Immunol* (2003) **4**(4):355–60. doi:10.1038/ni908
45. Holler PD, Kranz DM. Quantitative analysis of the contribution of TCR/pepMHC affinity and CD8 to T cell activation. *Immunity* (2003) **18**(2):255–64. doi:10.1016/S1074-7613(03)00019-0
46. Tuosto L, Acuto O. CD28 affects the earliest signaling events generated by TCR engagement. *Eur J Immunol* (1998) **28**(7):2131–42. doi:10.1002/(SICI)1521-4141(199807)28:07<2131::AID-IMMU2131>3.0.CO;2-Q
47. Iezzi G, Karjalainen K, Lanzavecchia A. The duration of antigenic stimulation determines the fate of naive and effector T cells. *Immunity* (1998) **8**(1):89–95. doi:10.1016/S1074-7613(00)80461-6
48. Rosenthal KM, Edwards LJ, Sabatino JJ Jr, Hood JD, Wasserman HA, Zhu C, et al. Low 2-dimensional CD4 T cell receptor affinity for myelin sets in motion delayed response kinetics. *PLoS ONE* (2012) **7**(3):e32562. doi:10.1371/journal.pone.0032562
49. Corr M, Slanetz AE, Boyd LF, Jelonek MT, Khilko S, al-Ramadi BK, et al. T cell receptor-MHC class I peptide interactions: affinity, kinetics, and specificity. *Science* (1994) **265**(5174):946–9. doi:10.1126/science.8052850
50. Matsui K, Boniface JJ, Steffner P, Reay PA, Davis MM. Kinetics of T-cell receptor binding to peptide/I-Ek complexes: correlation of the dissociation rate with T-cell responsiveness. *Proc Natl Acad Sci U S A* (1994) **91**(26):12862–6. doi:10.1073/pnas.91.26.12862
51. Davis MM, Boniface JJ, Reich Z, Lyons D, Hampl J, Arden B, et al. Ligand recognition by alpha beta T cell receptors. *Annu*

Rev Immunol (1998) **16**:523–44. doi:10.1146/annurev.immunol.16.1.523
52. Stone JD, Chervin AS, Kranz DM. T-cell receptor binding affinities and kinetics: impact on T-cell activity and specificity. *Immunology* (2009) **126**(2):165–76. doi:10.1111/j.1365-2567.2008.03015.x
53. McKeithan TW. Kinetic proofreading in T-cell receptor signal transduction. *Proc Natl Acad Sci U S A* (1995) **92**(11):5042–6. doi:10.1073/pnas.92.11.5042
54. Rabinowitz JD, Beeson C, Lyons DS, Davis MM, McConnell HM. Kinetic discrimination in T-cell activation. *Proc Natl Acad Sci U S A* (1996) **93**(4):1401–5. doi:10.1073/pnas.93.4.1401
55. Germain RN, Stefanova I. The dynamics of T cell receptor signaling: complex orchestration and the key roles of tempo and cooperation. *Annu Rev Immunol* (1999) **17**:467–522. doi:10.1146/annurev.immunol.17.1.467
56. Lyons DS, Lieberman SA, Hampl J, Boniface JJ, Chien Y, Berg LJ, et al. A TCR binds to antagonist ligands with lower affinities and faster dissociation rates than to agonists. *Immunity* (1996) **5**(1):53–61. doi:10.1016/S1074-7613(00)80309-X
57. van der Merwe PA. The TCR triggering puzzle. *Immunity* (2001) **14**(6):665–8. doi:10.1016/S1074-7613(01)00155-8
58. al-Ramadi BK, Jelonek MT, Boyd LF, Margulies DH, Bothwell AL. Lack of strict correlation of functional sensitization with the apparent affinity of MHC/peptide complexes for the TCR. *J Immunol* (1995) **155**(2):662–73.
59. Alam SM, Travers PJ, Wung JL, Nasholds W, Redpath S, Jameson SC, et al. T-cell-receptor affinity and thymocyte positive selection. *Nature* (1996) **381**(6583):616–20. doi:10.1038/381616a0
60. Kersh GJ, Kersh EN, Fremont DH, Allen PM. High- and low-potency ligands with similar affinities for the TCR: the importance of kinetics in TCR signaling. *Immunity* (1998) **9**(6):817–26. doi:10.1016/S1074-7613(00)80647-0
61. Alam SM, Davies GM, Lin CM, Zal T, Nasholds W, Jameson SC, et al. Qualitative and quantitative differences in T cell receptor binding of agonist and antagonist ligands. *Immunity* (1999) **10**(2):227–37. doi:10.1016/S1074-7613(00)80023-0
62. Rosette C, Werlen G, Daniels MA, Holman PO, Alam SM, Travers PJ, et al. The impact of duration versus extent of TCR occupancy on T cell activation: a revision of the kinetic proofreading model. *Immunity* (2001) **15**(1):59–70. doi:10.1016/S1074-7613(01)00173-X
63. Ma Z, Sharp KA, Janmey PA, Finkel TH. Surface-anchored monomeric agonist pMHCs alone trigger TCR with high sensitivity. *PLoS Biol* (2008) **6**(2):e43. doi:10.1371/journal.pbio.0060043
64. Tolentino TP, Wu J, Zarnitsyna VI, Fang Y, Dustin ML, Zhu C. Measuring diffusion and binding kinetics by contact area FRAP. *Biophys J* (2008) **95**(2):920–30. doi:10.1529/biophysj.107.114447
65. Wu J, Fang Y, Zarnitsyna VI, Tolentino TP, Dustin ML, Zhu C. A coupled diffusion-kinetics model for analysis of contact-area FRAP experiment. *Biophys J* (2008) **95**(2):910–9. doi:10.1529/biophysj.107.114439
66. Huppa JB, Axmann M, Mörtelmaier MA, Lillemeier BF, Newell EW, Brameshuber M, et al. TCR-peptide-MHC interactions in situ show accelerated kinetics and increased affinity. *Nature* (2010) **463**(7283):963–7. doi:10.1038/nature08746
67. Edwards LJ, Zarnitsyna VI, Hood JD, Evavold BD, Zhu C. Insights into T cell recognition of antigen: significance of two-dimensional kinetic parameters. *Front Immunol* (2012) **3**:86. doi:10.3389/fimmu.2012.00086
68. James JR, Vale RD. Biophysical mechanism of T-cell receptor triggering in a reconstituted system. *Nature* (2012) **487**(7405):64–9. doi:10.1038/nature11220
69. Zhu C, Jiang N, Huang J, Zarnitsyna VI, Evavold BD. Insights from in situ analysis of TCR-pMHC recognition: response of an interaction network. *Immunol Rev* (2013) **251**(1):49–64. doi:10.1111/imr.12016
70. Huang J, Zarnitsyna VI, Liu B, Edwards LJ, Jiang N, Evavold BD, et al. The kinetics of two-dimensional TCR and pMHC interactions determine T-cell responsiveness. *Nature* (2010) **464**(7290):932–6. doi:10.1038/nature08944
71. Zarnitsyna VI, Zhu C. Adhesion frequency assay for in situ kinetics analysis of cross-junctional molecular interactions at the cell-cell interface. *J Vis Exp* (2011) (57):e3519. doi:10.3791/3519
72. Chesla SE, Selvaraj P, Zhu C. Measuring two-dimensional receptor-ligand binding kinetics by micropipette. *Biophys J* (1998) **75**(3):1553–72. doi:10.1016/S0006-3495(98)74074-3
73. Chen W, Zarnitsyna VI, Sarangapani KK, Huang J, Zhu C. Measuring receptor-ligand binding kinetics on cell surfaces: from adhesion frequency to thermal fluctuation methods. *Cell Mol Bioeng* (2008) **1**(4):276–88. doi:10.1007/s12195-008-0024-8
74. Davis MM, Bjorkman PJ. T-cell antigen receptor genes and T-cell recognition. *Nature* (1988) **334**(6181):395–402. doi:10.1038/334395a0
75. Davis MM. T cell receptor gene diversity and selection. *Annu Rev Biochem* (1990) **59**:475–96. doi:10.1146/annurev.bi.59.070190.002355
76. Evavold BD, Allen PM. Separation of IL-4 production from Th cell proliferation by an altered T cell receptor ligand. *Science* (1991) **252**(5010):1308–10. doi:10.1126/science.1833816
77. Evavold BD, Sloan-Lancaster J, Allen PM. Antagonism of superantigen-stimulated helper T-cell clones and hybridomas by altered peptide ligand. *Proc Natl Acad Sci U S A* (1994) **91**(6):2300–4. doi:10.1073/pnas.91.6.2300
78. Sabatino JJ Jr, Huang J, Zhu C, Evavold BD. High prevalence of low affinity peptide-MHC II tetramer-negative effectors during polyclonal CD4+ T cell responses. *J Exp Med* (2011) **208**(1):81–90. doi:10.1084/jem.20101574
79. Zehn D, Lee SY, Bevan MJ. Complete but curtailed T-cell response to very low-affinity antigen. *Nature* (2009) **458**(7235):211–4. doi:10.1038/nature07657
80. Bettelli E, Pagany M, Weiner HL, Linington C, Sobel RA, Kuchroo VK. Myelin oligodendrocyte glycoprotein-specific T cell receptor transgenic mice develop spontaneous autoimmune optic neuritis. *J Exp Med* (2003) **197**(9):1073–81. doi:10.1084/jem.20021603
81. Xiong Y, Kern P, Chang H, Reinherz E. T cell receptor binding to a pMHCII ligand is kinetically distinct from and independent of CD4. *J Biol Chem* (2001) **276**(8):5659–67. doi:10.1074/jbc.M009580200
82. Alli R, Nguyen P, Geiger TL. Retrogenic modeling of experimental allergic encephalomyelitis associates T cell frequency but not TCR functional affinity with pathogenicity. *J Immunol* (2008) **181**(1):136–45.
83. Savage PA, Boniface JJ, Davis MM. A kinetic basis for T cell receptor repertoire selection during an immune response. *Immunity* (1999) **10**(4):485–92. doi:10.1016/S1074-7613(00)80048-5
84. Price DA, Brenchley JM, Ruff LE, Betts MR, Hill BJ, Roederer M, et al. Avidity for antigen shapes clonal dominance in CD8+ T cell populations specific for persistent DNA viruses. *J Exp Med* (2005) **202**(10):1349–61. doi:10.1084/jem.20051357
85. Corse E, Gottschalk RA, Krogsgaard M, Allison JP. Attenuated T cell responses to a high-potency ligand in vivo. *PLoS Biol* (2010) **8**(9):doi:10.1371/journal.pbio.1000481
86. Konkel JE, Frommer F, Leech MD, Yagita H, Waisman A, Anderton SM. PD-1 signalling in CD4(+) T cells restrains their clonal expansion to an immunogenic stimulus, but is not critically required for peptide-induced tolerance. *Immunology* (2010) **130**(1):92–102. doi:10.1111/j.1365-2567.2009.03216.x
87. Alli R, Nguyen P, Geiger TL. Altered differentiation, diminished pathogenicity, and regulatory activity of myelin-specific T cells expressing an enhanced affinity TCR. *J Immunol* (2011) **187**(11):5521–31. doi:10.4049/jimmunol.1102202
88. Hebeisen M, Baitsch L, Presotto D, Baumgaertner P, Romero P, Michielin O, et al. SHP-1 phosphatase activity counteracts increased T cell receptor affinity. *J Clin Invest* (2013) **123**(3):1044–56. doi:10.1172/JCI65325
89. van Gisbergen KP, Klarenbeek PL, Kragten NA, Unger PP, Nieuwenhuis MB, Wensveen FM, et al. The costimulatory molecule CD27 maintains clonally diverse CD8(+) T cell responses of low antigen affinity to protect against viral variants. *Immunity* (2011) **35**(1):97–108. doi:10.1016/j.immuni.2011.04.020

90. Caserta S, Kleczkowska J, Mondino A, Zamoyska R. Reduced functional avidity promotes central and effector memory CD4 T cell responses to tumor-associated antigens. *J Immunol* (2010) **185**(11):6545–54. doi:10.4049/jimmunol.1001867
91. McMahan RH, McWilliams JA, Jordan KR, Dow SW, Wilson DB, Slansky JE. Relating TCR-peptide-MHC affinity to immunogenicity for the design of tumor vaccines. *J Clin Invest* (2006) **116**(9):2543–51.
92. Corse E, Gottschalk RA, Allison JP. Strength of TCR-peptide/MHC interactions and in vivo T cell responses. *J Immunol* (2011) **186**(9):5039–45. doi:10.4049/jimmunol.1003650
93. Baumgartner CK, Yagita H, Malherbe LP. A TCR affinity threshold regulates memory CD4 T cell differentiation following vaccination. *J Immunol* (2012) **189**(5):2309–17. doi:10.4049/jimmunol.1200453
94. Malherbe L, Mark L, Fazilleau N, McHeyzer-Williams LJ, McHeyzer-Williams MG. Vaccine adjuvants alter TCR-based selection thresholds. *Immunity* (2008) **28**(5):698–709. doi:10.1016/j.immuni.2008.03.014
95. Baumgartner CK, Malherbe LP. Regulation of CD4 T-cell receptor diversity by vaccine adjuvants. *Immunology* (2010) **130**(1):16–22. doi:10.1111/j.1365-2567.2010.03265.x

17

Beyond the antigen receptor: editing the genome of T-cells for cancer adoptive cellular therapies

Angharad Lloyd, Owen N. Vickery and Bruno Laugel*

Institute of Infection and Immunity, Cardiff University School of Medicine, Cardiff, Wales, UK

Edited by:
Michael Sitkovsky, Northeastern University, USA

Reviewed by:
Balbino Alarcon, Consejo Superior de Investigaciones Cientificas, Spain
Edward John Collins, The University of North Carolina, USA

****Correspondence:***
Bruno Laugel, Institute of Infection and Immunity, Cardiff University School of Medicine, Henry Wellcome Building, Heath Park, Cardiff, CF14 4XN, Wales, UK
e-mail: laugelbf@cardiff.ac.uk

Recent early stage clinical trials evaluating the adoptive transfer of patient CD8$^+$ T-cells re-directed with antigen receptors recognizing tumors have shown very encouraging results. These reports provide strong support for further development of the therapeutic concept as a curative cancer treatment. In this respect combining the adoptive transfer of tumor-specific T-cells with therapies that increase their anti-tumor capacity is viewed as a promising strategy to improve treatment outcome. The *ex vivo* genetic engineering step that underlies T-cell re-direction offers a unique angle to combine antigen receptor delivery with the targeting of cell-intrinsic pathways that restrict T-cell effector functions. Recent progress in genome editing technologies such as protein- and RNA-guided endonucleases raise the possibility of disrupting gene expression in T-cells in order to enhance effector functions or to bypass tumor immune suppression. This approach would avoid the systemic administration of compounds that disrupt immune homeostasis, potentially avoiding autoimmune adverse effects, and could improve the efficacy of T-cell based adoptive therapies.

Keywords: T-cells, genome editing, cancer, cell therapies, immune checkpoints

INTRODUCTION

Although there is still controversy over the role of the immune system in protecting the organism against the development of neoplasms in a natural setting (1) it is well accepted that artificial immunity can efficiently contain and even eradicate established tumors (2). Harnessing the anti-tumor potential of T-cells, and particularly CD8$^+$ T-cells, is a promising approach for curative cancer treatment. Because of their relative ease of administration and documented low toxicities therapeutic vaccines that trigger T-cell responses are a very attractive approach. However, even though they efficiently induce antigen-specific immunity, the clinical benefit of cancer vaccines has so far been limited (3). In contrast adoptive cell therapies (ACT), where T-cells are modified *ex vivo* and re-infused in a patient's circulation, are more difficult to implement and require important infrastructural investment. Yet a number of studies have now reported long-term remissions or tumor clearance (4–6), warranting further development of the therapeutic concept.

While conferring the immune system with the ability to recognize tumors through vaccination or ACT is a pre-requisite for the induction of efficient anti-tumor responses it is likely insufficient to achieve long-term clinical benefit in a majority of patients. An increasing body of evidence points to the necessity of combining different therapeutic approaches in order to improve treatment outcome (7, 8). For instance several small-molecule compounds that target oncogenic pathways also enhance tumor destruction by immune mechanisms, e.g., by sensitizing cancer cells to cytolysis (9, 10). The coordinated delivery of these compounds with immunotherapies is expected to improve clinical responses in an additive or even synergistic manner. Similarly the combination of immune-based therapies also holds great potential. Monoclonal antibodies (mAbs) blocking immune checkpoint receptors have recently emerged as promising therapeutics and many believe that the recent marketing authorization of Ipilimumab, targeting CTLA-4, heralds great strides in this area. Immune checkpoint receptor blocking agents are currently marketed or developed as single therapies but are expected to achieve maximal efficacy in combination with immune stimulatory approaches such as vaccination or ACTs (11, 12). Although generic treatment combinations will undoubtedly provide some degree of clinical benefit it is the prospect of developing personalized therapies tailored to individual needs that holds the greatest potential to improve clinical outcome in cancer therapy. The heterogenous nature of similar tumor histologies as well as individual genetic variability are believed to account for the varied response levels to generic treatments and the wider availability of prognostic tools should help define adequate treatment options that improve patient response. With respect to cancer vaccines or ACTs information about the nature of the immune checkpoint pathway(s) relevant to a tumor would be particularly useful in order to counteract immune suppression.

T-cell-based ACTs rely on the infusion in a patient's circulation of *ex vivo* expanded tumor-infiltrating lymphocytes (TILs) or peripheral blood T-cells transduced with viral vectors expressing a tumor-specific antigen receptor. This engineering step offers the opportunity to transfer additional genetic material conferring T-cells with enhanced anti-tumor activity. Targeted genome editing relying on viral gene transfer could readily be combined with the delivery of antigen receptors at little additional cost in one unique therapeutic entity. This approach would avoid the drawbacks associated with combining treatment modalities of different nature requiring distinct administration regimens, e.g., cellular therapy and mAb injection. In addition cell-intrinsic disruption of immune checkpoints in tumor-specific T-cells is likely to display a better safety profile than the systemic administration of blocking agents. Recently developed gene targeting technologies such as zinc-finger proteins (ZFPs), transcription activator-like proteins (TALs), and RNA-guided endonucleases (RGENs) could thus be harnessed in order to silence the expression of T-cell-intrinsic genes that restrain their anti-tumor potential.

MAIN TEXT

TECHNICAL ASPECTS AND CHALLENGES TO THE MODULATION OF GENE EXPRESSION IN T-CELLS

RNA interference (RNAi) often is the technique of choice to silence gene expression in somatic cells and lentivirus-mediated RNAi is a good option for sustained and efficient silencing. Most lentiviral RNAi systems express short-hairpin RNAs (shRNAs) from RNApolIII promoters, which drive high levels of transcription using precise initiation and termination sites. A recurrent problem of lentivirus-mediated RNAi, which is particularly salient in T-cells (13), is that the constant generation of shRNAs interferes with endogenous miRNA biogenesis and can result in the deregulation of gene expression (14, 15). This issue has prompted investigators to seek alternative methods to silence gene expression (16).

Recently developed genome editing technologies based on DNA-targeting proteins have the potential to revolutionize ACTs by offering convenient tools to alter gene expression. TAL effector-nucleases (TALENs) and ZFP-nucleases (ZFNs) effect complete gene knockout (**Figure 1A**) and are promising alternatives to RNAi for therapeutic applications (17–19). TALs are bacterial DNA-binding proteins consisting of near identical 34 amino-acid modules that bind one nucleotide with high affinity. The variable 12th and 13th amino-acids of TALs, called repeat-variable di-nucleotide confers base specificity (NN → G/A, NI → A, NG → T, NK → G, HD → C, and NS → A/T/C/G) and TAL arrays that target a nucleotide sequence can be generated by assembling individual modules (17, 20). ZFPs are eukaryotic DNA-binding proteins. Cys2-His2 fingers, which are used for genome editing, are the most common ZFP motif (21) and are each specific for a nucleotide triplet. Artificial ZFP domains that target specific DNA sequences, usually 9–18 nt long, can be constructed by assembling individual fingers (18). ZFPs and TALs have similar modular configurations but TALs can in theory target any stretch of nucleotides beginning with a thymidine whereas some structural incompatibilities between individual ZFP modules due to overlapping DNA-binding domains make the assembly

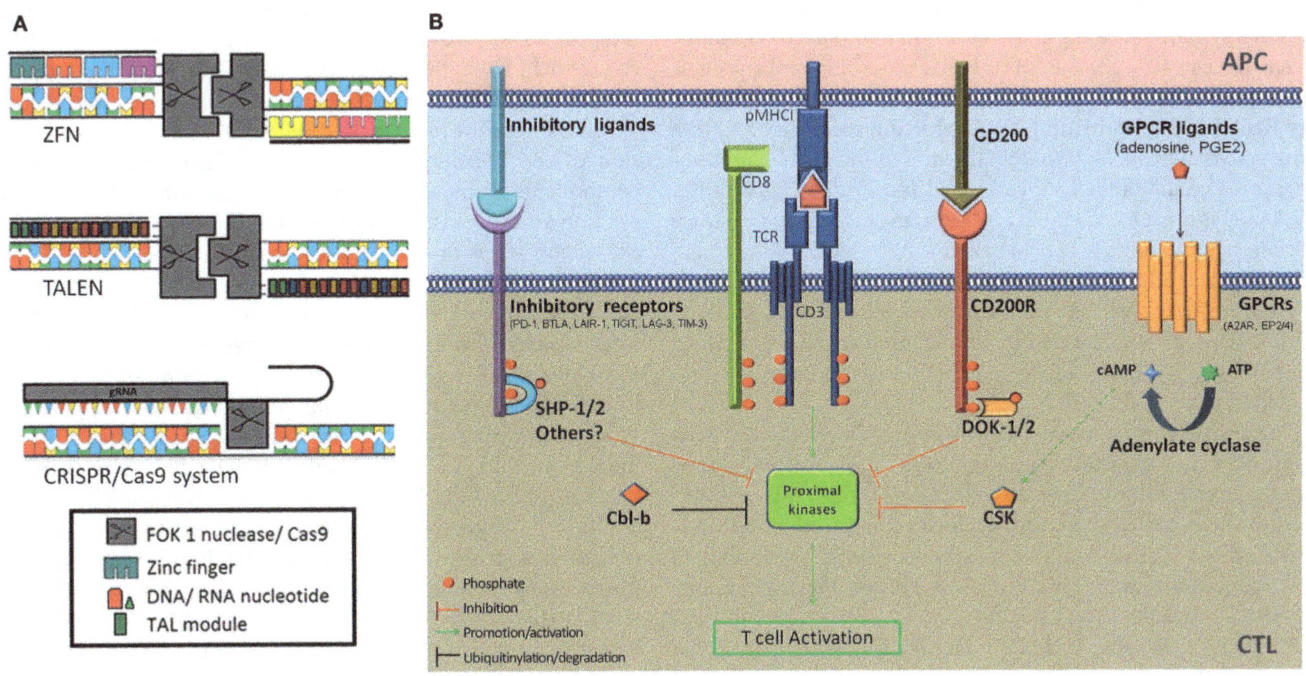

FIGURE 1 | (A) Schematic diagram of the ZFN, TALEN, and CRISPR/Cas9 genome editing tools. **(B)** Inhibition of T-cell activation by immune checkpoint receptors and downstream signaling proteins. Several co-inhibitory receptors (PD-1, BTLA, and LAIR-1) inhibit T-cell signaling by recruiting the SHP-1 and/or SHP-2 tyrosine phosphatases at proximity of the TCR signaling complex via ITIMs and ITSMs. This results in the dephosphorylation of proximal kinases downstream of TCR triggering. In addition PD-1 ligation was shown to induce increased expression of the Cbl-b E3 ubiquitin ligase, which targets signaling molecules for degradation. Activation of the CD200R leads to the recruitment of DOK2 and RasGAP to its intra-cellular domain, resulting in the inhibition of downstream MAP kinases. The adenosine receptor 2A and PGE2 receptors EP2 and EP4 modulate T-cell activation through mobilization of the cAMP-PKAI-CSK pathway. CSK phosphorylates the inhibitory C-terminal tyrosine residue of Src kinases and negatively regulates TCR signaling. A2AR, adenosine A2a receptor; APC, antigen-presenting cell; BTLA-4, B- and T-lymphocyte attenuator; Cbl-b, casitas B-cell lymphoma; CTL, cytotoxic T-lymphocyte; DOK-1/2, docking protein 1/2; EP2/4, prostaglandin E receptor 2/4; Erk, extra-cellular signal regulated kinases; ITIM, immunoreceptor tyrosine-based inhibition motif; ITSM, immunoreceptor tyrosine-based switch motif; GPCR, G-protein coupled receptor; LAG-3, lymphocyte-activation gene 3; LAIR-1, leukocyte-associated immunoglobulin-like receptor 1; Lck, lymphocyte-specific protein tyrosine kinase; MHC1, major histocompatibility complex class 1; PD-1, programed death receptor 1; PD1-L1, programed death receptor 1-ligand 1; SHP-1, Src homology 2 domain containing protein tyrosine phosphatase; TCR, T-cell receptor; TIGIT, T-cell immunoreceptor with Ig and ITIM domains; TIM-3, T-cell immunoglobulin domain and mucin domain 3.

of oligomeric ZFPs error-prone and narrow down the diversity of possible target DNA sequences. A successful and popular application of these technologies is the fusion of customized ZFPs or TALs to the catalytic domain of the restriction nuclease Fok1 (ZFNs and TALENs). Fok1 nucleases catalyze DNA double strand breaks (DSBs) when they dimerize (22). TALENs and ZFNs are therefore designed in pairs that target adjacent sequences on opposite DNA strands, thereby promoting Fok1 dimerization, separated by a spacer region where DNA cleavage occurs. Non-homologous end joining (NHEJ) repair of DSBs results in insertions or deletions at the DNA cleavage site (17, 23) and bi-allelic frameshift mutations that result in complete knockout occur at low frequencies (18, 24). The overall efficiency of the approach is sufficient to generate knockout cells following appropriate selection procedures. Of note TALEN design is more flexible as they can accommodate spacers of different lengths (25) whereas ZFNs strictly require 5–7 nt (26). Taking this into account, as well as structural constraints mentioned above, it is estimated that the frequency of target sequences is 1 in 500 bp for ZFNs and 1 in 35 bp for TALENs (20).

RNA-guided endonucleases provide a distinct and attractive alternative to genome editing compared with protein-guided nucleases. The functions of clustered regularly interspaced short palindromic repeats (CRISPR) and CRISPR-associated (Cas) proteins as a system providing adaptive immunity to bacteria against bacteriophages (27, 28) was recently harnessed for genome engineering (29, 30). The Cas9 nuclease binds to a short complementary RNA (crRNA) providing DNA-targeting specificity and to a trans-activating crRNA (tracRNA), required for crRNA processing, expressed individually or combined as a chimeric guide RNA (gRNA) (**Figure 1A**). CRISPR-Cas9 systems displayed a cleavage efficiency comparable (31) or superior (32) to TALENs in human cells. The clear advantage of RGEN is that it can be easily adapted to target different genomic sequences by customizing the synthetic crRNA/gRNA delivered in combination with Cas9 (33). In comparison ZFNs and TALENs require extensive engineering and validation steps.

The delivery of genome editing agents to T-cells is a crucial aspect of their successful application to ACTs. Because nuclease-based genome editing relies on generating transmissible mutations, protein- or RNA-guided nucleases only need to be transiently expressed. In fact transient expression probably minimizes off-target DNA cleavage (34). Provasi et al. have used integration-deficient lentiviruses as well as adenoviruses in order to modify the genome of T-cells with ZFNs (35). Of note it was recently shown that, due to their very repetitive nature, TAL arrays were incompatible with efficient reverse transcription required for the delivery of genetic material using lentiviruses (36), thereby limiting the range of delivery methods for TALENs.

APPLICATION OF THERAPEUTIC GENOME EDITING TO T-CELLS

Crucially therapies based on T-cell genome editing have already entered clinical development. A phase II clinical trial based on preventing the expression of the CCR5 gene, acting as a co-receptor for HIV in $CD4^+$ T-cells, using ZFNs (37) was recently initiated for the treatment of HIV/AIDS (NCT01252641). The safety results will be of huge importance for ZFN-based therapies and for genome editing in T-cells in general. Moreover a recent study provided proof of concept for the combination of TCR gene delivery with genome editing by using ZFNs specific for the endogenous constant TCR gene segments in order to prevent mispairing with ectopic TCR chains (35). The success of this approach provides a good rationale for wider applications of ZFN genome editing to T-cells.

Enhancing the anti-tumor potential of $CD8^+$ T-cells through genome editing can be done in many ways. Here we will focus on disrupting the expression of genes that inhibit T-cell functions as a result of the suppressive activity of the tumor microenvironment. T-cell inhibitory pathways targeted by genome editing in the context cancer ACTs should meet several criteria. First, their mechanism of action should be strictly cell-intrinsic. Second, they should be relevant to effector T-cells as opposed to naive T-cells. For instance CTLA-4 does not meet these two criteria since it works at least partly by reducing the availability of co-stimulatory molecules on the surface of antigen-presenting cells during the priming of naive T-cells (38). Finally, since only anti-tumor T-cells are modified, one of the advantages of this approach is that it allows targeting ubiquitous suppressive pathways whose systemic blockade or inhibition might result in serious adverse effects. Because it is clinically validated the most obvious target is probably PDCD1: the gene encoding the co-inhibitory receptor PD-1. PD-1 is expressed on activated T-cells and its engagement by its two known ligands PD-L1 and PD-L2 inhibits proximal signaling events triggered by TCR stimulation through recruitment of the phosphatase SHP-2 (39) and increased expression of the E3 ubiquitin ligase Cbl-b (40), which impair key components of the TCR signaling cascade through dephosphorylation and proteasomal degradation (**Figure 1B**). High cellular expression levels of PD-1 are characteristic of exhausted $CD8^+$ T-cells in chronic viral infections as well as TILs and correlate with impaired effector functions (41). Histological analyses have revealed that numerous tumor types express one or both PD-1 ligands (42, 43), prompting the targeting of this pathway in order to augment anti-tumor immunity. PD-1 blockade has shown promising objective response rates in a range of cancer indications and it is anticipated that PD-1 blocking agents will be approved for marketing authorization as mono-therapies. In addition these therapeutics are evaluated in combination with cancer vaccines, small-molecule signaling inhibitors, tumor-targeting mAbs, and cytokine therapy (http://clinicaltrials.gov/ct2/results?term=pd1&Search=Search). The combination of PD-1 blockade with these treatments, as well as with cancer ACTs, is expected to further enhance anti-tumor activity (11). Several other co-inhibitory receptors expressed by T-cells qualify as targets for gene editing coupled with antigen receptor delivery (**Table 1; Figure 1B**). *In vivo* and *in vitro* pre-clinical data strongly support the development of reagents targeting TIM-3 and LAG-3. Dual targeting of PD-1 and TIM-3 or LAG-3 with mAbs synergistically enhanced anti-tumor responses (44) and pre-clinical evaluations of a soluble Fc-LAG3 complex, which has now entered clinical development, were promising (45). Other targets are currently under similar evaluation procedures and might expand the list of druggable co-inhibitory receptors for cancer immunotherapy (**Table 1; Figure 1B**).

Table 1 | Potential immune checkpoint receptor targets for genome editing in the context of cancer adoptive cellular therapies.

	Name (gene)	Function	Ligand	Intra-cellular signaling/second messengers	Recognition motif	References
Co-inhibitory receptors	PD-1 (CD279)	Inhibition of T-cell activation and promotion of tolerance	PD-L1 (B7-H1) PD-L2 (B7-DC)	SHP-1 SHP-2	ITIM ITSM	Keir et al. (56), Parry et al. (57)
	LAG-3 (CD223)	Down regulation of T-cell cytokine secretion and proliferation	MHCII	–	–	Pardoll (12), Turnis et al. (58)
	BTLA (CD272)	Suppression of T-cell response	HVEM	SHP-2	ITIM	Murphy et al. (59), Watanabe et al. (60)
	OX2R (CD200R)	Inhibits T-cell function	CD200	DOK2	NPxY	Kretz-Rommel et al. (61), Moreaux et al. (62), Pallasch et al. (63)
	TIM-3	Down regulation of T-cell cytokine secretion and proliferation	Galectin 9 Phosphatidylserine	–	–	Pardoll (12), Zhu et al. (64)
	TIGIT	Inhibition of T-cell activation	VR, PVRL2, and PVRL3	–	ITIM	Joller et al. (65)
	LAIR-1	Inhibits cytotoxic activity	Collagen	SHP-1 SHP-2	ITIM	Lebbink et al. (66), Meyaard (67)
Receptors for soluble regulatory mediators	PGE2 receptors EP2/4	Inhibition of T-cell activity	PGE2	Adenylyl cyclase cAMP	–	Mahic et al. (68), Oberprieler et al. (53)
	Adenosine receptor 2A (A2AR)	Blocks T-cell activity	Adenosine	Adenylyl cyclase cAMP	–	Pardoll (12), Ohta et al. (50), Raskovalova et al. (69)

Non-extensive list of immune checkpoint receptors known to impair anti-tumor T-cell immunity in a cell-intrinsic manner. The relevant intra-cellular signaling and second messenger pathways, when known, are indicated.

The presence of cognate ligands within the tumor microenvironment is a crucial aspect for targeting co-inhibitory receptors and other immune checkpoint receptors. In the case of PD-1 retrospective analysis of patient biopsies in the phase Ib clinical trial assessing the blocking mAb BMS-936558 showed that the objective response rate in patients whose tumors expressed PD-L1 reached 36% compared with 18% in the entire cohort and 0% among patients with PD-L1-negative tumors (46). These striking results highlight the importance of prognosis and patient stratification for the design of appropriate cancer immunotherapies based on PD-1 inhibition. Such a strong correlation is still to be established for other immune checkpoint receptors but it is tempting to speculate that similar principles are applicable. However, even though their relevance in tumor immunity is established, it is not entirely clear what the actual ligands for several co-inhibitory receptors are in the context of anti-tumor immunity. More fundamental and clinical investigations are required in order to unambiguously identify relevant inhibitory ligands and assess their presence in the tumor environment.

Several soluble regulatory mediators also act as immune checkpoints in anti-tumor immunity. For instance high levels of extracellular adenosine are found in the vicinity of many solid tumors because of the hypoxic environment, a well-known environmental factor promoting adenosine release. Suppressive adenosine is also generated through direct dephosphorylation of extracellular adenosine nucleotides by the cell-surface nucleotidases CD39 and CD73 expressed by regulatory T-cells (T_{regs}) and some tumors, e.g., ovarian carcinomas (47, 48). The adenosine receptor 2A (A2AR), belonging to the G-protein coupled receptor family (GPCRs), is expressed on T-cells and has been identified as a target for immunotherapy for over a decade (12, 49–51). The A2AR inhibits T-cell activation through the cAMP-PKAI-CSK pathway (**Figure 1B**) and pre-clinical *in vivo* models have shown that A2AR knock-down or antagonism in adoptively transferred T-cells dramatically increased anti-tumor immunity (50). Inhibiting adenosine-mediated immune suppression is therefore believed to be an efficient strategy for cancer immunotherapies. Yet because adenosine receptors are ubiquitously expressed and involved in many physiological processes, especially in neurotransmission, classical antagonistic approaches are likely to result in a number of side effects. Such systemic adverse effects could be avoided in the context of adoptive T-cell therapies through T-cell-intrinsic gene editing or the *in vitro* selection of desensitized and irresponsive T-cells (52). Similarly, prostaglandin E2 (PGE2) directly suppresses T-cell activation through the cAMP second messenger pathway in effector/memory $CD8^+$ T-cells (53). Tumor-associated T_{regs} as well as colorectal cancer cells express high levels of immunosuppressive PGE2 (54). Interfering with EP2/EP4 receptors expression in T-cells may therefore enhance their anti-tumor potential.

A broader, possibly riskier, alternative to targeting individual immune checkpoint receptors would be interfering with the expression of downstream molecules conveying intra-cellular inhibitory signals. For instance several co-inhibitory receptors use the tyrosine phosphatases SHP-1 and/or SHP-2 to inhibit T-cell activation (**Figure 1B**). Inhibition of SHP-1/2 expression may therefore confer resistance to several checkpoint pathways used by tumors. Stromnes and colleagues reported that conditional knockout of SHP-1 in mature murine CD8$^+$ T-cells improved effector cell functions and tumor clearance in an adoptive transfer setting similar to cancer ACTs without resulting in autoimmune toxicity, thereby providing a good rationale for such an approach (55).

CONCLUDING REMARKS

T-cell based ACTs that rely on the re-infusion of patient T-cells expressing an artificial antigen receptor is an epitome of personalized medicine. These therapies require the identification of specific tumor antigens and/or patient HLA-type and would undoubtedly benefit from further prognostic analysis and subsequent treatment customization. Based on recent successes in cancer immunotherapy, immune checkpoint receptors that suppress T-cells represent a particularly attractive class of targets for such an approach. We believe that enhancing the anti-tumor potential of re-directed T-cells by targeting inhibitory pathways through genome editing can further improve the efficacy of cancer ACTs. Moreover cell-intrinsic inhibition of these pathways may display an advantageous safety profile compared with immune checkpoint blockade relying on the systemic administration of mAbs, recombinant proteins, or small molecules.

The field of genome editing is currently buzzing with new ideas and technologies that make the application of targeted gene knockout and gene correction a tantalizing prospect for the development of customized ACTs in regenerative medicine and immunotherapy. However, numerous potential pitfalls must be assessed in pre-clinical development. At this point ZFNs are the most advanced technology for genome editing and have already entered clinical development. However, their complicated and labor-intensive design, construction, and validation are major drawbacks for their widespread use in non-specialized laboratories, which often rely on commercial reagents. TALENs, on the other hand, are much more user-friendly and several toolboxes that allow investigators to generate custom reagents are available at low cost. With regard to T-cell based cancer ACTs, however, the incompatibility of TALENs with retroviral delivery, often used to express ectopic TCRs or CARs, might be problematic. Finally, CRISPR-Cas9 genome editing may prove to be the holy grail of genome editing but the current lack of hindsight on this technology does not allow concluding on its use yet. Thorough assessment of the respective advantages and drawbacks of each technology as well as pre-clinical feasibility and safety studies are warranted to validate genome editing applied to cancer ACTs.

REFERENCES

1. Schreiber RD, Old LJ, Smyth MJ. Cancer immunoediting: integrating immunity's roles in. *Science* (2011) **331**(6024):1565–70. doi:10.1126/science.1203486
2. Mellman I, Coukos G, Dranoff G. Cancer immunotherapy comes of age. *Nature* (2011) **480**:480–9. doi:10.1038/nature10673
3. Klebanoff CA, Acquavella N, Yu Z, Restifo NP. Therapeutic cancer vaccines: are we there yet? *Immunol Rev* (2011) **239**:27–44. doi:10.1111/j.1600-065X.2010.00979.x
4. Porter DL, Levine BL, Kalos M, Bagg A, June CH. Chimeric antigen receptor-modified T cells in chronic lymphoid leukemia. *N Engl J Med* (2011) **365**:725–33. doi:10.1056/NEJMoa1103849
5. Robbins PF, Morgan RA, Feldman SA, Yang JC, Sherry RM, Dudley ME, et al. Tumor regression in patients with metastatic synovial cell sarcoma and melanoma using genetically engineered lymphocytes reactive with NY-ESO-1. *J Clin Oncol* (2011) **29**:917–24. doi:10.1200/JCO.2010.32.2537
6. Rosenberg SA, Yang JC, Sherry RM, Kammula US, Hughes MS, Phan GQ, et al. Durable complete responses in heavily pre-treated patients with metastatic melanoma using T-cell transfer immunotherapy. *Clin Cancer Res* (2011) **17**:4550–7. doi:10.1158/1078-0432.CCR-11-0116
7. Blank CU, Hooijkaas AI, Haanen JB, Schumacher TN. Combination of targeted therapy and immunotherapy in melanoma. *Cancer Immunol Immunother* (2011) **60**:1359–71. doi:10.1007/s00262-011-1079-2
8. Vanneman M, Dranoff G. Combining immunotherapy and targeted therapies in cancer treatment. *Nat Rev Cancer* (2012) **12**:237–51. doi:10.1038/nrc3237
9. Noh KH, Kang TH, Kim JH, Pai SI, Lin KY, Hung CF, et al. Activation of Akt as a mechanism for tumor immune evasion. *Mol Ther* (2009) **17**:439–47. doi:10.1038/mt.2008.255
10. Boni A, Cogdill AP, Dang P, Udayakumar D, Njauw CN, Sloss CM, et al. Selective BRAFV600E inhibition enhances T-cell recognition of melanoma without affecting lymphocyte function. *Cancer Res* (2010) **70**:5213–9. doi:10.1158/0008-5472.CAN-10-0118
11. Martinez Forero I, Okada H, Topalian SL, Gajewski TF, Korman AJ, Melero I. Workshop on immunotherapy combinations. Society for immunotherapy of cancer annual meeting Bethesda, November 3, 2011. *J Transl Med* (2012) **10**:108. doi:10.1186/1479-5876-10-108
12. Pardoll DM. The blockade of immune checkpoints in cancer immunotherapy. *Nat Rev Cancer* (2012) **12**:252–64. doi:10.1038/nrc3239
13. An DS, Qin FX, Auyeung VC, Mao SH, Kung SK, Baltimore D, et al. Optimization and functional effects of stable short hairpin RNA expression in primary human lymphocytes via lentiviral vectors. *Mol Ther* (2006) **14**:494–504. doi:10.1016/j.ymthe.2006.05.015
14. Yi R, Doehle BP, Qin Y, Macara IG, Cullen BR. Overexpression of exportin 5 enhances RNA interference mediated by short hairpin RNAs and microRNAs. *RNA* (2005) **11**:220–6. doi:10.1261/rna.7233305
15. Castanotto D, Sakurai K, Lingeman R, Li H, Shively L, Aagaard L, et al. Combinatorial delivery of small interfering RNAs reduces RNAi efficacy by selective incorporation into RISC. *Nucleic Acids Res* (2007) **35**:5154–64. doi:10.1093/nar/gkm543
16. Couto LB, High KA. Viral vector-mediated RNA interference. *Curr Opin Pharmacol* (2010) **10**:534–42. doi:10.1016/j.coph.2010.06.007
17. Sanjana NE, Cong L, Zhou Y, Cunniff MM, Feng G, Zhang F. A transcription activator-like effector toolbox for genome engineering. *Nat Protoc* (2012) **7**:171–92. doi:10.1038/nprot.2011.431
18. Urnov FD, Rebar EJ, Holmes MC, Zhang HS, Gregory PD. Genome editing with engineered zinc finger nucleases. *Nat Rev Genet* (2010) **11**:636–46. doi:10.1038/nrg2842
19. Hwang WY, Fu Y, Reyon D, Maeder ML, Tsai SQ, Sander JD, et al. Efficient genome editing in zebrafish using a CRISPR-Cas system. *Nat Biotechnol* (2013) **31**:227–9. doi:10.1038/nbt.2501
20. Cermak T, Doyle EL, Christian M, Wang L, Zhang Y, Schmidt C, et al. Efficient design and assembly of custom TALEN and other TAL effector-based constructs for DNA targeting. *Nucleic Acids Res* (2011) **39**:e82. doi:10.1093/nar/gkr218
21. Wolfe SA, Nekludova L, Pabo CO. DNA recognition by Cys2His2 zinc finger proteins. *Annu Rev Biophys Biomol Struct* (2000) **29**:183–212. doi:10.1146/annurev.biophys.29.1.183
22. Hockemeyer D, Soldner F, Beard C, Gao Q, Mitalipova M, DeKelver RC, et al. Efficient targeting of expressed and silent genes in human ESCs and iPSCs using zinc-finger nucleases. *Nat Biotechnol* (2009) **27**:851–7. doi:10.1038/nbt.1562
23. Kim Y, Kweon J, Kim A, Chon JK, Yoo JY, Kim HJH, et al. A library of TAL effector nucleases spanning the human genome. *Nat Biotechnol* (2013) **31**:251–8. doi:10.1038/nbt.2517
24. Urnov FD, Miller JC, Lee YL, Beausejour CM, Rock JM, Augustus S, et al. Highly efficient endogenous human gene correction using designed zinc-finger nucleases. *Nature* (2005) **435**:646–51. doi:10.1038/nature03556
25. Miller JC, Tan S, Qiao G, Barlow KA, Wang J, Xia DF, et al. A TALE nuclease architecture for efficient genome editing. *Nat Biotechnol* (2011) **29**:143–8. doi:10.1038/nbt.1755

26. Christian M, Cermak T, Doyle EL, Schmidt C, Zhang F, Hummel A, et al. Targeting DNA double-strand breaks with TAL effector nucleases. *Genetics* (2010) **186**:757–61. doi:10.1534/genetics.110.120717
27. Brouns SJ, Jore MM, Lundgren M, Westra ER, Slijkhuis RJ, Snijders AP, et al. Small CRISPR RNAs guide antiviral defense in prokaryotes. *Science* (2008) **321**:960–4. doi:10.1126/science.1159689
28. Jinek M, Chylinski K, Fonfara I, Hauer M, Doudna JA, Charpentier E. A programmable dual-RNA-guided DNA endonuclease in adaptive bacterial immunity. *Science* (2012) **337**:816–21. doi:10.1126/science.1225829
29. Cong L, Ran FA, Cox D, Lin S, Barretto R, Habib N, et al. Multiplex genome engineering using CRISPR/Cas systems. *Science* (2013) **339**:819–23. doi:10.1126/science.1231143
30. Mali P, Yang L, Esvelt KM, Aach J, Guell M, DiCarlo JE, et al. RNA-guided human genome engineering via Cas9. *Science* (2013) **339**:823–6. doi:10.1126/science.1232033
31. Habib N, Hsu PD, Wu X, Jiang W, Luciano A, Cong L, et al. Multiplex genome engineering using CRISPR/Cas systems. *Science* (2013) **339**:819–23. doi:10.1126/science.1231143
32. Ding Q, Regan SN, Xia Y, Oostrom LA, Cowan CA, Musunuru K. Enhanced efficiency of human pluripotent stem cell genome editing through replacing TALENs with CRISPRs. *Cell Stem Cell* (2013) **12**:393–4. doi:10.1016/j.stem.2013.03.006
33. van der Oost J. Molecular biology. New tool for genome surgery. *Science* (2013) **339**:768–70. doi:10.1126/science.1234726
34. Lombardo A, Genovese P, Beausejour CM, Colleoni S, Lee YL, Kim KA, et al. Gene editing in human stem cells using zinc finger nucleases and integrase-defective lentiviral vector delivery. *Nat Biotechnol* (2007) **25**:1298–306. doi:10.1038/nbt1353
35. Provasi E, Genovese P, Lombardo A, Magnani Z, Liu PQ, Reik A, et al. Editing T cell specificity towards leukemia by zinc finger nucleases and lentiviral gene transfer. *Nat Med* (2012) **18**:807–15. doi:10.1038/nm.2700
36. Holkers M, Maggio I, Liu J, Janssen JM, Miselli F, Mussolino C, et al. Differential integrity of TALE nuclease genes following adenoviral and lentiviral vector gene transfer into human cells. *Nucleic Acids Res* (2012) **41**(5):e63. doi:10.1093/nar/gks1446
37. Perez EE, Wang J, Miller JC, Jouvenot Y, Kim KA, Liu O, et al. Establishment of HIV-1 resistance in CD4+ T cells by genome editing using zinc-finger nucleases. *Nat Biotechnol* (2008) **26**:808–16. doi:10.1038/nbt1410
38. Qureshi OS, Zheng Y, Nakamura K, Attridge K, Manzotti C, Schmidt EM, et al. Trans-endocytosis of CD80 and CD86: a molecular basis for the cell-extrinsic function of CTLA-4. *Science* (2011) **332**:600–3. doi:10.1126/science.1202947
39. Freeman GJ, Long AJ, Iwai Y, Bourque K, Chernova T, Nishimura H, et al. Engagement of the PD-1 immunoinhibitory receptor by a novel B7 family member leads to negative regulation of lymphocyte activation. *J Exp Med* (2000) **192**:1027–34. doi:10.1084/jem.192.7.1027
40. Karwacz K, Bricogne C, Macdonald D, Arce F, Bennett CL, Collins M, et al. PD-L1 co-stimulation contributes to ligand-induced T cell receptor down-modulation on CD8+ T cells. *EMBO Mol Med* (2011) **3**:581–92. doi:10.1002/emmm.201100165
41. Wherry EJ. T cell exhaustion. *Nat Immunol* (2011) **12**:492–9. doi:10.1038/ni.2035
42. Topalian SL, Drake CG, Pardoll DM. Targeting the PD-1/B7-H1(PD-L1) pathway to activate anti-tumor immunity. *Curr Opin Immunol* (2012) **24**:207–12. doi:10.1016/j.coi.2011.12.009
43. Zitvogel L, Kroemer G. Targeting PD-1/PD-L1 interactions for cancer immunotherapy. *Oncoimmunology* (2012) **1**:1223–5. doi:10.4161/onci.21335
44. Woo SR, Turnis ME, Goldberg MV, Bankoti J, Selby M, Nirschl CJ, et al. Immune inhibitory molecules LAG-3 and PD-1 synergistically regulate T-cell function to promote tumoral immune escape. *Cancer Res* (2012) **72**:917–27. doi:10.1158/0008-5472.CAN-11-1620
45. Fougeray S, Brignone C, Triebel F. A soluble LAG-3 protein as an immunopotentiator for therapeutic vaccines: preclinical evaluation of IMP321. *Vaccine* (2006) **24**:5426–33. doi:10.1016/j.vaccine.2006.03.050
46. Topalian SL, Hodi FS, Brahmer JR, Gettinger SN, Smith DC, McDermott DF, et al. Safety, activity, and immune correlates of anti-PD-1 antibody in cancer. *N Engl J Med* (2012) **366**:2443–54. doi:10.1056/NEJMoa1200690
47. Jin D, Fan J, Wang L, Thompson LF, Liu A, Daniel BJ, et al. CD73 on tumor cells impairs antitumor T-cell responses: a novel mechanism of tumor-induced immune suppression. *Cancer Res* (2010) **70**:2245–55. doi:10.1158/0008-5472.CAN-09-3109
48. Häusler SF, Montalbán del Barrio I, Strohschein J, Anoop Chandran P, Engel JB, Hönig A, et al. Ectonucleotidases CD39 and CD73 on OvCA cells are potent adenosine-generating enzymes responsible for adenosine receptor 2A-dependent suppression of T cell function and NK cell cytotoxicity. *Cancer Immunol Immunother* (2011) **60**:1405–18. doi:10.1007/s00262-011-1040-4
49. Ohta A, Sitkovsky M. Role of G-protein-coupled adenosine receptors in downregulation of inflammation and protection from tissue damage. *Nature* (2001) **414**:916–20. doi:10.1038/414916a
50. Ohta A, Gorelik E, Prasad SJ, Ronchese F, Lukashev D, Wong MKK, et al. A2A adenosine receptor protects tumors from antitumor T cells. *Proc Natl Acad Sci USA* (2006) **103**:13132–7. doi:10.1073/pnas.0605251103
51. Sitkovsky M, Ohta A. Targeting the hypoxia-adenosinergic signaling pathway to improve the adoptive immunotherapy of cancer. *J Mol Med (Berl)* (2013) **91**:147–55. doi:10.1007/s00109-013-1001-9
52. Ohta A, Kjaergaard J, Sharma S, Mohsin M, Goel N, Madasu M, et al. In vitro induction of T cells that are resistant to A2 adenosine receptor-mediated immunosuppression. *Br J Pharmacol* (2009) **156**:297–306. doi:10.1111/j.1476-5381.2008.00019.x
53. Oberprieler NG, Lemeer S, Kalland ME, Torgersen KM, Heck AJ, Tasken K. High-resolution mapping of prostaglandin E2-dependent signaling networks identifies a constitutively active PKA signaling node in CD8+CD45RO+ T cells. *Blood* (2010) **116**:2253–65. doi:10.1182/blood-2010-01-266650
54. Mosenden R, Tasken K. Cyclic AMP-mediated immune regulation – overview of mechanisms of action in T cells. *Cell Signal* (2011) **23**:1009–16. doi:10.1016/j.cellsig.2010.11.018
55. Stromnes IM, Fowler C, Casamina CC, Georgopolos CM, McAfee MS, Schmitt TM, et al. Abrogation of SRC homology region 2 domain-containing phosphatase 1 in tumor-specific T cells improves efficacy of adoptive immunotherapy by enhancing the effector function and accumulation of short-lived effector T cells in vivo. *J Immunol* (2012) **189**:1812–25. doi:10.4049/jimmunol.1200552
56. Keir ME, Butte MJ, Freeman GJ, Sharpe AH. PD-1 and its ligands in tolerance and immunity. *Annu Rev Immunol* (2008) **26**:677–704. doi:10.1146/annurev.immunol.26.021607.090331
57. Parry RV, Chemnitz JM, Frauwirth KA, Lanfranco AR, Braunstein I, Kobayashi SV, et al. CTLA-4 and PD-1 receptors inhibit T-cell activation by distinct mechanisms. *Mol Cell Biol* (2005) **25**:9543–53. doi:10.1128/MCB.25.21.9543-9553.2005
58. Turnis ME, Korman AJ, Drake CG, Vignali DA. Combinatorial immunotherapy: PD-1 may not be LAG-ing behind any more. *Oncoimmunology* (2012) **1**:1172–4. doi:10.4161/onci.20593
59. Murphy KM, Nelson CA, Sedý JR. Balancing co-stimulation and inhibition with BTLA and HVEM. *Nat Rev Immunol* (2006) **6**:671–81. doi:10.1038/nri1917
60. Watanabe N, Gavrieli M, Sedy JR, Yang J, Fallarino F, Loftin SK, et al. BTLA is a lymphocyte inhibitory receptor with similarities to CTLA-4 and PD-1. *Nat Immunol* (2003) **4**:670–9. doi:10.1038/ni944
61. Kretz-Rommel A, Qin F, Dakappagari N, Ravey EP, McWhirter J, Oltean D, et al. CD200 expression on tumor cells suppresses antitumor immunity: new approaches to cancer immunotherapy. *Mian Yi Xue Za Zhi* (2007) **178**:5595–605.
62. Moreaux J, Veyrune JL, Reme T, De Vos J, Klein B. CD200: a putative therapeutic target in cancer. *Biochem Biophys Res Commun* (2008) **366**:117–22. doi:10.1016/j.bbrc.2007.11.103
63. Pallasch CP, Ulbrich S, Brinker R, Hallek M, Uger RA, Wendtner C-M. Disruption of T cell suppression in chronic lymphocytic leukemia by CD200 blockade. *Leuk Res* (2009) **33**:460–4. doi:10.1016/j.leukres.2008.08.021
64. Zhu C, Anderson AC, Schubart A, Xiong H, Imitola J, Khoury SJ, et al. The Tim-3 ligand galectin-9 negatively regulates T helper type 1 immunity. *Nat Immunol* (2005) **6**:1245–52. doi:10.1038/ni1271
65. Joller N, Hafler JP, Brynedal B, Kassam N, Spoerl S, Levin

SD, et al. Cutting edge: TIGIT has T cell-intrinsic inhibitory functions. *Mian Yi Xue Za Zhi* (2011) **186**:1338–42. doi:10.4049/jimmunol.1003081

66. Lebbink RJ, de Ruiter T, Adelmeijer J, Brenkman AB, van Helvoort JM, Koch M, et al. Collagens are functional, high affinity ligands for the inhibitory immune receptor LAIR-1. *J Exp Med* (2006) **203**:1419–25. doi:10.1084/jem.20052554
67. Meyaard L. The inhibitory collagen receptor LAIR-1 (CD305). *J Leukoc Biol* (2008) **83**:799–803. doi:10.1189/jlb.0907609
68. Mahic M, Yaqub S, Johansson CC, Taskén K, Aandahl EM. FOXP3+CD4+CD25+ adaptive regulatory T cells express cyclooxygenase-2 and suppress effector T cells by a prostaglandin E2-dependent mechanism. *Mian Yi Xue Za Zhi* (2006) **177**:246–54.
69. Raskovalova T, Lokshin A, Huang X, Su Y, Mandic M, Zarour HM, et al. Inhibition of cytokine production and cytotoxic activity of human antimelanoma specific CD8+ and CD4+ T lymphocytes by adenosine-protein kinase A type I signaling. *Cancer Res* (2007) **67**:5949–56. doi:10.1158/0008-5472.CAN-06-4249

18

Molecular insights for optimizing T cell receptor specificity against cancer

Michael Hebeisen[1], Susanne G. Oberle[2,3], Danilo Presotto[1], Daniel E. Speiser[1,4], Dietmar Zehn[2,3] and Nathalie Rufer[1,4]*

[1] Department of Oncology, Lausanne University Hospital Center (CHUV), University of Lausanne, Lausanne, Switzerland
[2] Swiss Vaccine Research Institute, Epalinges, Switzerland
[3] Division of Immunology and Allergy, Department of Medicine, Lausanne University Hospital (CHUV), Lausanne, Switzerland
[4] Ludwig Center for Cancer Research, University of Lausanne, Lausanne, Switzerland

Edited by:
Bruno Laugel, Cardiff University, UK

Reviewed by:
Cyrille J. Cohen, Bar-Ilan University, Israel
David Escors, University College London, UK

***Correspondence:**
Nathalie Rufer, Department of Oncology, Lausanne University Hospital, c/o HO, niv 5, Avenue Pierre-Decker 4, CH-1011 Lausanne, Switzerland
e-mail: nathalie.rufer@unil.ch

Cytotoxic CD8 T cells mediate immunity to pathogens and they are able to eliminate malignant cells. Immunity to viruses and bacteria primarily involves CD8 T cells bearing high affinity T cell receptors (TCRs), which are specific to pathogen-derived (non-self) antigens. Given the thorough elimination of high affinity self/tumor-antigen reactive T cells by central and peripheral tolerance mechanisms, anti-cancer immunity mostly depends on TCRs with intermediate-to-low affinity for self-antigens. Because of this, a promising novel therapeutic approach to increase the efficacy of tumor-reactive T cells is to engineer their TCRs, with the aim to enhance their binding kinetics to pMHC complexes, or to directly manipulate the TCR-signaling cascades. Such manipulations require a detailed knowledge on how pMHC-TCR and co-receptors binding kinetics impact the T cell response. In this review, we present the current knowledge in this field. We discuss future challenges in identifying and targeting the molecular mechanisms to enhance the function of natural or TCR-affinity optimized T cells, and we provide perspectives for the development of protective anti-tumor T cell responses.

Keywords: cytotoxic T cells, TCR-affinity, melanoma, immunotherapy, TCR engineering, TCR signaling, T cell activating receptors, T cell inhibitory receptors

QUANTITATIVE ASPECTS OF ANTIGEN RECOGNITION BY CD8 T LYMPHOCYTES

Cytotoxic CD8 T lymphocytes recognize through their T cell receptors (TCRs) an antigenic peptide that is presented by MHC class I molecules (peptide-MHC, pMHC) on the surface of an infected or transformed cell. TCR triggering activates in T cells a signaling cascade, which leads to the release of effector molecules and to the cytolytic elimination of the cell that stimulated the T cell. The efficiency of triggering a T cell response critically depends on how well a TCR binds to a stimulating pMHC complex and stronger interactions are thought to cause more vigorous T cell activation than weaker interactions (Stone et al., 2009; Zehn et al., 2009). The dissociation constant K_D is a physical parameter that is generally used to describe the strength with which a TCR binds to a given pMHC complex (Zehn et al., 2012) and to which we usually refer to as the affinity of TCR and pMHC interaction.

Peripheral CD8 T cells express TCRs that only weakly react with self-peptide presenting pMHC and the K_D values of these interactions are in the range of 100–10 μM (Cole et al., 2007). In contrast, TCRs that interact with foreign-peptide presenting MHC with a K_D of up to 1 μM are frequently found among T cells that respond to pathogens (Davis et al., 1998). In fact, it is well established that immune responses to pathogen are dominated by cytotoxic T cells that express high affinity TCRs (**Figure 1**), and these cells are thought to be superior in executing effector function than low affinity T cells (Speiser et al., 1992; Alexander-Miller et al., 1996). Nonetheless, recent observations indicate that also a larger number of lower affinity T cell clones participate in immune responses. Moreover, it is well established that anti-tumor immune responses critically rely on lower affinity T cells, as most high affinity self/tumor-antigen specific T cells are usually thoroughly eliminated by both central and peripheral tolerance mechanisms. Within the subsequent sections, we will present key findings regarding the biology of cytotoxic CD8 T cells that respond with high or low affinity to antigen, we will describe how differences in affinity impact the outcome of a T cell response, and we will discuss several strategies to bypass the limitation that are linked to T cell responses mediated by low affinity T cells.

EVIDENCE FOR THE PARTICIPATION OF LOW AFFINITY CD8 T CELLS IN IMMUNE RESPONSES TO PATHOGENS

To characterize how TCR–pMHC affinity impacts T cells in an infection, we expressed in pathogens a set of altered peptide ligands that gradually differ in the strength of binding to the OT-1 TCR. By infecting mice with pathogens expressing these ligands, we can mimic high, intermediate, or low affinity stimulation, as it would be the case with polyclonal cytotoxic T cells of which some respond with high and others with low affinity to pathogen-derived antigen (Zehn et al., 2009). Unexpectedly, we found that the OT-1 T cells initially responded similarly to pMHC complexes that very differently stimulated the OT-1 TCR. Even very low affinity complexes induced the same initial rapid T cell proliferation as high affinity ones. Low affinity-stimulated OT-1 CD8 T cells were early on phenotypically indistinguishable from cells stimulated by

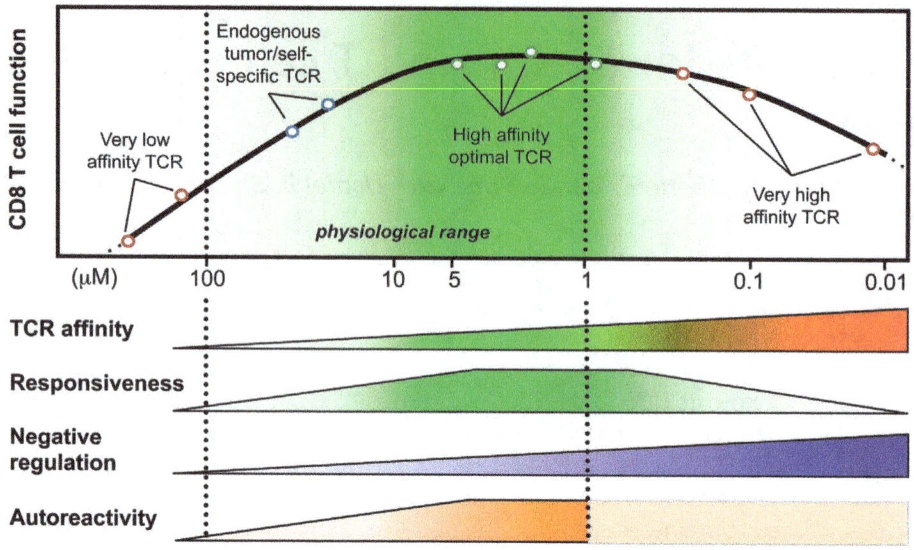

FIGURE 1 | Model integrating the relationship between T cell responsiveness (e.g., cell signaling, gene expression, and functionality) and TCR-affinity (in K_D, μM) of human CD8 T lymphocytes engineered with anti-tumor TCR variants of optimized affinities (Irving et al., 2012; Hebeisen et al., 2013; Zhong et al., 2013). Optimal/maximal T cell effectiveness is observed with cells expressing affinities in the upper natural limit (K_D from 5 to 1 μM; dark green). Negative regulation mechanisms may counteract T cell responsiveness in T cells bearing very high affinities (depicted as blue gradients) (Corse et al., 2010; Slansky and Jordan, 2010; Hebeisen et al., 2013). Moreover, Zhong et al. (2013) recently described an affinity threshold (K_D around 10 μM) for maximal anti-tumor activity and autoreactivity (depicted as orange gradients).

high affinity complexes. Expression of effector molecules such as granzyme B, as well as effector and memory T cell functions were surprisingly efficient (Zehn and Bevan, 2006; Enouz et al., 2012). It has also been shown that very low affinity stimulated T cells support pathogen elimination (Turner et al., 2008). Together, these findings indicate that lower affinity CD8 T cells fully participate in the immune response.

However, there is a major difference between low and high affinity CD8 T cells. Namely, the former undergo fewer rounds of division and decline in numbers faster than high affinity stimulated T cells. Thus, while undergoing full differentiation, low affinity primed effector T cells reach lower numbers. Therefore the high affinity T cells dominate in numbers at the time when T cell expansion is at its maximum.

Given their low numbers, one may question the importance of low affinity CD8 T cells. The large numbers of high affinity T cells at the peak of the immune response have so far distracted from exploring the relevance of low affinity T cells during infection. Several kinetic aspects may suggest that low affinity T cells could perhaps be more important than previously appreciated. In the naïve T cell repertoire, high affinity T cell clones specific to any given antigen are rare. In contrast, it is likely that low affinity T cell clones are more frequent. As low and high affinity clones expand equally at the beginning, there should be a larger number of low than high affinity effector T cells in the early phase of the T cell response, as we found in our experiments. The dominance of high affinity CD8 T cells develops later, because these cells overgrow the lower affinity T cells in the late T cell expansion phase (Zehn et al., 2009). Importantly, we noticed that low affinity T cells leave secondary lymphoid organs earlier than high affinity T cells, suggesting that the earliest wave of effector T cells that enter peripheral organs predominately consists of low affinity T cells. Thus, the critical early phase of pathogen elimination may be primarily achieved by low affinity cytolytic T cells (Zehn et al., 2009).

The number of low affinity T cells responding to one particular epitope is perhaps small. However, there could be many unknown epitopes recognized by low affinity T cells, which cumulatively might result in a reasonably sized T cell population. These considerations suggest that low affinity CD8 T cells play a more important role during infection than previously anticipated, which may have been underestimated in the past.

ANTI-SELF AND -TUMOR IMMUNE RESPONSES ARE FREQUENTLY MEDIATED BY LOW AFFINITY CD8 T CELLS

Anti-tumor immune response targets tumor-associated antigens such as cancer testis antigens (e.g., NY-ESO-1 or MAGEs) expressed by several tumors or differentiation antigens (e.g., Melan-A/MART-1, gp100, or tyrosinase) expressed in melanoma cells (Romero et al., 2002; Van Der Bruggen et al., 2002; Boon et al., 2006). Most of these antigens are expressed in the thymus (Kyewski and Klein, 2006) and accordingly, T cells with high affinity become negatively selected. As a backup, tumor-antigen reactive T cells can be eliminated in the periphery through mechanisms of peripheral tolerance (Kurts et al., 1997). However, it has been convincingly shown, that these mechanisms spare cytotoxic T cells that react with lower affinity to self- or tumor-antigens (von Herrath et al., 1994; Zehn and Bevan, 2006; McMahan and Slansky, 2007; Turner et al., 2008). Although, it is still often rather difficult to judge how effectively lower affinity CD8 T cells execute effector T cell functions, several strong line of evidence indicate that low affinity auto-reactive T cells are able to eliminate tumors and play a critical role in autoimmunity (von Herrath et al., 1994; Zehn and Bevan, 2006; McMahan and Slansky, 2007; Bulek et al., 2012). In fact, it becomes more and more clear that most self/tumor-specific cytotoxic T cells express low affinity TCRs and there is increasing evidence that the self/tumor-specific T cells are indeed capable to destroy cancer cells *in vivo* (Boon et al., 2006; Rosenberg et al., 2008). Moreover, it has been shown that self/tumor-antigen specific CD8 T cells can undergo considerable clonal expansion in cancer patients, differentiate to memory and effector cells, and persist during several years at relatively high frequencies (Speiser et al., 2011; Baitsch et al., 2012). These observations are well in line with the aforementioned findings that low affinity CD8 T cells participating in the response to pathogens may have great implications for anti-cancer immunity.

However, researchers must still deal with several challenges associated with activating low affinity CD8 T cells. For example, these cells require higher numbers of presented pMHC complexes than high affinity T cells before they become activated and for mounting an effector T cell response. Also, requirements for interactions with DCs by CD8 T cells of low TCR affinities are likely higher, to achieve sufficient TCR triggering and co-stimulation (Liechtenstein et al., 2012; Chen and Flies, 2013). Furthermore, lower affinity CD8 T cells undergo, as mentioned above, shorter clonal expansion following stimulation than high affinity T cells which means that fewer of such cells will be obtained following vaccination. Given these limitations, we need to find better ways to more effectively activate these T cells, to enhance their function, and to selectively interfere with the mechanisms, which prevent these cells from responding to tumors. One possible way to do this is to alter the kinetics with which the TCR of a tumor-specific T cell binds to its peptide-pMHC complex. Another approach would be to manipulate the signaling cascades downstream of the TCR.

TCR-AFFINITY OPTIMIZATION AGAINST CANCER ANTIGENS

Immunotherapy aims at mobilizing the body's immune cells to fight against tumor cells in a highly specific manner. There are two biological strategies to achieve immune activity: active immunization with the use of vaccination and passive immunization. A form of passive immunotherapy is the adoptive cell transfer (ACT) of autologous T lymphocytes to patients with metastatic cancer (Restifo et al., 2012). This approach uses autologous TIL (tumor infiltrating lymphocytes), which are isolated from metastatic lesions, expanded *in vitro*, and selected for tumor reactivity. Remarkably, about 50 to 70% of patients with metastatic melanoma experience objective clinical responses, and up to 20% even have complete and durable responses (Rosenberg et al., 2011). Nevertheless, further improvements are necessary.

A limiting factor is the relatively low affinity of tumor-antigen reactive T cells. For improvement, T cells can be engineered with TCRs of increased affinity for tumor-antigens before transfer to patients (**Figure 1**). Indeed, this approach may augment the functional and protective capacity of tumor-antigen reactive CD8 T cells (Robbins et al., 2008, 2011; Bendle et al., 2009; Bowerman et al., 2009; Chervin et al., 2009; Johnson et al., 2009). In turn, TCR engineering also bears the risk that the normal tissue could be harmed. It has been demonstrated that T cells, whose TCR binds to pMHC complexes with very high affinities ($K_D < 1$ nM) lose antigen specificity and can become cross-reactive or alloreactive (Holler et al., 2003; Zhao et al., 2007; Robbins et al., 2008). Importantly, genetically engineered T lymphocytes expressing very high affinity self/tumor-specific TCRs also target normal tissues expressing the cognate antigen (e.g., melanocytes in the skin, eye, and ear for Melan-A-specific T cells and neurons for MAGE-A3-specific T cells), and can mount harmful cytotoxic immune responses *in vivo* (Johnson et al., 2009; Morgan et al., 2013). Moreover, TCR mispairing between introduced and endogenous TCR α and β chains has also been shown to lead to off-target toxicity (Bendle et al., 2010; van Loenen et al., 2010). Therefore, TCR optimization through affinity alteration must include the evaluation of optimal T cell responsiveness and lack of cross-reactivity to ensure the safety of TCR-engineered T cells in clinical trials. Moreover, it must further include the development of new strategies to minimize the extent of mispairing (reviewed in Govers et al., 2010; Daniel-Meshulam et al., 2012), as elegantly shown by Aggen et al. (2012), describing the use of stabilized VαVβ single-chain TCRs (scTv; **Figure 2**). Unfortunately, unexpected auto-reactive responses may never be completely excluded. In that regard, it is important to further study the tissue distribution of self/tumor-antigen expression, to optimize the choice of antigens targeted by ACT therapy (e.g., cancer testis versus differentiation antigens) (Offringa, 2009).

TCR-AFFINITY THRESHOLD FOR MAXIMAL ANTI-TUMOR CD8 T CELL RESPONSE

During recent years we established a panel of human CD8 T cells expressing engineered TCRs of optimized affinities against the tumor-antigen NY-ESO-1 presented in the context of HLA-A2. They were obtained through structure-based rational predictions (Zoete and Michielin, 2007; Zoete et al., 2010). The functional potential of these T cells (Schmid et al., 2010; Irving et al., 2012) showed that T cells expressing TCRs with affinities in the upper natural range (K_D from 5 to 1 μM) displayed greater biological responses when compared to those expressing intermediate affinity wild-type TCR (K_D at 21.4 μM) or very low affinity ($K_D > 100$ μM) (**Figure 1**). Unexpectedly, we noticed that T cells which express TCRs beyond the natural affinity range ($K_D < 1$ μM) showed a severe decline in their gene expression profile, signaling, and functionality (Irving et al., 2012; Hebeisen et al., 2013), despite retaining their antigen specificity and showing no broad cross-reactivity as observed in other studies (Holler et al., 2003). Major findings revealed that maximal T cell effectiveness was limited by at least two mechanisms (**Figure 1**). The first one was characterized by the preferential expression of the inhibitory receptor programed cell death-1 (PD-1) within T cells of the highest TCR affinities and this correlated in those cells with full functional recovery upon PD-1 ligand 1 (PD-L1) blockade (Hebeisen et al., 2013). The second one contrasted to PD-1 expression with the gradual upregulation of the Src homology 2 domain-containing phosphatase 1 (SHP-1) in CD8 T cells with increasing TCR affinities. Consequently, pharmacological inhibition allowed further incremental gaining of cell function in

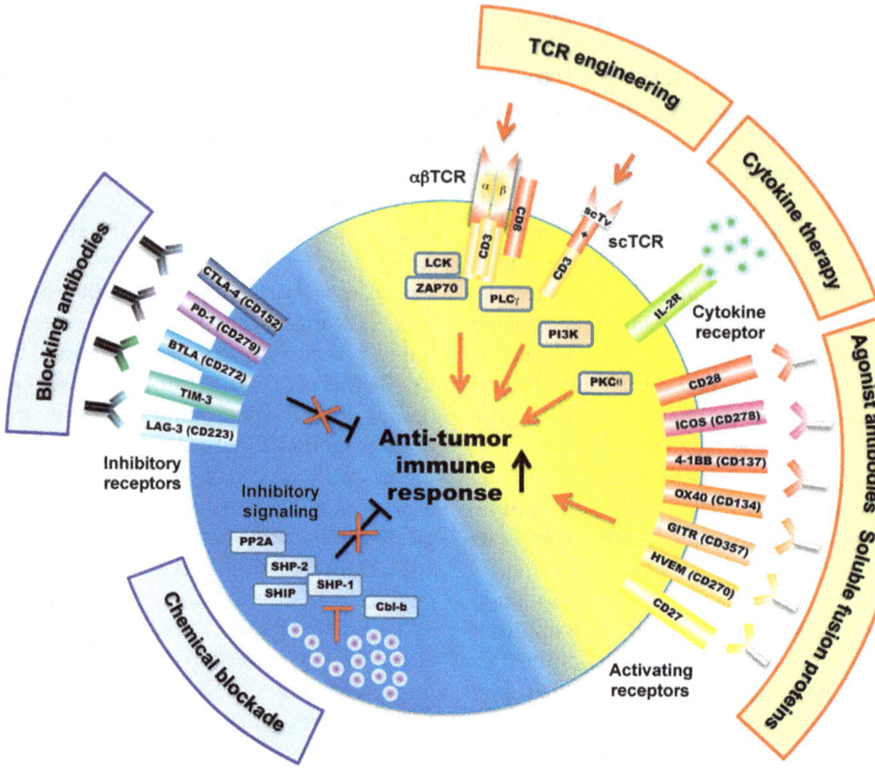

FIGURE 2 | Overview of mechanisms and potential therapeutic targets as a strategy to improve tumor-antigen reactive T lymphocytes. These include a large variety of receptors (e.g., engineered TCRs, activating/inhibitory surface receptors, cytokine receptor) as well as TCR-downstream signaling molecules (e.g., SHP-1, SHP-2, PP2A) that regulate T cell activation, signaling, and function (e.g., killing, cytokine secretion) against cancer antigens. Of note, the scTv single VαVβ chain TCRs may be linked to intracellular signaling domains such as Lck and CD28, independently of the CD3 subunits (Aggen et al., 2012).

all engineered T cells, according to their TCR-binding affinities (Hebeisen et al., 2013).

Our observations provide new evidence that T cell activation and signaling may be limited to a given affinity threshold for the TCR-pMHC interaction and that above this threshold, T cells may not develop productive functions. They also nicely fit with other *in vitro* and *in vivo* studies that reported maximal T cell responses at an optimal TCR–pMHC off rate (k_{off}) or K_{D} while functional attenuation was observed when kinetic parameters extended above the natural range (Kalergis et al., 2001; Gonzalez et al., 2005; McMahan et al., 2006; Carreno et al., 2007; Corse et al., 2010; Thomas et al., 2011). Furthermore, Krogsgaard and colleagues (Zhong et al., 2013) recently evaluated the TCR-affinity threshold defining the optimal balance between effective anti-tumor activity and autoimmunity *in vivo*, using human melanoma gp100$_{209-217}$–specific TCRs spanning within the physiological affinity range. Their results show the presence of an affinity threshold (around 10 μM) for maximal anti-tumoral activity and autoreactivity, suggesting that a relatively low-affinity threshold is necessary for the immune system to avoid self-damage (Zhong et al., 2013). Altogether, we and others propose that the rational design of improved self-specific TCRs for adoptive T cell therapy may not need to be optimized beyond the natural TCR-affinity range to achieve optimal T cell function and avoidance of unpredictable risk of cross-reactivity (Schmid et al., 2010; Slansky and Jordan, 2010).

Recently, Liddy et al. (2012) described the use of novel reagents termed immune-mobilizing monoclonal TCRs (or ImmTACs) against tumor-antigens including NY-ESO-1, which are fused to a humanized CD3-specific single-chain αβ fragment (scFv). These ImmTACs comprise TCRs of picomolar affinity range and allow to effectively redirect T cells to kill *in vivo* cancer cells expressing very low surface epitope densities. In line with previous studies from the same group (Li et al., 2005; Dunn et al., 2006), soluble monomeric TCRs possessing affinity ≈10^6-fold higher than native TCRs showed a remarkable high degree of specificity for the cognate pMHC molecules. Possibly, soluble monomeric TCRs may allow circumventing the two major limitations associated with TCR engineering within CD8 T cells. First, the loss of target cell specificity associated with T cells expressing extremely high affinity TCRs ($K_{\text{D}} < 1$ nM) (Zhao et al., 2007; Robbins et al., 2008). And second, the functional defects of T cells with supraphysiological TCR affinities ($K_{\text{D}} < 1$ μM) (Kalergis et al., 2001; Gonzalez et al., 2005; McMahan et al., 2006; Corse et al., 2010; Thomas et al., 2011).

At present, what remains intriguing is how super affine TCRs modulate cell activation and responsiveness. One likely explanation is that in contrast to soluble TCRs, the cellular TCR expression integrates and potentiates the effect of several variables/parameters including TCR density, multivalent TCR clustering, and basal cell activation state (Stone et al., 2009). Furthermore, several observations including ours (Hebeisen et al., 2013) now indicate that T cell activation and signaling is also finely tuned by the proximal TCR-signaling complex as well as by activatory or inhibitory co-receptors, and will be discussed in detail below.

LOW AND HIGH AFFINITY ANTIGEN RECOGNITION DEPENDS ON THE PROXIMAL TCR-SIGNALING COMPLEX

The TCR complex is composed of the TCR αβ chains, which are directly involved in the pMHC recognition, and of the invariant CD3 proteins, that contain in their cytosolic domains the immunoreceptor tyrosine-based activation motifs (ITAM) (Hedrick et al., 1984; Malissen et al., 1984; Letourneur and Klausner, 1992). TCR triggering elicits a series of membrane-associated events, leading to the transduction of signal across the plasma membrane and phosphorylation of key residues in the TCR-associated CD3 ITAM domains (Stefanova et al., 2003; James and Vale, 2012). Phosphorylation of CD3ζ-associated ITAM is mediated by the Src family kinases Lck and Fyn (Acuto et al., 2008) and form docking sites for several protein tyrosine kinases (PTKs) including the Syk-family kinase ζ-associated protein of 70 kDa, ZAP-70. Activation of ZAP-70 by Lck in turns results in phosphorylation and activation of other proteins and recruitment of adaptors (e.g., LAT and SLP-76). This initiates the formation of multi-molecular signalosomes, leading to the subsequent generation of secondary messengers and of multiple distal signaling cascades (Acuto et al., 2008; Smith-Garvin et al., 2009).

CD8 T cells may further adapt these signaling pathways to different stimulation conditions and different requirements for antigen sensitivity. Several lines of evidence indicate that differential patterns of CD3ζ ITAM phosphorylation directly modulate TCR-pMHC mediated downstream signaling and that ITAMs can act as both positive (ITAMs) and negative (inhibitory ITAMi) cell signaling regulators (Blank et al., 2009). For instance, resting peripheral T cells have a constitutive pattern of phosphorylated ITAMs, and incomplete CD3ζ ITAM phosphorylation after TCR triggering can by itself become inhibitory depending on the nature of the TCR ligand (Kersh et al., 1999). Thus, it is of great importance to further explore whether distinct CD3ζ ITAM phosphorylation states could also influence cell activation and responsiveness along the range of TCR-affinity and particularly in engineered CD8 T cells of supraphysiological affinity TCRs.

Lck represents another key regulatory element involved in the modulation of proximal TCR activation and signaling, and Lck activation stage may currently be viewed as a sensor of the strength of TCR engagement. On the one hand, weak binding of the TCR triggers Lck-dependent activation and recruitment of SHP-1, which in a classical feedback loop inactivates Lck and downregulates TCR signaling. On the other hand, stronger TCR activation induces an Erk-dependent Lck phosphorylation that impairs the inhibitory SHP-1 recruitment and in contrast reinforces TCR signaling by decreasing the threshold of T cell activation (Stefanova et al., 2003). Interestingly, as mentioned above, we recently used a panel of CD8 T cells engineered with TCRs of incremental affinities for an NY-ESO-1 derived peptide and saw that SHP-1 phosphatase was upregulated in a TCR-affinity-dependent manner, with the highest levels in T cells of the supraphysiological TCRs (Hebeisen et al., 2013). These observations further suggests that SHP-1 may play a dual role and restricts not only T cell signaling at the very low range of TCR stimulation (e.g., antagonist ligands) as described by Stefanova et al. (2003), but also at the higher range.

Other phosphatases have been shown to act on the proximal TCR signaling such as Lyp, a PTPN22 encoded phosphatase, and together with Csk inhibit T cell activation, likely through dephosphorylation of the activating tyrosine on Lck and ZAP-70 (Cloutier and Veillette, 1999). The importance of PTPN22 is highlighted by the observation that PTPN22 deficient mice have augmented TCR-induced phosphorylation and activation (Hasegawa et al., 2004). Furthermore, a point mutation in PTPN22 has been found associated with several autoimmune diseases (Mustelin et al., 2005). The precise role of PTPN22 in T cell activation remains unknown and there is contradictory data on the effect of the polymorphism found in autoimmune patients and whether or not it causes a loss or gain of function (Vang et al., 2005).

These TCR-affinity-dependent feedback mechanisms are likely part of a tunable instrument that enables T cells to adapt their reactivity to different stimulatory conditions, and we have just began to understand how those are achieved. For instance specific microRNAs such as miR-181a are thought to be critical in augmenting TCR-signaling sensitivity during positive selection in the thymus (Li et al., 2007). The expression of miR-181a has been shown to decrease the amount of several phosphatases, resulting in an elevated steady-state level of phosphorylated proteins of the TCR-signaling cascade and therefore a reduction in the TCR-signaling threshold (Li et al., 2007; Ebert et al., 2009). TCR activation and signaling transduction may also be negatively regulated by SHP-1 phosphatase and contributes to the settings of threshold during thymocyte selection (Plas et al., 1996; Acuto et al., 2008). Moreover, SHP-1 and SHP-2 can be recruited by multiple inhibitory surface receptors in T cells, and inhibit TCR signaling through dephosphorylation of proximal targets including Lck and ZAP-70 (Lorenz, 2009). In line with this concept, Yokosuka et al. (2012) recently showed that ITIM-containing PD-1 could directly inhibit TCR-mediated signaling by recruiting SHP-2 phosphatase in a TCR stimulation strength-dependent manner.

CYTOTOXIC CD8 T CELL RESPONSES ARE REGULATED BY ACTIVATING AND INHIBITORY SURFACE RECEPTORS

Co-stimulatory and inhibitory membrane receptors have great influence on T cell responses (Chen and Flies, 2013). T cell co-stimulation prevents T cell anergy, a state of unresponsiveness that is induced after TCR stimulation in absence of co-stimulation (**Figure 2**). This was first observed when studying co-stimulation via CD28 that binds to its ligands B7.1 (CD80) and B7.2 (CD86) expressed on antigen-presenting cells (APC). This interaction also lowers the threshold for T cell activation, thus allowing increased IL-2 production and promoting cell proliferation and survival (Sharpe and Freeman, 2002). CD28 ligation stimulates T cell function by activating phosphoinositol-3-kinase (PI3K) and protein kinase C theta (PKCθ), and the downstream Akt, mTOR, and Ras signaling pathways, which eventually synergize with TCR signaling (Smith-Garvin et al., 2009). T cell activation also leads to surface expression of CTLA-4, which has a much higher binding avidity to B7.1 and B7.2, and thus outcompetes CD28 (Greene et al., 1996). Possibly, this may be the main reason for CTLA-4 mediated T cell inhibition. In addition, it has been shown that CTLA-4 directly triggers inhibitory signaling by interacting with SHP-1, SHP-2, and PP2A phosphatases, with the consequence of down-regulating TCR-signaling pathway (Scalapino and Daikh, 2008). CTLA-4 inhibition also occurs indirectly via retro-signaling through B7.1 and B7.2 and production of IDO in APCs (Grohmann et al., 2002) or by a process of trans-endocytosis of its ligands (B7.1 and B7.2) from APC (Qureshi et al., 2011). CTLA-4 may preferentially inhibit T cells with strong TCR signaling, as suggested by observations that accumulation of CTLA-4 at the immunological synapse depended on the strength of TCR triggering (Egen et al., 2002).

Programed death-1 is also highly upregulated in T cells following TCR stimulation, similarly to CTLA-4. Expression of PD-1 is not restricted to T cells, suggesting a broader role in immune regulation (Greenwald et al., 2005). PD-1 interacts with the two ligands PD-L1 and PD-L2, expressed non-redundantly in different tissues and cell types. CTLA-4-deficient mice have lymphoproliferative disorders and early fatal multi-organ tissue destruction (Tivol et al., 1995; Waterhouse et al., 1995), whereas PD-1-deficient mice spontaneously develop milder forms of autoimmune diseases (Nishimura et al., 2001). Based on the observed differential expression of CTLA-4 and PD-1 ligands, it is assumed that CTLA-4 plays a preferential role in limiting T cell function early during thymocyte development and in secondary lymphoid structures, whereas PD-1 may mediate inhibition in the periphery, for example in maintaining long-term peripheral tolerance to self-antigens by preventing activation of self-reactive T cells that have escaped negative selection (Fife and Pauken, 2011). TCR down-modulation through TCR/CD28 signaling transduction represents a fundamental process regulating the initial events of T cell activation. Recently, the interaction of PD-L1 on DCs and PD-1 on CD8 T cells has been shown to contribute to ligand-induced TCR down-modulation (Karwacz et al., 2011). Furthermore, interference with PD-L1/PD-1 signaling inhibited TCR down-modulation, leading to hyper-activated and proliferative CD8 T cells in an arthritis model (Karwacz et al., 2011).

In humans, a regulatory polymorphism in PD-1 is associated with susceptibility to systemic lupus erythematosus and multiple sclerosis (Prokunina et al., 2002; Kroner et al., 2005), while polymorphisms of the CTLA-4 have been linked to multiple autoimmune diseases including asthma, systemic lupus erythematosus, Graves' disease, and autoimmune thyroid diseases (Kristiansen et al., 2000). The induction of PD-L1 ligand expression was observed in several tumor cells as a mechanism of cancer immune evasion (Schreiber et al., 2011). A specific polymorphism of CTLA-4 was found to be protective for autoimmune disease, but associated with risk of multiple types of cancer (Sun et al., 2009).

Members of the tumor necrosis factor receptor (TNFR) superfamily represent further important co-stimulatory molecules, mediating survival signals to T cells after initial CD28-B7 interactions (Acuto and Michel, 2003) (**Figure 2**). Multiple members of TNFR/TNF ligand pairs have been shown to directly impact T cell function following TCR activation, namely OX40/OX40L, 4-1BB/4-1BBL, GITR/GITRL, CD27/CD70, and CD30/CD30L (Watts, 2005). These receptors and their ligands are expressed on a variety of immune and non-immune cells and are inducible and non-ubiquitous, suggesting that they are involved in modulating and coordinating global immune responses (Croft, 2009). Intense translational and clinical research in this field aims at modulating T cell function in pathological settings such as autoimmunity and cancer (**Figure 2**). TNFR/TNF family member ligation often induces bi-directional activating signaling pathways in both the APC and the T cell. The recruitment of TNFR-associated factors (TRAF) activate the NF-κB signaling pathway and increase the expression of anti-apoptotic molecules, thus promoting the survival of CD4 and CD8 T cells (Croft, 2009). Like CD28, TNFR signaling can also synergize with the TCR pathway to promote cell cycle progression and cytokine production. Finally, ligation of OX40 and 4-1BB may concomitantly block the generation of inducible regulatory T cells (Tregs), and may inhibit their suppressive activity (So et al., 2008).

A particularly unique and interesting member of the TNFR superfamily is HVEM (Herpes virus entry molecule). It binds to the TNFR ligands LIGHT and lymphotoxin Ltα3, which are predominantly co-stimulatory and pro-inflammatory in T cells. Curiously, HVEM also binds to BTLA and CD160, which are structurally similar to PD-1 and CTLA-4 and transduce inhibitory signals, in part through recruitment of SHP-1 and SHP-2 phosphatases (Watanabe et al., 2003; Sedy et al., 2005). The individual effects of HVEM interaction with its different ligands are particularly complex to elucidate since both receptor and ligands can be expressed on the same T cell, as well as on other immune and epithelial cell types (Shui et al., 2011). *Hvem*$^{-/-}$ and *Btla*$^{-/-}$ T cells were found to be hyper-responsive to TCR stimulation *in vitro*. Furthermore, *Hvem*$^{-/-}$ and *Btla*$^{-/-}$ knockout mice had enhanced susceptibility to autoimmune diseases, suggesting a predominant inhibitory role in T cells during inflammatory conditions (Watanabe et al., 2003; Wang et al., 2005). BTLA was found to inhibit tumor-antigen specific cytotoxic T cells in melanoma patients (Derre et al., 2010). HVEM may also interact in *cis* with BTLA expressed by the same cell, likely interfering with HVEM activation by other ligands (Ware and Sedy, 2011). Therefore HVEM seems to mediate immune stimulation or inhibition in a switch-like, bi-directional, and context-dependent mode, suggesting that HVEM/LIGHT/CD160/BTLA interactions represent an important regulatory network for controlling immune responses.

Together, combined TCR and CD28/TNFR triggering primes CD8 T cells, followed by positive and negative regulation. The latter involves CTLA-4, PD-1, and BTLA. This highlights the intricate regulatory network that controls the immune system in health and disease (**Figure 2**). These mechanisms can be exploited therapeutically in patients with infectious or malignant diseases, as well as in autoimmunity and transplantation (Fife and Bluestone, 2008; del Rio et al., 2010).

ACTIVATORY OR INHIBITORY T CELL SIGNALS MAY BE TARGETED FOR THERAPEUTIC IMPROVEMENTS OF CANCER THERAPIES

Since cytotoxic CD8 T cells and T-helper type 1 [Th1] cells have the potential to eliminate cancer cells and to mediate long-term protection from disease (Sallusto et al., 2010), it is important to increase the functions of these anti-cancer T cells in cancer patients. As mentioned above, basic immunology characterized a number of interesting pathways that can be targeted to enhance the performance of tumor-specific CD8 T cells. Some approaches have already reached clinical application, but most still need to be tested in clinical trials. The therapy that seems most efficient for melanoma patients is the adoptive transfer of autologous tumor-antigen specific T cells (Rosenberg, 2011). Molecular modification of T cells before transfer may eventually increase the clinical efficacy, despite that this is currently not the case (Speiser, 2013). Several small-scale clinical studies suggested clinical usefulness of inserting TCRs (Rosenberg, 2011) or chimeric antigen receptors (Porter et al., 2011; Kochenderfer and Rosenberg, 2013). Hopefully, larger patient numbers will soon benefit thanks to steady improvements of these techniques (Thomas et al., 2010; Di Stasi et al., 2011; Linnemann et al., 2011; Ochi et al., 2011).

Not only antigen receptors but also co-receptors can be targeted therapeutically (**Figure 2**). Receptors that inhibit T cell functions are particularly attractive. Ipilimumab (Yervoy ®) is a monoclonal antibody that blocks the inhibitory receptor CTLA-4. It was recently approved for the treatment of metastatic melanoma, as it improves the clinical outcome, likely due to enhanced numbers and functions of tumor-specific T cells (Hodi et al., 2010). More recently, remarkable benefit for patients with advanced kidney cancer, non-small-cell lung cancer, and melanoma (Ribas, 2012) was demonstrated due to treatment with antibodies against PD-1 (Topalian et al., 2012) or its ligand PD-L1 (Brahmer et al., 2012). Likely, these results represent real therapeutic progress, despite significant toxicity linked to autoimmune reactions. Also, antibodies that block LAG-3, TIM-3, B7-H3, or B7-H4 are under development (Pardoll, 2012). Certainly, the clinical oncology landscape will change during the next years due to these novel approaches.

In addition to the targeting of cell surface receptors, intracellular mechanisms may be considered. In the complex signaling network downstream of the TCR, there are several possibilities. Interventions are for example possible at the level of E3 ligases (Hoyne, 2011) (**Figure 2**). As therapeutic targets, the SHP protein tyrosine phosphatases have been proposed (Irandoust et al., 2009). A member of a new class of SHP-1 inhibitors is the tyrosine phosphatase inhibitor-1 (TPI-1) that has been shown to inhibit the growth of transplanted tumor cells in mice together with enhanced cytokine production by T cells (Kundu et al., 2010). However, optimal targeting is challenged by the fact that SHP-1 and many other signal transducers are widely expressed. For example, hematopoietic tumors are suppressed by SHP-1 (Lopez-Ruiz et al., 2011), thus precluding this approach for such diseases. Therefore, novel drugs are needed that promote TCR signaling more specifically, suggesting a drug development similar to what is pursued for optimizing the well known tyrosine kinase inhibitors (De Roock et al., 2011; Goldstraw et al., 2011; Cascone and Heymach, 2012). In parallel to approaches targeting TCR pathways, further immune cells and functions can be supported therapeutically, such as e.g., B cells, adhesion- and homing-receptors, or cytokines (Scott et al., 2010; Miller and Rhoades, 2012; Nylander and Hafler, 2012).

Most likely, we are only at the beginning of understanding the enormous potential that is associated with the therapeutic approaches discussed here. Significant progress is yet to come, despite that immunotherapy has already become standard therapy for some cancer patients. Besides, antibodies blocking CTLA, anti-PD-1, and anti-PD-L1 mAb treatments and adoptive T cell therapy are promising. Novel therapies need to be improved and validated. Furthermore, it is important to learn predicting which therapy is most suitable for which patient. Potentially predictive parameters are the frequencies of tumor-reactive T cells, their ability to migrate to tumor sites, their affinity for antigen recognition, status of effector function, and presence of inhibitory regulatory circuits. More precise knowledge on correlates of protection, and immune monitoring techniques for their characterization in individual patients will support the progress of T cell based therapy against cancer.

REFERENCES

Acuto, O., Di Bartolo, V., and Michel, F. (2008). Tailoring T-cell receptor signals by proximal negative feedback mechanisms. *Nat. Rev. Immunol.* 8, 699–712. doi:10.1038/nri2397

Acuto, O., and Michel, F. (2003). CD28-mediated co-stimulation: a quantitative support for TCR signalling. *Nat. Rev. Immunol.* 3, 939–951. doi:10.1038/nri1248

Aggen, D. H., Chervin, A. S., Schmitt, T. M., Engels, B., Stone, J. D., Richman, S. A., et al. (2012). Single-chain ValphaVbeta T-cell receptors function without mispairing with endogenous TCR chains. *Gene Ther.* 19, 365–374. doi:10.1038/gt.2011.104

Alexander-Miller, M. A., Leggatt, G. R., and Berzofsky, J. A. (1996). Selective expansion of high- or low-avidity cytotoxic T lymphocytes and efficacy for adoptive immunotherapy. *Proc. Natl. Acad. Sci. U.S.A.* 93, 4102–4107. doi:10.1073/pnas.93.9.4102

Baitsch, L., Fuertes-Marraco, S. A., Legat, A., Meyer, C., and Speiser, D. E. (2012). The three main stumbling blocks for anticancer T cells. *Trends Immunol.* 33, 364–372. doi:10.1016/j.it.2012.02.006

Bendle, G. M., Haanen, J. B., and Schumacher, T. N. (2009). Preclinical development of T cell receptor gene therapy. *Curr. Opin. Immunol.* 21, 209–214. doi:10.1016/j.coi.2009.02.007

Bendle, G. M., Linnemann, C., Hooijkaas, A. I., Bies, L., de Witte, M. A., Jorritsma, A., et al. (2010). Lethal graft-versus-host disease in mouse models of T cell receptor gene therapy. *Nat. Med.* 16, 565–570. doi:10.1038/nm.2128

Blank, U., Launay, P., Benhamou, M., and Monteiro, R. C. (2009). Inhibitory ITAMs as novel regulators of immunity. *Immunol. Rev.* 232, 59–71. doi:10.1111/j.1600-065X.2009.00832.x

Boon, T., Coulie, P. G., van den Eynde, B. J., and van der Bruggen, P. (2006). Human T cell responses against melanoma. *Annu. Rev. Immunol.* 24, 175–208. doi:10.1146/annurev.immunol.24.021605.090733

Bowerman, N. A., Crofts, T. S., Chlewicki, L., Do, P., Baker, B. M., Christopher Garcia, K., et al. (2009). Engineering the binding properties of the T cell receptor:peptide:MHC ternary complex that governs T cell activity. *Mol. Immunol.* 46, 3000–3008. doi:10.1016/j.molimm.2009.06.012

Brahmer, J. R., Tykodi, S. S., Chow, L. Q., Hwu, W. J., Topalian, S. L., Hwu, P., et al. (2012). Safety and activity of anti-PD-L1 antibody in patients with advanced cancer. *N. Engl. J. Med.* 366, 2455–2465. doi:10.1056/NEJMoa1200694

Bulek, A. M., Cole, D. K., Skowera, A., Dolton, G., Gras, S., Madura, F., et al. (2012). Structural basis for the killing of human beta cells by CD8(+) T cells in type 1 diabetes. *Nat. Immunol.* 13, 283–289. doi:10.1038/ni.2206

Carreno, L. J., Bueno, S. M., Bull, P., Nathenson, S. G., and Kalergis, A. M. (2007). The half-life of the T-cell receptor/peptide-major histocompatibility complex interaction can modulate T-cell activation in response to bacterial challenge. *Immunology* 121, 227–237. doi:10.1111/j.1365-2567.2007.02561.x

Cascone, T., and Heymach, J. V. (2012). Targeting the angiopoietin/Tie2 pathway: cutting tumor vessels with a double-edged sword? *J. Clin. Oncol.* 30, 441–444. doi:10.1200/JCO.2011.38.7621

Chen, L., and Flies, D. B. (2013). Molecular mechanisms of T cell co-stimulation and co-inhibition. *Nat. Rev. Immunol.* 13, 227–242. doi:10.1038/nri3405

Chervin, A. S., Stone, J. D., Holler, P. D., Bai, A., Chen, J., Eisen, H. N., et al. (2009). The impact of TCR-binding properties and antigen presentation format on T cell responsiveness. *J. Immunol.* 183, 1166–1178. doi:10.4049/jimmunol.0900054

Cloutier, J. F., and Veillette, A. (1999). Cooperative inhibition of T-cell antigen receptor signaling by a complex between a kinase and a phosphatase. *J. Exp. Med.* 189, 111–121. doi:10.1084/jem.189.1.111

Cole, D. K., Pumphrey, N. J., Boulter, J. M., Sami, M., Bell, J. I., Gostick, E., et al. (2007). Human TCR-binding affinity is governed by MHC class restriction. *J. Immunol.* 178, 5727–5734.

Corse, E., Gottschalk, R. A., Krogsgaard, M., and Allison, J. P. (2010). Attenuated T cell responses to a high-potency ligand in vivo. *PLoS Biol.* 8:e1000481. doi:10.1371/journal.pbio.1000481

Croft, M. (2009). The role of TNF superfamily members in T-cell function and diseases. *Nat. Rev. Immunol.* 9, 271–285. doi:10.1038/nri2526

Daniel-Meshulam, I., Ya'akobi, S., Ankri, C., and Cohen, C. J. (2012). How (specific) would like your T-cells today? Generating T-cell therapeutic function through TCR-gene transfer. *Front. Immunol.* 3:186. doi:10.3389/fimmu.2012.00186

Davis, M. M., Boniface, J. J., Reich, Z., Lyons, D., Hampl, J., Arden, B., et al. (1998). Ligand recognition by alpha beta T cell receptors. *Annu. Rev. Immunol.* 16, 523–544. doi:10.1146/annurev.immunol.16.1.523

De Roock, W., De Vriendt, V., Normanno, N., Ciardiello, F., and Tejpar, S. (2011). KRAS, BRAF, PIK3CA, and PTEN mutations: implications for targeted therapies in metastatic colorectal cancer. *Lancet Oncol.* 12, 594–603. doi:10.1016/S1470-2045(10)70209-6

del Rio, M. L., Lucas, C. L., Buhler, L., Rayat, G., and Rodriguez-Barbosa, J. I. (2010). HVEM/LIGHT/BTLA/CD160 cosignaling pathways as targets for immune regulation. *J. Leukoc. Biol.* 87, 223–235. doi:10.1189/jlb.0809590

Derre, L., Rivals, J. P., Jandus, C., Pastor, S., Rimoldi, D., Romero, P., et al. (2010). BTLA mediates inhibition of human tumor-specific CD8+ T cells that can be partially reversed by vaccination. *J. Clin. Invest.* 120, 157–167. doi:10.1172/JCI40070

Di Stasi, A., Tey, S. K., Dotti, G., Fujita, Y., Kennedy-Nasser, A., Martinez, C., et al. (2011). Inducible apoptosis as a safety switch for adoptive cell therapy. *N. Engl. J. Med.* 365, 1673–1683. doi:10.1056/NEJMoa1106152

Dunn, S. M., Rizkallah, P. J., Baston, E., Mahon, T., Cameron, B., Moysey, R., et al. (2006). Directed evolution of human T cell receptor CDR2 residues by phage display dramatically enhances affinity for cognate peptide-MHC without increasing apparent cross-reactivity. *Protein Sci.* 15, 710–721. doi:10.1110/ps.051936406

Ebert, P. J., Jiang, S., Xie, J., Li, Q. J., and Davis, M. M. (2009). An endogenous positively selecting peptide enhances mature T cell responses and becomes an autoantigen in the absence of microRNA miR-181a. *Nat. Immunol.* 10, 1162–1169. doi:10.1038/ni.1797

Egen, J. G., Kuhns, M. S., and Allison, J. P. (2002). CTLA-4: new insights into its biological function and use in tumor immunotherapy. *Nat. Immunol.* 3, 611–618. doi:10.1038/ni0702-611

Enouz, S., Carrié, L., Merkler, D., Bevan, M. J., and Zehn, D. (2012). Autoreactive T cells bypass negative selection and respond to self-antigen stimulation during infection. *J. Exp. Med.* 209, 1769–1779.

Fife, B. T., and Bluestone, J. A. (2008). Control of peripheral T-cell tolerance and autoimmunity via the CTLA-4 and PD-1 pathways. *Immunol. Rev.* 224, 166–182. doi:10.1111/j.1600-065X.2008.00662.x

Fife, B. T., and Pauken, K. E. (2011). The role of the PD-1 pathway in autoimmunity and peripheral tolerance. *Ann. N. Y. Acad. Sci.* 1217, 45–59. doi:10.1111/j.1749-6632.2010.05919.x

Goldstraw, P., Ball, D., Jett, J. R., Le Chevalier, T., Lim, E., Nicholson, A. G., et al. (2011). Non-small-cell lung cancer. *Lancet* 378, 1727–1740. doi:10.1016/S0140-6736(10)62101-0

Gonzalez, P. A., Carreno, L. J., Coombs, D., Mora, J. E., Palmieri, E., Goldstein, B., et al. (2005). T cell receptor binding kinetics required for T cell activation depend on the density of cognate ligand on the antigen-presenting cell. *Proc. Natl. Acad. Sci. U.S.A.* 102, 4824–4829. doi:10.1073/pnas.0500922102

Govers, C., Sebestyen, Z., Coccoris, M., Willemsen, R. A., and Debets, R. (2010). T cell receptor gene therapy: strategies for optimizing transgenic TCR pairing. *Trends. Mol. Med.* 16, 77–87. doi:10.1016/j.molmed.2009.12.004

Greene, J. L., Leytze, G. M., Emswiler, J., Peach, R., Bajorath, J., Cosand, W., et al. (1996). Covalent dimerization of CD28/CTLA-4 and oligomerization of CD80/CD86 regulate T cell costimulatory interactions. *J. Biol. Chem.* 271, 26762–26771. doi:10.1074/jbc.271.43.26762

Greenwald, R. J., Freeman, G. J., and Sharpe, A. H. (2005). The B7 family revisited. *Annu. Rev. Immunol.* 23, 515–548. doi:10.1146/annurev.immunol.23.021704.115611

Grohmann, U., Orabona, C., Fallarino, F., Vacca, C., Calcinaro, F., Falorni, A., et al. (2002). CTLA-4-Ig regulates tryptophan catabolism in vivo. *Nat. Immunol.* 3, 1097–1101. doi:10.1038/ni846

Hasegawa, K., Martin, F., Huang, G., Tumas, D., Diehl, L., and Chan, A. C. (2004). PEST domain-enriched tyrosine phosphatase (PEP) regulation of effector/memory T cells. *Science* 303, 685–689. doi:10.1126/science.1092138

Hebeisen, M., Baitsch, L., Presotto, D., Baumgaertner, P., Romero, P., Michielin, O., et al. (2013). SHP-1 phosphatase activity counteracts increased T cell receptor affinity. *J. Clin. Invest.* 123, 1044–1056. doi:10.1172/JCI65325

Hedrick, S. M., Cohen, D. I., Nielsen, E. A., and Davis, M. M. (1984). Isolation of cDNA clones encoding T cell-specific membrane-associated proteins. *Nature* 308, 149–153. doi:10.1038/308149a0

Hodi, F. S., O'Day, S. J., McDermott, D. F., Weber, R. W., Sosman, J. A., Haanen, J. B., et al. (2010). Improved survival with ipilimumab in patients with metastatic melanoma. *N. Engl. J. Med.* 363, 711–723. doi:10.1056/NEJMoa1003466

Holler, P. D., Chlewicki, L. K., and Kranz, D. M. (2003). TCRs with high affinity for foreign pMHC show self-reactivity. *Nat. Immunol.* 4, 55–62. doi:10.1038/ni863

Hoyne, G. F. (2011). Mechanisms that regulate peripheral immune responses to control organ-specific autoimmunity. *Clin. Dev. Immunol.* 2011, 294968. doi:10.1155/2011/294968

Irandoust, M., van den Berg, T. K., Kaspers, G. J., and Cloos, J. (2009). Role of tyrosine phosphatase inhibitors in cancer treatment with emphasis on SH2 domain-containing tyrosine phosphatases (SHPs). *Anticancer Agents Med. Chem.* 9, 212–220. doi:10.2174/187152009787313864

Irving, M., Zoete, V., Hebeisen, M., Schmid, D., Baumgartner, P., Guillaume, P., et al. (2012). Interplay between T cell receptor binding kinetics and the level of cognate peptide presented by major histocompatibility complexes governs CD8+ T cell responsiveness. *J. Biol. Chem.* 287, 23068–23078. doi:10.1074/jbc.M112.357673

James, J. R., and Vale, R. D. (2012). Biophysical mechanism of T-cell receptor triggering in a reconstituted system. *Nature* 487, 64–69. doi:10.1038/nature11220

Johnson, L. A., Morgan, R. A., Dudley, M. E., Cassard, L., Yang, J. C., Hughes, M. S., et al. (2009). Gene therapy with human and mouse T-cell receptors mediates cancer regression and targets normal tissues expressing cognate antigen. *Blood* 114, 535–546. doi:10.1182/blood-2009-03-211714

Kalergis, A. M., Boucheron, N., Doucey, M. A., Palmieri, E., Goyarts, E. C., Vegh, Z., et al. (2001). Efficient T cell activation requires an optimal dwell-time of interaction between the TCR and the pMHC complex. *Nat. Immunol.* 2, 229–234. doi:10.1038/85286

Karwacz, K., Bricogne, C., MacDonald, D., Arce, F., Bennett, C. L., Collins, M., et al. (2011). PD-L1 co-stimulation contributes to ligand-induced T cell receptor down-modulation on CD8+ T cells. *EMBO Mol. Med.* 3, 581–592. doi:10.1002/emmm.201100165

Kersh, E. N., Kersh, G. J., and Allen, P. M. (1999). Partially phosphorylated T cell receptor zeta molecules can inhibit T cell activation. *J. Exp. Med.* 190, 1627–1636. doi:10.1084/jem.190.11.1627

Kochenderfer, J. N., and Rosenberg, S. A. (2013). Treating B-cell cancer with T cells expressing anti-CD19 chimeric antigen receptors.

Nat. Rev. Clin. Oncol. 10, 267–276. doi:10.1038/nrclinonc.2013.46

Kristiansen, O. P., Larsen, Z. M., and Pociot, F. (2000). CTLA-4 in autoimmune diseases – a general susceptibility gene to autoimmunity? *Genes Immun.* 1, 170–184. doi:10.1038/sj.gene.6363655

Kroner, A., Mehling, M., Hemmer, B., Rieckmann, P., Toyka, K. V., Maurer, M., et al. (2005). A PD-1 polymorphism is associated with disease progression in multiple sclerosis. *Ann. Neurol.* 58, 50–57. doi:10.1002/ana.20514

Kundu, S., Fan, K., Cao, M., Lindner, D. J., Zhao, Z. J., Borden, E., et al. (2010). Novel SHP-1 inhibitors tyrosine phosphatase inhibitor-1 and analogs with preclinical antitumor activities as tolerated oral agents. *J. Immunol.* 184, 6529–6536. doi:10.4049/jimmunol.0903562

Kurts, C., Kosaka, H., Carbone, F. R., Miller, J. F., and Heath, W. R. (1997). Class I-restricted cross-presentation of exogenous self-antigens leads to deletion of autoreactive CD8(+) T cells. *J. Exp. Med.* 186, 239–245. doi:10.1084/jem.186.2.239

Kyewski, B., and Klein, L. (2006). A central role for central tolerance. *Annu. Rev. Immunol.* 24, 571–606. doi:10.1146/annurev.immunol.23.021704.115601

Letourneur, F., and Klausner, R. D. (1992). Activation of T cells by a tyrosine kinase activation domain in the cytoplasmic tail of CD3 epsilon. *Science* 255, 79–82. doi:10.1126/science.1532456

Li, Q. J., Chau, J., Ebert, P. J., Sylvester, G., Min, H., Liu, G., et al. (2007). miR-181a is an intrinsic modulator of T cell sensitivity and selection. *Cell* 129, 147–161. doi:10.1016/j.cell.2007.03.008

Li, Y., Moysey, R., Molloy, P. E., Vuidepot, A. L., Mahon, T., Baston, E., et al. (2005). Directed evolution of human T-cell receptors with picomolar affinities by phage display. *Nat. Biotechnol.* 23, 349–354. doi:10.1038/nbt1070

Liddy, N., Bossi, G., Adams, K. J., Lissina, A., Mahon, T. M., Hassan, N. J., et al. (2012). Monoclonal TCR-redirected tumor cell killing. *Nat. Med.* 18, 980–987. doi:10.1038/nm.2764

Liechtenstein, T., Dufait, I., Lanna, A., Breckpot, K., and Escors, D. (2012). Modulating co-stimulation during antigen presentation to enhance cancer immunotherapy. *Immunol. Endocr. Metab. Agents Med. Chem.* 12, 224–235. doi:10.2174/187152212802001875

Linnemann, C., Schumacher, T. N., and Bendle, G. M. (2011). T-cell receptor gene therapy: critical parameters for clinical success. *J. Invest. Dermatol.* 131, 1806–1816. doi:10.1038/jid.2011.160

Lopez-Ruiz, P., Rodriguez-Ubreva, J., Cariaga, A. E., Cortes, M. A., and Colas, B. (2011). SHP-1 in cell-cycle regulation. *Anticancer Agents Med. Chem.* 11, 89–98. doi:10.2174/187152011794941154

Lorenz, U. (2009). SHP-1 and SHP-2 in T cells: two phosphatases functioning at many levels. *Immunol. Rev.* 228, 342–359. doi:10.1111/j.1600-065X.2008.00760.x

Malissen, M., Minard, K., Mjolsness, S., Kronenberg, M., Goverman, J., Hunkapiller, T., et al. (1984). Mouse T cell antigen receptor: structure and organization of constant and joining gene segments encoding the beta polypeptide. *Cell* 37, 1101–1110. doi:10.1016/0092-8674(84)90444-6

McMahan, R. H., McWilliams, J. A., Jordan, K. R., Dow, S. W., Wilson, D. B., and Slansky, J. E. (2006). Relating TCR-peptide-MHC affinity to immunogenicity for the design of tumor vaccines. *J. Clin. Invest.* 116, 2543–2551.

McMahan, R. H., and Slansky, J. E. (2007). Mobilizing the low-avidity T cell repertoire to kill tumors. *Semin. Cancer Biol.* 17, 317–329. doi:10.1016/j.semcancer.2007.06.006

Miller, A. E., and Rhoades, R. W. (2012). Treatment of relapsing-remitting multiple sclerosis: current approaches and unmet needs. *Curr. Opin. Neurol.* 25(Suppl.), S4–S10. doi:10.1097/01.wco.0000413319.87092.19

Morgan, R. A., Chinnasamy, N., Abate-Daga, D., Gros, A., Robbins, P. F., Zheng, Z., et al. (2013). Cancer regression and neurological toxicity following anti-MAGE-A3 TCR gene therapy. *J. Immunother.* 36, 133–151. doi:10.1097/CJI.0b013e3182829903

Mustelin, T., Vang, T., and Bottini, N. (2005). Protein tyrosine phosphatases and the immune response. *Nat. Rev. Immunol.* 5, 43–57. doi:10.1038/nri1530

Nishimura, H., Okazaki, T., Tanaka, Y., Nakatani, K., Hara, M., Matsumori, A., et al. (2001). Autoimmune dilated cardiomyopathy in PD-1 receptor-deficient mice. *Science* 291, 319–322. doi:10.1126/science.291.5502.319

Nylander, A., and Hafler, D. A. (2012). Multiple sclerosis. *J. Clin. Invest.* 122, 1180–1188. doi:10.1172/JCI58649

Ochi, T., Fujiwara, H., Okamoto, S., An, J., Nagai, K., Shirakata, T., et al. (2011). Novel adoptive T-cell immunotherapy using a WT1-specific TCR vector encoding silencers for endogenous TCRs shows marked antileukemia reactivity and safety. *Blood* 118, 1495–1503. doi:10.1182/blood-2011-02-337089

Offringa, R. (2009). Antigen choice in adoptive T-cell therapy of cancer. *Curr. Opin. Immunol.* 21, 190–199. doi:10.1016/j.coi.2009.02.006

Pardoll, D. M. (2012). The blockade of immune checkpoints in cancer immunotherapy. *Nat. Rev. Cancer* 12, 252–264. doi:10.1038/nrc3239

Plas, D. R., Johnson, R., Pingel, J. T., Matthews, R. J., Dalton, M., Roy, G., et al. (1996). Direct regulation of ZAP-70 by SHP-1 in T cell antigen receptor signaling. *Science* 272, 1173–1176. doi:10.1126/science.272.5265.1173

Porter, D. L., Levine, B. L., Kalos, M., Bagg, A., and June, C. H. (2011). Chimeric antigen receptor-modified T cells in chronic lymphoid leukemia. *N. Engl. J. Med.* 365, 725–733. doi:10.1056/NEJMoa1103849

Prokunina, L., Castillejo-Lopez, C., Oberg, F., Gunnarsson, I., Berg, L., Magnusson, V., et al. (2002). A regulatory polymorphism in PDCD1 is associated with susceptibility to systemic lupus erythematosus in humans. *Nat. Genet.* 32, 666–669. doi:10.1038/ng1020

Qureshi, O. S., Zheng, Y., Nakamura, K., Attridge, K., Manzotti, C., Schmidt, E. M., et al. (2011). Trans-endocytosis of CD80 and CD86: a molecular basis for the cell-extrinsic function of CTLA-4. *Science* 332, 600–603. doi:10.1126/science.1202947

Restifo, N. P., Dudley, M. E., and Rosenberg, S. A. (2012). Adoptive immunotherapy for cancer: harnessing the T cell response. *Nat. Rev. Immunol.* 12, 269–281. doi:10.1038/nri3191

Ribas, A. (2012). Tumor immunotherapy directed at PD-1. *N. Engl. J. Med.* 366, 2517–2519. doi:10.1056/NEJMe1205943

Robbins, P. F., Li, Y. F., El-Gamil, M., Zhao, Y., Wargo, J. A., Zheng, Z., et al. (2008). Single and dual amino acid substitutions in TCR CDRs can enhance antigen-specific T cell functions. *J. Immunol.* 180, 6116–6131.

Robbins, P. F., Morgan, R. A., Feldman, S. A., Yang, J. C., Sherry, R. M., Dudley, M. E., et al. (2011). Tumor regression in patients with metastatic synovial cell sarcoma and melanoma using genetically engineered lymphocytes reactive with NY-ESO-1. *J. Clin. Oncol.* 29, 917–924. doi:10.1200/JCO.2010.32.2537

Romero, P., Valmori, D., Pittet, M. J., Zippelius, A., Rimoldi, D., Levy, F., et al. (2002). Antigenicity and immunogenicity of Melan-A/MART-1 derived peptides as targets for tumor reactive CTL in human melanoma. *Immunol. Rev.* 188, 81–96. doi:10.1034/j.1600-065X.2002.18808.x

Rosenberg, S. A. (2011). Cell transfer immunotherapy for metastatic solid cancer – what clinicians need to know. *Nat. Rev. Clin. Oncol.* 8, 577–585. doi:10.1038/nrclinonc.2011.116

Rosenberg, S. A., Dudley, M. E., and Restifo, N. P. (2008). Cancer immunotherapy. *N. Engl. J. Med.* 359, 1072. doi:10.1056/NEJMc081511

Rosenberg, S. A., Yang, J. C., Sherry, R. M., Kammula, U. S., Hughes, M. S., Phan, G. Q., et al. (2011). Durable complete responses in heavily pretreated patients with metastatic melanoma using T-cell transfer immunotherapy. *Clin. Cancer Res.* 17, 4550–4557. doi:10.1158/1078-0432.CCR-11-0116

Sallusto, F., Lanzavecchia, A., Araki, K., and Ahmed, R. (2010). From vaccines to memory and back. *Immunity* 33, 451–463. doi:10.1016/j.immuni.2010.10.008

Scalapino, K. J., and Daikh, D. I. (2008). CTLA-4: a key regulatory point in the control of autoimmune disease. *Immunol. Rev.* 223, 143–155. doi:10.1111/j.1600-065X.2008.00639.x

Schmid, D. A., Irving, M. B., Posevitz, V., Hebeisen, M., Posevitz-Fejfar, A., Sarria, J. C., et al. (2010). Evidence for a TCR affinity threshold delimiting maximal CD8 T cell function. *J. Immunol.* 184, 4936–4946. doi:10.4049/jimmunol.1000173

Schreiber, R. D., Old, L. J., and Smyth, M. J. (2011). Cancer immunoediting: integrating immunity's roles in cancer suppression and promotion. *Science* 331, 1565–1570. doi:10.1126/science.1203486

Scott, D. L., Wolfe, F., and Huizinga, T. W. (2010). Rheumatoid arthritis. *Lancet* 376, 1094–1108. doi:10.1016/S0140-6736(10)60826-4

Sedy, J. R., Gavrieli, M., Potter, K. G., Hurchla, M. A., Lindsley, R. C., Hildner, K., et al. (2005). B and T lymphocyte attenuator regulates T cell activation through interaction with herpesvirus entry mediator. *Nat. Immunol.* 6, 90–98. doi:10.1038/ni1144

Sharpe, A. H., and Freeman, G. J. (2002). The B7-CD28 superfamily. *Nat. Rev. Immunol.* 2, 116–126. doi:10.1038/nri727

Shui, J. W., Steinberg, M. W., and Kronenberg, M. (2011). Regulation of inflammation, autoimmunity, and infection immunity by HVEM-BTLA signaling. *J. Leukoc. Biol.* 89, 517–523. doi:10.1189/jlb.0910528

Slansky, J. E., and Jordan, K. R. (2010). The Goldilocks model for TCR-too much attraction might not be best for vaccine design. *PLoS Biol.* 8:e1000482. doi:10.1371/journal.pbio.1000482

Smith-Garvin, J. E., Koretzky, G. A., and Jordan, M. S. (2009). T cell activation. *Annu. Rev. Immunol.* 27, 591–619. doi:10.1146/annurev.immunol.021908.132706

So, T., Lee, S. W., and Croft, M. (2008). Immune regulation and control of regulatory T cells by OX40 and 4-1BB. *Cytokine Growth Factor Rev.* 19, 253–262. doi:10.1016/j.cytogfr.2008.04.003

Speiser, D. E. (2013). Hit parade for adoptive cell transfer therapy: the best T cells for superior clinical responses. *Cancer Discov.* 3, 379–381. doi:10.1158/2159-8290.CD-13-0064

Speiser, D. E., Kyburz, D., Stubi, U., Hengartner, H., and Zinkernagel, R. M. (1992). Discrepancy between in vitro measurable and in vivo virus neutralizing cytotoxic T cell reactivities. Low T cell receptor specificity and avidity sufficient for in vitro proliferation or cytotoxicity to peptide-coated target cells but not for in vivo protection. *J. Immunol.* 149, 972–980.

Speiser, D. E., Wieckowski, S., Gupta, B., Iancu, E. M., Baumgaertner, P., Baitsch, L., et al. (2011). Single cell analysis reveals similar functional competence of dominant and nondominant CD8 T-cell clonotypes. *Proc. Natl. Acad. Sci. U.S.A.* 108, 15318–15323. doi:10.1073/pnas.1105419108

Stefanova, I., Hemmer, B., Vergelli, M., Martin, R., Biddison, W. E., and Germain, R. N. (2003). TCR ligand discrimination is enforced by competing ERK positive and SHP-1 negative feedback pathways. *Nat. Immunol.* 4, 248–254. doi:10.1038/ni895

Stone, J. D., Chervin, A. S., and Kranz, D. M. (2009). T-cell receptor binding affinities and kinetics: impact on T-cell activity and specificity. *Immunology* 126, 165–176. doi:10.1111/j.1365-2567.2008.03015.x

Sun, T., Hu, Z., Shen, H., and Lin, D. (2009). Genetic polymorphisms in cytotoxic T-lymphocyte antigen 4 and cancer: the dialectical nature of subtle human immune dysregulation. *Cancer Res.* 69, 6011–6014. doi:10.1158/0008-5472.CAN-09-0176

Thomas, S., Stauss, H. J., and Morris, E. C. (2010). Molecular immunology lessons from therapeutic T-cell receptor gene transfer. *Immunology* 129, 170–177. doi:10.1111/j.1365-2567.2009.03227.x

Thomas, S., Xue, S. A., Bangham, C. R., Jakobsen, B. K., Morris, E. C., and Stauss, H. J. (2011). Human T cells expressing affinity-matured TCR display accelerated responses but fail to recognize low density of MHC-peptide antigen. *Blood* 118, 319–329. doi:10.1182/blood-2010-12-326736

Tivol, E. A., Borriello, F., Schweitzer, A. N., Lynch, W. P., Bluestone, J. A., and Sharpe, A. H. (1995). Loss of CTLA-4 leads to massive lymphoproliferation and fatal multiorgan tissue destruction, revealing a critical negative regulatory role of CTLA-4. *Immunity* 3, 541–547. doi:10.1016/1074-7613(95)90125-6

Topalian, S. L., Hodi, F. S., Brahmer, J. R., Gettinger, S. N., Smith, D. C., McDermott, D. F., et al. (2012). Safety, activity, and immune correlates of anti-PD-1 antibody in cancer. *N. Engl. J. Med.* 366, 2443–2454. doi:10.1056/NEJMoa1200690

Turner, M. J., Jellison, E. R., Lingenheld, E. G., Puddington, L., and Lefrancois, L. (2008). Avidity maturation of memory CD8 T cells is limited by self-antigen expression. *J. Exp. Med.* 205, 1859–1868. doi:10.1084/jem.20072390

Van Der Bruggen, P., Zhang, Y., Chaux, P., Stroobant, V., Panichelli, C., Schultz, E. S., et al. (2002). Tumor-specific shared antigenic peptides recognized by human T cells. *Immunol. Rev.* 188, 51–64. doi:10.1034/j.1600-065X.2002.18806.x

van Loenen, M. M., de Boer, R., Amir, A. L., Hagedoorn, R. S., Volbeda, G. L., Willemze, R., et al. (2010). Mixed T cell receptor dimers harbor potentially harmful neoreactivity. *Proc. Natl. Acad. Sci. U.S.A.* 107, 10972–10977. doi:10.1073/pnas.1005802107

Vang, T., Congia, M., Macis, M. D., Musumeci, L., Orru, V., Zavattari, P., et al. (2005). Autoimmune-associated lymphoid tyrosine phosphatase is a gain-of-function variant. *Nat. Genet.* 37, 1317–1319. doi:10.1038/ng1673

von Herrath, M. G., Dockter, J., and Oldstone, M. B. (1994). How virus induces a rapid or slow onset insulin-dependent diabetes mellitus in a transgenic model. *Immunity* 1, 231–242. doi:10.1016/1074-7613(94)90101-5

Wang, Y., Subudhi, S. K., Anders, R. A., Lo, J., Sun, Y., Blink, S., et al. (2005). The role of herpesvirus entry mediator as a negative regulator of T cell-mediated responses. *J. Clin. Invest.* 115, 711–717. doi:10.1172/JCI200522982

Ware, C. F., and Sedy, J. R. (2011). TNF superfamily networks: bidirectional and interference pathways of the herpesvirus entry mediator (TNFSF14). *Curr. Opin. Immunol.* 23, 627–631. doi:10.1016/j.coi.2011.08.008

Watanabe, N., Gavrieli, M., Sedy, J. R., Yang, J., Fallarino, F., Loftin, S. K., et al. (2003). BTLA is a lymphocyte inhibitory receptor with similarities to CTLA-4 and PD-1. *Nat. Immunol.* 4, 670–679. doi:10.1038/ni944

Waterhouse, P., Penninger, J. M., Timms, E., Wakeham, A., Shahinian, A., Lee, K. P., et al. (1995). Lymphoproliferative disorders with early lethality in mice deficient in Ctla-4. *Science* 270, 985–988. doi:10.1126/science.270.5238.985

Watts, T. H. (2005). TNF/TNFR family members in costimulation of T cell responses. *Annu. Rev. Immunol.* 23, 23–68. doi:10.1146/annurev.immunol.23.021704.115839

Yokosuka, T., Takamatsu, M., Kobayashi-Imanishi, W., Hashimoto-Tane, A., Azuma, M., and Saito, T. (2012). Programmed cell death 1 forms negative costimulatory microclusters that directly inhibit T cell receptor signaling by recruiting phosphatase SHP2. *J. Exp. Med.* 209, 1201–1217. doi:10.1084/jem.20112741

Zehn, D., and Bevan, M. J. (2006). T cells with low avidity for a tissue-restricted antigen routinely evade central and peripheral tolerance and cause autoimmunity. *Immunity* 25, 261–270. doi:10.1016/j.immuni.2006.06.009

Zehn, D., King, C., Bevan, M. J., and Palmer, E. (2012). TCR signaling requirements for activating T cells and for generating memory. *Cell. Mol. Life Sci.* 69, 1565–1575. doi:10.1007/s00018-012-0965-x

Zehn, D., Lee, S. Y., and Bevan, M. J. (2009). Complete but curtailed T-cell response to very low-affinity antigen. *Nature* 458, 211–214. doi:10.1038/nature07657

Zhao, Y., Bennett, A. D., Zheng, Z., Wang, Q. J., Robbins, P. F., Yu, L. Y., et al. (2007). High-affinity TCRs generated by phage display provide CD4+ T cells with the ability to recognize and kill tumor cell lines. *J. Immunol.* 179, 5845–5854.

Zhong, S., Malecek, K., Johnson, L. A., Yu, Z., de Miera, E., Darvishian, F., et al. (2013). T-cell receptor affinity and avidity defines antitumor response and autoimmunity in T-cell immunotherapy. *Proc. Natl. Acad. Sci. U.S.A.* 110, 6973–6978. doi:10.1073/pnas.1221609110

Zoete, V., Irving, M. B., and Michielin, O. (2010). MM-GBSA binding free energy decomposition and T cell receptor engineering. *J. Mol. Recognit.* 23, 142–152. doi:10.1002/jmr.1005

Zoete, V., and Michielin, O. (2007). Comparison between computational alanine scanning and per-residue binding free energy decomposition for protein-protein association using MM-GBSA: application to the TCR-p-MHC complex. *Proteins* 67, 1026–1047. doi:10.1002/prot.21395

19

APECED: is this a model for failure of T cell and B cell tolerance?

Nicolas Kluger[1], Annamari Ranki[1] and Kai Krohn[2]*

[1] *Department of Dermatology, Allergology and Venereology, Institute of Clinical Medicine, Skin and Allergy Hospital, Helsinki University Central Hospital, University of Helsinki, Helsinki, Finland*
[2] *Clinical Research Institute HUCH Ltd, Helsinki, Finland*

Edited by:
Rosa Bacchetta, Fondazione Centro San Raffaele Del Monte Tabor, Italy

Reviewed by:
Rosa Bacchetta, Fondazione Centro San Raffaele Del Monte Tabor, Italy
Mario Abinun, Newcastle upon Tyne Hospitals NHS Foundation Trust, UK

Correspondence:
Kai Krohn, Clinical Research Institute HUCH Ltd, Salmentaantie 751, 36450 Salmentaka, Finland.
e-mail: kai.krohn@nic.fi

In APECED, the key abnormality is in the T cell defect that may lead to tissue destruction chiefly in endocrine organs. Besides, APECED is characterized by high-titer antibodies against a wide variety of cytokines that could partly be responsible for the clinical symptoms during APECED, mainly chronic mucocutaneous candidiasis, and linked to antibodies against Th17 cells effector molecules, IL-17 and IL-22. On the other hand, the same antibodies, together with antibodies against type I interferons may prevent the patients from other immunological diseases, such as psoriasis and systemic lupus erythematous. The same effector Th17 cells, present in the lymphocytic infiltrate of target organs of APECED, could be responsible for the tissue destruction. Here again, the antibodies against the corresponding effector molecules, anti-IL-17 and anti-IL-22 could be protective. The occurrence of several effector mechanisms ($CD4^+$ Th17 cell and $CD8^+$ CTL and the effector cytokines IL-17 and IL-22), and simultaneous existence of regulatory mechanisms ($CD4^+$ Treg and antibodies neutralizing the effect of the effector cytokines) may explain the polymorphism of APECED. Almost all the patients develop the characteristic manifestations of the complex, but temporal course and severity of the symptoms vary considerably, even among siblings. The autoantibody profile does not correlate with the clinical picture. One could speculate that a secondary homeostatic balance between the harmful effector mechanisms, and the favorable regulatory mechanisms, finally define both the extent and severity of the clinical condition in the *AIRE* defective individuals. The proposed hypothesis that in APECED, in addition to strong tissue destructive mechanisms, a controlling regulatory mechanism does exist, allow us to conclude that APECED could be treated, and even cured, with immunological manipulation.

Keywords: AIRE, APECED, endocrine disorders, interleukin 17, interleukin 22, IPEX, T regulatory cells

INTRODUCTION

Autoimmune polyendocrinopathy syndrome type 1 (APS-1) or autoimmune polyendocrinopathy–candidiasis–ectodermal dystrophy syndrome (APECED; OMIM 240300) is a rare recessively inherited disorder (Perheentupa, 2002; Betterle and Zanchetta, 2003; Perheentupa, 2006; Husebye et al., 2009). It is caused by mutations in the autoimmune regulator (*AIRE*) gene located on locus 21q22.3 (Bjorses et al., 1996; Nagamine et al., 1997; The Finnish–German APECED Consortium, 1997). APECED displays a worldwide distribution, but specific clusters of high prevalence of the disease are observed among Finns (1:25,000; Ahonen et al., 1990) and Sardinians 1 (1:14,500; Rosatelli et al., 1998; Meloni et al., 2012). It is characterized by the variable association of autoimmune endocrine [hypoparathyroidism (HP), Addison's disease (AD), hypothyroidism, gonadal insufficiency, insulin-dependent diabetes mellitus, atrophic gastritis, and Biermer's disease] and non-endocrine disorders (keratitis, malabsorption, vitiligo, and alopecia areata) and a specific predisposition to chronic mucocutaneous candidiasis (CMC). A definite diagnosis of APECED is made upon one of the following criteria: (i) the presence of at least two of three major clinical features: CMC, HP, and AD, or (ii) one disease component if a sibling has already a definite diagnosis, or (iii) disease-causing mutations in both alleles of the *AIRE* gene. However, APECED being highly variable in its presentation, the classical triad may be complete only after years of evolution and diagnose may be therefore missed. Besides, APECED may appear during adolescence or in the young adult (Husebye et al., 2009). Therefore, criteria for a probable APECED have been defined as follows: (i) presence of one of CMC, HP, AD (before 30 years of age) and at least one of the minor components chronic diarrhea, keratitis, periodic rash with fever, severe constipation, autoimmune hepatitis, vitiligo, alopecia, enamel

Abbreviations: AADC, aromatic L-amino acid decarboxylase; AD, Addison's disease; AE, autoimmune enteropathy; APS-1, autoimmune polyendocrinopathy syndrome type 1; APECED, autoimmune polyendocrinopathy–candidiasis–ectodermal dystrophy; CMC, chronic mucocutaneous candidiasis; EECs, enteroendocrine cells; GI, gastro-intestinal; HP, hypoparathyroidism; IPEX, immune dysregulation, polyendocrinopathy, enteropathy and X-linked; IF, intrinsic factor; IL-1, interleukin-1; IL-17, interleukin-17; IL-22, interleukin-22; mTECs, thymic medullary epithelial cells; NALP-5, NACHT leucine-rich-repeat protein 5; PE, promiscuous expression; PTH, parathormone; SLE, systemic lupus erythematosus; TH, tyrosine hydroxylase; TPH, tryptophan hydroxylase; TRIMs, tripartite motif-containing proteins; TSA, tissue-specific antigens.

hypoplasia, (ii) any component and anti-interferon antibodies, or (iii) any component and antibodies against NACHT leucine-rich repeat protein 5 (NALP5), AADC, tryptophan hydroxylase (TPH), or TH (Husebye et al., 2009).

FROM CIRCULATING AUTOIMMUNE ANTIBODIES TO *AIRE, FOXP3,* APECED, AND IPEX

Our knowledge of the nature of the condition now called APS-1 or APECED has increased simultaneously with the general development of immunology and autoimmunity. Since the condition was clearly defined in the end of 1950s and early 1960s, the characteristic clinical picture, the immunological abnormalities and the relationship to other autoimmune endocrine diseases were defined in late 1960s and early 1970s. Furthermore, the genetics of APECED, and the fact that the syndrome was caused by a recessive gene defect – as opposed to the HLA-linked genetics seen in the other solitarily occurring endocrine diseases – were characterized in the 1980s and the target antigens in the organs affected by APECED were molecularly defined in 1990s. A landmark stage in the study of APECED was reached in 1997, when the long sought APECED gene was cloned by two independent groups (Nagamine et al., 1997; The Finnish–German APECED Consortium, 1997). Finally, a new phase in APECED research occurred during the first decennium of 2000, when the autoantibodies toward soluble mediators if immune response were characterized (Meager et al., 2006; Kisand et al., 2011).

The notion that several diseases affecting endocrine organs and earlier defined as idiopathic, were in fact caused by an autoimmune response toward self antigens, became apparent when novel immunological methods became available in 1950s and early 1960s (Blizzard et al., 1963). The association of the three conditions, candidiasis, HP, and AD that were later judged to be the hallmarks of APECED was clearly stated by the groups of Blizzard and Maclaren (Blizzard et al., 1963; Brun, 1978; Neufeld et al., 1981). These groups also defined two clearly distinct syndromes with several associated autoimmune diseases: autoimmune polyglandular syndrome type 1 (PGS-1) and polyglandular syndrome type 2 (PGS-2). The nomenclature was later changed to APS-1 and APS-2, and the former further to APECED (Ahonen et al., 1990; Perheentupa, 2002, 2006; Betterle and Zanchetta, 2003).

Pioneering studies in this field were made especially with the use of immunohistochemistry, demonstrating antibodies reacting with gastric parietal cells in chronic gastritis (Walder et al., 1963; Irvine et al., 1965) and intrinsic factor (IF) in pernicious anemia (Schwartz, 1961; Jeffries et al., 1962), with thyroid epithelial cells in various forms of thyroid diseases (Witebsky et al., 1957; Irvine et al., 1962; Doniach and Roitt, 1964), with the beta cells of Langerhans islands in diabetes mellitus (Kaldany, 1979; Bottazzo et al., 1980), and adrenal cortical cells in AD (Blizzard et al., 1962).

Blizzard's group noticed that the two polyglandular syndromes, APS-1 and APS-2, differed in their HLA haplotypes (Neufeld et al., 1981). Further studies on the HLA haplotypes revealed that the genetic basis of APS-2, but also of the other isolated forms of endocrine autoimmune diseases found in APS-1, were in the HLA haplotype of the patients. In contrast, APS-1 was shown not to be linked to HLA, and studies with large patient material, collected by Perheentupa's group in Finland, clearly stated that APS-1 was linked to a recessively inherited gene defect (Ahonen et al., 1990; Perheentupa, 2002, 2006). The autoimmune endocrinopathies could thus be grouped on the basis of their genetic background in two distinct categories: those linked to HLA variation and the one, APS-1 caused by a single mutated gene (**Table 1**). At that stage, however, the responsible gene, the APECED gene, was not yet identified. Once identified, the APECED gene was renamed as *AIRE* in 1997 (Nagamine et al., 1997; The Finnish–German APECED Consortium, 1997).

Another immunopathy, termed originally as autoimmune enteropathy (AIE) and later identified as immune dysregulation, polyendocrinopathy, enteropathy and X-linked (IPEX), was described in the 1980s and 1990s (Powell et al., 1982). This disorder was later shown to be caused by a defect in a single gene, *FOXP3* (Bennett et al., 2000). IPEX and APECED are two examples of immune deficiency diseases disclosing both disturbed tolerance and autoimmune phenomena (Moraes-Vasconcelos et al., 2008). Traditionally, reviews tend to associate both IPEX and APECED because of common features. However, both clinical manifestations and predisposition to infections are rather different when comparing both diseases (Moraes-Vasconcelos et al., 2008).

AIRE GENE, MUTATIONS, AND MECHANISM OF ACTION

AIRE is expressed in thymus, lymph nodes, and fetal liver, and encodes a protein with two putative zinc fingers and other motifs suggestive of a transcriptional regulator (Nagamine et al., 1997; The Finnish–German APECED Consortium, 1997). The *AIRE* gene, approximately 13 kb in length, contains 14 exons that encode a polypeptide of 545 amino acids. The AIRE protein functions as a transcription factor (Fierabracci, 2011; Gardner et al., 2009). AIRE is expressed in the thymic medullary epithelial cells (mTECs, **Figure 1**) and in cells of the monocyte/dendritic cell lineage (Kogawa et al., 2002). mTECs through the expression of MHC class II express a wide array of tissue-restricted antigens (TRAs) derived from different organs in the body. TRAs include self-proteins with patterns of expression restricted to a single or small handful of organs. Thymic expression of TRA serves as an important source of self-antigens to allow the negative selection of autoreactive T cells. Collectively, mTEC and thymic monocyte/dendritic cells play a crucial role in establishing self-tolerance by eliminating autoreactive T cells (negative selection) and/or by producing immunoregulatory FOXP3$^+$ T cells, which prevent CD4$^+$ T cell-mediated organ-specific autoimmune diseases. Collectively, several studies in mouse and man have shown that AIRE regulates thymic expression of several genes of ectopic peripheral proteins including many TRAs. Thus, AIRE dysfunction leads to a decrease in the expression of TRAs in the thymus, and consequently, autoreactive T cell clones escape into the periphery (Derbinski et al., 2005; Moraes-Vasconcelos et al., 2008; Gardner et al., 2009; Fierabracci, 2011)

The most common *AIRE* mutation, the "Finnish mutation," R257X, affects 82% of Finnish *APECED* alleles (Nagamine et al., 1997; The Finnish–German APECED Consortium, 1997). Interestingly, this mutation occurs also in 70% of the Russian APECED patients studied (Orlova et al., 2010). The same mutation, R257X was also detected in Swiss patients on a different haplotype with closely linked polymorphic markers (Nagamine et al., 1997) and in

Table 1 | Key laboratory findings in the different autoimmune endocrine diseases.

Diagnosis	Clinical findings	Autoantibodies	HLA	Gene defect	Cellular immune response
APECED (APS-1)	Candidiasis and multiple failure of most endocrine organs and non-endocrine autoimmunity	Against all affected organs	No association (?)	Close to 100 mutations described in the *AIRE* gene	CTL against affected organs? Failure in Treg population
APS-2	Addison's disease with insulin-dependant type I diabetes or thyroid diseases	Against adrenal cortex, pancreatic beta cells, thyroid	Risk haplotypes HLA DR3: DRB1*0301, DQA1*0501, DQB1*0201 DR4 DR1, DR7, DR13, and DR14: protective (Betterle and Zanchetta, 2003)	No single gene defect	CTL against affected organs?
Addison's disease	Low levels of gluco- and mineralocorticoid High ACTH, low cortisol, high renin, low aldosterone, subnormal cortisol response to ACTH test: hyponatremia, hyperkalemia	Against P450c21, P450scc	HLA-DRB1-DQA1-DQB1 HLA-DR3	No single gene defect	CTL against affected organs?
IPEX	Enteropathy, diabetes skin disease (mainly eczema), failure to thrive, thyroiditis, recurrent infections	Against enterocytes (autoimmune enteropathy-related 75-kDa antigen) pancreatic-islet cells, insulin, and glutamic acid decarboxilase (GAD), and thyroid (antithyroid microsomal antibodies)	No association	Defective *FOXP3* gene	Impaired function of regulatory T cells, defective IL-2, IFN-γ, and TNF-α production. Increased production of IL-17

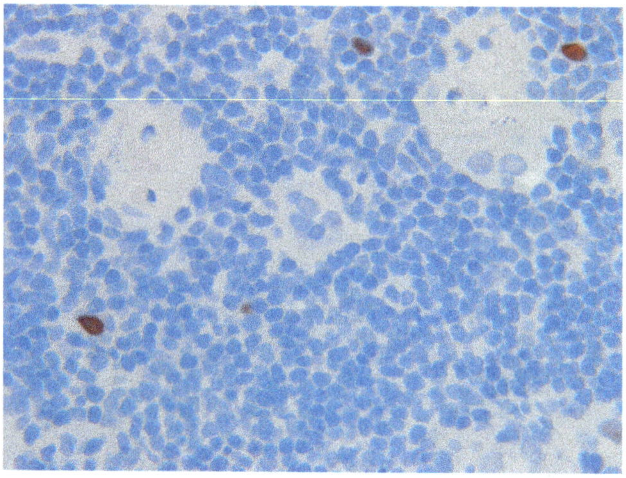

FIGURE 1 | Medullary epithelia cells in thymus, expressing the AIRE proteins (reddish brown), in close vicinity of the Hassall's corpuscles (HC) where auto-reactive T cells are thought to be destroyed. Note cell debris in HC. Magnification 1:40. AIRE was demonstrated with specific monoclonal antibody at 1:2,000 dilution.

northern Italian *APECED* patients. Nonsense mutation R139X was found as the predominant haplotype among Sardinian patients (18/20 independent alleles; Rosatelli et al., 1998). Other hotspots have been identified such as the Y85C missense mutation in an isolated Iranian Jewish community (Zlotogora and Shapiro, 1992; Björses et al., 2000). A 13-bp deletion in exon 8 [1085–1097(del)] is ubiquitous and can be found in Norwegians, but also Anglo–Saxons descendant (Zlotogora and Shapiro, 1992) and south Americans (Moraes-Vasconcelos et al., 2008). Today, over 60 different mutations have been described throughout the coding region of AIRE (Akirav et al., 2011).

CLINICAL PICTURE OF APECED

The clinical picture of APECED is characterized by sequentially occurring diseases, with great variation among the patients as to the severity and time course of the various conditions. In most cases, the affected individual starts suffering from CMC in early infancy or childhood. In most cases, the next organs to be affected are the parathyroid glands, followed by AD and at puberty, hypogonadism mainly in female teens or young adults. Additional clinical features are less common, and include diabetes type I, hypothyroidism, atrophic gastritis with or without pernicious anemia (Biermer's disease), cutaneous manifestations (alopecia areata, vitiligo, transient skin rash during fever episodes, non-infectious nail dysplasia), ocular symptoms (keratoconjunctivitis, dry eye, iridocyclitis, cataract, retinal detachment, and optic atrophy; Merenmies and Tarkkanen, 2000), enamel dysplasia, hyposplenism/asplenia (implying vaccination against *Streptococcus pneumonia, Haemophilus influenzae*, and Hepatitis B as well as antibiotic prophylaxis), autoimmune hepatitis, tubulo-interstitial nephritis, or organized pneumonitis. Involvement of the gastrointestinal (GI) tract may be responsible for chronic diarrhea, constipation, and malabsorption leading sometimes to malnutrition. GI involvement is difficult to assess as it can be due to numerous various causes that may be associated or follow each other during the life of the patients.

CANDIDIASIS

Chronic mucocutaneous candidiasis infection by *Candida albicans* is one of the major characteristic of APECED, usually one of first symptoms and most likely the most disabling features of APECED. CMC is naturally not specific for APECED but any child with CMC should be suspected of APECED. According to the Finnish experience, almost all adults with APECED display symptoms of CMC, up to 70% of the patients at the age of 10, up to 94% at age of 20, and 97% at the age of 30 (Perheentupa, 2002, 2006; Betterle and Zanchetta, 2003; Husebye et al., 2009). However, the course and severity vary widely. Oral candidiasis affects the tongue, the buccal mucosa, the gingival, and the pharynx. It ranges in severity from mild form with redness, soreness, angular cheilitis, pseudomembranous lesions, erosions, ulceration and pain to severe chronic inflammation with dysphagia, and development of hyperkeratotic plaques. In the absence of active antimycotic treatment and careful follow-up, chronic oral candidiasis may lead to the development of squamous cell carcinoma with potential lethality by metastatic dissemination. *Candida* esophagitis has been reported to affect 15–22% of the patients (Perheentupa, 2006; Kisand et al., 2011) with pain while swallowing, retrosternal pain, and dysphagia (Ahonen et al., 1990; Husebye et al., 2009). Chronic esophagitis can lead to local stricture and exceptional esophageal cancer (Rautemaa et al., 2007).

Intestinal candidiasis may cause chronic diarrhea. It should be stressed that esophageal and intestinal candidiasis may occur without any active oral candidiasis. Genital candidiasis affects mainly women with pruritus and vaginal whitish discharge while genital candidiasis seems less frequent in males, possibly underreported due to discrete signs of balanitis. Lastly, *Candida* may affect the nails with chronic paronychia and onychomycosis (Collins et al., 2006). Fingernails are more commonly affected than toenails and the thumbs are the commonest digit affected. This can be explained as infection occurs during the "thumbsucking" period. Management of candidiasis in APECED patients implies an excellent oral hygiene with a careful and regular dental follow-up. Candidiasis should be treated aggressively with antimicrobial therapy and regular prophylaxis should be given.

Any clinically suspicious, chronic thickening or erosion of the mucosa that does not heal should be biopsied to rule out a potential underlying lesion of squamous cell carcinoma. Any difficulties in swallowing or eating or retrosternal pain should prompt to perform esophagoscopy (Rautemaa et al., 2007).

HYPOPARATHYOIDISM

Hypoparathyroidism is one of the first endocrine features of APECED. Symptoms are related to hypocalcemia, muscle cramps, paresthesia, clumsiness, seizures, and diarrhea. The diagnosis is simply based on blood calcium, phosphorus, and parathormone (PTH) levels: hypocalcemia, hyperphosphatemia, inadapted normal/low PTH without any kidney failure. It is considered that APECED should be systematically considered in cases of primary HP (Husebye et al., 2009). Antibodies against NALP5 as well as against the calcium-sensing receptor of parathyroid epithelial cell have been identified in APECED patients (Gavalas et al., 2007; Kemp et al., 2009, 2010). Patients who are free of HP need an annual monitoring of blood calcium and phosphorus levels. Management of HP relies on daily oral supplementation of vitamin D derivatives and calcium.

GASTRITIS AND PERNICIOUS ANEMIA

Chronic gastritis, with or without concomitant pernicious anemia belongs to the APECED complex but is found only in a fraction of cases. In non-APECED population, two types of chronic gastritis occur, divided by Strickland into type A and B gastritis. Type A gastritis was known to be caused by autoimmunity while the B gastritis was suspected to be the results of environmental factors. In early 1980s, it was shown by Warren and Marshall (1984) that the major environmental factor was in fact a chronic infection with *Helicobacterium pylori.*

The type A chronic gastritis, with and without pernicious anemia that occur in non-APECED individuals, is clearly linked to certain HLA risk haplotypes, in analogy to isolated AD. In APECED patients, the chronic gastritis differs from the above also in time of occurrence and the speed of the progression. In non-APECED patients, the time needed for progression from the early stage of gastritis, the superficial form to diffuse gastritis, to atrophic gastric and to full gastric atrophy is a slow process, taking up several decennia. Also, the process usually starts in the adult life. In contrast, an APECED-associated gastritic process is much faster and can start in the first decennium of life. Thus, one of the authors of this review was able to follow such a gastric process in two 8-year-old girls with sequential gastric biopsies and could see how, within the time period of only 2 months, the superficial process lead to complete gastric atrophy of the fundus and corpus (K. Krohn, personal experience).

The target molecule for the parietal cell antibodies were shown to be the sodium-potassium channel molecule of the parietal cells on corpus and fundal part of the stomach (Karlsson et al., 1988). In antral gastritis, the antigen are the gastrin-producing cells (Uibo and Krohn, 1984).

Pernicious anemia is the end stage of the gastric immunological destruction, caused partly by the lack of IF, that in addition to the hydrochloric acid is the main product of parietal cells, but also by the autoantibodies recognizing this vitamin B12-binding protein. There are two types of antibodies to IF: one blocking vitamin B12 binding to IF and another type, binding to the IF molecule without interfering with vitamin B12 binding (Toh et al., 1997). Both antibody types prevent the binding of IF to its receptor on the ileal mucosa and subsequent translocation of the vitamin B12 from ileum to circulation.

ADDISON'S DISEASE

Adrenocortical failure or AD, described by Thomas Addison in the ninetieth century, is considered one of the three hallmarks of APECED, but it occurs also as a solitary disease, or as part of the APS-2 complex. Today, in western word, most cases of AD are caused by autoimmunity, but adrenal cortical destruction and subsequent cortical failure can be caused by several other factors, notably by secondary tuberculosis or other chronic infections. In retrospect, the cases described by Thomas Addison were most likely caused by tuberculosis.

The clinical signs and symptoms of AD are mostly similar in APECED and in solitary AD as well as in APS-2 complex. These include decreased levels of gluco- and mineralocorticoids and elevated ACTH concentrations. The most severe consequence of AD is the life-threatening Addisonian crisis, characterized by general fatigue, dizziness, diarrhea, and death, if the patient is not quickly substituted with corticosteroids, mainly hydrocortisol.

Autoantibodies to adrenal cortex are the characteristic immunological feature in AD, be it part of APECED or APS-2 or the solitary form. These antibodies can be easily demonstrated by immunofluorescence. However, in APECED, but not in the other forms of AD, the autoantibodies are precipitating, and this phenomenon can be demonstrated by Ouchterlony's immunodiffusion (Andrada et al., 1968; Krohn et al., 1974; Heinonen et al., 1976). In immunodiffusion with APECED serum against adrenal homogenate three precipitating lines were observed, and one of these were shown to represent a mitochondrial antigen while the two others were microsomal.

The nature of the adrenal cortical autoantigens were revealed in early 1990s and shown to be the three main steroidogenic enzymes, P450c17, P450c21, and P450scc (Krohn et al., 1974; Winqvist et al., 1993; Uibo et al., 1994a,b). These three enzymes were also shown to be the ones that could be precipitated by immunodiffusion. The autoantibodies against these three steroidogenic enzymes clearly distinguish the three clinical conditions with adrenal failure: antibodies to all three can be found only in APECED, while in solitary AD and in APS-1, only antibodies to P450c21 are seen. Furthermore, in non-autoimmune AD, caused by tumors or chronic infections, such antibodies do not occur.

GONADAL FUNCTIONS

Autoimmune oophoritis is responsible for an ovarian insufficiency that may be dramatic for female patients as insufficiency starting in teenagers and young adults. Patients may have either a primary amenorrhea with no or arrested puberty. Other patients develop premature menopause. The diagnosis is confirmed by sexual hormones status; elevated plasma levels of follicle stimulating hormone (FSH) and luteinizing hormone (LH) and low estrogen levels. Autoantibodies against side-chain cleavage enzyme have been related to ovarian insufficiency (Soderbergh et al., 2004) and also steroidogenic enzymes antibodies against cytochrome p450 21-hydroxylase (CYP21A2), cytochrome p450 17α-hydroxylase (CYP17), and cytochrome p450 side-chain cleavage enzyme (CYP11A1).

In female patients, hormonal substitution by estrogen needs to be initiated during puberty. It is strongly advised not to delay pregnancy. In case of hypogonadism, embryo donation has been tried with success.

In males, testicular failure is less common and occurs later. The prevalence of hypogonadism in males is three times lower (8–28%) than in females (35–70%; Perheentupa, 2006). It leads to clinical hypogonadism or isolated azoospermia (Husebye et al., 2009). It has been hypothesized that the blood–testis barrier protects the Leydig cells from an autoimmune attack. However, the physiopathogenic link between circulating autoantibodies and hypogonadism is far from being clear. The two steroidogenic enzymes, p450scc and p450c17, are the main antigens in gonadal failure linked to APECED, but other potential antigenic targets have been identified such as testis-expressed protein TSGA10 (Reimand et al., 2008). However, despite autoantibodies directed against TSGA10 in 7% of the APECED patients, no correlation could be found with gonadal failure (Reimand et al., 2008). One should not forget that the origin of gonadal dysfunction may be related to an authentic-specific autoimmune attack but also be related to other hormonal dysfunction such as AD, pituitary insufficiency, dysthyroidism, or diabetes for instance. Besides, Schaller et al. (2008) suggested that lack of AIRE might affect fertility by disrupting scheduled apoptosis of testicular germ cells. In this respect, the recent hypothesis presented by Matsumoto (2011) that the function of AIRE in thymus would not be in the regulation of transcription but rather in the development and differentiation of the medullary epithelial cells is of primary interest

OTHER ENDOCRINE DISORDERS

Various other endocrine disorders have been described such diabetes type I mellitus, hypothyroidism, and pituitary failure, the latter diagnosed by a growth hormone deficiency. The diagnosis and management of these conditions does not differ from the standard guidelines for each disorder separately (Perheentupa, 2002; Betterle and Zanchetta, 2003; Husebye et al., 2009).

OTHER NON-ENDOCRINE DISORDERS

Enamel hypoplasia affect mainly permanent teeth (Perheentupa, 2006), but also deciduous teeth (Pavlic and Waltimo-Sirén, 2009). Pavlic and Waltimo-Sirén (2009) recently suggested that an inadequate process of enamel formation might affect all ameloblasts in phase. Ameloblasts have an epithelial origin with parenchymal cells of endocrine origin. It is speculated that ameloblasts or secreted protein in the extracellular matrix may be the target of autoantibodies leading to hypoplasia. Thereby, APECED would be the first model of dental hard tissue autoimmune disease (Pavlic and Waltimo-Sirén, 2009).

Ocular manifestations affect 25% of the patients and include mainly keratitis that can lead to blindness. It is assumed that the origin of keratitis is the result of autoimmunity against corneal epithelium (Merenmies and Tarkkanen, 2000; Perheentupa, 2006). However, to our knowledge no specific antibodies have been identified in APECED patients. Only antibodies against OBP1 have been found in the AIRE mouse model against lacrimal glands (DeVoss et al., 2010).

Hyposplenism or asplenia is often diagnosed upon the development of thrombocytosis, circulating Howell–Jolly bodies, abdominal ultrasound imaging or in case of severe *S. pneumoniae* infection (Pollak et al., 2009). Destruction of the spleen in APECED has been related to an autoimmune attack against the spleen (Perheentupa, 2002, 2006; Betterle and Zanchetta, 2003; Husebye et al., 2009) although the exact mechanism remains obscure. Again, the mechanisms proposed by Schaller et al. (2008) and by Matsumoto (2011) are of interest, as AIRE expression has also been described in lymphoid tissue and skin. A speculative hypothesis to the evolution of splenic atrophy could thus be disturbance of differentiation, due to lack of AIRE expression.

Various types of GI manifestations are common in APECED patients. These include chronic diarrhea that can be related to HP, severe constipation. Intestinal infection by candida and giardia especially, pancreatic insufficiency and autoimmune enteropathy. Several autoreactive circulating antibodies directed toward intestinal components have been described. Ekwall et al. (1998) identified TPH as an intestinal autoantigen in APECED patients. TPH is expressed in serotonin-producing cells in the central nervous system and in the intestine. In their series of 80 patients, they were able to relate "GI symptoms" to the presence of circulating TPH antibodies and also to the total absence of enterochromaffin cells in the mucosa of small bowel. These enteroendocrine cells (EECs) are scattered through the intestinal mucosa, from the gastric body and antrum to the rectum. They play a key role in growth of the gut, blood flow, motility, secretion of pancreatic enzymes, bile, and bicarbonate-rich fluid (Posovszky et al., 2012). TPH antibodies were found in 89% of the APECED patients with GI symptoms and in 34% of those without (Ekwall et al., 1998). Antibodies can precede clinical symptoms (Ekwall et al., 1998). Conversely, TPH autoantibodies are absent in other inflammatory or autoimmune intestinal diseases. Additionally, Sköldberg et al. (2003) identified also autoantibodies against histidine decarboxylase expressed by EEC – like cells in the gastric mucosa. It is noteworthy, that it is not a routine procedure to perform EECs staining on intestinal biopsies in case of diarrhea or malabsorption, as stressed by Ohsie et al. (2009). Besides, several studies showed repeatedly that EECs were lacking in the intestinal mucosa and were related to chronic diarrhea (Padeh et al., 1997; Ward et al., 1999; Oliva-Hemker et al., 2006; Posovszky et al., 2012).

Tubulo-interstitial nephritis, life-threatening autoimmune bronchiolitis and other rare manifestations have also been reported in APECED (Perheentupa, 2002, 2006; Betterle and Zanchetta, 2003; Husebye et al., 2009). The main identified autoantibodies are summarized in **Table 2**.

TREATMENT

Management of APECED relies in education of the patients to know his disease, education of the local physician, and the knowledge that new components of the disease may develop during life. Psychological support is strongly recommended as this disease impairs greatly the quality of life of the patients (Perheentupa, 2006). Except candidiasis treatment that has been explained previously, treatment of APECED relies mostly on hormone replacement therapy according to affected organs (thyroid, parathyroid, pancreas, etc.). In some rare and potentially lethal situations, however, patients may require corticosteroid treatment in association with immunosuppressive therapies. These rare situations include autoimmune hepatitis, especially its fulminant form, which may be lethal and therefore prompt immunosuppressive therapy is needed (Obermayer-Straub et al., 2001). The same is true for interstitial nephritis and bronchiolitis in association to APECED. Immunosuppressive therapies have been also proposed in case of severe intestinal malabsorption with efficacy (Padeh et al., 1997; Ward et al., 1999). Very recently, Rituximab, a chimeric monoclonal antibody targeting B cell lymphocytes

Table 2 | Main identified target of autoimmune antibodies in APECED patients.

Diagnosis	Main identified circulating autoantibodies
Addison's disease	21 hydroxylase, 17α hydroxylase
	Side-chain cleavage enzyme antibodies
	(or steroid cell antibodies)
Hypoparathyroidism	NALP5, Ca^{2+} sensing receptor
Hypothyroidism	Thyroperoxydase
	Thyroglobuline
Hypogonadism	17α hydroxylase
	Side-chain cleavage enzyme antibodies
	(or steroid cell antibodies)
Diabetes type I	Glutamic acid decarboxylase 65-kDa isoform
	(GAD65)
	Insulin
	Tyrosine phosphatase (IA2)
Pituitary insufficiency	Tudor Domain containing protein 6 (TDRD6)
Atrophic gastritis/	Intrinsic factor, gastric parietal cell
Biermer's disease	
Intestine	Glutamic acid decarboxylase 65-kDa isoform
	(GAD65)
	Histidine decarboxylase
	Tryptophan hydroxylase
Autoimmune hepatitis	Aromatic L-amino acid decarboxylase (AADC)
	Cytochrome P450 1A2
	Cytochrome P450 2A6
	Cytochrome P450 1A1
	Cytochrome P450 2B6
Vitiligo	Transcription factors: SOX 9, SOX 10, aromatic
	L-amino acid decarboxylase (AADC)
Alopecia areata	Tyrosine hydroxylase
Nephropathy	Antibody against tubular basement membrane
	(Hannigan et al., 1996)
Pulmonary disease	Potassium channel regulatory protein (KCNRG)
Eye	OBP1*
Non-tissue specific**	IFN-α, IFN-β, IFN-ω, IL-22, IL-17F, IL-17A

Identified in a mouse model $AIRE^{-/-}$.
***Main non-tissue-specific antibodies according to Kisand et al. (2011).*

expressive CD20 has been successfully used in a young patient with bronchiolitis (Popler et al., 2012). The rationale for Rituximab use in APECED is supported by the presence of B cell infiltrates in the affected organs (Gavanescu et al., 2008).

AUTOANTIBODIES TOWARD INTERFERONS AND CYTOKINES

At the beginning of this millennium, the antibody responses to the main target organs affected in APECED, and the responsible target antigens were fairly well characterized. A new period in APECED studies started along the publication by Meager et al. (2006), describing high-titer antibodies to several type I interferons in practically all APECED patients studied. This anti-interferon response was exceptionally strong, since serum titers up to 1:1,000,000, and clearly exceeding the titers seen against organ-specific antigens, were found.

Furthermore, high-titer antibodies were seen against the two main mediators secreted by Th17 cells, interleukin-17 and interleukin-22 (IL-17 and IL-22). Responses with lower titers were occasionally seen against other interleukins, too. In our own as yet unpublished observations we have detected occasional high-titer responses against several other interleukins and chemokines, as well, but in contrast to the aforementioned responses, these responses are not characteristic to all APECED patients but rather occur occasionally in only a few patients.

The significance of these novel findings are still unclear, but some information concerning the role of IL-17/IL-22 antibodies in the chronic candida infections, characteristic for APECED, has been obtained. Th17 cells secrete IL-17 and IL-22, which are cytokines with potent antifungal properties (Engelhardt and Grimbacher, 2012) and the occurrence of autoantibodies against IL-17/IL-22 were reported to closely correlate to the presence of candida infection (Kisand et al., 2011; Engelhardt and Grimbacher, 2012). However, recent evidence points to a new interaction between AIRE and dectin-1, a pattern-recognition receptor that is important in antifungal innate immunity. Pedroza et al. (2012) recently showed that AIRE participates in the dectin-1 signaling pathway, and thus, missing AIRE activity could contribute to fungal susceptibility through this pathway. Dectin-1 is expressed on phagocytes and was recently shown to induce a non-canonical caspase-8 inflammasome in response to fungal and mycobacterial infection (Gringhuis et al., 2012). The activation of the dectin signaling pathway also leads to expression of IL-17 and 22 and defensins, however. Besides, other mechanisms such Dominant-negative mutations in STAT3, gain of mutation of STAT1, mutations in IL-17F and IL-17R may be alternate causes of CMC (Engelhardt and Grimbacher, 2012).

The significance of the antibody response toward interferons and other cytokines is presently also unclear. One could speculate that some of these antibodies against type I interferons as well as reacting with IL-17 and IL-22 might have a protective function. As pointed out by Waterfield and Anderson (2011), antibodies to type I interferons do not seem to lead to increased susceptibility to viral infections. This resistance might be due to redundancy and it has to be seen whether this anti-interferon response is directed only toward certain members of the interferon family. While Th17 cell response and the release of soluble IL-17 and IL-22 are evidently necessary for the defense against mucocutaneous candida infection, the same cytokines have a role in the development of psoriasis. Similarly, interferons are known to be involved in the pathogenesis of several conditions, and one such chronic ailment is the autoimmune diseases belonging to the systemic lupus erythematosus (SLE) complex. Anti-interferon alpha antibodies are currently being tested as a therapeutic mean against SLE (Merrill et al., 2011). In order to be able to find out if the antibodies against interferons and other cytokines could have a protective role in APECED, large APECED patient cohorts have to be studied in order to find out whether, e.g., psoriasis and SLE are significantly less common in APECED patients than in the general population.

The reason for the antibody response toward soluble immune mediators is still unclear, and we do not yet know what exactly elicits them and thus, only speculative scenarios can be presented. It is conceivable to hypothesize, however, that the tissue destruction preceding the failure of the endocrine organs may have a role. Tissue destruction, be it caused by trauma, viral infection or autoimmune attack, would probably lead not only to the release of potential tissue-specific autoantigens and thus, to autoantibody formation against these proteins, but could also lead to an inflammatory response and production of several mediators of inflammation. One key group of molecules in this respect is the acute phase proteins, notably those belonging to the IL-1 group.

It is generally believed that the destruction of the endocrine organs in APECED is caused by the autoreactive $CD8^+$ cytotoxic T cells, although definitive evidence for this mechanism is still lacking (Betterle and Zanchetta, 2003; Moraes-Vasconcelos et al., 2008). This hypothesis is reinforced by the examination of microscopic examinations of samples, sometimes obtained postmortem. Indeed, parathyroid, adrenal glands, or ovaries pathology disclosed also atrophy and lymphocytic infiltration that suggest lymphocytic aggression of the organs leading to atrophy and dysfunction (Betterle and Zanchetta, 2003). This is also stressed, indirectly, by the analysis of the AIRE-deficient mouse model, who develop also a lymphocytic infiltration in some inner organs along with atrophy (Ramsey et al., 2002).

However, cell destruction caused by an immune response against the endocrine organ would in fact lead to a similar situation that is thought to happen in viral infections. In fact, several autoimmune diseases, such as diabetes type I or chronic autoimmune liver diseases are thought to be a consequence of preceding viral infection: enterovirus infection in the case of diabetes type I and hepatitis B in the case of chronic active hepatitis. In viral infections, a specific group of intracellular regulatory molecules, TRIMs (tripartite motif-containing proteins), have been shown to have a key role in eliciting an autoimmune or auto inflammatory consequence (Jefferies et al., 2011).

The TRIM protein family is a form of RING domain containing E3 ligases and they exert a variety of biological functions, related to immunity and inflammation (Jefferies et al., 2011). Specifically, of the more than 20 different TRIM proteins, some seem to up-regulate the expression of type I interferons and proinflammatory cytokines, notable interleukin-1beta (IL-1beta). Furthermore, the same mediators of immune response and inflammation are in some cases known to up-regulate the expression of TRIMs. Thus, a vicious circle can theoretically occur and this in turn could lead to autoimmunity. So far, overexpression of TRIMs, or an autoimmune response toward them, has been shown to be linked to autoimmune and autoinflammatory processes in Sjögren's syndrome or rheumatoid arthritis (Jefferies et al., 2011).

Presently, we have no information how the occurrence of autoantibodies toward the interferons and other mediators of immune response might affect the aforementioned vicious circle, but it is conceivable to speculate that such an antibody response could have an balancing effect. One could thus form a hypothesis, that in APECED, the primary defect outside thymus, where the autoreactive T cells are not destroyed, would be the cell destruction of the endocrine organs by cell-mediated immune response, followed by release of cellular components taken up by professional antigen presenting cells and further stimulating the activation of $CD4^+$ Th-cells and finally resulting in an autoantibody response to these organ-specific antigens. However, simultaneous overexpression of TRIMs and subsequent up-regulation of a variety of soluble mediators of immune response and inflammation, such as interferons and members of the IL-1 family would lead to autoantibody formation also against these cytokines. Lastly, one reason for the break of tolerance to immune mediators, and subsequent production of autoantibodies could be related the fact that AIRE expression seems to occur, in addition to thymic epithelial cells also outside thymus, notably in dendritic cells, that normally express also such mediators (Heath and Carbone, 2009)

The consequences of such cytokine-directed antibody response are still an open question. In case of the Th17 type interleukins (IL-17 and IL-22) there is convincing evidence that such antibodies are linked to the CMC. However, at least in some cases, the antibodies may have a balancing, down-regulating effect on the expression of the corresponding biologically active molecules but also, by regulating the immune response to target organs. Thus, it is possible to presume, that especially the antibodies to type I interferons might have a protective effect, as some chronic immune diseases, such as psoriasis and SLE, are rare or non-existing among APECED patients.

CELL-MEDIATED IMMUNE RESPONSES

Although it is now a generally accepted view that the consequence of the AIRE defect in APECED will lead to the escape of the potentially autoreactive T cells, there is in fact rather little direct evidence to show that the tissue destruction in the endocrine organs affected in APECED is caused by cytotoxic $CD8^+$ T cells. Furthermore, most studies describing the phenotype of the lymphocytes infiltrating affected organs is not from APECED patients directly, but from patients suffering of solitary lesions that are similar to the ones seen in APECED, such as solitary AD or diabetes. However, the solitary endocrine diseases, such as isolated thyroid disease or AD are remarkably similar in their clinical picture as well as immunological findings as those of APECED. Thus, in solitary AD and in APECED with adrenocortical failure, autoantibodies recognize the p450c21 steroidogenic enzyme. Interestingly, in this disease complex $CD8^+$ T cells that reach against specific T cell epitopes in p450c21 has been demonstrated (Bratland et al., 2009; Rottembourg et al., 2010) Likewise, in thyroid diseases, thyroglobulin and thyroid peroxidase are recognized by the autoantibodies, irrespective if the condition is occurring alone, in association of APS-2 or as part of the APECED complex. The similar synergism in terms of the nature of autoantigens occurs in chronic immunological liver diseases, too.

In chronic aggressive hepatitis the lymphocytic infiltrating cell population has been shown to be of the $CD8^+$ lineage (Si et al., 1984). In a murine model of Graves' disease, the $CD8^+$ cell population contains also the recently identified $CD8^+CD122^+$ T cells that are functionally similar to the $CD4^+CD25^+$ regulatory T cells (Ryan et al., 2005). Furthermore, studies in thyroid and other affected organs show that one of the main cell population in the lymphocytic infiltrate are in fact the $CD4^+$ Th17 cells that secrete as effector molecules, the cytokines IL-17 and IL-22. In experimental autoimmune diseases, the balance between the Th17 effector cells and the two regulatory T cells, $CD8^+CD122^+$ and $CD4^+CD25^+$, seems to regulate both the occurrence and severity of tissue destruction and functional failure.

There could thus be two distinct mechanisms operating in the pathogenesis of autoimmunity in the endocrinopathies: one mediated by soluble effector molecules, such as IL-17 and IL-22 as well as type I interferons, and an other one mediated by effector T cells, which are either of the $CD8^+$ CTL cell or of the Th17 effector cell lineage. To counteract these, again two distinct biological processes would occur: the production of autoantibodies and secondly, the emergency of the regulatory T cells. As to the regulatory T cell response, it is to note that one key immunological failure in APECED, is the dysregulation of the Treg cell maturation (Ryan et al., 2005; Kekäläinen et al., 2007; Saitoh et al., 2007; Laakso et al., 2010, 2011; Wolff et al., 2010).

In normal thymus, Treg maturation follows a preprogrammed scheme, and the immature $CD8^+CD4^+FOXP3^+$ seems to be prone to apoptosis, whereas the more mature form $CD4^+CD8^-FOXP3^+$ cells form the active Treg population (Lehtoviita et al., 2009). According to Endharti et al. (2011) the $CD8^+CXCR3^+$ Tregs in humans are functionally similar to murine $CD8^+CD122^+$ Tregs. Furthermore, in APECED patients the recent thymic emigrant (RTE) pool of Treg cells shift to the activated pool and the RTE reservoir is depleted. Most importantly, in APECED patients these cells express less FOXP3 than in the healthy controls (Laakso et al., 2010). Thus, in APECED the newly formed Treg cells have a developmental defect and their function is therefore impaired. Data concerning the $CD8^+$ regulatory T cells in APECED patients is missing, however.

The finding that the regulatory T cell population in APECED is functionally defective and that the expression of the key molecule for Treg function, the FOXP3 is impaired, is consistent with clinical findings in IPEX syndrome, caused by a defect in the function of the FOXP3 gene. However, it should be noted that the effect of FOXP3 mutations in Treg population also in the IPEX patients is highly variable. Also, in contrast to APECED there seems to be a genotype–phenotype correlation in IPEX, as different mutations are associated in variable clinical picture, that show differences in severity as well in the types of clinical components that are present (Torgerson et al., 2007; d'Hennezel et al., 2009) A consistent finding in IPEX is however the inability of the $CD4^+CD25$ high Tregs to suppress the function of autologous effector T cells (Bacchetta et al., 2006). There are, thus, several differences in the clinical picture of APECED and IPEX, but both conditions show clear immune destruction of at least some endocrine organs. Both conditions also share some similarities in the GI symptoms.

The proposed hypothesis that in APECED both tissue destructive mechanisms and controlling regulatory mechanisms exist raises a question whether APECED could be treated or even cured by immunological manipulations. To find an answer for this question is one of the further challenges for APECED research

ACKNOWLEDGMENTS

The study was financially supported by the European Science Foundation (ESF) and the Sigrid Juselius foundation (to Nicolas Kluger). We thank Professors Jaakko Perheentupa, Adrian Hayday, and Pärt Peterson, as well as Drs Kai Kisand, Annalisa Macagno, and Edward Stuart for stimulating discussions.

REFERENCES

Ahonen, P., Myllarniemi, S., Sipila, I., and Perheentupa, J. (1990). Clinical variation of autoimmune polyendocrinopathy–candidiasis–ectodermal dystrophy (APECED) in a series of 68 patients. *N. Engl. J. Med.* 322, 1829–1836.

Akirav, E. M., Ruddle, N. H., and Herold, K. C. (2011). The role of AIRE in human autoimmune disease. *Nat. Rev. Endocrinol.* 7, 25–33.

Andrada, J. A., Bigazzi, P. L., Andrada, E., Milgrom, F., and Witebsky, E. (1968). Serological investigations on Addison's disease. *JAMA* 206, 1535–1541.

Bacchetta, R., Passerini, L., Gambineri, E., Dai, M., Allan, S. E., Perroni, L., Dagna-Bricarelli, F., Sartirana, C., Matthes-Martin, S., Lawitschka, A., Azzari, C., Ziegler, S. F., Levings, M. K., and Roncarolo, M. G. (2006). Defective regulatory and effector T cell functions in patients with FOXP3 mutations. *J. Clin. Invest.* 116, 1713–1722.

Bennett, C. L., Yoshioka, R., Kiyosawa, H., Barker, D. F., Fain, P. R., Shigeoka, A. O., and Chance, P. F. (2000). X-Linked syndrome of polyendocrinopathy, immune dysfunction, and diarrhea maps to Xp11.23–Xq13.3. *Am. J. Hum. Genet.* 66, 461–468.

Betterle, C., and Zanchetta, R. (2003). Update on autoimmune polyendocrine syndromes (APS). *Acta Biomed.* 74, 9–33.

Bjorses, P., Alltonen, J., Vikman, A., Perheentupa, J., Ben-Zion, G., Chiumello, G., Dahl, N., Heidemen, P., Hoorweg-Nijman, J. J., Mathivon, L., Mullis, P. E., Pohl, M., Ritzen, M., Romeo, G., Shapiro, M. S., Smith, C. S., Solyom, J., Zlotogora, J., and Peltonen, L. (1996). Genetic homogeneity of autoimmune polyglandular disease type I. *Am. J. Hum. Genet.* 59, 879–886.

Björses, P., Halonen, M., Palvimo, J. J., Kolmer, M., Aaltonen, J., Ellonen, P., Perheentupa, J., Ulmanen, I., and Peltonen, L. (2000). Mutations in the AIRE gene: effects on subcellular location and transactivation function of the autoimmune polyendocrinopathy-candidiasis-ectodermal dystrophy protein. *Am. J. Hum. Genet.* 66, 378–392.

Blizzard, R. M., Tomasi, T. B., and Christy, N. P. (1963). Autoantibodies against thyroid and adrenal tissue in a patient with mutiple, primary endocrine deficiencies. *J. Clin. Endocrinol. Metab.* 23, 1179–1180.

Blizzard, R. M., Chandler, R. W., Kyle, M. A., and Hung, W. (1962). Adrenal antibodies in Addison's disease. *Lancet* 2, 901–903.

Bottazzo, G. F., Dean, B. M., Gorsuch, A. N., Cudworth, A. G., and Doniach, D. (1980). Complement-fixing islet-cell antibodies in type-I diabetes: possible monitors of active beta-cell damage. *Lancet* 1, 668–672.

Bratland, E., Skinningsrud, B., Undlien, D. E., Mozes, E., and Husebye, E. S. (2009). T cell responses to steroid cytochrome P450 21-hydroxylase in patients with autoimmune primary adrenal insufficiency. *J. Clin. Endocrinol. Metab.* 12, 5117–5124.

Brun, J. M. (1978). Auto-immune juvenile polyendocrinopathy (author's transl). *Ann. Endocrinol. (Paris)* 39, 463–481.

Collins, S. M., Dominguez, M., Ilmarinen, T., Costigan, C., and Irvine, A. D. (2006). Dermatological manifestations of autoimmune polyendocrinopathy-candidiasis-ectodermal dystrophy syndrome. *Br. J. Dermatol.* 154, 1088–1093.

Derbinski, J., Gäbler, J., Brors, B., Tierling, S., Jonnakuty, S., Hergenhahn, M., Peltonen, L., Walter, J., and Kyewski, B. (2005). Promiscuous gene expression in thymic epithelial cells is regulated at multiple levels. *J. Exp. Med.* 202, 33–45.

DeVoss, J. J., LeClair, N. P., Hou, Y., Grewal, N. K., Johannes, K. P., Lu, W., Yang, T., Meagher, C., Fong, L., Strauss, E. C., and Anderson, M. S. (2010). An autoimmune response to odorant binding protein 1a is associated with dry eye in the Aire-deficient mouse. *J. Immunol.* 184, 4236–4246.

d'Hennezel, E., Ben-Shoshan, M., Ochs, H. D., Torgerson, T. R., Russell, L. J., Lejtenyi, C., Noya, F. J., Jabado, N., Mazer, B., and Piccirillo, C. A. (2009). FOXP3 forkhead domain mutation and regulatory T cells in the IPEX syndrome. *N. Engl. J. Med.* 361, 1710–1713.

Doniach, D., and Roitt, I. M. (1964). An evaluation of gastric and thyroid auto-immunity in relatation to hematologic auto-immunity. *Semin. Hematol.* 1, 313–343.

Ekwall, O., Hedstrand, H., Grimelius, L., Haavik, J., Perheentupa, J., Gustafsson, J., Husebye, E., Kämpe, O., and Rorsman, F. (1998). Identification of tryptophan hydroxylase as an intestinal autoantigen. *Lancet* 352, 279–283.

Endharti, A. T., Okuno, Y., Shi, Z., Misawa, N., Toyokuni, S., Ito, M., Isobe, K., and Suzuki, H. (2011). CD8+CD122+ regulatory T cells (Tregs) and CD4+ Tregs cooperatively prevent and cure CD4+ cell-induced colitis. *J. Immunol.* 186, 41–52.

Engelhardt, K. R., and Grimbacher, B. (2012). Mendelian traits causing susceptibility to mucocutaneous fungal infections in human subjects. *J. Allergy Clin. Immunol.* 129, 294–305.

Fierabracci, A. (2011). Recent insights into the role and molecular mechanisms of the autoimmune regulator (AIRE) gene in autoimmunity. *Autoimmu. Rev.* 10, 137–143.

Gardner, J. M., Fletcher, A. L., Anderson, M. S., and Turley, S. J. (2009). AIRE in the thymus and beyond. *Curr. Opin. Immunol.* 21, 582–589.

Gavalas, N. G., Kemp, E. H., Krohn, K. J., Brown, E. M., Watson, P. F., and Weetman, A. P. (2007). The calcium-sensing receptor is a target of autoantibodies in patients with autoimmune polyendocrine syndrome type 1. *J. Clin. Endocrinol. Metab.* 92, 2107–2114.

Gavanescu, I., Benoist, C., and Mathis, D. (2008). B cells are required for Aire-deficient mice to develop multi-organ autoinflammation: a therapeutic approach for APECED patients. *Proc. Natl. Acad. Sci. U.S.A.* 105, 13009–13014.

Gringhuis, S. I., Kaptein, T. M., Wevers, B. A., Theelen, B., van der Vlist, M., Boekhout, T., and Geijtenbeek, T. B. (2012). Dectin-1 is an extracellular pathogen sensor for the induction and processing of IL-1β via a noncanonical caspase-8 inflammasome. *Nat. Immunol.* 13, 246–254.

Hannigan, N. R., Jabs, K., Perez-Atayde, A. R., and Rosen, S. (1996). Autoimmune interstitial nephritis and hepatitis in polyglandular autoimmune syndrome. *Pediatr. Nephrol.* 10, 511–514.

Heath, W. R., and Carbone, F. R. (2009). Dendritic cell subsets in primary and secondary T cell responses at body surfaces. *Nat. Immunol.* 10, 1237–1244.

Heinonen, E., Krohn, K., Perheentupa, J., Aro, A., and Pelkonen, R. (1976). Association of precipitating anti-adrenal anti-adrenal antibodies with moniliasis-polyendocrinopathy syndrome. *Ann. Clin. Res.* 8, 262–265.

Husebye, E. S., Perheentupa, J., Rautemaa, R., and Kämpe, O. (2009). Clinical manifestations and management of patients with autoimmune polyendocrine syndrome type I. *J. Intern. Med.* 265, 514–529.

Irvine, W. J., Davies, S. H., Teitelbaum, S., Delamore, I. W., and Williams, A. W. (1965). The clinical and pathological significance of gastric parietal cell antibody. *Ann. N. Y. Acad. Sci.* 124, 657–691.

Irvine, W. J., MacGregor, A. G., and Stuart, A. E. (1962). The prognostic significance of thyroid antibodies in the management of thyrotoxicosis. *Lancet* 2, 843–847.

Jefferies, C., Wynne, C., and Higgs, R. (2011). Antiviral TRIMs: friend or foe in autoimmune and autoinflammatory disease? *Nat. Rev. Immunol.* 11, 617–625.

Jeffries, G. H., Hoskins, D. W., and Sleisenger, M. H. (1962). Antibody to intrinsic factor in serum from patients with pernicious anemia. *J. Clin. Invest.* 41, 1106–1115.

Kaldany, A. (1979). Autoantibodies to islet cells in diabetes mellitus. *Diabetes* 28, 102–105.

Karlsson, F. A., Burman, P., Lööf, L., and Mårdh, S. (1988). Major parietal cell antigen in autoimmune gastritis with pernicious anemia is the acid-producing H+,K+-adenosine triphosphatase of the stomach. *J. Clin. Invest.* 81, 475–479.

Kekäläinen, E., Tuovinen, H., Joensuu, J., Gylling, M., Franssila, R., Pöntynen, N., Talvensaari, K., Perheentupa, J., Miettinen, A., and Arstila, T. P. (2007). A defect of regulatory T cells in patients with autoimmune polyendocrinopathy-candidiasis-ectodermal dystrophy. *J. Immunol.* 178, 1208–1215.

Kemp, E. H., Gavalas, N. G., Akhtar, S., Krohn, K. J., Pallais, J. C., Brown, E. M., Watson, P. F., and Weetman, A. P. (2010). Mapping of human autoantibody binding sites on the calcium-sensing receptor. *J. Bone Miner. Res.* 25, 132–140.

Kemp, E. H., Gavalas, N. G., Krohn, K. J., Brown, E. M., Watson, P. F., and Weetman, A. P. (2009). Activating autoantibodies against the calcium-sensing receptor detected in two patients with autoimmune polyendocrine syndrome type 1. *J. Clin. Endocrinol. Metab.* 94, 4749–4756.

Kisand, K., Lilic, D., Casanova, J. L., Peterson, P., Meager, A., and Willcox, N. (2011). Mucocutaneous candidiasis and autoimmunity against cytokines in APECED and thymoma patients: clinical and pathogenetic implications. *Eur. J. Immunol.* 41, 1517–1527.

Kogawa, K., Nagafuchi, S., Katsuta, H., Kudoh, J., Tamiya, S., Sakai, Y., Shimizu, N., and Harada, M. (2002). Expression of AIRE gene in peripheral monocyte/dendritic cell lineage. *Immunol. Lett.* 80, 195–198.

Krohn, K., Perheentupa, J., and Heinonen, E. (1974). Precipitating anti-adrenal antibodies in Addison's disease. *Clin. Immunol. Immunopathol.* 3, 59–68.

Laakso, S. M., Laurinolli, T. T., Rossi, L. H., Lehtoviita, A., Sairanen, H., Perheentupa, J., Kekäläinen, E., and Arstila, T. P. (2010). Regulatory T cell defect in APECED patients is associated with loss of naive FOXP3(+) precursors and impaired activated population. *J. Autoimmun.* 35, 351–357.

Laakso, S. M., Kekäläinen, E., Rossi, L. H., Laurinolli, T. T., Mannerström, H., Heikkilä, N., Lehtoviita, A., Perheentupa, J., Jarva, H., and Arstila, T. P. (2011). IL-7 dysregulation and loss of CD8+ T cell homeostasis in the monogenic human disease autoimmune polyendocrinopathy-candidiasis-ectodermal dystrophy. *J. Immunol.* 187, 2023–2030.

Lehtoviita, A., Rossi, L. H., Kekäläinen, E., Sairanen, H., and Arstila, T. P. (2009). The CD4(+)CD8(+) and CD4(+) subsets of FOXP3(+) thymocytes differ in their response to growth factor deprivation or stimulation. *Scand. J. Immunol.* 70, 377–383.

Matsumoto, M. (2011). Contrasting models for the roles of Aire in the differentiation program of epithelial cells in the thymic medulla. *Eur. J. Immunol.* 41, 12–17.

Meager, A., Visvalingam, K., Peterson, P., Möll, K., Murumägi, A., Krohn, K., Eskelin, P., Perheentupa, J., Husebye, E., Kadota, Y., and Willcox, N. (2006). Anti-interferon autoantibodies in autoimmune polyendocrinopathy syndrome type 1. *PLoS Med.* 3, e289. doi: 10.1371/journal.pmed.0030289

Meloni, A., Willcox, N., Meager, A., Atzeni, M., Wolff, A. S., Husebye, E. S., Furcas, M., Rosatelli, M. C., Cao, A., and Congia, M. (2012). Autoimmune polyendocrine syndrome type 1: an extensive longitudinal study in Sardinian patients. *J. Clin. Endocrinol. Metab.* 97, 1114–1124.

Merenmies, L., and Tarkkanen, A. (2000). Chronic bilateral keratitis in autoimmune polyendocrinopathy-candidiadis-ectodermal dystrophy (APECED). A long-term follow-up and visual prognosis. *Acta Ophthalmol. Scand.* 78, 532–535.

Merrill, J. T., Wallace, D. J., Petri, M., Kirou, K. A., Yao, Y., White, W. I., Robbie, G., Levin, R., Berney, S. M., Chindalore, V., Olsen, N., Richman, L,. Le, C., Jallal, B., and White, B.; Lupus Interferon Skin Activity (LISA) Study Investigators. (2011). Safety profile and clinical activity of sifalimumab, a fully human anti-interferon α monoclonal antibody, in systemic lupus erythematosus: a phase I, multicentre, double-blind randomised study. *Ann. Rheum. Dis.* 70, 1905–1913.

Moraes-Vasconcelos, D., Costa-Carvalho, B. T., Torgerson, T. R., and Ochs, H. D. (2008). Primary immune deficiency disorders presenting as autoimmune diseases: IPEX and APECED. *J. Clin. Immunol.* 28, S11–S19.

Nagamine, K., Peterson, P., Scott, H. S., Kudoh, J., Minoshima, S., Heino, M., Krohn, K. J., Lalioti, M. D., Mullis, P. E., Antonarakis, S. E., Kawasaki, K., Asakawa, S., Ito, F., and Shimizu, N. (1997). Positional cloning of the APECED gene. *Nat. Genet.* 17, 393–398.

Neufeld, M., Maclaren, N. K., and Blizzard, R. M. (1981). Two types of autoimmune Addison's disease associated with different polyglandular autoimmune (PGA) syndromes. *Medicine (Baltimore)* 60, 355–362.

Obermayer-Straub, P., Perheentupa, J., Braun, S., Kayser, A., Barut, A., Loges, S., Harms, A., Dalekos, G., Strassburg, C. P., and Manns, M. P. (2001). Hepatic autoantigens in patients with autoimmune polyendocrinopathy-candidiasis-ectodermal dystrophy. *Gastroenterology* 121, 668–677.

Ohsie, S., Gerney, G., Gui, D., Kahana, D., Martín, M. G., and Cortina, G. (2009). A paucity of colonic enteroendocrine and/or enterochromaffin cells characterizes a subset of patients with chronic unexplained diarrhea/malabsorption. *Hum. Pathol.* 40, 1006–1014.

Oliva-Hemker, M., Berkenblit, G. V., Anhalt, G. J., and Yardley, J. H. (2006). Pernicious anemia and widespread absence of gastrointestinal endocrine cells in a patient with autoimmune polyglandular syndrome type I and malabsorption. *J. Clin. Endocrinol. Metab.* 91, 2833–2838.

Orlova, E. M., Bukina, A. M., Kuznetsova, E. S., Kareva, M. A., Zakharova, E. U., Peterkova, V. A., and Dedov, I. I. (2010). Autoimmune polyglandular syndrome type 1 in Russian patients: clinical variants and autoimmune regulator mutations. *Horm. Res. Paediatr.* 73, 449–457.

Padeh, S., Theodor, R., Jonas, A., and Passwell, J. H. (1997). Severe malabsorption in autoimmune polyendocrinopathy-candidosis-ectodermal dystrophy syndrome successfully treated with immunosuppression. *Arch. Dis. Child.* 76, 532–534.

Pavlic, A., and Waltimo-Sirén, J. (2009). Clinical and microstructural aberrations of enamel of deciduous and permanent teeth in patients with autoimmune polyendocrinopathy-candidiasis-ectodermal dystrophy. *Arch. Oral Biol.* 54, 658–665.

Pedroza, L. A., Kumar, V., Sanborn, K. B., Mace, E. M., Niinikoski, H., Nadeau, K., Vasconcelos Dde, M., Perez, E., Jyonouchi, S., Jyonouchi, H., Banerjee, P. P., Ruuskanen, O., Condino-Neto, A., and Orange, J. S. (2012). Autoimmune regulator (AIRE) contributes to Dectin-1-induced TNF-α production and complexes with caspase recruitment domain-containing protein 9 (CARD9), spleen tyrosine kinase (Syk), and Dectin-1. *J. Allergy Clin. Immunol.* 129, 464–472, 472.e1–3.

Perheentupa, J. (2002). APS-I/APECED: the clinical disease and therapy. *Endocrinol. Metab. Clin. North Am.* 31, 295–320, vi.

Perheentupa, J. (2006). Autoimmune polyendocrinopathy-candidiasis-ectodermal dystrophy. *J. Clin. Endocrinol. Metab.* 91, 2843–2850.

Pollak, U., Bar-Sever, Z., Hoffer, V., Marcus, N., Scheuerman, O., and Garty, B. Z. (2009). Asplenia and functional hyposplenism in autoimmune polyglandular syndrome type 1. *Eur. J. Pediatr.* 168, 233–235.

Popler, J., Alimohammadi, M., Kämpe, O., Dalin, F., Dishop, M. K., Barker, J. M., Moriarty-Kelsey, M., Soep, J. B., and Deterding, R. R. (2012). Autoimmune polyendocrine syndrome type Utility of KCNRG autoantibodies as a marker of active pulmonary disease and successful treatment with rituximab. *Pediatr. Pulmonol.* 47, 84–87.

Posovszky, C., Lahr, G., von Schnurbein, J., Buderus, S., Findeisen, A., Schröder, C., Schütz, C., Schulz, A, Debatin, K. M., Wabitsch, M., and Barth, T. F. (2012). Loss of enteroendocrine cells in autoimmune-polyendocrine-candidiasis-ectodermal-dystrophy (APECED) syndrome with gastrointestinal dysfunction. *J. Clin. Endocrinol. Metab.* 97, E292–E300.

Powell, B. R., Buist, N. R., and Stenzel, P. (1982). A X-linked syndrome of diarrhea, polyendocrinopathy, and fatal infection in infancy. *J. Pediatr.* 100, 731–737.

Ramsey, C., Winqvist, O., Puhakka, L., Halonen, M., Moro, A., Kämpe, O., Eskelin, P., Pelto-Huikko, M., and Peltonen, L. (2002). Aire deficient mice develop multiple features of APECED phenotype and show altered immune response. *Hum. Mol. Genet.* 11, 397–409.

Rautemaa, R., Hietanen, J., Niissalo, S., Pirinen, S., and Perheentupa, J. (2007). Oral and oesophageal squamous cell carcinoma – a complication or component of autoimmune polyendocrinopathy-candidiasis-ectodermal dystrophy (APECED, APS-1). *Oral Oncol.* 43, 607–613.

Reimand, K., Perheentupa, J., Link, M., Krohn, K., Peterson, P., and Uibo, R. (2008). Testis-expressed protein TSGA10 an auto-antigen in autoimmune polyendocrine syndrome type I. *Int. Immunol.* 20, 39–44.

Rosatelli, M. C., Meloni, A., Meloni, A., Devoto, M., Cao, A., Scott, H. S., Peterson, P., Heino, M., Krohn, K. J., Nagamine, K., Kudoh, J., Shimizu, N., and Antonarakis, S. E. (1998). A common mutation in Sardinian autoimmune polyendocrinopathy-candidiasis-ectodermal dystrophy patients. *Hum. Genet.* 103, 428–434.

Rottembourg, D., Deal, C., Lambert, M., Mallone, R., Carel, J. C., Lacroix, A., Caillat-Zucman, S., and le Deist, F. (2010). 21-Hydroxylase epitopes are targeted by CD8 T cells in autoimmune Addison's disease. *J. Autoimmun.* 35, 309–315.

Ryan, K. R., Lawson, C. A., Lorenzi, A. R., Arkwright, P. D., Isaacs, J. D., and Lilic, D. (2005) CD4+CD25+ T-regulatory cells are decreased in patients with autoimmune polyendocrinopathy candidiasis ectodermal dystrophy. *J. Allergy Clin. Immunol.* 116, 1158–1159.

Saitoh, O., Abiru, N., Nakahara, M., and Nagayama, Y. (2007). CD8+CD122+ T cells, a newly identified regulatory T subset, negatively regulate Graves' hyperthyroidism in a murine model. *Endocrinology* 148, 6040–6046.

Schaller, C. E., Wang, C. L., Beck-Engeser, G., Goss, L., Scott, H. S., Anderson, M. S., and Wabl, M. (2008). Expression of Aire and the early wave of apoptosis in spermatogenesis. *J. Immunol.* 180, 1338–1343.

Schwartz, M. (1961). Antibodies to intrinsic factor. *Acta Allergol.* 16, 263–266.

Si, L., Whiteside, T. L., Van Thiel, D. H., and Rabin, B. S. (1984). Lymphocyte subpopulations at the site of "piecemeal" necrosis in end stage chronic liver diseases and rejecting liver allografts in cyclosporine-treated patients. *Lab. Invest.* 50, 341–347.

Sköldberg, F., Portela-Gomes, G. M., Grimelius, L., Nilsson, G., Perheentupa, J., Betterle, C., Husebye, E. S., Gustafsson, J., Rönnblom, A., Rorsman, F., and Kämpe, O. (2003). Histidine decarboxylase, a pyridoxal phosphate-dependent enzyme, is an autoantigen of gastric enterochromaffin-like cells. *J. Clin. Endocrinol. Metab.* 88, 1445–1452.

Soderbergh, A., Myhre, A. G., Ekwall, O., Gebre-Medhin, G., Hedstrand, H., Landgren, E., Miettinen, A., Eskelin, P., Halonen, M., Tuomi, T., Gustafsson, J., Husebye, E. S., Perheentupa, J., Gylling, M., Manns, M. P., Rorsman, F., Kämpe, O., and Nilsson, T. (2004). Prevalence and clinical associations of 10 defined autoantibodies in autoimmune polyendocrine syndrome type I. *J. Clin. Endocrinol. Metab.* 89, 557–562.

The Finnish–German APECED Consortium. (1997). An autoimmune disease, APECED, caused by mutations in a novel gene featuring two PHD-type zinc-finger domains. *Nat. Genet.* 17, 399–403.

Toh, B. H., van Driel, I. R., and Gleeson, P. A. (1997). Pernicious anemia. *N. Engl. J. Med.* 337, 1441–1448.

Torgerson, T. R., Linane, A., Moes, N., Anover, S., Mateo, V., Rieux-Laucat, F., Hermine, O., Vijay, S., Gambineri, E., Cerf-Bensussan, N., Fischer, A., Ochs, H. D., Goulet, O., and Ruemmele, F. M. (2007). Severe food allergy as a variant of IPEX syndrome caused by a deletion in a noncoding region of the FOXP3 gene. *Gastroenterology* 132, 1705–1717.

Uibo, R., Aavik, E., Peterson, P., Perheentupa, J., Aranko, S., Pelkonen, R., and Krohn, K. J. (1994a). Autoantibodies to cytochrome P450 enzymes P450scc, P450c17, and P450c21 in autoimmune polyglandular disease types I and II and in isolated Addison's disease. *J. Clin. Endocrinol. Metab.* 78, 323–328.

Uibo, R., Perheentupa, J., Ovod, V., and Krohn, K. J. (1994b). Characterization of adrenal autoantigens recognized by sera from patients with autoimmune polyglandular syndrome (APS) type I. *J. Autoimmun.* 7, 399–411.

Uibo, R. M., and Krohn, K. J. (1984). Demonstration of gastrin cell autoantibodies in antral gastritis with avidin-biotin complex antibody technique. *Clin. Exp. Immunol.* 58, 341–347.

Walder, A. I., Lunseth, J. B., and Peter, E. T. (1963). Antibodies to the gastric parietal cell. *Surg. Forum* 14, 327–328.

Ward, L., Paquette, J., Seidman, E., Huot, C., Alvarez, F., Crock, P., Delvin, E., Kämpe, O., and Deal, C. (1999). Severe autoimmune polyendocrinopathy-candidiasis-ectodermal dystrophy in an adolescent girl with a novel AIRE mutation: response to immunosuppressive therapy. *J. Clin. Endocrinol. Metab.* 84, 844–852.

Warren, J. R., and Marshall, B. J. (1984). Unidentified curved bacilli in the stomach of patients with gastritis and peptic ulceration. *Lancet* 1, 1311–1315.

Waterfield, M., and Anderson, M. S. (2011). Autoimmunity's collateral damage: Immunodeficiency hints at autoreactivity to cytokines. *Nat. Med.* 17, 1054–1055.

Winqvist, O., Gustafsson, J., Rorsman, F., Karlsson, F. A., and Kämpe, O. (1993). Two different cytochrome P450 enzymes are the adrenal antigens in autoimmune polyendocrine syndrome type I and Addison's disease. *J. Clin. Invest.* 92, 2377–2385.

Witebsky, E., Rose, N. R., Paine, J. R., and Egan, R. W. (1957). Thyroid-specific autoantibodies. *Ann. N. Y. Acad. Sci.* 69, 669–677.

Wolff, A. S., Oftedal, B. E., Kisand, K., Ersvaer, E., Lima, K., and Husebye, E. S. (2010). Flow cytometry study of blood cell subtypes reflects autoimmune and inflammatory processes in autoimmune polyendocrine syndrome type I. *Scand. J. Immunol.* 71, 459–467.

Zlotogora, J., and Shapiro, M. S. (1992). Polyglandular autoimmune syndrome type I among Iranian Jews. *J. Med. Genet.* 29, 824–826.

20

The role of natural killer cells and CD8$^+$ T cells in hepatitis B virus infection

Anita Schuch*[1,2], *Alexander Hoh*[1,2,3] *and Robert Thimme*[1]

[1] *Department of Medicine II, University Hospital of Freiburg, Freiburg, Germany*
[2] *Faculty of Biology, University of Freiburg, Freiburg, Germany*
[3] *Spemann Graduate School of Biology and Medicine, University of Freiburg, Freiburg, Germany*

Edited by:
Lynn B. Dustin, University of Oxford, UK

Reviewed by:
John J. Miles, Queensland Institute of Medical Research, Australia
Mala K. Maini, University College London, UK

****Correspondence:***
Robert Thimme, Department of Medicine II, University Hospital of Freiburg, Hugstetter Street 55, Freiburg 79106, Germany
e-mail: robert.thimme@uniklinik-freiburg.de

Hepatitis B virus (HBV) infection is one of the main causes of chronic liver diseases that may progress to liver cirrhosis and hepatocellular carcinoma. Host immune responses are important factors that determine whether HBV infection is cleared or persists. Natural killer (NK) cells represent the main effector population of the innate immune system and are abundant in the human liver. Recently, it has been demonstrated that NK cells not only exhibit antiviral functions but may also regulate adaptive immune responses by deletion of HBV-specific CD8$^+$ T cells. It is well-established that HBV-specific CD8$^+$ T cells contribute to virus elimination. However, the mechanisms contributing to CD8$^+$ T cell failure in chronic HBV infection are not well-understood. In this review, we will summarize the current knowledge about NK cells and CD8$^+$ T cells and illustrate their contribution to viral clearance and persistence in HBV infection. Moreover, novel immunological *in vitro* model systems and techniques to analyze HBV-specific CD8$^+$ T cells, which are barely detectable using current multimer staining methods, will be discussed.

Keywords: natural killer cells, CD8$^+$ T cells, hepatitis B virus, functional dichotomy, T cell failure

INTRODUCTION

Hepatitis B virus (HBV) infection represents a major health care problem that affects around 350 million people worldwide, despite the availability of a prophylactic vaccine (1). The course of infection can be either acute or chronic, while persistence rate is considerably higher when HBV is acquired at birth or early infancy. Chronically infected patients are at risk of developing HBV-related diseases such as liver cirrhosis and hepatocellular carcinoma that account for 600,000 deaths annually (1). Although potent antiviral drugs such as nucleos(t)ide analogs and pegylated interferon-α (pegIFN-α) are available, treatment is rarely curative and patients often receive life-long therapy with the potential emergence of resistance and toxicity.

Natural killer (NK) cells, as part of the innate immune system, represent the first line of defense against viral infections. In addition to their antiviral effector functions, NK cells may also interact with and thereby negatively regulate HBV-specific CD8$^+$ T cells (2). CD8$^+$ T cells are thought to be the main effector cells since their experimental depletion delays the clearance of acute HBV infection in chimpanzees (3). Of note, persistent infection is characterized by impaired HBV-specific CD8$^+$ T cell responses (4). The mechanisms responsible for this CD8$^+$ T cell failure are less understood. Interestingly, different mechanisms that may lead to impaired and dysfunctional HBV-specific CD8$^+$ T cell responses in chronically infected patients have been reported. Therefore, it is plausible that at least a part of immune-mediated liver damage is due to immune cells other than virus-specific T cells (5).

In the present review, we will focus on the role of NK cells and HBV-specific CD8$^+$ T cells, which are thought to be responsible for both virus control and disease pathogenesis.

NK CELLS

Natural killer cells represent the main effector cell population involved in innate immune responses against intracellular pathogens and abnormal cells (6). They are enriched in the liver (7) and account for one-third of the intrahepatic lymphocytes compared to 5–15% in the peripheral blood (8).

Natural killer cells do not express recombination-dependent antigen-specific receptors, therefore it is assumed that stimulation of NK cells is antigen-independent (9). However, NK cells have several traits in common with CD8$^+$ T cells (10, 11): they share a common bipotential progenitor and exert similar killing mechanisms. Additionally, a number of cell surface molecules, referred to as "NK receptors" are also expressed on activated CD8$^+$ T cells. Furthermore, murine NK cells have been described to mediate long-lived hapten-specific recall responses leading to the assumption of a NK cell memory (12).

Natural killer cell activation is regulated by the interplay of several activating and inhibitory receptors (10, 13) and cytokines such as type I IFN, interleukin (IL)-2, IL-12, IL-15, and IL-18 (14, 15). The best characterized activating receptor on the surface of NK cells is NKG2D. This receptor recognizes molecules, that are expressed at low levels on most cells but are upregulated upon infection or stress, such as MICA, MICB, and RAET1 proteins (10, 16, 17). Furthermore, NKp46 (18), NKp44 (19), and NKp30 (20) are important receptors involved in target cell recognition and killing (21). Another important NK cell stimulatory receptor is CD16, also known as the Fc receptor FcγRIII, which triggers antibody-dependent cell cytotoxicity (22). Moreover, NK cells are regulated by inhibitory receptors, which are known to mainly engage major histocompatibility complex (MHC) class I molecules expressed on the surface of target cells (23). Some of these inhibitory markers belong to a distinct family of receptors termed killer cell immunoglobulin-like receptors (KIRs), which include both activating and inhibitory molecules (22). Additionally, the CD94/NKG2A heterodimeric receptor is often used as an inhibitory marker (24).

Depending on the distribution of activating versus inhibitory signals and the prevalent cytokine milieu NK cells display at least two effector functions: they are able to produce a variety of antiviral active and immunoregulatory cytokines such as IFN-γ, tumor necrosis factor (TNF), granulocyte–macrophage colony stimulating factor (GM-CSF), and IL-10 (25, 26) and they can directly kill target cells through the release of perforin and granzymes at immunological synapses (27). Since hepatocytes are considered to be relatively resistant to cytotoxicity of NK cells via the perforin/granzyme pathway, tumor-necrosis-factor-related-apoptosis-inducing ligand (TRAIL) is likely to play a major role in hepatocellular damage (28).

Based on their expression of CD56, two NK cell subpopulations can be defined: $CD56^{dim}$ and $CD56^{bright}$. $CD56^{dim}$ NK cells represent the major circulating subset and are regarded as developmentally mature. Furthermore, this subset is thought to exert mainly cytotoxic effector functions (29), although it has been shown that $CD56^{dim}$ NK cells are also able to produce large amounts of IFN-γ during the first hours after stimulation (30). By contrast, $CD56^{bright}$ NK cells represent an earlier stage of maturation. They comprise the minority in the peripheral blood and are considered as the main cytokine producers (29, 31–33). However, viral infections may alter these proportions, leading to a relative enrichment of the $CD56^{bright}$ population (34, 35).

Next to their antiviral function, NK cells have also been shown to regulate other immune cells thereby shaping both innate and adaptive immune responses. Indeed, various studies focused on the interaction between NK cells and innate immune cells such as monocyte-derived dendritic cells, plasmacytoid dendritic cells (pDCs), and macrophages. This crosstalk can modulate NK cell functions by direct cell-to-cell contact or the activity of soluble factors (36). For example, NK cell interaction with macrophages and DCs via CD40L/CD40 drives production of IL-12, which in turn not only induces NK cells to produce IFN-γ but also enhances NK cell cytotoxicity (37–39). Additionally, NK cell function can also be improved by type I IFN abundantly secreted by pDCs (40). Furthermore, NK cells can also interact with components of the adaptive immune system and may limit $CD8^+$ T cell responses, as it has been shown in LCMV infection (41–43).

Below, we will summarize the current knowledge about of NK cells in acute and chronic HBV infection and discuss their role in regulating HBV-specific $CD8^+$ T cell immunity.

NK CELLS IN ACUTE HBV INFECTION

Viral replication usually results in the activation of an innate immune response that is characterized by the rapid production of type I IFN. These cytokines induce the expression of interferon-stimulated genes (ISGs), which in turn exert several intracellular antiviral mechanisms to limit viral spread, including the upregulation of MHC I molecules on the surface of infected cells (44). However, HBV seems not to induce any detectable intrahepatic expression of ISGs in chimpanzees during the first weeks of infection and therefore has been postulated to be a "stealth virus" that does not activate the innate immune system (45). This assumption has been challenged *in vitro* by the finding that HBV replication elicits a strong and specific innate antiviral response in HepaRG cells with an upregulation of IFN-β and other ISGs resulting in a non-cytopathic clearance of HBV DNA (46). Furthermore, a significant reduction in HBV DNA has been reported in acutely infected chimpanzees long before the peak of T cell infiltration and liver damage, suggesting a contribution of non-cytopathic antiviral mechanisms to viral clearance (47). The influx of NK cells that recognize infected cells in the absence of MHC I expression has been suggested to contribute in this setting. Moreover, the induction of IFN-γ and TNF in the liver of chimpanzees during the described non-cytopathic pre-T cell phase of viral clearance supports this hypothesis, because these effector cytokines are produced not only by $CD8^+$ T cells but also by NK cells.

Since the incubation period of acute HBV infection is predominantly asymptomatic and therefore difficult to study, only limited and partially contradicting information about the role of NK cells during the early stages of infection is available in humans. One of the leading studies was performed during the preclinical phase in two subjects with acute HBV infection characterized by persistently normal alanine aminotransferase (ALT) levels (48). NK cells were promptly activated before peak viremia occurred, as indicated by the early increase of NK cells expressing the activation markers CD69 and NKG2D. According to this, the highest number of circulating NK cells was found at an early stage in the incubation period of patients with acute HBV infection (49).

However, an impaired NK cell function in patients with acute hepatitis B has also been reported. Indeed, Dunn et al. showed that NK cell activation in acutely HBV-infected patients is significantly inhibited compared to healthy subjects, especially during the time of peak viremia (50). High viral load was also associated with a reduction of rather non-cytolytic than cytolytic NK cell effector functions. In addition, type I IFN, IFN-λ1, and IL-15, essential activators of NK cells, were barely detectable in these patients, supporting the dogma of HBV being a stealth virus. However, IL-10 levels increased early in the course of infection and the highest concentration was found at the time of peak viremia when NK cell IFN-γ production was severely reduced. This suggests a role for IL-10 in the inhibition of NK cell antiviral responses. The authors confirmed *in vitro* that addition of exogenous IL-10 to activated NK cells induces significant suppression of NK cell-derived IFN-γ, while blocking of IL-10 restored NK cell effector function (50).

However, it has also been reported that NK cells exert higher cytolytic activity and IFN-γ production during acute HBV infection. This was concomitant with the elevated expression of activating receptors such as NKp46, and lower levels of inhibitory markers, e.g., NKG2A (34). Furthermore, NK cell activation, measured by the expression of CD69, CD38, and HLA-DR, was correlated positively with ALT levels and negatively with viral load, suggesting a close association of activated NK cells with liver necroinflammation and HBV clearance in acute HBV infection. In addition to the altered phenotype, the frequency and subset distribution was also modified in patients with acute hepatitis B, showing a significant enrichment of $CD56^{bright}$ NK cells (34, 35).

The discrepancy between these different studies may arise from the fact that disease progression in the analyzed patients was either asymptomatic or symptomatic in concert with normal and elevated ALT levels, respectively. Overall, these results point to an important role of NK cells that are activated during acute HBV infection but might be functionally suppressed.

NK CELLS IN CHRONIC HBV INFECTION

Studies regarding phenotype and function of NK cells during chronic HBV infection have revealed, in part, conflicting results. Several reports conclude that NK cells exhibit selective defects in their antiviral function. This functional dichotomy features a conserved or enhanced cytolytic activity (51, 52) and a diminished cytokine production (51, 53) that may contribute to viral persistence and implicate a role for NK cells in disease pathogenesis. The mechanisms leading to this functional impairment are still not fully understood but thought to be heterogeneous.

Hepatitis B virus infection may alter the activation status and receptor expression patterns on the surface of NK cells. Indeed, the expression of inhibitory receptors such as NKG2A is elevated while activating receptors, CD16 and NKp30, are downregulated (53, 54) and this correlates with serum HBV DNA load. Interestingly, antiviral therapy partially restores NK cell phenotype and functionality (53). However, these findings are controversial, since Bonorio et al. showed decreased levels of NKG2A-expressing NK cells in chronic HBV infection (55) and it was also reported, that HBV infection does not alter NKG2A expression on NK cells (35). In addition to classical NK cell receptors other co-inhibitory molecules involved in immune responses may impair NK cell function. Of note, T cell immunoglobulin- and mucin-domain-containing molecule-3 (Tim-3) has been shown to be upregulated on NK cells during HBV infection and *in vitro* blockade was able to enhance NK cell cytotoxicity (56).

An impaired NK cell activation and function may also arise from modified expression patterns of ligands for inhibitory and activating NK cell receptors. Indeed, it has been shown that the decreased expression of NKG2D ligands, MICA/B, on HBV-infected hepatocytes inhibits NK cell lysis (57).

Furthermore, the immunosuppressive cytokine environment in chronic HBV infection, created through high levels of IL-10, may inhibit the ability of NK cells to produce IFN-γ (58), as has already been shown in acutely infected patients (50). This defect persists in patients with chronic HBV infection receiving antiviral therapy, but can be reversed *in vitro* by specific blockade of IL-10 and transforming growth factor (TGF)-β (58).

In addition, the interaction with other immune cells may alter the reactivity of NK cells during persistent viral infection. For example, several studies have revealed that HBV interferes with pDCs, thereby modulating pDC-NK cell crosstalk *in vivo* and *in vitro* (59–61). Although circulating and intrahepatic pDCs from patients with chronic HBV infection showed a more activated phenotype, their ability to respond to toll-like receptor (TLR) 9 stimulation was significantly impaired (60). Moreover, patient-derived mature pDCs were poor activators of NK cell cytotoxic function due to their impaired IFN-α secretion and reduced OX40L expression. HBV seems not only to directly inhibit pDC maturation in a TLR9-dependent manner, but also to abrogate the supporting function of monocytes regarding IFN-α production by pDCs (59).

As mentioned above, NK cells may also exert regulatory functions (41–43). This is supported by a study in patients with chronic HBV infection, where *in vitro* depletion of NK cells increased HBV- but not CMV-specific $CD8^+$ T cell responses (2). Elevated expression of TRAIL receptor 2 (TRAIL-R2) renders HBV-specific $CD8^+$ T cells more susceptible to apoptosis by TRAIL-expressing NK cells. TRAIL-R2-expression patterns correlated with HBV DNA titer, thus the regulatory role of NK cells may be relevant during HBV flares. Longitudinal analysis of chronically HBV-infected patients already revealed a temporal correlation between ALT flares and TRAIL-expressing NK cells (62).

Taken together, these findings suggest that NK cells may exert a non-classical regulatory next to their classical antiviral function in HBV infection.

$CD8^+$ T CELLS

$CD8^+$ T cells are a major component of cellular adaptive immunity. They normally mediate protection against intracellular pathogens and tumor cells. In order to be properly activated, $CD8^+$ T cells require at least two signals: first, the recognition of their cognate antigen presented by MHC I molecules on antigen-presenting cells (APCs). This is mediated by the interaction of the antigen-specific T cell receptor (TCR) with peptide-MHC I complexes. Second, additional co-stimulatory signals have to be provided by the same APC to prevent anergy. Furthermore, different cytokine milieus may influence this activation process (63). Upon antigen-recognition, naïve $CD8^+$ T cells undergo clonal expansion and differentiate into cytotoxic effector and memory T cells (64). According to their differentiation status, they are characterized by distinct expression patterns of surface markers such as CD45RA, CD27, CD28, and CCR7 (65). Similar to NK cells, the effector functions of $CD8^+$ T cells comprise several mechanisms such as the secretion of cytokines (IFN-γ and TNF), the release of cytotoxic mediators (perforin/granzyme), and receptor-mediated induction of apoptosis (e.g., through TRAIL) (63). In the following, we will elaborate the current knowledge about phenotype and function of $CD8^+$ T cells in the context of acute and chronic HBV infection.

$CD8^+$ T CELLS IN ACUTE HBV INFECTION

Hepatitis B virus-specific $CD8^+$ T cells play a major role in controlling and resolving HBV infection. Indeed, strong HBV-specific $CD8^+$ T cell responses have been shown to correlate with viral clearance during acute infection (66). The antiviral role of $CD8^+$ T cells has been further confirmed by depletion studies in experimentally infected chimpanzees, where in the absence of $CD8^+$ T cells virus titer remained at high levels (3). Importantly, the re-appearance of $CD8^+$ T cells in the circulation coincided with a decrease in viremia and the onset of liver disease. However, it has been shown that virus-specific $CD8^+$ T cells are functionally impaired during the acute phase until infection is resolved (50, 66, 67). Furthermore, the mechanisms of $CD8^+$ T cell-mediated antiviral control are still debated.

Indeed, studies in the transgenic mouse model revealed that HBV-specific $CD8^+$ T cells are able to abolish viral replication in the liver while killing only a small fraction of hepatocytes (68). This was mediated by inflammatory cytokines such as IFN-γ and TNF. The contribution of non-cytolytic effector mechanisms has been further supported by findings in a cell culture model, where virus-specific $CD8^+$ T cells were able to inhibit HBV replication in HepG2 2.2.15 cells with only minimal cell lysis (69). Of note, the authors could show that particularly IFN-γ and TNF are responsible for HBV inactivation in target cells, since blocking of these two cytokines abrogated the non-cytolytic inhibition of virus replication. Furthermore, in acutely infected chimpanzees most of HBV DNA elimination has been shown to occur before the peak of T cell infiltration and liver injury, also suggesting non-cytolytic effector mechanisms like the secretion of IFN-γ and TNF (47). Still, the contribution of cytolytic effects is supported by several studies (3, 70).

The development of cell culture models permits the investigation of the relative importance of cytolytic versus non-cytolytic effector functions and their impact on the suppression of HBV replication (71). Various cell lines transfected with the HBV genome have been established, e.g., HepG2.117 (72), HepG2.2.15 (73), or HepAD38 (74). Although the secreted virions are infectious, these cell lines are still quite artificial, since none of them is susceptible for HBV infection. Until the recent discovery of human sodium taurocholate cotransporting polypeptide (hNTCP) as HBV entry receptor (75, 76) *in vitro* infection could only be conducted in primary human hepatocytes, primary tupaia hepatocytes, and in differentiated HepaRG cells. The latter was the first hepatoma cell line being susceptible to HBV and supporting the full viral replication cycle after DMSO-dependent differentiation (77). However, cultures of differentiated HepaRG cells represent a mixture of biliary-like epithelial cells and hepatocyte-like cells and only the latter subset was shown to be susceptible for HBV infection with an infection efficacy below 20% (78). Hepatoma cell lines such as HuH7 and HepG2 cells lack hNTCP expression and are therefore non-permissive to HBV infection. Of note, infection rates with up to 70% can be achieved when HepG2 cells are transduced with hNTCP (76). These novel cell lines may be useful not only to study the molecular virology of HBV but also to improve our understanding of the relative contribution of cytolytic and non-cytolytic effector functions to viral clearance.

$CD8^+$ T CELLS IN CHRONIC HBV INFECTION

In chronically HBV-infected individuals, virus-specific $CD8^+$ T cell responses are rarely detectable (5, 79–82). The profiles of HBV-specific $CD8^+$ T cell responses depend on the stage of disease and are highly influenced by the level of HBV replication. Indeed, circulating multispecific HBV-specific $CD8^+$ T cell responses are predominantly detectable *ex vivo* in patients with low viral load. In individuals with a high level of HBV replication ($>10^7$ copies/ml) virus-specific $CD8^+$ T cells were occasionally detectable only after *in vitro* expansion (81). However, the mechanisms responsible for the lack of functional $CD8^+$ T cell responses are not completely understood. It might be that virus-specific $CD8^+$ T cells are deleted. Indeed, the elevated intracellular expression of the pro-apoptotic protein Bcl2-interacting mediator (Bim) in HBV-specific $CD8^+$ T cells of chronically infected patients supports this hypothesis (83).

Furthermore, HBV-specific $CD8^+$ T cells may not or only insufficiently be primed by APCs and consequently may not expand upon antigen-encounter. Of note, several studies suggest a dysfunction of DCs in chronically HBV-infected patients, including reduced expression of co-stimulatory molecules, impaired cytokine secretion, and lower allostimulatory capacity compared to healthy subjects (84–87). According to this, HBV-specific $CD8^+$ T cells would be expected to display a naïve phenotype, characterized by high expression levels of CD45RA, CD27, CD28, and CCR7 (65).

In addition, it is possible that they are not traceable since the frequencies of virus-specific $CD8^+$ T cell responses are below the detection limit of conventional quantitative assays, as it has been shown in chronic HCV infection (Schmidt, unpublished data). New techniques for enumerating epitope-specific T cells from human peripheral blood based on the combination of tetramer staining, magnetic-bead enrichment, and multiparametric flow cytometry (88) may address at least the latter two possibilities.

Virus-specific $CD8^+$ T cells isolated from the peripheral blood of chronically HBV-infected patients are functionally impaired and seem to have lost most of their ability to proliferate and to produce cytokines, like IFN-γ (82). The reported $CD8^+$ T cell failure has been attributed to high levels of persisting viral antigens. Despite the constant presentation of viral peptides on MHC molecules, circulating sub-viral particles, comprised of soluble HBV surface antigen (HBsAg) along with HBeAg may drive chronic T cell stimulation. Particularly, the latter has been implicated in altering the reactivity of virus-specific $CD8^+$ T cells (89). Moreover, accessory HBsAg seroconversion has been reported to induce a more potent restoration of $CD8^+$ T cell responses than HBV viral load reduction alone (90).

$CD8^+$ T cell dysfunction in chronic HBV infection follows a well-established pattern with elevated expression of inhibitory molecules such as programmed death-1 (PD-1) (82, 91), cytotoxic T lymphocyte antigen 4 (CTLA-4) (92), Tim-3 (93, 94), and 2B4 (CD244) (95) on T cells. Furthermore, the expression of corresponding ligands such as PD ligand (PD-L)1 has been shown to be increased on hepatocytes (96). According to this, highly viremic HBV-infected patients show a more severely impaired $CD8^+$ T cell phenotype and T cell dysfunction is more profound in the liver than in the blood (91, 97). Blockade of these inhibitory pathways may at least partially restore HBV-specific $CD8^+$ T cell functionality, as it has been shown *in vitro* (82, 91, 92, 94, 95). The potential relevance of blocking the PD-1 pathway was demonstrated in the HBV mouse model where HBV-transgenic mice were treated with blocking antibodies for PD-L1 prior to the adoptive transfer of HBV-specific cytotoxic T cells (98). This treatment resulted in an increased number of IFN-γ-producing $CD8^+$ T cells in the liver and in a delayed suppression of these $CD8^+$ T cells. Furthermore, a recent study could show that *in vivo* blockade of the PD-1/PD-L1 pathway, together with entecavir treatment and DNA

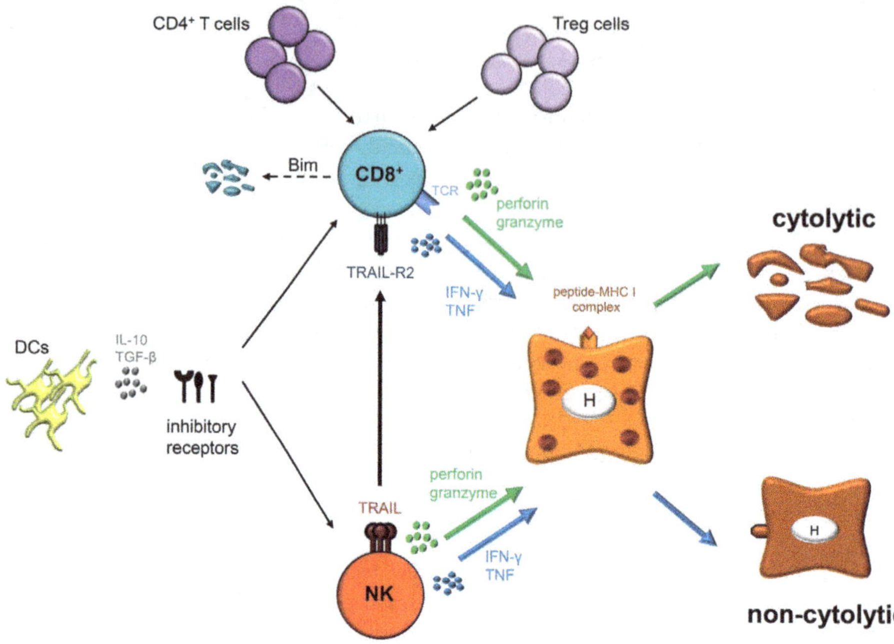

FIGURE 1 | Natural killer cells as well as HBV-specific CD8⁺ T cells exhibit their antiviral functions by cytolytic (perforin and granzyme) and/or non-cytolytic (IFN-γ and TNF) mechanisms. However, CD8⁺ T cells express antigen-specific T cell receptors (TCRs) that interact with peptide-MHC I complexes on infected hepatocytes (H) whereas NK cell activation is thought to be antigen-independent. Effector functions and phenotype of both cell types are modulated during acute and chronic HBV infection. Indeed, different mechanisms play a role in regulating both effector populations, such as DCs, immunoregulatory cytokines (IL-10 and/or TGF-β) and expression of several inhibitory receptors. Furthermore, lack of CD4⁺ T cell help and interaction with regulatory T (Treg) cells may lead to CD8⁺ T cell dysfunction in chronically HBV-infected patients resulting in Bim-mediated apoptosis. Importantly, NK cells are also able to inhibit antiviral T cell responses by deleting HBV-specific CD8⁺ T cells in a TRAIL-dependent manner.

vaccination, enhances virus-specific CD8 T cell responses in the woodchuck model, leading to sustained immunological control of viral infection (99).

The combined modulation of these inhibitory pathways along with the activation of co-stimulatory pathways might be beneficial (92, 95, 100, 101). However, a more detailed insight into the relative contribution of individual inhibitory pathways to HBV-specific CD8^{+} T cell dysfunction and concomitant the impact of inhibitory receptor blockade on restoration of CD8$_{+}$ T cell responses is necessary.

Moreover, the lack of CD4^{+} T cell help contributes to defective CD8^{+} T cell function (102). Increased regulatory T cell numbers 103–105), together with immunosuppressive cytokines such as IL-10 and TGF-β (50, 58, 106) impair virus-specific CD8$_{+}$ T cell responses. It has also been reported that increased intrahepatic arginase levels (67, 107) and hence the lack of arginine lead to a functional silencing of CD8^{+} T cells due to the downregulation of the CD3ζ-chain (108).

Collectively, these studies demonstrate that several mechanisms may contribute to the diminished frequency and function of virus-specific CD8^{+} T cells in the chronic phase of HBV infection and that combined modulation of different pathways may lead to a restoration of HBV-specific T cell responses.

CONCLUSION

CD8^{+} T cell responses play an important role in HBV infection and contribute not only to viral clearance but also to liver injury. In the setting of chronic infection, several mechanisms of T cell dysfunction including expression of inhibitory molecules and pro-apoptotic proteins, as well as suppressive cell subsets and cytokines favor viral persistence (**Figure 1**). In addition, even antivirally active NK cells, which exert a unique influence in the early defense against HBV are supposed to control CD8^{+} T cells, particularly during hepatic flares.

Cell culture models taking advantage of hepatoma cell lines that are transduced with the recently identified HBV entry receptor, hNTCP, may allow novel insights into HBV immunobiology and pathogenesis, revealing the relative contribution of cytolytic and non-cytolytic mechanisms to viral clearance. Furthermore, enrichment techniques could uncover whether HBV-specific CD8^{+} cells are actually deleted in chronically HBV-infected patients and could also elucidate the phenotype of the detectable virus-specific CD8^{+} T cells. A better understanding of the mechanisms leading to viral persistence may result in new therapeutic treatment strategies that aim to remedy the T cell defects described, thereby augmenting functional responses and decreasing antigen-unspecific liver damage.

REFERENCES

1. Honer Zu Siederdissen C, Cornberg M. The role of HBsAg levels in the current management of chronic HBV infection. *Ann Gastroenterol* (2014) **27**:105–12.
2. Peppa D, Gill US, Reynolds G, Easom NJ, Pallett LJ, Schurich A, et al. Up- regulation of a death receptor renders antiviral T cells susceptible to NK cell- mediated deletion. *J Exp Med* (2013) **210**:99–114. doi:10.1084/jem.20121172
3. Thimme R, Wieland S, Steiger C, Ghrayeb J, Reimann KA, Purcell RH, et al. CD8(+) T cells mediate viral clearance and disease pathogenesis during acute hepatitis B virus infection. *J Virol* (2003) **77**:68–76. doi:10.1128/JVI.77.1.68- 76.2003
4. Bertoletti A, Ferrari C. Innate and adaptive immune responses in chronic hepatitis B virus infections: towards restoration of immune control of viral infection. *Gut* (2012) **61**:1754–64. doi:10.1136/gutjnl-2011-301073
5. Maini MK, Boni C, Lee CK, Larrubia JR, Reignat S, Ogg GS, et al. The role of virus-specific CD8(+) cells in liver damage and viral control dur- ing persistent hepatitis B virus infection. *J Exp Med* (2000) **191**:1269–80. doi:10.1084/jem.191.8.1269
6. Doherty DG, O'Farrelly C. Innate and adaptive lymphoid cells in the human liver. *Immunol Rev* (2000) **174**:5–20. doi:10.1034/j.1600-0528.2002.017416.x
7. Gregoire C, Chasson L, Luci C, Tomasello E, Geissmann F, Vivier E, et al. The trafficking of natural killer cells. *Immunol Rev* (2007) **220**:169–82. doi:10.1111/j.1600-065X.2007.00563.x
8. Mackay IR. Hepatoimmunology: a perspective. *Immunol Cell Biol* (2002) **80**:36–44. doi:10.1046/j.1440-1711.2002.01063.x
9. Chen Y, Wei H, Gao B, Hu Z, Zheng S, Tian Z. Activation and function of hepatic NK cells in hepatitis B infection: an underinvestigated innate immune response. *J Viral Hepat* (2005) **12**:38–45. doi:10.1111/j.1365-2893.2005.00543.x
10. Lanier LL. NK cell recognition. *Annu Rev Immunol* (2005) **23**:225–74. doi:10. 1146/annurev.immunol.23.021704.115526
11. Lanier LL. Back to the future – defining NK cells and T cells. *Eur J Immunol* (2007) **37**:1424–6. doi:10.1002/eji.200737418
12. O'Leary JG, Goodarzi M, Drayton DL, Von Andrian UH. T cell- and B cell- independent adaptive immunity mediated by natural killer cells. *Nat Immunol* (2006) **7**:507–16. doi:10.1038/ni1332
13. Lanier LL. Up on the tightrope: natural killer cell activation and inhibition. *Nat Immunol* (2008) **9**:495–502. doi:10.1038/ni1581
14. Cooper MA, Fehniger TA, Caligiuri MA. The biology of human natural killer- cell subsets. *Trends Immunol* (2001) **22**:633–40. doi:10.1016/S1471-4906(01) 02060-9
15. Kimura K, Kakimi K, Wieland S, Guidotti LG, Chisari FV. Interleukin-18 inhibits hepatitis B virus replication in the livers of transgenic mice. *J Virol* (2002) **76**:10702–7. doi:10.1128/JVI.76.21.10702-10707.2002
16. Raulet DH. Roles of the NKG2D immunoreceptor and its ligands. *Nat Rev Immunol* (2003) **3**:781–90. doi:10.1038/nri1199
17. Raulet DH, Gasser S, Gowen BG, Deng W, Jung H. Regulation of ligands for the NKG2D activating receptor. *Annu Rev Immunol* (2013) **31**:413–41. doi:10.1146/annurev-immunol-032712-095951
18. Sivori S, Vitale M, Morelli L, Sanseverino L, Augugliaro R, Bottino C, et al. p46, a novel natural killer cell-specific surface molecule that mediates cell activation. *J Exp Med* (1997) **186**:1129–36. doi:10.1084/jem.186.7.1129
19. Vitale M, Bottino C, Sivori S, Sanseverino L, Castriconi R, Marcenaro E, et al. NKp44, a novel triggering surface molecule specifically expressed by acti- vated natural killer cells, is involved in non-major histocompatibility complex-restricted tumor cell lysis. *J Exp Med* (1998) **187**:2065–72. doi:10.1084/jem.187.12.2065
20. Pende D, Parolini S, Pessino A, Sivori S, Augugliaro R, Morelli L, et al. Identi- fication and molecular characterization of NKp30, a novel triggering receptor involved in natural cytotoxicity mediated by human natural killer cells. *J Exp Med* (1999) **190**:1505–16. doi:10.1084/jem.190.10.1505
21. Moretta L, Pietra G, Montaldo E, Vacca P, Pende D, Falco M, et al. Human NK cells: from surface receptors to the therapy of leukemias and solid tumors. *Front Immunol* (2014) **5**:87. doi:10.3389/fimmu.2014.00087
22. Campbell KS, Hasegawa J. Natural killer cell biology: an update and future directions. *J Allergy Clin Immunol* (2013) **132**:536–44. doi:10.1016/j.jaci.2013. 07.006
23. Moretta A, Bottino C, Vitale M, Pende D, Biassoni R, Mingari MC, et al. Recep- tors for HLA class-I molecules in human natural killer cells. *Annu Rev Immunol* (1996) **14**:619–48. doi:10.1146/annurev.immunol.14.1.619
24. Lazetic S, Chang C, Houchins JP, Lanier LL, Phillips JH. Human natural killer cell receptors involved in MHC class I recognition are disulfide-linked het- erodimers of CD94 and NKG2 subunits. *J Immunol* (1996) **157**:4741–5.
25. Biron CA, Nguyen KB, Pien GC, Cousens LP, Salazar-Mather TP. Natural killer cells in antiviral defense: function and regulation by innate cytokines. *Annu Rev Immunol* (1999) **17**:189–220. doi:10.1146/annurev. immunol.17.1.189
26. Guidotti LG, Chisari FV. Noncytolytic control of viral infections by the innate and adaptive immune response. *Annu Rev Immunol* (2001) **19**:65–91. doi:10.1146/annurev.immunol.19.1.65
27. Tang H, Li C, Wang L, Zhang H, Fan Z. Granzyme H of cytotoxic lymphocytes is required for clearance of the hepatitis B virus through cleavage of the hepatitis B virus X protein. *J Immunol* (2012) **188**:824–31. doi:10.4049/jimmunol.1102205
28. Mundt B, Kuhnel F, Zender L, Paul Y, Tillmann H, Trautwein C, et al. Involve- ment of TRAIL and its receptors in viral hepatitis. *FASEB J* (2003) **17**:94–6. doi:10.1096/fj.02-0537fje
29. Inngjerdingen M, Kveberg L, Naper C, Vaage JT. Natural killer cell subsets in man and rodents. *Tissue Antigens* (2011) **78**:81–8. doi:10.1111/j.1399-0039.2011.01714.x
30. De Maria A, Bozzano F, Cantoni C, Moretta L. Revisiting human natural killer cell subset function revealed cytolytic CD56(dim)CD16+ NK cells as rapid producers of abundant IFN-gamma on activation. *Proc Natl Acad Sci U S A* (2011) **108**:728–32. doi:10.1073/pnas.1012356108
31. Chan A, Hong DL, Atzberger A, Kollnberger S, Filer AD, Buckley CD, et al. CD56bright human NK cells differentiate into CD56dim cells: role of con- tact with peripheral fibroblasts. *J Immunol* (2007) **179**:89–94. doi:10.4049/ jimmunol.179.1.89
32. Ouyang Q, Baerlocher G, Vulto I, Lansdorp PM. Telomere length in human natural killer cell subsets. *Ann N Y Acad Sci* (2007) **1106**:240–52. doi:10.1196/ annals.1392.001
33. Romagnani C, Juelke K, Falco M, Morandi B, D'Agostino A, Costa R, et al. CD56brightCD16− killer Ig-like receptor-NK cells display longer telomeres and acquire features of CD56dim NK cells upon activation. *J Immunol* (2007) **178**:4947–55. doi:10.4049/jimmunol.178.8.4947
34. Zhao J, Li Y, Jin L, Zhang S, Fan R, Sun Y, et al. Natural killer cells are characterized by the concomitantly increased interferon-gamma and cyto- toxicity in acute resolved hepatitis B patients. *PLoS One* (2012) **7**:e49135. doi:10.1371/journal.pone.0049135
35. Lunemann S, Malone DF, Hengst J, Port K, Grabowski J, Deterding K, et al. Compromised function of natural killer cells in acute and chronic viral hepati- tis. *J Infect Dis* (2013) **209**(9):1362–73. doi:10.1093/infdis/jit561
36. Moretta A, Marcenaro E, Parolini S, Ferlazzo G, Moretta L. NK cells at the interface between innate and adaptive immunity. *Cell Death Differ* (2008) **15**:226–33. doi:10.1038/sj.cdd.4402170
37. Carbone E, Ruggiero G, Terrazzano G, Palomba C, Manzo C, Fontana S, et al. A new mechanism of NK cell cytotoxicity activation: the CD40-CD40 ligand interaction. *J Exp Med* (1997) **185**:2053–60. doi:10.1084/jem.185.12.2053
38. Nakajima A, Kodama T, Morimoto S, Azuma M, Takeda K, Oshima H, et al. Antitumor effect of CD40 ligand: elicitation of local and systemic antitumor responses by IL-12 and B7. *J Immunol* (1998) **161**:1901–7.
39. Rakhmilevich AL, Alderson KL, Sondel PM. T-cell-independent antitumor effects of CD40 ligation. *Int Rev Immunol* (2012) **31**:267–78. doi:10.3109/ 08830185.2012.698337
40. Della Chiesa M, Romagnani C, Thiel A, Moretta L, Moretta A. Multidirectional interactions are bridging human NK cells with plasmacytoid and monocyte-derived dendritic cells during innate immune responses. *Blood* (2006) **108**:3851–8. doi:10.1182/blood-2006-02-004028
41. Lang PA, Lang KS, Xu HC, Grusdat M, Parish IA, Recher M, et al. Natural killer cell activation enhances immune pathology and promotes chronic infection by limiting CD8+ T-cell immunity. *Proc Natl Acad Sci U S A* (2012) **109**:1210–5. doi:10.1073/pnas.1118834109
42. Waggoner SN, Cornberg M, Selin LK, Welsh RM. Natural killer cells act as rheostats modulating antiviral T cells. *Nature* (2012) **481**:394–8. doi:10.1038/ nature10624
43. Cook KD, Whitmire JK. The depletion of NK cells prevents T cell exhaustion to efficiently control disseminating virus infection. *J Immunol* (2013) **190**:641–9. doi:10.4049/jimmunol.1202448
44. Chisari FV, Isogawa M, Wieland SF. Pathogenesis of hepatitis B virus infection. *Pathol Biol (Paris)* (2010) **58**:258–66. doi:10.1016/j.patbio.2009.11.001
45. Wieland S, Thimme R, Purcell RH, Chisari FV. Genomic analysis of the host response to hepatitis B virus infection. *Proc Natl Acad Sci U S A* (2004) **101**:6669–74. doi:10.1073/pnas.0401771101
46. Lucifora J, Durantel D, Testoni B, Hantz O, Levrero M, Zoulim F. Control of hepatitis B virus replication by innate response of HepaRG cells. *Hepatology* (2010) **51**:63–72. doi:10.1002/hep.23230
47. Guidotti LG, Rochford R, Chung J, Shapiro M, Purcell R, Chisari FV. Viral clearance without destruction of infected cells during acute HBV infection. *Science* (1999) **284**:825–9. doi:10.1126/science.284.5415.825
48. Fisicaro P, Valdatta C, Boni C, Massari M, Mori C, Zerbini A, et al. Early

kinetics of innate and adaptive immune responses during hepatitis B virus infection. *Gut* (2009) **58**:974–82.doi:10.1136/gut.2008.163600

49. Webster GJ, Reignat S, Maini MK, Whalley SA, Ogg GS, King A, et al. Incubation phase of acute hepatitis B in man: dynamic of cellular immune mechanisms. *Hepatology* (2000) **32**:1117–24. doi:10.1053/jhep.2000.19324

50. Dunn C, Peppa D, Khanna P, Nebbia G, Jones M, Brendish N, et al. Temporal analysis of early immune responses in patients with acute hepatitis B virus infection. *Gastroenterology* (2009) **137**:1289–300. doi:10.1053/j.gastro.2009.06. 054

51. Oliviero B, Varchetta S, Paudice E, Michelone G, Zaramella M, Mavilio D, et al. Natural killer cell functional dichotomy in chronic hepatitis B and chronic hepatitis C virus infections. *Gastroenterology* (2009) **137**:1151–60. doi:10.1053/j.gastro.2009.05.047

52. Zhang Z, Zhang S, Zou Z, Shi J, Zhao J, Fan R, et al. Hypercytolytic activity of hepatic natural killer cells correlates with liver injury in chronic hepatitis B patients. *Hepatology* (2011) **53**:73–85. doi:10.1002/hep.23977

53. Tjwa ET, Van Oord GW, Hegmans JP, Janssen HL, Woltman AM. Viral load reduction improves activation and function of natural killer cells in patients with chronic hepatitis B. *J Hepatol* (2011) **54**:209–18. doi:10.1016/j.jhep.2010. 07.009

54. Nattermann J, Feldmann G, Ahlenstiel G, Langhans B, Sauerbruch T, Spengler U. Surface expression and cytolytic function of natural killer cell receptors is altered in chronic hepatitis C. *Gut* (2006) **55**:869–77. doi:10.1136/gut.2005. 076463

55. Bonorino P, Ramzan M, Camous X, Dufeu-Duchesne T, Thelu MA, Sturm N, et al. Fine characterization of intrahepatic NK cells expressing natural killer receptors in chronic hepatitis B and C. *J Hepatol* (2009) **51**:458–67. doi:10.1016/j.jhep.2009.05.030

56. Ju Y, Hou N, Meng J, Wang X, Zhang X, Zhao D, et al. T cell immunoglobulin- and mucin-domain-containing molecule-3 (Tim-3) mediates natural killer cell suppression in chronic hepatitis B. *J Hepatol* (2010) **52**:322–9. doi:10.1016/j. jhep.2009.12.005

57. Tang KF, Chen M, Xie J, Song GB, Shi YS, Liu Q, et al. Inhibition of hepatitis B virus replication by small interference RNA induces expression of MICA in HepG2.2.15 cells. *Med Microbiol Immunol* (2009) **198**:27–32. doi:10.1007/s00430-008-0101-6

58. Peppa D, Micco L, Javaid A, Kennedy PT, Schurich A, Dunn C, et al. Blockade of immunosuppressive cytokines restores NK cell antiviral function in chronic hepatitis B virus infection. *PLoS Pathog* (2010) **6**:e1001227. doi:10. 1371/journal.ppat.1001227

59. Woltman AM, Op Den Brouw ML, Biesta PJ, Shi CC, Janssen HL. Hepatitis B virus lacks immune activating capacity, but actively inhibits plasmacytoid dendritic cell function. *PLoS One* (2011) **6**:e15324. doi:10.1371/journal.pone. 0015324

60. Martinet J, Dufeu-Duchesne T, Bruder Costa J, Larrat S, Marlu A, Leroy V, et al. Altered functions of plasmacytoid dendritic cells and reduced cytolytic activity of natural killer cells in patients with chronic HBV infection. *Gastroenterology* (2012) **143**:1586–1596e1588. doi:10.1053/j.gastro.2012.08.046

61. Shi CC, Tjwa ET, Biesta PJ, Boonstra A, Xie Q, Janssen HL, et al. Hepatitis B virus suppresses the functional interaction between natural killer cells and plasmacytoid dendritic cells. *J Viral Hepat* (2012) **19**:e26–33. doi:10.1111/j. 1365-2893.2011.01496.x

62. Dunn C, Brunetto M, Reynolds G, Christophides T, Kennedy PT, Lampertico P, et al. Cytokines induced during chronic hepatitis B virus infection promote a pathway for NK cell-mediated liver damage. *J Exp Med* (2007) **204**:667–80. doi:10.1084/jem.20061287

63. Zhang N, Bevan MJ. CD8(+) T cells: foot soldiers of the immune system. *Immunity* (2011) **35**:161–8. doi:10.1016/j.immuni.2011.07.010

64. Youngblood B, Hale JS, Ahmed R. T-cell memory differentiation: insights from transcriptional signatures and epigenetics. *Immunology* (2013) **139**:277–84. doi:10.1111/imm.12074

65. Appay V, Van Lier RA, Sallusto F, Roederer M. Phenotype and function of human T lymphocyte subsets: consensus and issues. *Cytometry A* (2008) **73**:975–83. doi:10.1002/cyto.a.20643

66. Maini MK, Boni C, Ogg GS, King AS, Reignat S, Lee CK, et al. Direct ex vivo analysis of hepatitis B virus-specific CD8(+) T cells associated with the control of infection. *Gastroenterology* (1999) **117**:1386–96. doi:10.1016/S0016- 5085(99)70289-1

67. Sandalova E, Laccabue D, Boni C, Watanabe T, Tan A, Zong HZ, et al. Increased levels of arginase in patients with acute hepatitis B suppress antivi- ral T cells. *Gastroenterology* (2012) **143**:78–87e73. doi:10.1053/j.gastro.2012. 03.041

68. Guidotti LG, Ishikawa T, Hobbs MV, Matzke B, Schreiber R, Chisari FV. Intracel- lular inactivation of the hepatitis B virus by cytotoxic T lymphocytes. *Immunity* (1996) **4**:25–36. doi:10.1016/S1074-7613(00)80295-2

69. Phillips S, Chokshi S, Riva A, Evans A, Williams R, Naoumov NV. CD8(+) T cell control of hepatitis B virus replication: direct comparison between cytolytic and noncytolytic functions. *J Immunol* (2010) **184**:287–95. doi:10. 4049/jimmunol.0902761

70. Ando K, Guidotti LG, Wirth S, Ishikawa T, Missale G, Moriyama T, et al. Class I-restricted cytotoxic T lymphocytes are directly cytopathic for their target cells in vivo. *J Immunol* (1994) **152**:3245–53.

71. Dandri M, Lutgehetmann M, Petersen J. Experimental models and therapeu- tic approaches for HBV. *Semin Immunopathol* (2013) **35**:7–21. doi:10.1007/ s00281-012-0335-7

72. Sun D, Nassal M. Stable HepG2- and Huh7-based human hepatoma cell lines for efficient regulated expression of infectious hepatitis B virus. *J Hepatol* (2006) **45**:636–45. doi:10.1016/j.jhep.2006.05.019

73. Sells MA, Chen ML, Acs G. Production of hepatitis B virus particles in Hep G2 cells transfected with cloned hepatitis B virus DNA. *Proc Natl Acad Sci U S A* (1987) **84**:1005–9. doi:10.1073/pnas.84.4.1005

74. Ladner SK, Otto MJ, Barker CS, Zaifert K, Wang GH, Guo JT, et al. Inducible expression of human hepatitis B virus (HBV) in stably transfected hepatoblas- toma cells: a novel system for screening potential inhibitors of HBV replication. *Antimicrob Agents Chemother* (1997) **41**:1715–20.

75. Yan H, Zhong G, Xu G, He W, Jing Z, Gao Z, et al. Sodium taurocholate cotrans- porting polypeptide is a functional receptor for human hepatitis B and D virus. *Elife* (2012) **1**:e00049. doi:10.7554/eLife.00049

76. Ni Y, Lempp FA, Mehrle S, Nkongolo S, Kaufman C, Falth M, et al. Hepati- tis B and D viruses exploit sodium taurocholate co-transporting polypep- tide for species-specific entry into hepatocytes. *Gastroenterology* (2014) **146**:1070–1083e1076. doi:10.1053/j.gastro.2013.12.024

77. Gripon P, Rumin S, Urban S, Le Seyec J, Glaise D, Cannie I, et al. Infection of a human hepatoma cell line by hepatitis B virus. *Proc Natl Acad Sci U S A* (2002) **99**:15655–60. doi:10.1073/pnas.232137699

78. Hantz O, Parent R, Durantel D, Gripon P, Guguen-Guillouzo C, Zoulim F. Persistence of the hepatitis B virus covalently closed circular DNA in HepaRG human hepatocyte-like cells. *J Gen Virol* (2009) **90**:127–35. doi:10.1099/vir.0. 004861-0

79. Ferrari C, Penna A, Bertoletti A, Valli A, Antoni AD, Giuberti T, et al. Cellular immune response to hepatitis B virus-encoded antigens in acute and chronic hepatitis B virus infection. *J Immunol* (1990) **145**:3442–9.

80. Bertoletti A, Costanzo A, Chisari FV, Levrero M, Artini M, Sette A, et al. Cyto- toxic T lymphocyte response to a wild type hepatitis B virus epitope in patients chronically infected by variant viruses carrying substitutions within the epi- tope. *J Exp Med* (1994) **180**:933–43. doi:10.1084/jem.180.3.933

81. Webster GJ, Reignat S, Brown D, Ogg GS, Jones L, Seneviratne SL, et al. Lon- gitudinal analysis of CD8+ T cells specific for structural and nonstructural hepatitis B virus proteins in patients with chronic hepatitis B: implications for immunotherapy. *J Virol* (2004) **78**:5707–19. doi:10.1128/JVI.78.11.5707-5719. 2004

82. Boni C, Fisicaro P, Valdatta C, Amadei B, Di Vincenzo P, Giuberti T, et al. Char- acterization of hepatitis B virus (HBV)-specific T-cell dysfunction in chronic HBV infection. *J Virol* (2007) **81**:4215–25.doi:10.1128/JVI.02844-06

83. Lopes AR, Kellam P, Das A, Dunn C, Kwan A, Turner J, et al. Bim-mediated deletion of antigen-specific CD8 T cells in patients unable to control HBV infection. *J Clin Invest* (2008) **118**:1835–45.doi:10.1172/JCI33402

84. Wang FS, Xing LH, Liu MX, Zhu CL, Liu HG, Wang HF, et al. Dysfunction of peripheral blood dendritic cells from patients with chronic hepatitis B virus infection. *World J Gastroenterol* (2001) **7**:537–41.

85. Beckebaum S, Cicinnati VR, Dworacki G, Muller-Berghaus J, Stolz D, Harnaha J, et al. Reduction in the circulating pDC1/pDC2 ratio and impaired function of ex vivo-generated DC1 in chronic hepatitis B infection. *Clin Immunol* (2002) **104**:138–50. doi:10.1006/clim.2002.5245

86. van der Molen RG, Sprengers D, Binda RS, De Jong EC, Niesters HG, Kusters JG, et al. Functional impairment of myeloid and plasmacytoid den- dritic cells of patients with chronic hepatitis B. *Hepatology* (2004) **40**:738–46. doi:10.1002/hep.20366

87. Duan XZ, Zhuang H, Wang M, Li HW, Liu JC, Wang FS. Decreased numbers and impaired function of circulating dendritic cell subsets in patients with chronic hepatitis B infection (R2). *J Gastroenterol Hepatol* (2005) **20**:234–42. doi:10.1111/j.1440-1746.2004.03529.x

88. Alanio C, Lemaitre F, Law HK, Hasan M, Albert ML. Enumeration of human antigen-specific naive CD8+ T cells reveals conserved precursor frequencies. *Blood* (2010) **115**:3718–25. doi:10.1182/blood-2009-10-251124

89. Reignat S, Webster GJ, Brown D, Ogg GS, King A, Seneviratne SL, et al. Escaping high viral load exhaustion: CD8 cells with altered tetramer bind- ing in chronic hepatitis B virus infection. *J Exp Med* (2002) **195**:1089–101. doi:10.1084/jem.20011723

90. Boni C, Laccabue D, Lampertico P, Giuberti T, Vigano M, Schivazappa S, et al. Restored function of HBV-specific T cells after long-term effective therapy with nucleos(t)ide analogues. *Gastroenterology* (2012) **143**:963–73. doi:10.1053/j.gastro.2012.07.014

91. Fisicaro P, Valdatta C, Massari M, Loggi E, Biasini E, Sacchelli L, et al. Antivi- ral intrahepatic T-cell responses can be restored by blocking programmed death-1 pathway in chronic hepatitis B. *Gastroenterology* (2010) **138**:682–93. doi:10.1053/j.gastro.2009.09.052
92. Schurich A, Khanna P, Lopes AR, Han KJ, Peppa D, Micco L, et al. Role of the coinhibitory receptor cytotoxic T lymphocyte antigen-4 on apoptosis- prone CD8 T cells in persistent hepatitis B virus infection. *Hepatology* (2011) **53**:1494–503. doi:10.1002/hep.24249
93. Nebbia G, Peppa D, Schurich A, Khanna P, Singh HD, Cheng Y, et al. Upregula- tion of the Tim-3/ galectin-9 pathway of T cell exhaustion in chronic hepatitis B virus infection. *PLoS One* (2012) **7**:e47648. doi:10.1371/journal.pone.0047648
94. Wu W, Shi Y, Li S, Zhang Y, Liu Y, Wu Y, et al. Blockade of Tim-3 signaling restores the virus-specific CD8(+) T-cell response in patients with chronic hepatitis B. *Eur J Immunol* (2012) **42**:1180–91. doi:10.1002/eji.201141852
95. Raziorrouh B, Schraut W, Gerlach T, Nowack D, Gruner NH, Ulsenheimer A, et al. The immunoregulatory role of CD244 in chronic hepatitis B infection and its inhibitory potential on virus-specific CD8+ T-cell function. *Hepatology* (2010) **52**:1934–47. doi:10.1002/hep.23936
96. Muhlbauer M, Fleck M, Schutz C, Weiss T, Froh M, Blank C, et al. PD- L1 is induced in hepatocytes by viral infection and by interferon-alpha and -gamma and mediates T cell apoptosis. *J Hepatol* (2006) **45**:520–8. doi:10.1016/j.jhep.2006.05.007
97. Knolle PA, Thimme R. Hepatic immune regulation and its involvement in viral hepatitis infection. *Gastroenterology* (2014) **146**(5):1193–207. doi:10.1053/j.gastro.2013.12.036
98. Maier H, Isogawa M, Freeman GJ, Chisari FV. PD-1:PD-L1 interactions con- tribute to the functional suppression of virus-specific CD8+ T lymphocytes in the liver. *J Immunol* (2007) **178**:2714–20. doi:10.4049/jimmunol.178.5.2714
99. Liu J, Zhang E, Ma Z, Wu W, Kosinska A, Zhang X, et al. Enhancing virus- specific immunity in vivo by combining therapeutic vaccination and PD-L1 blockade in chronic hepadnaviral infection. *PLoS Pathog* (2014) **10**:e1003856. doi:10.1371/journal.ppat.1003856
100. Fisicaro P, Valdatta C, Massari M, Loggi E, Ravanetti L, Urbani S, et al. Com- bined blockade of programmed death-1 and activation of CD137 increase responses of human liver T cells against HBV, but not HCV. *Gastroenterology* (2012) **143**:1576–1585e1574. doi:10.1053/j.gastro.2012.08.041
101. Schurich A, Pallett LJ, Lubowiecki M, Singh HD, Gill US, Kennedy PT, et al. The third signal cytokine IL-12 rescues the anti-viral function of exhausted HBV- specific CD8 T cells. *PLoS Pathog* (2013) **9**:e1003208. doi:10.1371/journal.ppat. 1003208
102. Yang PL, Althage A, Chung J, Maier H, Wieland S, Isogawa M, et al. Immune effectors required for hepatitis B virus clearance. *Proc Natl Acad Sci U S A* (2010) **107**:798–802. doi:10.1073/pnas.0913498107
103. Stoop JN, van der Molen RG, Baan CC, van der Laan LJ, Kuipers EJ, Kusters JG, et al. Regulatory T cells contribute to the impaired immune response in patients with chronic hepatitis B virus infection. *Hepatology* (2005) **41**:771–8. doi:10.1002/hep.20649
104. Xu D, Fu J, Jin L, Zhang H, Zhou C, Zou Z, et al. Circulating and liver resi- dent CD4+CD25+ regulatory T cells actively influence the antiviral immune response and disease progression in patients with hepatitis B. *J Immunol* (2006) **177**:739–47. doi:10.4049/jimmunol.177.1.739
105. Yang G, Liu A, Xie Q, Guo TB, Wan B, Zhou B, et al. Association of CD4+CD25+Foxp3+ regulatory T cells with chronic activity and viral clear- ance in patients with hepatitis B. *Int Immunol* (2007) **19**:133–40. doi:10.1093/ intimm/dxl130
106. Das A, Ellis G, Pallant C, Lopes AR, Khanna P, Peppa D, et al. IL-10-producing regulatory B cells in the pathogenesis of chronic hepatitis B virus infection. *J Immunol* (2012) **189**:3925–35. doi:10.4049/jimmunol.1103139
107. Chisari FV. Regulation of human lymphocyte function by a soluble extract from normal human liver. *J Immunol* (1978) **121**:1279–86.
108. Das A, Hoare M, Davies N, Lopes AR, Dunn C, Kennedy PT, et al. Functional skewing of the global CD8 T cell population in chronic hepatitis B virus infec- tion. *J Exp Med* (2008) **205**:2111–24. doi:10.1084/jem.20072076

21

All PI3Kinase signaling is not mTOR: dissecting mTOR-dependent and independent signaling pathways in T cells

Christopher J. Gamper and Jonathan D. Powell*

Department of Oncology, Johns Hopkins University, Baltimore, MD, USA

Edited by:
Klaus Okkenhaug, Babraham Institute, UK

Reviewed by:
David A. Fruman, University of California, Irvine, USA
David K. Finlay, Trinity College Dublin, Ireland

****Correspondence:***
Jonathan D. Powell, Department of Oncology, Johns Hopkins University, 1650 Orleans St., CRB I, Rm. 443, Baltimore, MD 21212, USA.
e-mail: poweljo@jhmi.edu

The mechanistic target of rapamycin (mTOR) is emerging as playing a central role in regulating T cell activation, differentiation, and function. mTOR integrates diverse signals from the immune microenvironment to shape the outcome of T cell receptor (TCR) antigen recognition. Phosphatidylinositol 3-kinase (PI3K) enzymes are critical mediators of T cell activation through their generation of the second messenger phosphatidylinositol (3,4,5) triphosphate (PIP3). Indeed, PIP3 generation results in the activation of Protein Kinase B (PKB, also known as AKT), a key activator of mTOR. However, recent genetic studies have demonstrated inconsistencies between PI3K disruption and loss of mTOR expression with regard to the regulation of effector and regulatory T cell homeostasis and function. In this review, we focus on how PI3K activation directs mature CD4 T cell activation and effector function by pathways dependent on and independent of mTOR signaling. Importantly, what has become clear is that targeting both mTOR-dependent and mTOR-independent PI3K-induced signaling distally affords the opportunity for more selective regulation of T cell differentiation and function.

Keywords: mTOR pathway, PI3K, CD4 T cells, effector function, tolerance

INTRODUCTION

The Class IA phosphatidylinositol 3-kinase (PI3K) family consists of a heterodimeric complex of one of the 110-kDa catalytic subunits (p110α, β, δ) with a regulatory subunit (p85α, p55α, p50α, p85β, and p55γ), reviewed in Kane and Weiss (2003); Okkenhaug and Vanhaesebroeck (2003). Catalytic subunits are each encoded by separate genes, while the *pik3r1* gene generates p85α, p55α, and p50α from alternative promoters and the *pik3r2* and *pik3r3* genes encode p85β and p55γ, respectively. Details of receptor interactions with PI3Ks have recently been reviewed elsewhere (Okkenhaug and Fruman, 2010). Co-localization of catalytic subunits with regulatory subunits permits juxtaposition of catalytic subunits to the cell membrane in response to receptor ligation, increasing the local synthesis of phosphatidylinositol (3,4,5) triphosphate (PIP3). The p110α and β subunits are ubiquitously expressed while p110δ expression is restricted to hematopoietic cells. The Class IB PI3 Kinase family consists of a complex of the p110γ catalytic subunit and either the p101 or p84 regulatory subunits. This complex interacts with G-protein coupled receptors including chemokine receptors via binding to Gβ and γ regulatory proteins. Like p110δ, p110γ expression is restricted to hematopoietic cells. Accumulation of the PIP3 signaling intermediate is opposed by phosphatase and tensin homolog (PTEN) that converts PIP3 back to phosphatidylinositol (4,5) bisphosphate and Src homology 2 domain-containing inositol phosphatase (SHIP)1 and SHIP2 that hydrolyze PIP3 to phosphatidylinositol (3,4) bisphosphate (Okkenhaug and Fruman, 2010).

PIP3 acts as a second messenger to mediate downstream signaling by recruitment of pleckstrin homology (PH) domain containing proteins that bind to the high local concentrations of PIP3 generated by PI3Ks at the inner leaflet of the plasma membrane. Examples include the Tec family of tyrosine kinases that mediate signals to phospholipase C-γ (PLCγ), the 3-phosphoinositide-dependent protein kinase 1 (PDK1), and Protein Kinase B (PKB), also known as AKT [reviewed in Kane and Weiss (2003 Members of the Vav family of guanine nucleotide exchange factors that regulate cellular motility may also be recruited via PIP3 binding, although some data suggest recruitment may be indirect via other protein interactions. AKT binding to PIP3 induces a conformational change that renders it accessible to phosphorylation at residue T308 by PDK1 co-localized at the plasma membrane, resulting in activation of AKT serine/threonine kinase activity (Stokoe et al., 1997; Currie et al., 1999; Milburn et al., 2003 One critical substrate for activated AKT is tuberous sclerosis complex (TSC)-2. TSC2 functions with TSC1 as a GTPase activating complex for Ras homolog enriched in brain (Rheb). TSC2 is inactivated by phosphorylation, resulting in accumulation of GTP-bound Rheb that activates the mechanistic target of rapamycin (mTOR) that is in a complex with regulatory-associated protein of mTOR (Raptor) termed mTORC1. Activated mTORC1 phosphorylates and inhibits the eukaryotic initiation factor 4E-binding proteins (4E-BP1, 2, 3) and activates the p70 ribosomal S6 kinases (S6K1, 2), resulting in increased protein translation and upregulation of glycolysis, promoting cell growth and division [reviewed in Laplante and Sabatini (2012)]. In addition, mTORC1 activation is required for several key elements of T cell effector differentiation that are discussed in further detail below.

A second mTOR complex containing the rapamycin insensitive companion of TOR (Rictor) and the mammalian homolog of the yeast *SIN1* gene (mSIN1), termed mTORC2, is also critical to mediating PI3K signaling via AKT. Although the precise mechanisms underlying activation of mTORC2 remain incompletely understood, it was recently observed that physical association with ribosomes stimulates mTORC2 activity (Zinzalla et al., 2011) and that Rictor acetylation by p300 stimulates mTORC2 activity (Glidden et al., 2012). mTORC2 is strongly activated in T cells by costimulation and cytokines [reviewed in Cantrell (2002)]. mTORC2 has several substrates including serum- and glucocorticoid-induced protein kinase 1 (SGK1), protein kinase C-α (PKC-α), and importantly, AKT itself. Phosphorylation at residue S473 in the AKT hydrophobic motif modifies substrate specificity of AKT and enhances its kinase activity (Sarbassov et al., 2005; Facchinetti et al., 2008; Garcia-Martinez and Alessi, 2008). In particular, S473 phosphorylation is required to permit AKT to phosphorylate members of the Forkhead box family of transcription factors Foxo1 and Foxo3a (Jacinto et al., 2006). Foxo phosphorylation leads to the cytoplasmic retention of these transcription factors with resulting downregulation of target gene expression (Brownawell et al., 2001). In T cells, a key Foxo target is KLF2 that regulates expression of CD62L, the c–c chemokine receptor 7 (CCR7), and the sphingosine-1-phosphate receptor (S1P1R) which each control homing of lymphocytes into and out of secondary lymphoid tissues [reviewed in Finlay and Cantrell (2010)].

The signaling cascade from receptors through PI3K to mTOR described above appears to imply a linear relationship, and older studies utilizing small molecule inhibitors of either PI3Ks such as wortmannin or LY294002 or mTOR using rapamycin demonstrated similar profound inhibition of T cell function *in vitro* (Kay et al., 1991; Ward et al., 1995). However, recent analysis of the pathways using more specific inhibitors and genetic manipulation has identified a more complex signaling cascade with both overlapping and unique functions. Phenotypes of mice discussed in this review with targeted disruption of components of the PI3K or mTOR pathways are summarized in **Table 1** below.

INTERRUPTION OF THE PI3K/AKT/mTOR PATHWAY AT DIFFERENT LEVELS HAS DIFFERENTIAL EFFECTS ON T CELL ACTIVATION

A critical aspect to TCR signaling is its ability to activate PLCγ and generate the second messenger inositol triphosphate (IP3) that triggers Ca^{++} entry following activation. This Ca^{++} binds calmodulin and activates calcineurin, which dephosphorylates NF-AT transcription factors that translocate to the nucleus to activate transcription of genes that regulate both T cell activation/effector function and tolerance (Macian et al., 2002). Cyclosporine acts as a potent immunosuppressant by binding to cyclophilin and blocking activation of calcineurin and thus NF-AT. Rapamycin inhibits T cell activation by a different mechanism, by binding to FKBP12 and preventing association of Raptor and mTOR to form the mTORC1 complex. The importance of this difference is highlighted by the fact that activation of Th1 cells in the presence of rapamycin renders them subsequently anergic and incapable of proliferation and IL-2 secretion upon secondary stimulation after rapamycin is washed away, in a manner similar to Th1 cells stimulated through the T cell receptor (Signal 1) in the absence of costimulation via CD28 (Signal 2) (Powell et al., 1999). This occurs despite the fact that while rapamycin acutely inhibits T cell proliferation, it does not block initial IL-2 secretion. Cyclosporine, in contrast, blocks both proliferation and IL-2 secretion acutely but does not impair secondary stimulation after drug is removed. Rapamycin appears to promote anergy and tolerance by permitting normal TCR-mediated activation of *NF-AT* gene targets including the transcription factors Egr-2 and Egr-3 and their targets such as Cbl-b, DGKα, and Fas-L that limit T cell activation and promote apoptosis (Sanjuan et al., 2001; Macian et al., 2002; Safford et al., 2005; Zha et al., 2006). As these signaling pathways would predict, co-incubation of T cells with cyclosporine and rapamycin blocks rapamycin-induced anergy (Powell et al., 1999). That is, blocking proximal TCR-mediated signaling with cyclosporine mitigates the effects of blocking mTOR with rapamycin. We emphasize the consequences of blocking proximal signaling with cyclosporine and more distal signaling with rapamycin because a parallel can be drawn comparing genetic blockade of mTOR that promotes generation of regulatory T cells (Treg) and genetic blockade of proximal PI3K signaling that results in decreased Treg function *in vivo* (to be discussed in depth below).

The generation of mice with T cell conditional deletion of mTOR using a floxed allele crossed with a CD4-Cre transgenic mouse confirms the specificity of rapamycin for blocking mTOR-mediated signaling (Delgoffe et al., 2009). Stimulation of mTOR deficient T cells with anti CD3/CD28 induces robust, even slightly increased, proximal AKT T308 phosphorylation but it is unable to elicit S6K1 and AKT S473 phosphorylation. Like rapamycin treated T cells, mTOR deficient T cells show normal IL-2 secretion during primary stimulation but reduced proliferation. However, the consequence of activation of naïve T cells lacking mTOR is the inhibition of effector differentiation and the generation of Tregs.

Since PI3K is upstream of mTOR, the effect of a PI3K inhibitor would be predicted to mimic rapamycin. In fact, stimulation of T cells in the presence of wortmannin does acutely block proliferation, but IL-2 secretion is also inhibited, similar to cyclosporine (Ward et al., 1995). Despite this difference, the presence of wortmannin during T cell priming does result in anergy upon restimulation similar in magnitude to that achieved by costimulatory blockade with CTLA4-Ig which blocks B7/CD28 interactions (Taub et al., 1997). Importantly, subsequent work has demonstrated that wortmannin is not selective for PI3K as originally thought, but it can inhibit mTOR as well (Brunn et al., 1996), therefore it is not clear if the findings reported by Taub et al. merely mimic the effect of rapamycin-induced mTOR blockade. Clarification of distinctions between PI3K and mTOR-dependent signals has subsequently been provided by genetic analysis.

Initial work deleting individual PI3K regulatory subunits demonstrated significant functional redundancy in T cells, with no overt defects in T cell development and signaling after disruption of p85α and paradoxically enhanced TCR and IL-2-induced proliferation in p85β knockouts (Fruman et al., 1999; Suzuki

Table 1 | T cell phenotype and function in PI3K and mTOR pathway gene-targeted mice.

Gene	Phenotype	References
pik3r1 (p85$\alpha^{-/-}$, p55$\alpha^{-/-}$, p50$\alpha^{-/-}$)	Normal T cell development and proliferation	Fruman et al., 1999
pik3r1 (p85$\alpha^{-/-}$)	Normal T cell development and proliferation	Suzuki et al., 1999
pik3r2 (p85$\beta^{-/-}$)	Normal T cell development Enhanced proliferation to TCR stimulation or TCR + IL-2	Deane et al., 2004
r1ΔT/r2n (p85$\alpha^{-/-}$, p55$\alpha^{-/-}$, p50$\alpha^{-/-}$, p85$\beta^{-/-}$)	Normal T cell development Normal Th1 but reduced Th2 differentiation Impaired T-dependent antibody response Reduced Treg numbers, spontaneous autoimmunity	Oak et al., 2006 Deane et al., 2007
pik3cd (p110$\delta^{-/-}$, CD4-Cre;p110$\delta^{flox/flox}$, or OX40-Cre;p110$\delta^{flox/flox}$)	Normal T cell development and proliferation Impaired T-dependent antibody response	Clayton et al., 2002 Rolf et al., 2010
pik3cd (p110$\delta^{D910A/D910A}$)	Decreased peripheral T cell numbers CD3/CD28-induced proliferation and IL-2 normal Antigen-induced proliferation and IL-2 reduced Impaired Th1 and Th2 differentiation *in vitro* Reduced Th1 contact hypersensitivity Inappropriate Th1 differentiation to Th2 stimulus *in vivo* Reduced Th17 differentiation with attenuated EAE Reduced IL-10 production Impaired Treg function with autoimmune colitis Impaired T-dependent antibody response	Okkenhaug et al., 2002 Okkenhaug et al., 2006 Patton et al., 2006 Nashed et al., 2007 Liu et al., 2009 Rolf et al., 2010 Soond et al., 2010 Haylock-Jacobs et al., 2011
pik3cg (p110$\gamma^{-/-}$)	Normal T cell development Variably decreased or normal proliferation Variably decreased or normal cytokine production Abnormal trafficking to sites of inflammation Impaired trafficking to chemokines	Sasaki et al., 2000 Alcazar et al., 2007 Garcon et al., 2008 Martin et al., 2008 Thomas et al., 2008
pten (Lck-Cre;PTEN$^{flox/-}$ or OX40-Cre;PTEN$^{flox/flox}$)	Lymphoproliferative disorder (Lck-Cre) Enhanced T cell proliferation and cytokine production Spontaneous autoimmunity (Lck-Cre) Enhanced T cell help (OX40-Cre) Enhanced tumor rejection (OX40-Cre)	Suzuki et al., 2001 Soond et al., 2012
frap1 (CD4-Cre;mTOR$^{flox/flox}$)	Normal T cell development Reduced proliferation Normal initial IL-2 secretion Impaired Th1, Th2, and Th17 differentiation Spontaneous iTreg differentiation	Delgoffe et al., 2009
rheb (CD4-cre;rheb$^{flox/flox}$)	Normal T cell development Impaired Th1 and Th17 differentiation Normal Th2 and iTreg differentiation	Delgoffe et al., 2011
raptor (Lck-Cre;raptor$^{flox/flox}$)	Reduced peripheral T cell numbers Impaired Th17 differentiation	Kurebayashi et al., 2012
rictor (CD4-Cre;rictor$^{flox/flox}$ or proximal Lck-Cre;rictor$^{flox/flox}$)	Normal T cell development Variably decreased Th1 and Th17 differentiation Impaired Th2 differentiation Normal iTreg differentiation Impaired T-dependent antibody response	Lee et al., 2010 Delgoffe et al., 2011

et al., 1999; Deane et al., 2004); therefore the p85α and p85β knockouts were crossed to disrupt all Class IA PI3K activity. This was accomplished by crossing *pik3r1*$^{2loxP/2loxP}$ mice with *pik3r2*$^{-/-}$ mice and breeding these onto an Lck-Cre background to cause T cell specific deletion of both regulatory subunits (Deane et al., 2007). Resulting mice, termed r1ΔT/r2n, have normal generation of T cells, but such cells have profound decreases in expression of multiple PI3K catalytic subunits with greatly reduced p110β and undetectable p110α and p110δ. Such T cells demonstrate expected loss of CD3/CD28-induced AKT S473 phosphorylation. This may be due to impaired mTORC2 signaling but it is important to comment that recruitment of AKT to the cell membrane to be phosphorylated by PDK1 at T308 is predicted to be interrupted as well. Since T308 phosphorylation was not directly measured, it cannot formally be determined whether the loss of AKT S473 phosphorylation represents a lack of singly phosphorylated AKT substrate for mTORC2 or is a consequence of reduced mTORC2 activity. Also, phosphorylation of other mTORC2 substrates such as SGK1 and PKCα was not reported in this study. Similar data on AKT S473 phosphorylation in isolation without other measures of mTORC2 activity has been extensively reported in other systems described in this review. Thus, interpretation of relative levels of mTORC2 activity in some of these systems remains speculative but is helpful to consider when comparing phenotypes with systems where mTORC2 is selectively disrupted. Deane et al. unexpectedly provide evidence for preservation of some CD3/CD28-induced phosphorylation of ribosomal S6 at S235/236. While some data have suggested that this particular S6 phosphorylation site may be more dependent on RSK activity than mTOR activity upstream of S6K (Salmond et al., 2009), Deane et al. demonstrate that this S6 phosphorylation in r1ΔT/r2n T cells is blocked by rapamycin, supporting that in r1ΔT/r2n T cells some mTORC1 activity is preserved. TCR-induced calcium flux was modestly reduced in r1ΔT/r2n T cells and TCR-induced NF-κB activation as measured by IκB phosphorylation was significantly reduced, consistent with reduced activation of the Tec kinase/PLCγ pathway due to inefficient PIP3 generation. However, IκB phosphorylation could be normalized with CD28 costimulation. This partial preservation of CD3/CD28-induced signals including some mTOR activation may explain why proliferation is only slightly reduced while IL-2 and IFN-γ are more profoundly suppressed, which would not be predicted by the PI3K and rapamycin inhibitor studies described above and differs from the phenotype following T cell specific deletion of mTOR.

Since disruption of the regulatory subunits indirectly affects expression of multiple PI3K catalytic subunits, targeted deletion of individual catalytic subunits has been used to dissect how each one contributes to T cell activation with the rationale that a selective inhibitor of a T cell dominant PI3K isoform might have less off target effects in non-immune cells and be a more useful immunosuppressant. Two parallel approaches have been used to determine the role of the PI3K p110δ isoform in lymphocytes, simple gene deletion and targeted knock-in of a kinase inactive mutant p110δ D910A allele (Clayton et al., 2002; Okkenhaug et al., 2002). The latter mice were generated due to concern that deletion of individual regulatory or catalytic subunits appears to result in compensatory changes in expression of remaining *PI3K* genes. Also, the catalytically inactive protein could still function in a scaffolding capacity during assembly of receptor-induced signaling complexes (Okkenhaug et al., 2002). p110$\delta^{-/-}$ mice (completely deleted for p110δ) have normal peripheral T cell numbers but impaired T-dependent antibody production (Clayton et al., 2002). Subsequent work relying on T and B cell conditional deletion of a p110δ floxed allele demonstrated that loss of p110δ expression in T cells due to conditional deletion with Lck-Cre is sufficient to disrupt T-dependent antibody responses despite preserving essentially normal T cell numbers and normal T cell proliferation in response to CD3/CD28 stimulation. This is correlated with an absence of AKT S473 phosphorylation in response to stimulation with anti CD3 plus ICOS-L and significantly decreased expression of CD40L by activated p110$\delta^{-/--}$ T cells (Rolf et al., 2010). The p110$\delta^{D910A/D910A}$ mice demonstrate normal cellularity of the thymus but have about a 50% reduction in mature T cell numbers and a decreased frequency of CD44^{high} effector T cells in the periphery. Phosphorylation of AKT on S473 is severely reduced after CD3 crosslinking, however T cell proliferation and IL-2 secretion when stimulated with anti CD3/CD28 coated beads was the same as WT mice. This stands in contrast to the diminished proliferation and IL-2 secretion that was seen when p110$\delta^{D910A/D910A}$ were crossed to a TCR Tg and stimulated with cognate peptide/APC, indicating that strength of stimulation may compensate in some manner for loss of efficient PIP3 generation in such cells, perhaps via activation of p110γ as discussed below (Alcazar et al., 2007). Similar to r1ΔT/r2n mice, mTOR-independent TCR signaling to induce NF-κB activation was reduced in p110$\delta^{D910A/D910A}$ T cells but NF-κB activation normalized when CD28 costimulation was provided (Okkenhaug et al., 2006). In summary, loss of the individual p110δ subunit or all class IA PI3Ks results in consistent inhibition of AKT S473 phosphorylation implying decreased mTORC2 activity, but TCR-induced proliferation may be relatively spared, depending on the strength of the TCR stimulation. Loss of IL-2 production also appeared to be more severe in the absence of all Class IA PI3K expression. These effects differ from the effects of rapamycin treatment or deletion of mTOR where proliferation is more severely inhibited, initial IL-2 production is preserved, but recall cytokine responses are diminished. Mechanisms underlying these differences may relate to CD4 T cell effector differentiation and are discussed in the next section.

There are conflicting data on the coupling of p110γ to TCR signaling. In one report, T cells from p110$\gamma^{-/-}$ mice have reduced anti CD3 and anti CD3/CD28-induced proliferation, IL-2 production, and IFN-γ production (Sasaki et al., 2000), to some extent resembling T cell anergy. However, while the addition of exogenous IL-2 can rescue Th1 cell anergy induced by rapamycin (Powell et al., 1999), supplementation of IL-2 only partially corrects the defective proliferation of p110$\gamma^{-/-}$ T cells in response to anti CD3/CD28 (Alcazar et al., 2007). Furthermore, p110$\gamma^{-/-}$ T cells demonstrate reduced AKT S473 and mitogen activated protein kinase (MAPK) phosphorylation after stimulation with anti CD3 or anti CD3/CD28, correlating with decreased F-actin polymerization and impaired formation of stable conjugates between T cells and peptide loaded APCs (Alcazar et al., 2007). These data stand in contrast to studies which examined early signaling events in p110$\gamma^{-/-}$ T cells following TCR binding to cognate peptide on APC. Recruitment of an AKT PH domain-GFP fusion protein to the immunologic synapse following stimulation with peptide loaded APC is normal in T cells lacking p110γ while it is impaired in p110$\delta^{D910A/D910A}$ T cells and CD28$^{-/-}$ T cells (Garcon et al., 2008). Likewise, proliferation, downregulation of CD62L, and upregulation of CD44 in response to antigen *in vivo* is normal in CD4 T cells lacking p110γ (Thomas et al., 2008). Proliferation of CD8 T cells lacking p110γ was also normal in response to antigen pulsed APC *in vitro* and vaccinia virus expressing a model antigen *in vivo* (Martin et al., 2008). The mechanism underlying differences between the normal proliferation to antigen but reduced proliferation to anti CD3/CD28 crosslinking in p110$\gamma^{-/-}$ T cells as compared to the reduced proliferation to antigen but near normal proliferation to anti CD3/CD28 in T cells lacking normal p110δ remains incompletely understood, but it may be related to increased susceptibility of p110$\gamma^{-/-}$ T cells to activation induced cell death as p110$\gamma^{-/-}$ thymocytes showed enhanced death compared to WT when exposed to anti CD3 in the presence of adenosine receptor agonists (Sasaki et al., 2000). It will be interesting to see if preservation of antigen induced mTOR activation contributes to the proliferation seen from p110$\gamma^{-/-}$ T cells.

Deletion of PTEN in tumors is associated with constitutive accumulation of PIP3 and appears to promote proliferation and tumor survival, thus it was not surprising when mice with T cell conditional deletion of PTEN were found to develop a lymphoproliferative disorder and die prematurely of CD4 T cell lymphomas (Suzuki et al., 2001). Prior to the onset of lymphoma, peripheral T cells from such mice demonstrate enhanced proliferation, IL-2 secretion, IFN-γ secretion, and AKT S473 phosphorylation after CD3/CD28 stimulation. T cells demonstrate a spontaneous activated, CD69 high phenotype and are autoreactive. Furthermore, such mice develop autoimmunity and hypergammaglobulinemia due to aberrant self-tolerance. This immunopathology appears strongly related to the timing of loss of PTEN expression because conditional deletion of PTEN after completion of thymic negative selection using OX40-Cre, which results in deletion in mature peripheral T cells after initial activation, does not lead to development of autoreactive cells or systemic autoimmunity despite increased lymph node cellularity (Soond et al., 2012). OX40-Cre PTEN null T cells do exhibit enhanced CD3-induced proliferation and IFN-γ production compare to WT. Furthermore, consistent with an exaggerated AKT/mTOR activation state, such mice develop an increased secondary contact hypersensitivity recall response.

NAÏVE CD4 T CELLS REQUIRE PI3K-INDUCED mTOR-DEPENDENT AND mTOR-INDEPENDENT SIGNALS

Naïve CD4 T cells acquire restricted patterns of cytokine expression or regulatory function as a consequence of cytokine exposure or strength of antigenic stimulation during the period of initial activation. Specific patterns of cytokine expression are associated with master transcriptional regulators in the different lineages: Th1 cells express Tbet and IFN-γ; Th2 cells express GATA3 and IL-4, IL-5, and IL-13; Th17 cells express ROR-γT and IL-17A/F; Treg express FoxP3 and suppress other T cell responses [reviewed in Weaver et al. (2006)]. More recently an additional subset termed T follicular helper (Tfh) cell was identified that supports generation of T-dependent antibody production and is dependent on expression of the transcription factor Bcl6 and marked by surface ICOS and CXCR5 and secretion of IL-21 [reviewed in Crotty (2011)]. A requirement for mTOR activation in helper T cell differentiation was initially suggested by the observation that rapamycin inhibition of mTOR promotes *de novo* expression of FoxP3 by naïve T cells and promotes expansion of Tregs *in vitro* (Battaglia et al., 2005). Such rapamycin-induced FoxP3+ cells are functional Tregs capable of suppressing pancreatic allograft rejection *in vivo*. Additional evidence of a critical role for mTOR signals in promoting effector function and inhibiting Treg generation comes from the mice with conditional deletion of mTOR in T cells. Following initial activation, a high proportion of mTOR deficient T cells spontaneously become inducible FoxP3+ Tregs and Th effector differentiation to Th1, Th2, and Th17 fates *in vitro* is severely impaired (Delgoffe et al., 2009).

Mice with individual T cell conditional deletion of either mTORC1 or mTORC2 have provided surprising insight into non-overlapping roles for each of these complexes in normal T cell effector differentiation. Selective loss of mTORC1 following Rheb deletion results in CD4 T cells incapable of Th1 and Th17 differentiation but preserves the ability to make Th2 cells in response to IL-4 stimulation (Delgoffe et al., 2011). More recently, T cell conditional deletion of Raptor was shown to impair Th17 differentiation but Th1 differentiation was preserved (Kurebayashi et al., 2012). Conversely, deletion of Rictor with resulting loss of mTORC2 causes loss of Th2 differentiation, with variable effects on Th1 and Th17 differentiation depending on the timing of Cre expression in the thymus based on the particular Cre transgenic line that the floxed Rictor allele is crossed to (Lee et al., 2010; Delgoffe et al., 2011). T cell-dependent antibody production in mice with mTORC1 deficient T cells is normal but mice with mTORC2 deficient T cells have decreased antibody titers in both mouse lines, although enumeration of Tfh was not performed. As Th17 cells contribute significantly to the pathology of a murine model for multiple sclerosis, experimental autoimmune encephalitis (EAE), the Rheb deficient T cell mice were compared to WT in the EAE system. Rheb deficiency in T cells results in lower EAE severity scores than WT despite all mice developing some symptoms. This correlates with fewer T cells infiltrating the spinal cord and a lower frequency of IL-17 and IFN-γ secretion by T cells extracted from spinal cords of the Rheb deficient T cell mice. Strikingly, 60% of the Rheb deficient T cell mice immunized to induce EAE develop ataxia consistent with "non-classical EAE" that has been observed with induction of Th2 cells in other reports (Wensky et al., 2005). Rheb deficient mice with ataxia have T cell infiltrates in their cerebellum that produce Th2 cytokines *in vitro* in response to antigen (Delgoffe et al., 2011). Treg number and function are normal following T cell conditional deletion of Rheb and Rictor, but Rictor deficient T cells that only have mTORC1 demonstrate enhanced sensitivity to rapamycin in promoting expression of FoxP3 *in vitro* (Delgoffe et al., 2011). The observation that prolonged incubation of cells with higher doses of rapamycin blocks mTORC2 assembly serves to explain both this enhanced sensitivity of Rictor deficient T cells to rapamycin and the fact that loss of both mTORC1 and mTORC2 by deletion of mTOR is necessary to mimic the effect of rapamycin on promoting Tregs (Sarbassov et al., 2006).

Based on the regulation of mTOR by PI3K, the PI3K knockout models should recapitulate the effects of mTOR deletion on effector differentiation. However, just as the mTORC1 and mTORC2 deficient T cells demonstrated unexpected effector phenotypes, disruption of PI3K proximal signaling has also provided surprises. T cells from the r1ΔT/r2n mice lacking all p85 regulatory subunits and having low or absent p110α, β, and δ catalytic subunit expression supported normal Th1 polarization but Th2 cultures had decreased IL-4 and increased IFN-γ. This is consistent with the report above from Delgoffe et al. noting selective loss of IL-4 expression from T cells deficient in mTORC2 and the relative preservation of mTORC1-dependent S6 phosphorylation over mTORC2-dependent AKT S473 phosphorylation that Deane et al. report in the r1ΔT/r2n mice. However, the frequency of $CD4^+CD25^+FoxP3^+$ natural Tregs in the spleen was significantly decreased in r1ΔT/r2n mice despite normal thymic Treg numbers. This is in contrast to normal Treg numbers in the periphery of mice with T cells lacking Rictor (Lee et al., 2010; Delgoffe et al., 2011). T-dependent B cell responses to NP-Ova were impaired and germinal centers following vaccination were decreased but antiviral responses to mouse hepatitis virus were normal (Deane et al., 2007). In addition, the mice were noted to develop spontaneous autoimmunity with corneal opacities and eye lesions found to resemble Sjögren's syndrome. On necropsy the r1ΔT/r2n mice were noted to have a predominantly CD4 T cell infiltrate into lacrimal and salivary lands with lymphadenopathy, splenomegaly, and anti-nuclear and anti SSA autoantibodies (Oak et al., 2006). A mechanistic link between decreased Tregs and autoimmunity was speculated upon but not formally tested in this report. These clinical findings arise in the mice despite the biochemical profile with loss of AKT S473 phosphorylation that resembles the Rictor deficient T cell mice that lack autoimmunity. This serves to highlight the importance of additional PI3K signaling pathways distinct from the AKT/mTOR axis in the maintenance and function of Tregs.

Further characterization of the $p110\delta^{D910A/D910A}$ mice demonstrated that Th1 and Th2 differentiation *in vitro* is markedly reduced (Okkenhaug et al., 2006). Interestingly, when *in vivo* Th2 differentiation was examined following immunization with Ova/Alum, $p110\delta^{D910A/D910A}$ mice exhibit decreased Th2 responses and inappropriate Th1 responses. That is, splenocytes have decreased Ova specific IL-4, IL-5, and IL-13 secretion but enhanced Ova specific IFN-γ and CXCL10 secretion, and the mice demonstrate a reduction in Th2-dependent allergic airway inflammation *in vivo*. This appears to be secondary to defective IL-10 production by $p110\delta^{D910A/D910A}$ T cells because neutralization of IL-10 *in vitro* during Ova stimulation enhances WT splenocyte IFN-γ production and addition of IL-10 suppresses $p110\delta^{D910A/D910A}$ splenocyte IFN-γ production (Nashed et al., 2007). Phosphorylation of mTORC1 substrates is not described in these manuscripts to see if the phenotype is related to imbalance of mTORC1 versus mTORC2, as is ostensibly predicted by the Rictor conditional deletion data above.

Th17 differentiation is also partially p110δ-dependent. IL-17A production from Th17 culture *in vitro* is strongly inhibited by the p110δ isoform specific inhibitor IC87114 while IFN-γ production in Th1 culture is only modestly decreased. Likewise, induction of Th17 cells in $p110\delta^{D910A/D910A}$ mice *in vivo* in EAE is decreased while Th1 responses are spared, resulting in less severe clinical symptoms (Haylock-Jacobs et al., 2011). This preservation of Th1 cytokine expression resembles the phenotype noted for the r1ΔT/r2n mice and to some degree the Rictor T cell deficient mice noted above (Deane et al., 2007; Delgoffe et al., 2011).

Despite the preferential Th1 phenotype under a typical Th2 stimulus and in the EAE model above, Th1-driven contact hypersensitivity responses in $p110\delta^{D910A/D910A}$ mice are reduced (Soond et al., 2010). This would lead to a prediction that such mice would have increased susceptibly to the Th1-sensitive pathogen *Leishmania major*. However, while $p110\delta^{D910A/D910A}$ mice have diminished T cell proliferation, IFN-γ, and TNF-α production to *Leishmania* antigens after infection, consistent with impaired Th1 function, the clinical outcome of infectious challenge is actually enhanced resistance, smaller lesion size, and more rapid parasite clearance. This was found to correlate with impaired generation of IL-10 producing Treg and recruitment of such Tregs to sites of infection in $p110\delta^{D910A/D910A}$ mice (Liu et al., 2009). Adoptive transfer of WT Tregs to $p110\delta^{D910A/D910A}$ mice reverses their *Leishmania* resistance, supporting the hypothesis that Treg dysfunction permits the inefficient $p110\delta^{D910A/D910A}$ Th1 response to be sufficient to clear infection. Additional evidence for functional Treg deficiency in the $p110\delta^{D910A/D910A}$ mice comes from their spontaneous development of autoimmune colitis. Such mice have 50% reduction in Treg frequency in the periphery compared to WT and no detectable IL-10 secretion by cultured Tregs. This is associated with reduced *in vitro* suppression compared to WT Tregs and an inability of $p110\delta^{D910A/D910A}$ Tregs to suppress colitis induced by adoptive transfer of naïve T cells into $RAG1^{-/-}$ mice (Patton et al., 2006). In contrast to these autoimmune findings in mice with proximal PI3K defects, to date, no spontaneous autoimmune phenotype has been reported in mice with T cell conditional disruption of mTORC1, mTORC2, or both (Delgoffe et al., 2009, 2011; Lee et al., 2010).

Reminiscent of the mice with T cells lacking mTORC2 complexes and the r1ΔT/r2n mice, $p110\delta^{D910A/D910A}$ mice demonstrate abnormal T-dependent antibody responses. Such mice are largely devoid of germinal centers in spleen and lymph nodes (Okkenhaug et al., 2002). This appears to be due to a requirement for p110δ expression in Tfh, rather than B cells, based on subsequent conditional deletion experiments. Mice bearing $p110\delta^{2loxP/2loxP}$ alleles were crossed with CD4-Cre to delete p110δ during the double positive thymocyte stage or Ox40-Cre to delete p110δ in peripheral T cells after their initial activation. In both types of mice, PD-1+ CXCR5+ Tfh are decreased 10-fold and 5-fold, respectively with corresponding decreases in the number of germinal center B cells and the number of germinal centers per follicle within lymph nodes. Mechanistically, this correlates with decreased ICOS-induced AKT S473 phosphorylation and reduced expression of factors critical for T cell-dependent B cell help including CD40L, IL-21, IL-4, and c-Maf in T cells lacking p110δ expression (Rolf et al., 2010). A detailed Tfh phenotype has not been reported following T cell conditional deletion of Rictor, however the data from the PI3K deficient mice would predict that Tfh effector cytokines might be reduced.

Despite the controversy surrounding whether p110γ is coupled directly to TCR or CD28, it is clear that loss of p110γ impacts T cell effector function. Both CD4 and CD8 $p110\gamma^{-/-}$ T cells have defective effector T cell migration *in vivo* that correlates with impaired migratory responses to chemokines *in vitro* (Martin et al., 2008; Thomas et al., 2008). Expression of granzyme B and IFN-γ appears normal in $p110\gamma^{-/-}$ CD8 effector T cells generated *in vivo* by antigen exposure (Martin et al., 2008). Effector differentiation of $p110\gamma^{-/-}$ CD4 T cells *in vivo* has not been fully described and impaired footpad swelling induced by LCMV and impaired T-dependent antibody responses in p110$\gamma^{-/-}$ mice may be related to loss of p110γ expression in cells other that CD4 T cells (Sasaki et al., 2000). Anti CD3/CD28 induced phosphorylation of AKT S473 is decreased in p110$\gamma^{-/-}$ T cells, suggesting that CD4 effector differentiation may be abnormal in a manner analogous to mTOR or mTORC2 deficient T cells but in light of partial functional redundancy of p110δ activity in such cells, direct measurement of mTOR substrate phosphorylation in response to antigen or anti CD3/CD28 will ultimately need to be performed to address whether the p110$\gamma^{-/-}$ phenotype is mTOR related.

In contrast to immune dysregulation associated with Treg dysfunction after reducing PI3K activity, enhancing PI3K function by PTEN deletion in the OX40-Cre T cell conditional model not only enhances IFN-γ production *in vitro*, but also results in enhanced Th1 effector function *in vivo* by several measures. PTEN deletion in T cells increases contact hypersensitivity reactions. Adoptively transferred OX40-Cre PTEN floxed OT2 TCR Tg T cells secrete more IL-2 and IFN-γ after activation by infection with attenuated *Listeria* expressing ovalbumin and support better expansion of endogenous ovalbumin-specific CD8 T cells than WT OT2 cells. In addition, adoptively transferred OX40-Cre PTEN floxed OT2 T cells are better at rejecting syngeneic tumor expressing ovalbumin antigen (Soond et al., 2012). These findings are consistent with a robust Th1 response in the presence of increased PI3K/AKT/mTOR activity, but experiments to dissect if any findings were exclusively due to enhanced mTOR activity await experiments culturing PTEN null T cells or treating Ox40-Cre PTEN floxed mice with rapamycin or mTOR kinase inhibitors.

A MODEL FOR PI3K/AKT/mTOR REGULATION OF T CELL EFFECTOR FUNCTION

In an effort to propose a unifying model to explain the varied phenotypes arising from blockade of the PI3K/AKT/mTOR axis at different points, it is useful to consider experiments that disrupt more proximal and distal signaling events in T cells. Premature interruption of CD3/CD28 signaling or activation by very low doses of cognate peptide in CD4 T cells promotes expression of FoxP3 that is further enhanced by exposure to PI3K inhibitors and rapamycin (Kang et al., 2008; Sauer et al., 2008). Through use of dose responses to selective PI3K inhibitors, Sauer et al. attribute FoxP3 induction to inhibition of PI3Kα and δ upstream of AKT and mTOR. These findings raise a paradox: small molecule inhibitors of PI3K, AKT, and mTOR all result in a similar phenotype, promoting induction of FoxP3 expression following activation of naïve CD4 T cells, but the phenotypes of mice with genetic lesions resulting in loss of T cell PI3K expression demonstrate inefficient Treg production and decreased Treg function. Furthermore, mice with T cell conditional deletion of mTOR phenocopy the small molecule inhibitors and generate Tregs at the expense of effector helper T cells. These observations serve to highlight that there are mTOR-dependent effects of PI3K, mediated by AKT, that are necessary to suppress FoxP3 expression and promote normal effector function and that there are mTOR-independent effects of PI3K, some of which are necessary for normal inducible Treg differentiation. This is shown schematically in **Figure 1**, and details of the potential mechanisms for this effect are discussed below.

There are several potential mechanisms, currently largely speculative, to explain how loss of PI3K enzymatic activity, with associated decreased mTOR activity, may result in fewer and less functional Tregs. First, PI3K-dependent accumulation of PIP3 results in localization of other families of signaling molecules near the immunologic synapse including Vav guanine nucleotide exchange factors for Ras related GTPases Rac and Rho that control cell motility and Tec family tyrosine kinases that mediate PLCγ activation [reviewed in Cantrell (2001)]. A role for such pathways in T cell activation and effector cytokine expression is well established, but a direct connection between PI3K, Tec, Vav, and Treg function is incompletely characterized. However, disruption of other molecules downstream, including the Bcl-10 and PKCθ components of the NF-κB signaling pathway distal to the Tec family kinases, impairs generation of Tregs (Schmidt-Supprian et al., 2004). Also, Tregs normally have elevated levels of PTEN expression. This is associated with defective phosphorylation of AKT S473 in response to IL-2 stimulation in Tregs as compared to effector T cells and with defective Treg proliferation in response to TCR stimulation in the presence of IL-2 without concurrent CD28 ligation (Bensinger et al., 2004). Conditional deletion of PTEN in T cells does not affect generation of Tregs, the amount of FoxP3 they express, or the suppressive capacity of Tregs, but it does result in enhanced Treg proliferation in response to IL-2 or TCR stimulation (Walsh et al., 2006). Taken together, these data suggest that the Treg defects following loss of PI3K expression might be due to differential sensitivity of Tregs to decreased levels of PIP3 compared to effector cells due to high Treg PTEN expression. Preferential inhibition of Treg proliferation and suppressor cytokine production would be predicted to result in an enhanced ratio of effector T cells to Tregs and autoimmunity in the PI3K deficient mice. Such hypotheses await further experimental evaluation.

Another paradox that arises comparing T cells lacking PI3K with those lacking mTOR is how do PI3K null cells promote some effector function if they are unable to activate mTOR? It is important to remember that other inputs in addition to TCR and CD28-induced PI3K/AKT are able to activate mTOR. In particular, chemokine receptors via p110γ, cellular energy stores by regulating the adenosine monophosphate-dependent kinase (AMPK) pathway, cytoplasmic amino acids via the Ras-related small GTPase Rag proteins, and hypoxia via the hypoxia-induced factor protein regulated in the development of DNA damage response 1 (REDD1)/hypoxia-induced factor 1α (HIF1α) pathway, ERK and RSK downstream of Ras, and phosphatidic acid produced by phospholipase D are potent regulators of mTOR activation [reviewed in Laplante and Sabatini (2012); Waickman and Powell (2012)]. The capacity of these inputs to regulate mTOR activation in T cells is reflected by the ability of 2-deoxyglucose (2-DG) mimicking glucose deprivation, 5-aminoimidazole-4-carboxamide ribonucleoside (AICAR) mimicking cellular energy depletion, and n-acetyl leucine (NALA) mimicking amino acid depletion to result in anergy when present during CD3/CD28 stimulation of T cells, analogous to rapamycin treatment (Zheng et al., 2009). The

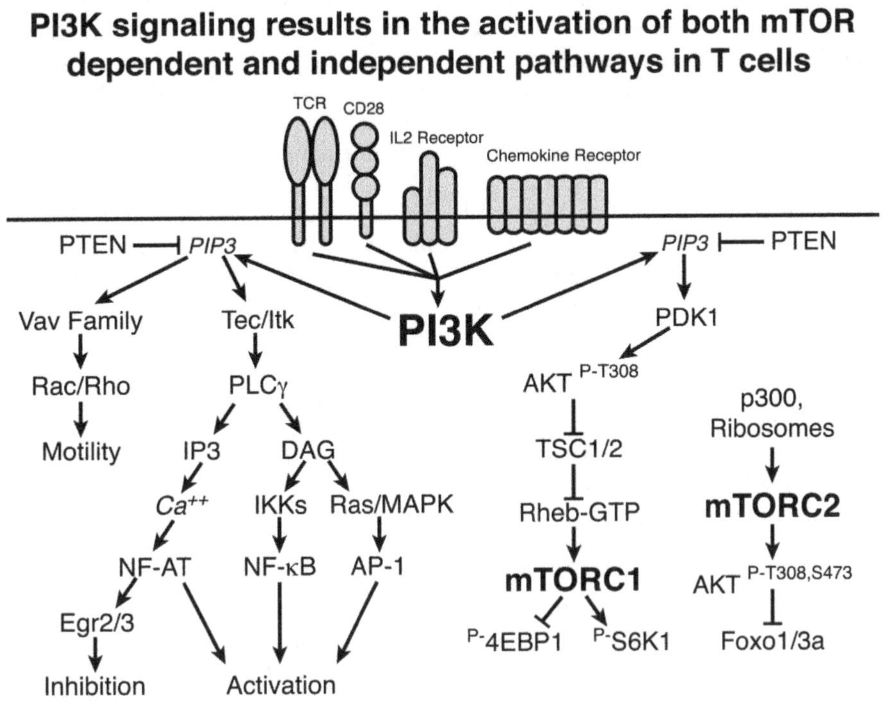

FIGURE 1 | PI3K signaling results in the activation of both mTOR-dependent and independent pathways in T cells. A schematic representation of PI3K signaling is shown demonstrating mTOR-independent and mTOR-dependent signaling cascades. Lines with arrows indicate activating signals and lines with bars indicate inhibitory signals. Importantly, this graphic does not include all of the nuanced inputs that are discussed in the text. Rather, these pathways represent connections and not absolute requirements for signaling. For example, while elimination of p110δ or all PI3K regulatory subunits leads to decreased NF-κB, such a deficit can be overcome by the addition of CD28 signaling. Overall, PI3K-induced mTOR-independent signaling can influence both the activation and inhibition of T cells as well as the generation and function of Tregs. The PI3K-induced mTOR-dependent pathways can influence CD4 effector differentiation and function as well as inhibit the generation of Tregs.

presence of normal energy, amino acids, and normoxia to promote mTOR activation is therefore consistent with the reported preservation of some mTORC1 activity in the r1ΔT/r2n mice (Deane et al., 2007). This relative increase in mTORC1 activity over mTORC2 activity in these mice supports the observed relative preservation of Th1 cytokine production over Th2 cytokines, analogous to the Rictor deficient T cell mice noted above (Lee et al., 2010; Delgoffe et al., 2011).

Finally, there are two mTOR-dependent pathways that can negatively regulate FoxP3 expression whose loss may explain the increased FoxP3 expression in mTOR null T cells. First, HIF1α is induced by mTORC1 and has been shown to directly bind to FoxP3 protein and promote its ubiquitination and degradation (Dang et al., 2011). Second, the Foxo transcription factors directly bind to and transactivate the FoxP3 promoter, and they are inactivated in an mTORC2-dependent manner following phosphorylation by doubly phosphorylated activated AKT, leading to nuclear export of the Foxos [reviewed in Coffer and Burgering (2004)]. The importance of the latter pathway to Tregs is seen following T cell conditional deletion of Foxo1 and Foxo3. Individually they have overlapping function in T cells to maintain naïve T cells in quiescence, but their simultaneous deletion in T cells results in functional Treg deficiency with early fatal autoimmunity that can be prevented by adoptive transfer of WT Treg (Ouyang et al., 2010). The fact that an increase in Tregs was observed following deletion of mTOR but not in the Rheb and Rictor T cell conditional knockouts suggests that loss of both of these pathways is necessary to result in enhanced generation of FoxP3+ Tregs (Lee et al., 2010; Delgoffe et al., 2011).

DISTAL INHIBITION OF THE PI3K/AKT/mTOR AXIS SHOULD YIELD MORE RELIABLE BLOCKADE OF T CELL MEDIATED PATHOLOGY

Based on the data and model above, treatment with mTOR inhibitors for immunologic diseases would be predicted to not only suppress immune responses but also potentially promote tolerance by fostering anergy and the induction of Treg. For example, in a mouse model of non-myeloablative peripheral blood stem cell transplantation, we found that treatment with cyclosporine led to eventual graft rejection while treatment with rapamycin led to stable mixed chimerism, even after the rapamycin was stopped. Such engrafted mice had negative mixed lymphocyte reactions to both donor and recipient target cells, indicating tolerance was achieved (Powell et al., 2005). This preclinical data served as the basis for a trial of human transplantation to treat sickle cell anemia with matched sibling donors that specifically avoided use of standard calcineurin inhibitors for graft versus host disease (GVHD) prophylaxis. Patients received alemtuzumab for T cell depletion, low dose total body irradiation, and peripheral blood stem cell transplant with rapamycin for GVHD prophylaxis. Nine of ten patients engrafted with mixed donor chimerism sufficient to abrogate symptoms of sickle cell disease, and patients that have tapered off their immunosuppression have demonstrated stable engraftment, consistent with donor-specific tolerance (Hsieh et al., 2009).

In contrast to the effects of mTOR blockade, loss of PI3K expression in T cells leads to consequences on both Treg and effector T cell function, with the net effect of enhanced or suppressed immune responses *in vivo* strongly dependent on the context. A recent study examined PI3K inhibition as a means of suppressing cardiac allograft rejection (Ying et al., 2012). Transplanting male hearts into female mice results in HY antigen driven chronic allograft rejection that is mitigated if the hearts are transplanted into $p110\delta^{D910A/D910A}$ female recipients. Splenocytes from both rejecting WT and non-rejecting $p110\delta^{D910A/D910A}$ recipient mice proliferate equally well to HY peptide, however, indicating that the absence of rejection in $p110\delta^{D910A/D910A}$ recipients is not due to tolerance. Instead, defective trafficking appears to prevent rejection, as adoptive transfer of HY specific TCR Tg T cells demonstrates reduced localization of the $p110\delta^{D910A/D910A}$ HY-specific T cells into male allografts despite normal trafficking of adoptively transferred cells to other tissues. Based on this, the authors tested the selective PI3K p110δ inhibitor IC87114 and found it also prevents rejection by blocking localization of alloreactive cells to the graft but fails to induce tolerance. The inability of proximal PI3K blockade to induce transplant tolerance resembles the inability of cyclosporine to promote engraftment in the stem cell transplant model discussed above and stands in contrast to the tolerance induced by rapamycin in that model.

Interestingly, the capacity for proximal PI3K blockade to potentiate immune function in specific contexts may nicely synergize with the broader ability of PI3K blockade inhibit tumor cell proliferation to make PI3K inhibitors particularly well suited to cancer treatment, reviewed in So and Fruman (2012). To this end, mice were given subcutaneous implants of different syngeneic tumors and then treated with immunotherapy in the presence or absence of ZSTK474, a pan-class I PI3K inhibitor. It was found that this drug both inhibits tumor growth and has the ability to enhance the efficacy of immunotherapy (Marshall et al., 2012). The authors did not assess whether impaired Treg function contributed to tumor clearance, but they demonstrate that inhibition of PI3K is sufficient to suppress DC secretion of IL-10 while permitting secretion of IL-12. This appears to result in enhanced Th1 immunity since neutralization of IFN-γ *in vivo* by blocking antibody abrogated the protection afforded by immunotherapy plus ZSTK474. In this regard, we would predict that mTOR inhibition in the absence of proximal PI3K blockade might also have directs effects on inhibiting tumor growth but would serve to limit development of anti-tumor immunity.

SUMMARY

By employing genetic analysis it has become clear that in T cells what initially appeared to be a straightforward connection between components of the PI3K signaling cascade via AKT to mTOR is substantially more complex. We have only been able to show a small subset of data published on the topic to illustrate this point and apologize to authors for whom we were not able to include their work. While inhibiting PI3K and mTOR interferes with T cell effector function, what has become clear is that through the inhibition of distal targets in these signaling pathways, selective effects can be achieved. For example, a drug that blocks mTORC2 might be helpful to treat Th2-mediated asthma without blunting Th17 and Th1-mediated antifungal and antibacterial responses. Conversely, an mTORC1 selective drug, unlike rapamycin that can inhibit mTORC2 under prolonged exposure to higher doses, might be helpful in a disease like multiple sclerosis mediated by Th17 and Th1 cells but might permit effective vaccine responses to seasonal influenza by preserving Tfh function. As the PI3K-induced mTOR-independent pathways in T cells become more precisely defined, blockade of nodes distal in the pathway might avoid unintended effects that interfere with function of Treg. Finally, it may turn out that concomitant distal inhibition of both mTOR-dependent and independent pathways will lead to the most robust and precise clinical outcomes.

ACKNOWLEDGMENTS

We are grateful to Robert Hagan and Emily Heikamp for their thoughtful comments on this manuscript.

REFERENCES

Alcazar, I., Marques, M., Kumar, A., Hirsch, E., Wymann, M., Carrera, A. C., et al. (2007). Phosphoinositide 3-kinase gamma participates in T cell receptor-induced T cell activation. *J. Exp. Med.* 204, 2977–2987.

Battaglia, M., Stabilini, A., and Roncarolo, M. G. (2005). Rapamycin selectively expands CD4+CD25+FoxP3+ regulatory T cells. *Blood* 105, 4743–4748.

Bensinger, S. J., Walsh, P. T., Zhang, J., Carroll, M., Parsons, R., Rathmell, J. C., et al. (2004). Distinct IL-2 receptor signaling pattern in CD4+CD25+ regulatory T cells. *J. Immunol.* 172, 5287–5296.

Brownawell, A. M., Kops, G. J., Macara, I. G., and Burgering, B. M. (2001). Inhibition of nuclear import by protein kinase B (Akt) regulates the subcellular distribution and activity of the forkhead transcription factor AFX. *Mol. Cell. Biol.* 21, 3534–3546.

Brunn, G. J., Williams, J., Sabers, C., Wiederrecht, G., Lawrence, J. C. Jr., and Abraham, R. T. (1996). Direct inhibition of the signaling functions of the mammalian target of rapamycin by the phosphoinositide 3-kinase inhibitors, wortmannin and LY294002. *EMBO J.* 15, 5256–5267.

Cantrell, D. (2002). Protein kinase B (Akt) regulation and function in T lymphocytes. *Semin. Immunol.* 14, 19–26.

Cantrell, D. A. (2001). Phosphoinositide 3-kinase signalling pathways. *J. Cell Sci.* 114, 1439–1445.

Clayton, E., Bardi, G., Bell, S. E., Chantry, D., Downes, C. P., Gray, A., et al. (2002). A crucial role for the p110delta subunit of phosphatidylinositol 3-kinase in B cell development and activation. *J. Exp. Med.* 196, 753–763.

Coffer, P. J., and Burgering, B. M. (2004). Forkhead-box transcription factors and their role in the immune system. *Nat. Rev. Immunol.* 4, 889–899.

Crotty, S. (2011). Follicular helper CD4 T cells (TFH). *Annu. Rev. Immunol.* 29, 621–663.

Currie, R. A., Walker, K. S., Gray, A., Deak, M., Casamayor, A., Downes, C. P., et al. (1999). Role of phosphatidylinositol 3 4, 5-trisphosphate in regulating the activity and localization of 3-phosphoinositide-dependent protein kinase-1. *Biochem. J.* 337(Pt 3), 575–583.

Dang, E. V., Barbi, J., Yang, H. Y., Jinasena, D., Yu, H., Zheng, Y., et al. (2011). Control of T(H)17/T(reg) balance by hypoxia-inducible factor 1. *Cell* 146, 772–784.

Deane, J. A., Kharas, M. G., Oak, J. S., Stiles, L. N., Luo, J., Moore, T. I., et al. (2007). T-cell function is partially maintained in the absence of class IA phosphoinositide 3-kinase signaling. *Blood* 109, 2894–2902.

Deane, J. A., Trifilo, M. J., Yballe, C. M., Choi, S., Lane, T. E., and Fruman, D. A. (2004). Enhanced T cell proliferation in mice lacking the p85beta subunit of phosphoinositide 3-kinase. *J. Immunol.* 172, 6615–6625.

Delgoffe, G. M., Kole, T. P., Zheng, Y., Zarek, P. E., Matthews, K. L., Xiao, B., et al. (2009). The mTOR kinase differentially regulates effector and regulatory T cell lineage commitment. *Immunity* 30, 832–844.

Delgoffe, G. M., Pollizzi, K. N., Waickman, A. T., Heikamp, E., Meyers, D. J., Horton, M. R., et al. (2011). The kinase mTOR regulates the differentiation of helper T cells through the selective activation of signaling by mTORC1 and mTORC2. *Nat. Immunol.* 12, 295–303.

Facchinetti, V., Ouyang, W., Wei, H., Soto, N., Lazorchak, A., Gould, C., et al. (2008). The mammalian target of rapamycin complex 2 controls folding and stability of Akt and protein kinase C. *EMBO J.* 27, 1932–1943.

Finlay, D., and Cantrell, D. (2010). Phosphoinositide 3-kinase and the mammalian target of rapamycin pathways control T cell migration. *Ann. N.Y. Acad. Sci.* 1183, 149–157.

Fruman, D. A., Snapper, S. B., Yballe, C. M., Davidson, L., Yu, J. Y., Alt, F. W., et al. (1999). Impaired B cell development and proliferation in absence of phosphoinositide 3-kinase p85alpha. *Science* 283, 393–397.

Garcia-Martinez, J. M., and Alessi, D. R. (2008). mTOR complex 2 (mTORC2) controls hydrophobic motif phosphorylation and activation of serum- and glucocorticoid-induced protein kinase 1 (SGK1). *Biochem. J.* 416, 375–385.

Garcon, F., Patton, D. T., Emery, J. L., Hirsch, E., Rottapel, R., Sasaki, T., et al. (2008). CD28 provides T-cell costimulation and enhances PI3K activity at the immune synapse independently of its capacity to interact with the p85/p110 heterodimer. *Blood* 111, 1464–1471.

Glidden, E. J., Gray, L. G., Vemuru, S., Li, D., Harris, T. E., and Mayo, M. W. (2012). Multiple site acetylation of Rictor stimulates mammalian target of rapamycin complex 2 (mTORC2)-dependent phosphorylation of Akt protein. *J. Biol. Chem.* 287, 581–588.

Haylock-Jacobs, S., Comerford, I., Bunting, M., Kara, E., Townley, S., Klingler-Hoffmann, M., et al. (2011). PI3Kdelta drives the pathogenesis of experimental autoimmune encephalomyelitis by inhibiting effector T cell apoptosis and promoting Th17 differentiation. *J. Autoimmun.* 36, 278–287.

Hsieh, M. M., Kang, E. M., Fitzhugh, C. D., Link, M. B., Bolan, C. D., Kurlander, R., et al. (2009). Allogeneic hematopoietic stem-cell transplantation for sickle cell disease. *N. Engl. J. Med.* 361, 2309–2317.

Jacinto, E., Facchinetti, V., Liu, D., Soto, N., Wei, S., Jung, S. Y., et al. (2006). SIN1/MIP1 maintains rictor-mTOR complex integrity and regulates Akt phosphorylation and substrate specificity. *Cell* 127, 125–137.

Kane, L. P., and Weiss, A. (2003). The PI-3 kinase/Akt pathway and T cell activation: pleiotropic pathways downstream of PIP3. *Immunol. Rev.* 192, 7–20.

Kang, J., Huddleston, S. J., Fraser, J. M., and Khoruts, A. (2008). De novo induction of antigen-specific CD4+CD25+Foxp3+ regulatory T cells *in vivo* following systemic antigen administration accompanied by blockade of mTOR. *J. Leukoc. Biol.* 83, 1230–1239.

Kay, J. E., Kromwel, L., Doe, S. E., and Denyer, M. (1991). Inhibition of T and B lymphocyte proliferation by rapamycin. *Immunology* 72, 544–549.

Kurebayashi, Y., Nagai, S., Ikejiri, A., Ohtani, M., Ichiyama, K., Baba, Y., et al. (2012). PI3K-Akt-mTORC1-S6K1/2 Axis Controls Th17 Differentiation by Regulating Gfi1 Expression and Nuclear Translocation of RORgamma. *Cell Rep.* 1, 360–373.

Laplante, M., and Sabatini, D. M. (2012). mTOR signaling in growth control and disease. *Cell* 149, 274–293.

Lee, K., Gudapati, P., Dragovic, S., Spencer, C., Joyce, S., Killeen, N., et al. (2010). Mammalian target of rapamycin protein complex 2 regulates differentiation of Th1 and Th2 cell subsets via distinct signaling pathways. *Immunity* 32, 743–753.

Liu, D., Zhang, T., Marshall, A. J., Okkenhaug, K., Vanhaesebroeck, B., and Uzonna, J. E. (2009). The p110delta isoform of phosphatidylinositol 3-kinase controls susceptibility to *Leishmania major* by regulating expansion and tissue homing of regulatory T cells. *J. Immunol.* 183, 1921–1933.

Macian, F., Garcia-Cozar, F., Im, S. H., Horton, H. F., Byrne, M. C., and Rao, A. (2002). Transcriptional mechanisms underlying lymphocyte tolerance. *Cell* 109, 719–731.

Marshall, N. A., Galvin, K. C., Corcoran, A. M., Boon, L., Higgs, R., and Mills, K. H. (2012). Immunotherapy with PI3K inhibitor and Toll-like receptor agonist induces IFN-gamma+IL−17+ polyfunctional T cells that mediate rejection of murine tumors. *Cancer Res.* 72, 581–591.

Martin, A. L., Schwartz, M. D., Jameson, S. C., and Shimizu, Y. (2008). Selective regulation of CD8 effector T cell migration by the p110 gamma isoform of phosphatidylinositol 3-kinase. *J. Immunol.* 180, 2081–2088.

Milburn, C. C., Deak, M., Kelly, S. M., Price, N. C., Alessi, D. R., and Van Aalten, D. M. (2003). Binding of phosphatidylinositol 3 4, 5-trisphosphate to the pleckstrin homology domain of protein kinase B induces a conformational change. *Biochem. J.* 375, 531–538.

Nashed, B. F., Zhang, T., Al-Alwan, M., Srinivasan, G., Halayko, A. J., Okkenhaug, K., et al. (2007). Role of the phosphoinositide 3-kinase p110delta in generation of type 2 cytokine responses and allergic airway inflammation. *Eur. J. Immunol.* 37, 416–424.

Oak, J. S., Deane, J. A., Kharas, M. G., Luo, J., Lane, T. E., Cantley, L. C., et al. (2006). Sjogren's syndrome-like disease in mice with T cells lacking class 1A phosphoinositide-3-kinase. *Proc. Natl. Acad. Sci. U.S.A.* 103, 16882–16887.

Okkenhaug, K., Bilancio, A., Farjot, G., Priddle, H., Sancho, S., Peskett, E., et al. (2002). Impaired B and T cell antigen receptor signaling in p110delta PI 3-kinase mutant mice. *Science* 297, 1031–1034.

Okkenhaug, K., and Fruman, D. A. (2010). PI3Ks in lymphocyte signaling and development. *Curr. Top. Microbiol. Immunol.* 346, 57–85.

Okkenhaug, K., Patton, D. T., Bilancio, A., Garcon, F., Rowan, W. C., and Vanhaesebroeck, B. (2006). The p110delta isoform of phosphoinositide 3-kinase controls clonal expansion and differentiation of Th cells. *J. Immunol.* 177, 5122–5128.

Okkenhaug, K., and Vanhaesebroeck, B. (2003). PI3K in lymphocyte development, differentiation and activation. *Nat. Rev. Immunol.* 3, 317–330.

Ouyang, W., Beckett, O., Ma, Q., Paik, J. H., Depinho, R. A., and Li, M. O. (2010). Foxo proteins cooperatively control the differentiation of Foxp3+ regulatory T cells. *Nat. Immunol.* 11, 618–627.

Patton, D. T., Garden, O. A., Pearce, W. P., Clough, L. E., Monk, C. R., Leung, E., et al. (2006). Cutting edge: the phosphoinositide 3-kinase p110 delta is critical for the function of CD4+CD25+Foxp3+ regulatory T cells. *J. Immunol.* 177, 6598–6602.

Powell, J. D., Fitzhugh, C., Kang, E. M., Hsieh, M., Schwartz, R. H., and Tisdale, J. F. (2005). Low-dose radiation plus rapamycin promotes long-term bone marrow chimerism. *Transplantation* 80, 1541–1545.

Powell, J. D., Lerner, C. G., and Schwartz, R. H. (1999). Inhibition of cell cycle progression by rapamycin induces T cell clonal anergy even in the presence of costimulation. *J. Immunol.* 162, 2775–2784.

Rolf, J., Bell, S. E., Kovesdi, D., Janas, M. L., Soond, D. R., Webb, L. M., et al. (2010). Phosphoinositide 3-kinase activity in T cells regulates the magnitude of the germinal center reaction. *J. Immunol.* 185, 4042–4052.

Safford, M., Collins, S., Lutz, M. A., Allen, A., Huang, C. T., Kowalski, J., et al. (2005). Egr-2 and Egr-3 are negative regulators of T cell activation. *Nat. Immunol.* 6, 472–480.

Salmond, R. J., Emery, J., Okkenhaug, K., and Zamoyska, R. (2009). MAPK, phosphatidylinositol 3-kinase, and mammalian target of rapamycin pathways converge at the level of ribosomal protein S6 phosphorylation to control metabolic signaling in CD8 T cells. *J. Immunol.* 183, 7388–7397.

Sanjuan, M. A., Jones, D. R., Izquierdo, M., and Merida, I. (2001). Role of diacylglycerol kinase alpha in the attenuation of receptor signaling. *J. Cell Biol.* 153, 207–220.

Sarbassov, D. D., Ali, S. M., Sengupta, S., Sheen, J. H., Hsu, P. P., Bagley, A. F., et al. (2006). Prolonged rapamycin treatment inhibits mTORC2 assembly and Akt/PKB. *Mol. Cell* 22, 159–168.

Sarbassov, D. D., Guertin, D. A., Ali, S. M., and Sabatini, D. M. (2005). Phosphorylation and regulation of Akt/PKB by the rictor-mTOR complex. *Science* 307, 1098–1101.

Sasaki, T., Irie-Sasaki, J., Jones, R. G., Oliveira-Dos-Santos, A. J., Stanford, W. L., Bolon, B., et al. (2000). Function of PI3Kgamma in thymocyte development, T cell activation, and neutrophil migration. *Science* 287, 1040–1046.

Sauer, S., Bruno, L., Hertweck, A., Finlay, D., Leleu, M., Spivakov, M., et al. (2008). T cell receptor signaling controls Foxp3 expression via PI3K, Akt, and mTOR. *Proc. Natl. Acad. Sci. U.S.A.* 105, 7797–7802.

Schmidt-Supprian, M., Tian, J., Grant, E. P., Pasparakis, M., Maehr, R., Ovaa, H., et al. (2004). Differential dependence of CD4+CD25+ regulatory and natural killer-like T cells on signals leading to NF-kappaB activation. *Proc. Natl. Acad. Sci. U.S.A.* 101, 4566–4571.

So, L., and Fruman, D. A. (2012). PI3K signalling in B- and T-lymphocytes: new developments and therapeutic advances. *Biochem. J.* 442, 465–481.

Soond, D. R., Bjorgo, E., Moltu, K., Dale, V. Q., Patton, D. T., Torgersen, K. M., et al. (2010). PI3K p110delta regulates T-cell cytokine production during primary and secondary immune responses in mice and humans. *Blood* 115, 2203–2213.

Soond, D. R., Garcon, F., Patton, D. T., Rolf, J., Turner, M., Scudamore, C., et al. (2012). Pten loss in CD4 T cells enhances their helper function but does not lead to autoimmunity or lymphoma. *J. Immunol.* 188, 5935–5943.

Stokoe, D., Stephens, L. R., Copeland, T., Gaffney, P. R., Reese, C. B., Painter, G. F., et al. (1997). Dual role of phosphatidylinositol-3 4, 5-trisphosphate in the activation of protein kinase B. *Science* 277, 567–570.

Suzuki, A., Yamaguchi, M. T., Ohteki, T., Sasaki, T., Kaisho, T., Kimura, Y., et al. (2001). T cell-specific loss of Pten leads to defects in central and peripheral tolerance. *Immunity* 14, 523–534.

Suzuki, H., Terauchi, Y., Fujiwara, M., Aizawa, S., Yazaki, Y., Kadowaki, T., et al. (1999). Xid-like immunodeficiency in mice with disruption of the p85alpha subunit of phosphoinositide 3-kinase. *Science* 283, 390–392.

Taub, D. D., Murphy, W. J., Asai, O., Fenton, R. G., Peltz, G., Key, M. L., et al. (1997). Induction of alloantigen-specific T cell tolerance through the treatment of human T lymphocytes with wortmannin. *J. Immunol.* 158, 2745–2755.

Thomas, M. S., Mitchell, J. S., Denucci, C. C., Martin, A. L., and Shimizu, Y. (2008). The p110gamma isoform of phosphatidylinositol 3-kinase regulates migration of effector CD4 T lymphocytes into peripheral inflammatory sites. *J. Leukoc. Biol.* 84, 814–823.

Waickman, A. T., and Powell, J. D. (2012). Mammalian target of rapamycin integrates diverse inputs to guide the outcome of antigen recognition in T cells. *J. Immunol.* 188, 4721–4729.

Walsh, P. T., Buckler, J. L., Zhang, J., Gelman, A. E., Dalton, N. M., Taylor, D. K., et al. (2006). PTEN inhibits IL-2 receptor-mediated expansion of CD4+ CD25+ Tregs. *J. Clin. Invest.* 116, 2521–2531.

Ward, S. G., Wilson, A., Turner, L., Westwick, J., and Sansom, D. M. (1995). Inhibition of CD28-mediated T cell costimulation by the phosphoinositide 3-kinase inhibitor wortmannin. *Eur. J. Immunol.* 25, 526–532.

Weaver, C. T., Harrington, L. E., Mangan, P. R., Gavrieli, M., and Murphy, K. M. (2006). Th17, an effector CD4 T cell lineage with regulatory T cell ties. *Immunity* 24, 677–688.

Wensky, A. K., Furtado, G. C., Marcondes, M. C., Chen, S., Manfra, D., Lira, S. A., et al. (2005). IFN-gamma determines distinct clinical outcomes in autoimmune encephalomyelitis. *J. Immunol.* 174, 1416–1423.

Ying, H., Fu, H., Rose, M. L., McCormack, A. M., Sarathchandra, P., Okkenhaug, K., et al. (2012). Genetic or pharmaceutical blockade of phosphoinositide 3-kinase p110delta prevents chronic rejection of heart allografts. *PLoS ONE* 7:e32892. doi: 10.1371/journal.pone.0032892

Zha, Y., Marks, R., Ho, A. W., Peterson, A. C., Janardhan, S., Brown, I., et al. (2006). T cell anergy is reversed by active Ras and is regulated by diacylglycerol kinase-alpha. *Nat. Immunol.* 7, 1166–1173.

Zheng, Y., Delgoffe, G. M., Meyer, C. F., Chan, W., and Powell, J. D. (2009). Anergic T cells are metabolically anergic. *J. Immunol.* 183, 6095–6101.

Zinzalla, V., Stracka, D., Oppliger, W., and Hall, M. N. (2011). Activation of mTORC2 by association with the ribosome. *Cell* 144, 757–768.

22

Regulation of T cell homeostasis and responses by *Pten*

Ryan H. Newton and Laurence A. Turka*

Department of Medicine, Beth Israel Deaconess Medical Center, Harvard Medical School, Boston, MA, USA

Edited by:
Klaus Okkenhaug, Babraham Institute, UK

Reviewed by:
Hergen Spits, University of Amsterdam, Netherlands
Klaus Okkenhaug, Babraham Institute, UK

****Correspondence:***
Laurence A. Turka, Department of Medicine, Beth Israel Deaconess Medical Center, Harvard Medical School, 330 Brookline Ave., Boston, MA 02215, USA.
e-mail: lturka@bidmc.harvard.edu

The generation of lipid products catalyzed by PI3K is critical for normal T cell homeostasis and a productive immune response. PI3K can be activated in response to antigen receptor, co-stimulatory, cytokine, and chemokine signals. Moreover, dysregulation of this pathway frequently occurs in T cell lymphomas and is implicated in lymphoproliferative autoimmune disease. Akt acts as a central mediator of PI3K signals, downstream of which is the mTOR pathway, controlling cell growth and metabolism. Members of the Foxo family of transcription factors are also regulated by Akt, thus linking control over homing and migration of T cells, as well cell cycle entry, apoptosis, and DNA damage and oxidative stress responses, to PI3K signaling. PTEN, first identified as a tumor suppressor gene, encodes a lipid phosphatase that, by catalyzing the reverse of the PI3K "reaction," directly opposes PI3K signaling. However, PTEN may have other functions as well, and recent reports have suggested roles for PTEN as a tumor suppressor independent of its effects on PI3K signaling. Through the use of models in which *Pten* is deleted specifically in T cells, it is becoming increasingly clear that control over autoimmunity and lymphomagenesis by PTEN involves multi-faceted functions of this molecule at multiple stages within the T cell compartment.

Keywords: Pten, T cells, autoimmunity, lymphoma

INTRODUCTION

Class 1A PI3Ks are directly linked to lymphocyte activation mainly through receptor tyrosine kinases, such as the antigen and cytokine receptors (Engelman et al., 2006; Huang and Sauer, 2010; So and Fruman, 2012). Class 1A PI3Ks, hereafter referred to as PI3K, are comprised of a catalytic subunit of 110 kDa (of which there are three isoforms) that generates phosphatidylinositol 3,4,5 phosphate (PIP3) from its main substrate phosphatidylinositol 4,5 phosphate (PIP2), and a regulatory subunit (of which there are five isoforms). *Pten* encodes a protein with a lipid phosphatase function that directly opposes PI3K signaling by dephosphorylating PIP3 at the 3′ position to generate PIP2. Cells lacking PTEN have elevated levels of PIP3 and constitutive activation of PI3K signaling pathways (Stambolic et al., 1998; Cantley and Neel, 1999). With increasing age, mice heterozygous for *Pten* develop T cell lymphomas and cancers in multiple tissues, and develop a lethal polyclonal autoimmune disorder, similar to that seen in Fas-deficient mice (Di Cristofano et al., 1998, 1999; Podsypanina et al., 1999; Suzuki et al., 2001). Germline mutations in *PTEN* occur in a group of autosomal dominant syndromes known as the PTEN hamartoma tumor syndromes, which include Cowden syndrome, Proteus syndrome, Proteus-like syndrome, and Bannayan–Riley–Ruvalcaba syndrome, demonstrating the importance of PTEN as a tumor suppressor. Consistent with this, genomic amplification and mutation of either PI3K or Akt has been reported in a large number of cancers as well (Samuels et al., 2004; Lee et al., 2005; Carpten et al., 2007; Jaiswal et al., 2009), although the role of PTEN as a tumor suppressor is now believed to involve more than its ability to oppose PI3K signaling. While disruption of regulation by PTEN has the overt phenotype of cancer progression, PTEN also plays an important role in maintaining T cell tolerance at multiple stages within the T cell compartment.

ACTIVATION AND REGULATION OF PI3K CLASS 1A IN T LYMPHOCYTES

Upon ligation of the T cell receptor (TCR) in the presence of co-stimulatory molecules, PI3K recruitment and activation leads to the production of lipid products which in turn recruit downstream PH-domain containing targets such as PDK1 and Akt (see **Figure 1**). Ultimately, these events lead to activation of the mTOR pathway and inactivation of members of the Foxo family, inducing growth and proliferation of T cells and acquisition of effector function (for review, see Engelman et al., 2006; Finlay and Cantrell, 2010; So and Fruman, 2012). In the absence of PTEN, TCR stimulation alone results in hyperactivation of the PI3K pathway, resulting in effective cytokine production and proliferation independent of co-stimulation (Buckler et al., 2006). Thus, put another way, negative regulation of PI3K signaling by PTEN enforces the requirement for co-stimulation in naïve T cells. However, the notion that PI3K signaling is required for co-stimulation to mediate its effects has been challenged by the generation of mice which lack all isoforms of the regulatory subunit of class 1A PI3K in T cells (Deane et al., 2007). T cells from these mice are able to proliferate under co-stimulatory conditions in the absence of detectable Akt signaling. These mice also maintained a normal anti-viral response upon MHV infection, although *in vivo* T helper function to B cell antibody responses was impaired. Whether the relative lack of defects is due to the fact that lack of PI3K was genetic, rather than acquired, is not known. However, these studies indicate that potential therapies targeting PI3K for inflammatory diseases and cancer may not compromise all aspects of cellular immunity, and further suggest that PI3K signaling has specialized functions in the context of T cell activation.

PI3K activation is critical for optimal responses of T cells to cytokines which utilize the common gamma chain. For example,

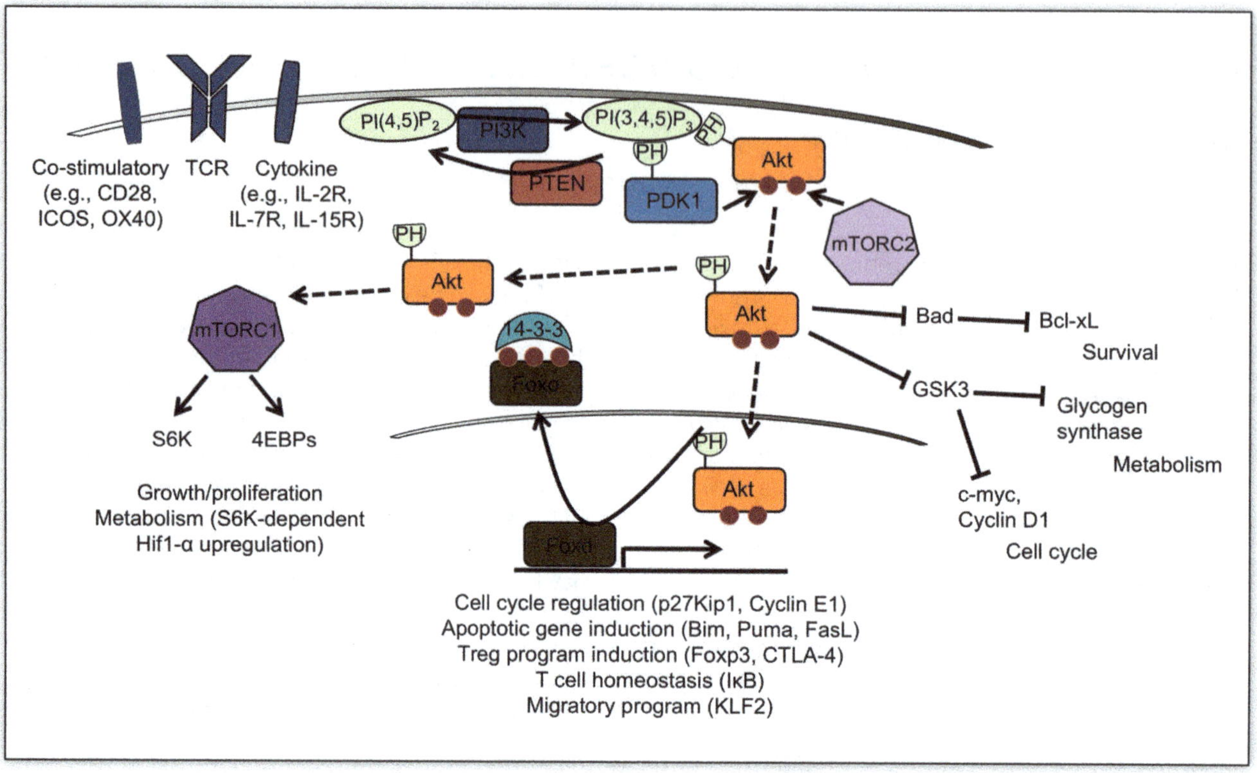

FIGURE 1 | PTEN/PI3K signaling in mature T cells. Class 1A PI3Ks are activated by receptor tyrosine kinases that drive co-stimulatory, T cell receptor (TCR), and cytokine signaling pathways. PTEN directly opposes PI3K signaling by converting PI(3,4,5)P3 to PI(4,5)P2. Through their PH-domains, PDK1 and Akt bind PIP3, enabling Akt to be phosphorylated by PDK1 on Ser308. Full activation of Akt requires phosphorylation on Ser473 by mTORC2. Akt can then target downstream substrates such as Foxos in the nucleus, leading to their inactivation and export from the nucleus. This results in attenuation of a Foxo-dependent gene program normally acting to promote pathways involved in, but not limited to, T cell homeostasis (in resting T cells), apoptosis (upon, for example, cytokine withdrawal), Treg induction, and homing to secondary lymphoid organs (in circulating, naïve T cells). Akt also targets TSC2 and Pras40 (not shown), negative regulators of mTORC1, allowing for activation of mTORC1. Activation of S6K and 4EBPs by mTORC1 results in increased protein translation, allowing growth and proliferation, and upregulation of Hif-1α, important for glycolytic metabolism. Inhibitory targeting of Bad and GSK3 also contribute to Akt's effect on cell cycle, survival and metabolism.

engagement of the IL-2R on activated T cells results in activation of the Jak/Stat pathway, as well as the PI3K and MAPK pathways, and the combination of these signals is required for the observed proliferation and cell survival in response to IL-2. Thus, appropriate responses to TCR ligation and cytokines require downregulation of PTEN, which is constitutively expressed in naïve T cells. This normally occurs as a consequence of TCR stimulation itself, which terminates detectable PTEN expression within 24–48 h. The importance of this is demonstrated by two findings. First, retroviral mediated "enforced" expression of PTEN renders activated IL-2R$^+$ T cells unable to fully respond to IL-2 stimulation. Second, regulatory T cells, which normally do not divide in response to IL-2 alone, have complete responses and signaling to IL-2 restored solely by genetic ablation of *Pten* (Bensinger et al., 2004; Walsh et al., 2006; Locke et al., 2009). This demonstrates that control of PI3K through PTEN plays an important role not only in modulating the degree of activation signals within lymphocytes, but in maintaining traits of a specific lineage.

PI3K-related signals can modulate ongoing responses as well. Deletion of *Pten*, or expression of constitutively active myristoylated-Akt, within the CD8$^+$ T cell compartment inhibits the development and survival of memory CD8$^+$ T cells (Hand et al., 2010). On the contrary, Akt is required for a transcriptional program leading to upregulation of cytolytic effector, chemokine, and adhesion molecules (Macintyre et al., 2011). Conditional deletion of *Pten* using OX40-Cre has demonstrated that PTEN plays a critical role in limiting the expansion of Tfh cells and in maintaining control over GC reactions, indicating that T cell intrinsic roles of PTEN are crucial for maintaining global levels of tolerance (Rolf et al., 2010). Lastly, the promotion of iTreg generation and maintenance by PD-L1 is associated with downregulation of Akt signaling and concomitant upregulation of PTEN expression (Francisco et al., 2009). These examples all provide evidence that the balance of Akt signaling within multiple stages of development and differentiation states helps determine cellular fate.

PTEN also has been shown to play an important role in central tolerance and in regulating proliferation of developing cells in the thymus (Suzuki et al., 2001; Hagenbeek et al., 2004). In the absence of IL-7R and pre-TCR signaling, loss of Pten allows cells to bypass the β-selection checkpoint, indicating that PI3K signaling is crucial for the ongoing development of early T cell precursors. Interestingly, thymic cellularity and subset percentages are relatively unperturbed prior to tumor development, which likely occurs at the DP stage during thymic maturation, suggesting that secondary events emerge in this context of Pten loss to promote transformation (discussed below; Hagenbeek et al., 2004; Hagenbeek and Spits, 2008; Xue et al., 2008; Guo et al., 2011).

SIGNALING DOWNSTREAM OF Pten-PI3K-Akt: A CRITICAL ROLE FOR Foxos

Members of the Foxo family of transcription factors play a critical role in DNA damage and oxidative stress responses (Tran et al., 2002; Miyamoto et al., 2007; Tothova et al., 2007; Choi et al., 2009) and in preventing entry into cell cycle (Medema et al., 2000), acting as bona fide tumor suppressors as demonstrated in hematopoietic and epithelial tissues (Coffer, 2003; Accili and Arden, 2004; Paik et al., 2007). It is becoming increasingly appreciated that Foxos play important roles within the T cell compartment as well, regulating homing (Fabre et al., 2008; Sinclair et al., 2008; Finlay et al., 2009; Kerdiles et al., 2009; Finlay and Cantrell, 2010), survival (Hedrick, 2009; Kerdiles et al., 2009; Dejean et al., 2011), and the development and function of effector and memory subsets (Kerdiles et al., 2010; Ouyang et al., 2010; Rao et al., 2012). In quiescent cells, Foxos are active within the nucleus, where they maintain the pattern of chemokine and adhesion molecule expression, and expression of the IL-7R, needed for the migration and survival of circulating T cells (Fabre et al., 2008; Finlay et al., 2009; Kerdiles et al., 2010). Akt phosphorylation on Ser473, mediated by mTORC2, is critical for Foxo inactivation, implicating mTOR in control over Foxos, and placing PTEN upstream in this pathway. Importantly, mTORC2 has been shown to be critical for the phenotype in models of PTEN loss. Prostate cancer caused by conditional *Pten* deletion in prostate epithelium requires mTORC2, and deletion of one copy of *Rictor*, required for mTORC2 complex assembly and activity, was sufficient to protect *Pten* heterozygous mice from prostate cancer (Guertin et al., 2009).

The role of Foxos in T cells was first described using mice in which retroviral gene-trap targeting of embryonic stem cells was used to generate a null *Foxo3* allele, although the authors could not rule out the possibility that undetectable levels of a truncated form of Foxo3 was produced (Lin et al., 2004). These mice exhibited spontaneous lymphoproliferation and multi-organ lymphocyte infiltration, indicating that Foxo3 is important for the control of T cell tolerance and homeostasis. This hyper-activated phenotype was correlated with decreased expression of IκBε and IκBβ, leading to increased NF-κB activation. As IKKβ has been shown to phosphorylate and inactivate Foxos (Hu et al., 2004), this implicates Foxos in a critical negative feedback loop that may serve to limit inflammatory responses in certain settings, and is potentially important in the context of tumors which maintain low levels of Akt activation. Other studies using *Foxo3*-deficient strains did not find the same immunological defects (Hosaka et al., 2004; Dejean et al., 2009), attesting first to the redundancy of members of this family and, second, to the possibility of dominant-negative effects of undetected Foxo3 gene products in the aforementioned mice. T cell-specific loss of Foxo1 was shown to severely disrupt T cell homeostasis, resulting in multi-organ lymphocyte infiltration as well as exocrine pancreatitis and hind limb paralysis (Kerdiles et al., 2010). This was attributed to a defect in both the development and function of $Foxp3^+$ regulatory T cells, and this phenotype was exacerbated by combined deletion of *Foxo1* and *Foxo3* (Kerdiles et al., 2010; Ouyang et al., 2010). More recently, Foxo3a has been mechanistically linked to anergy induction in T cells through upregulation of Sirt1 (Gao et al., 2012). IL-2 was shown to reverse T cell anergy through the PI3K pathway by inactivation of Foxos, which prevented transcriptional upregulation of Sirt1.

In mouse embryonic fibroblasts and lymphoid cells, growth factor and cytokine withdrawal upregulates BH3-only pro-apoptotic mediators Puma and Bim in a Foxo3a-dependent manner that requires downregulation of PI3K/Akt signaling (You et al., 2006). These findings strongly support the idea that impaired downregulation of PI3K activity, as seen in T cells lacking PTEN, results in survival effects and apoptotic resistance in response to cytokine deprivation through inactivation of Foxo family members. FasL has been shown to be another important target of Foxo (Brunet et al., 1999). Given that *Pten* heterozygous mice display decreased sensitivity to Fas-mediated AICD, similar to *lpr* and *gld* mice (Van Parijs and Abbas, 1996), constitutive inactivation of Foxos due to loss of PTEN is likely a partial mechanism underlying the phenotype observed in these mice. Additionally, the finding that a deficiency in Foxos is sufficient to drive the development of hemangiomas, similar to what is seen in patients with Cowden disease and Bannayan–Zonana syndrome, and thymic lymphomas, similar to mice with a T cell-specific deletion of *Pten*, as well suggests that inactivation of Foxos may be critical for the phenotype brought on by loss of *Pten* (Paik et al., 2007).

LYMPHOMA AND DYSREGULATED IMMUNE FUNCTION IN THE ABSENCE OF PTEN

Genetic studies in mice expressing conditional alleles of *Pten* have been crucial for studying the tissue specific role of PTEN in tumorigenesis. Deletion of *Pten* during hematopoiesis using Mx-1-Cre results in myeloproliferative disease and transplantable leukemia, and has shown that PTEN is required for maintaining the hematopoietic stem cell (HSC) compartment (Yilmaz et al., 2006; Lee et al., 2010). Similar to the Mx-1-Cre model of PTEN loss, Vec-Cre-mediated PTEN loss, in which nearly 40% of fetal liver HSCs were subject to deletion of *Pten*, led to impaired HSC self-renewal and the development of a myeloproliferative disorder followed by leukemia (Guo et al., 2008). It is notable that this phenotype shares striking similarity to mice in which all six alleles of *Foxo1/3a/4* were deleted by Mx-1-Cre (Tothova et al., 2007), and to $Foxo3a^{-/-}$ mice (Miyamoto et al., 2007). Importantly, this study reported the same t(14;15) chromosomal translocation (seen within a subset of human T-ALL), in all blast-crisis samples analyzed from these mice, suggesting a critical genomic destabilizing event potentially independent of PTEN's role in controlling PI3K/Akt signaling. Similarly, this translocation, involving the *c-myc* and *TCRα/δ* loci and resulting in constitutively high levels of c-myc, was found to recur with 100% incidence in T cell lymphomas from mice in which *Pten* was deleted specifically in T cells (CD4-Cre × $Pten^{fl/fl}$ mice, hereafter referred to as PTEN-ΔT mice; Liu et al., 2010). Thus, well after T lineage commitment in mice subject to lymphoma and lymphoproliferative autoimmune disease, PTEN is critical to prevent the emergence of the same genetic abnormality present in HSCs that correlates with the selective pressure of these cells for the development of leukemia.

A deficiency in *Rag1* or *TCRα* prevented the t(14;15) translocation event in PTEN-ΔT mice, but did not inhibit malignant transformation, although lymphomagenesis developed with delayed onset and was primarily restricted to the thymus (Liu et al., 2010). Interestingly, mature T cells from 3-week-old PTEN-ΔT mice that had not undergone transformation, when transferred into either immunocompetent or immunoincompetent recipients, did not develop a malignant phenotype throughout the duration of the host's life, suggesting that malignancy arises within the thymus after a period of latency in these mice, consistent with an earlier report demonstrating that transplanted $Pten^{-/-}$ thymocytes gave rise to T cell lymphomas in immunodeficient recipients (Hagenbeek and Spits, 2008). Supporting this, PTEN-ΔT mice thymectomized at 3 weeks of age did not develop lymphoma, although later in life these mice exhibited signs of systemic autoimmunity. Thus, within distinct developmental stages, PTEN is required for the prevention of lymphoma and autoimmunity.

In the context of DNA damage, loss of PTEN enables cells to bypass the normal G2/M checkpoint enforced by CHK1 as a result of Akt-mediated CHK1 sequestration in the cytoplasm (Puc et al., 2005). Akt has also been shown to promote prosurvival responses following DNA double-strand breaks (DSBs; Bozulic et al., 2008). It is possible that secondary mutations or other genetic alterations occurred in $Rag1^{-/-}$ or $TCR\alpha^{-/-}$ × PTEN-ΔT mice as a result of genetic instability due to PTEN loss, and that hyper-active Akt maintains the survival of these cells that would normally undergo apoptosis. Spectral karyotyping analyses, however, failed to detect any chromosomal translocations in these mice to support this idea. Induction of the Notch pathway in malignant cells from these mice, however, was shown to increase cellular levels of c-myc, suggesting that PI3K and c-myc cooperate in multiple models of PTEN loss to promote lymphomagenesis and lymphoproliferative autoimmune disorder.

Disruption of Foxo function has been shown to accelerate c-myc-driven lymphomagenesis (Bouchard et al., 2007), and constitutively active mutants of Foxo3a resistant to inactivation by Akt directly repress multiple target genes of c-myc and block c-myc-dependent proliferation and transformation (Bouchard et al., 2004; Jensen et al., 2011). Together, this offers the possibility that c-myc and PI3K cooperate in tumorigenesis through inactivation of Foxos. Whether or not restoration of Foxo signaling in mice lacking PTEN in T cells has an effect on metabolism, survival, infiltrative capacity, lymphomagenesis, or the prevention of autoimmunity remains to be seen.

A recent study in which $Pten^{fl/fl}$ × CD4-Cre mice were crossed to $PDK1^{fl/fl}$ mice has shown that while lymphoma did not develop in this model of T cell-specific *Pten* deletion, PDK1/Akt signaling was dispensable for the survival, proliferation and differentiation of T cell progenitors, and *in vivo* expansion of peripheral T cells (Finlay et al., 2009). The mechanism for control of cell metabolism independent of PDK1 is unclear in these mice, although thymocyte proliferation in the absence of PTEN was shown to require RhoA-dependent pathways, and a dependence on c-myc, which was recently shown to play a pivotal role in T cell metabolism following activation (Wang et al., 2011), was not ruled out. Mice which express a single hypomorphic *PDK1* allele similarly prevented a wide range of tumors when crossed to *Pten* heterozygous mice, indicating that the requirement for PDK1 in the context of tumor formation brought on by loss of PTEN is not limited to its role in controlling migratory capacity of T cells (Bayascas et al., 2005). Additionally, deletion of S6K1 in the Mx-1-Cre model of Pten loss resulted in delayed development of leukemia, indicating that an mTORC1-mediated pathway, in this context shown to involve induction of a Hif-1α-dependent glycolytic program, contributes to leukemogenesis in Pten-deficient cells (Tandon et al., 2011).

Akt-INDEPENDENT ROLES OF PTEN

PTEN nuclear function, independent of its lipid phosphatase activity, has been shown to contribute to its tumor-suppressive effects and, in particular, in maintaining genomic stability. Control of DNA stability and DSB repair has in part been attributed to interaction of PTEN with an integral kinetochore protein, CENP-C. Mutants originally identified in Cowden disease patients demonstrated that the C-terminus of PTEN, but not the phosphatase domain, was required for interaction with centromeres and with CENP-C, and that DNA instability and DSBs could be prevented by a phosphatase-dead PTEN mutant which retained its ability to bind to CENP-C (Shen et al., 2007). Additionally, nuclear exclusion of PTEN, but not a phosphatase-inactive mutant, was shown to impair the tumor-suppressive APC-CDH1 nuclear complex, again demonstrating tumor-suppressive capability of catalytically inactive PTEN (Song et al., 2011). Additional protein–protein interactions within the nucleus, independent of PTEN catalytic activity, have been shown to increase the activity and stability of p53 (Li et al., 2006; Salmena et al., 2008), and upregulate expression of Rad51, an essential component of the DSB repair machinery (Baker, 2007; Shen et al., 2007). A lysine to glutamate mutation in PTEN (K289E) identified in a Cowden syndrome family, which lead to a dramatic decrease in nuclear import without disrupting phosphatase activity or membrane localization of PTEN, as well strongly supports the idea that nuclear PTEN can be critical for tumor suppression independent of its role in opposing PI3K signaling in certain contexts (Trotman et al., 2007; See **Figure 2**).

Inactivation of PTEN phosphatase activity is sufficient to abrogate its tumor-suppressive effects, emphasizing the importance of PTEN's role in downregulation of PI3K signaling. This has been demonstrated by a subset of Cowden disease patients that harbor a missense mutation at a cysteine residue (C124) critical for phosphatase activity. A C124S mutant has been shown to form a stable complex with PIP3, potentially protecting it from dephosphorylation by other lipid phosphatases to account for higher cellular levels of PIP3 compared to conditions in which PTEN is completely absent (Myers et al., 1998). As well, the importance of Akt activity in tumor development induced by loss of PTEN has been reported in a number of studies (Stiles et al., 2002;

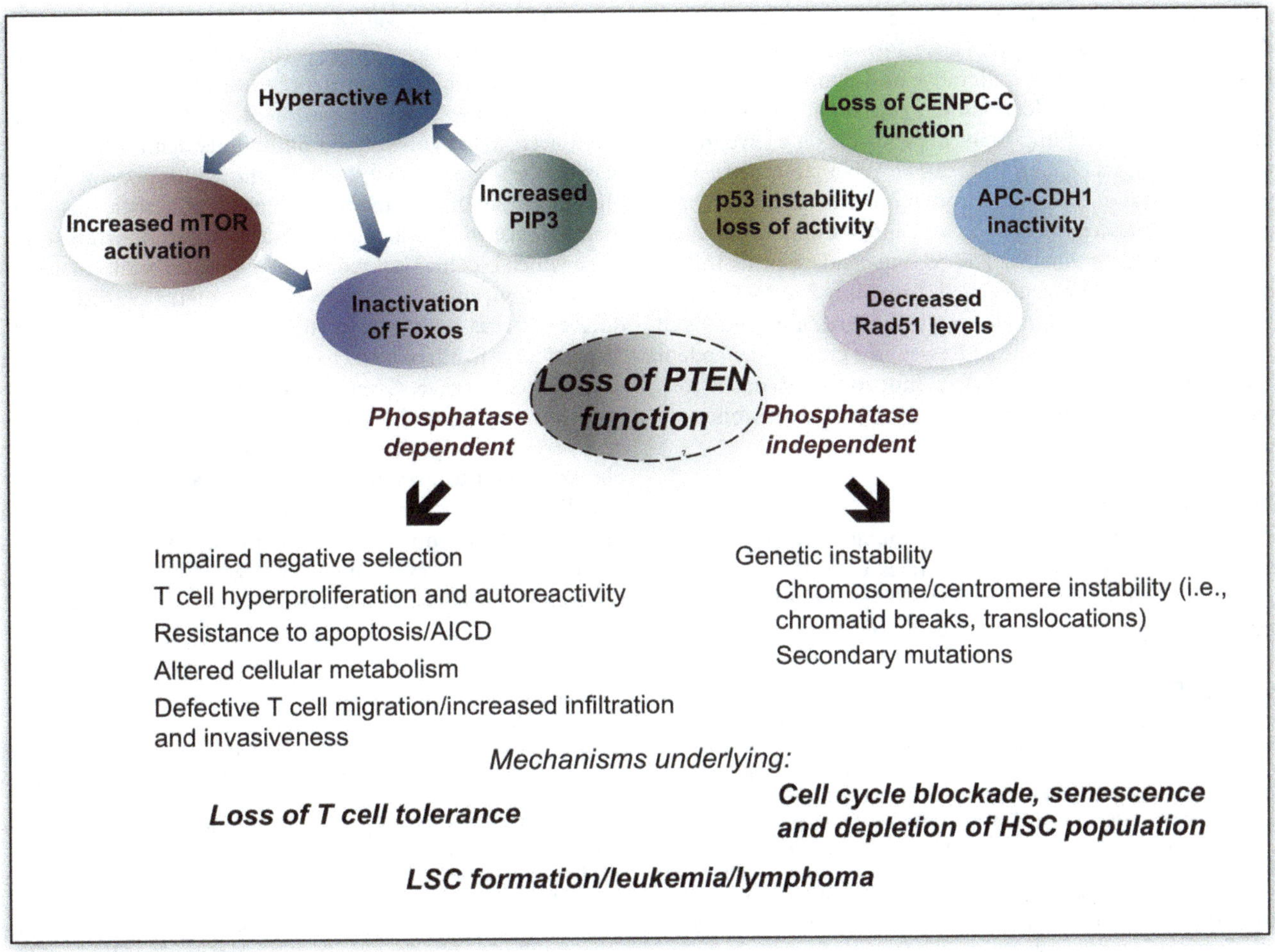

FIGURE 2 | Molecular and phenotypic consequences of loss of PTEN phosphatase-dependent and -independent functions during hematopoiesis and within the T cell compartment. Loss of PTEN phosphatase activity results in increased levels of PIP3, causing hyperactivation of the Akt pathway and subsequent activation of the mTOR pathway, and inactivation of the Foxo family of transcription factors. Disruption of PTEN phosphatase-independent function accounts for loss of much of its nuclear activity, compromising genetic stability and DSB repair, leading to chromatid breaks and translocations. That mature T cells do not undergo transformation, and that lymphoma in T cell-specific PTEN knockout mice is of thymic origin, suggests that PTEN phosphatase-independent function contributes less to the phenotype at the mature T cell stage, and that loss of T cell tolerance can likely be attributed to loss of PTEN phosphatase activity. Whether depletion of hematopoietic stem cells (HSCs) and development of leukemia stem cells (LSCs), as well lymphomagenesis, depends on the absence of PTEN phosphatase activity (which likely maintains survival of genetically aberrant cells), PTEN phosphatase-independent activity (promoting genetic instability), or both, remains an open question.

Bayascas et al., 2005; Chen et al., 2006). Constitutive Akt activation in T cells and thymocytes has been shown to be sufficient to drive autoimmunity and lymphoma (Rathmell et al., 2003) and thymomas (Malstrom et al., 2001), respectively, and bone marrow chimera experiments have demonstrated that enforced expression of constitutively active Akt in HSCs was sufficient for the development of myeloproliferative disease, T cell lymphoma, or AML (Kharas et al., 2010).

PTEN-ΔT mice crossed onto the *Rag1*$^{-/-}$ background, which do not harbor the t(14;15) translocation, potentially serve as an example in which Akt signaling is not sufficient to drive cancer progression (Liu et al., 2010). *In vitro* studies using malignant cells from these mice demonstrated a dependence on Notch, suggesting that Akt at the very least must cooperate with other oncogenic pathways to allow tumor growth in this model, similar to what has been suggested in an MMTV-myrAkt breast cancer model with respect to tumorigenesis induced by loss of PTEN (Blanco-Aparicio et al., 2007). In contrast to this, in a model of Notch-induced tumorigenesis, genetic loss of *Pten* induced an oncogene addiction switch that rendered T-ALL cells resistant to Notch inhibition through GSIs and dependent on PI3K/Akt signaling to maintain tumor growth (Palomero et al., 2007). Thus, the reliance on Akt signaling differs among models of PTEN loss. This idea is perhaps emphasized by the observation that PTEN-ΔT mice, regardless of whether the t(14;15) translocation event occurs, maintain constitutively high levels of c-myc.

The reliance on c-myc in the context of PTEN loss remains an important question. In tumors driven by inducible c-myc activation in a zebrafish model of T-ALL, constitutive activation of the Akt pathway through genetic disruption of *Pten* or transgenic expression of Akt2 rendered cells in this model independent of c-myc for tumor progression (Gutierrez et al., 2011). Conversely, conditional genetic disruption of both *Pten* and *c-myc* in mice, while still subject to myeloproliferative and lymphoproliferative disorders, prevented the development of hematopoietic malignancies, highlighting an important dependence on c-myc in this context of PTEN loss (Zhang et al., 2011). Whether loss of PTEN allows the survival of cells that, through other mechanisms, have acquired genetic aberrations, such as translocations resulting in constitutive c-myc, or whether PTEN, independent of its role in PI3K downregulation, prevents genetic instability that collaborates with dysregulation of PI3K to allow cancer progression, remains an open question that needs to be addressed in a context-dependent manner, with consideration of what function of PTEN is lost, changes in levels of expression, and in which tissues abnormal growth originates.

FUTURE DIRECTIONS

Pten is the one of the most frequently mutated or lost genes in human cancer. Given the emerging roles of PI3K in immune system regulation, it is possible that PTEN is also playing a prominent role in the prevention of autoimmune disease and inflammatory/lymphoproliferative syndromes. The finding that PTEN did not play a role in lymphomagenesis in mature T cells from mice which lack PTEN specifically in T cells suggested that PTEN has a specific function in preventing lymphoma within a distinct time frame in this compartment. That these non-malignant T cells were able to provoke autoimmunity demonstrates that well beyond the stage at which Pten is required for prevention of lymphomagenesis in this model, PTEN plays a critical role in the maintenance of T cell tolerance. It will be important to determine which biochemical requirements PTEN fulfills in each stage of protection, and whether these requirements are distinct within different stages from cells of the same lineage, or whether lack of particular features leads to different outcomes depending on developmental stage. Given the importance of PI3K signaling in both normal immunity and the development of cancer, it will be interesting to see how closely PTEN's role as a lipid phosphatase is tied to prevention of disease, and how integral PI3K signaling remains throughout disease progression. Uncovering the specific biochemical functions of PTEN within these contexts will be key to the development of targeted therapies for the prevention and treatment of T cell malignancies and autoimmune disease.

REFERENCES

Accili, D., and Arden, K. C. (2004). FoxOs at the crossroads of cellular metabolism, differentiation, and transformation. *Cell* 117, 421–426.

Baker, S. J. (2007). PTEN enters the nuclear age. *Cell* 128, 25–28.

Bayascas, J. R., Leslie, N. R., Parsons, R., Fleming, S., and Alessi, D. R. (2005). Hypomorphic mutation of PDK1 suppresses tumorigenesis in PTEN(+/−) mice. *Curr. Biol.* 15, 1839–1846.

Bensinger, S. J., Walsh, P. T., Zhang, J., Carroll, M., Parsons, R., Rathmell, J. C., Thompson, C. B., Burchill, M. A., Farrar, M. A., and Turka, L. A. (2004). Distinct IL-2 receptor signaling pattern in CD4+CD25+ regulatory T cells. *J. Immunol.* 172, 5287–5296.

Blanco-Aparicio, C., Renner, O., Leal, J. F., and Carnero, A. (2007). PTEN, more than the AKT pathway. *Carcinogenesis* 28, 1379–1386.

Bouchard, C., Lee, S., Paulus-Hock, V., Loddenkemper, C., Eilers, M., and Schmitt, C. A. (2007). FoxO transcription factors suppress Myc-driven lymphomagenesis via direct activation of Arf. *Genes Dev.* 21, 2775–2787.

Bouchard, C., Marquardt, J., Bras, A., Medema, R. H., and Eilers, M. (2004). Myc-induced proliferation and transformation require Akt-mediated phosphorylation of FoxO proteins. *EMBO J.* 23, 2830–2840.

Bozulic, L., Surucu, B., Hynx, D., and Hemmings, B. A. (2008). PKBalpha/Akt1 acts downstream of DNA-PK in the DNA double-strand break response and promotes survival. *Mol. Cell* 30, 203–213.

Brunet, A., Bonni, A., Zigmond, M. J., Lin, M. Z., Juo, P., Hu, L. S., Anderson, M. J., Arden, K. C., Blenis, J., and Greenberg, M. E. (1999). Akt promotes cell survival by phosphorylating and inhibiting a Forkhead transcription factor. *Cell* 96, 857–868.

Buckler, J. L., Walsh, P. T., Porrett, P. M., Choi, Y., and Turka, L. A. (2006). Cutting edge: T cell requirement for CD28 costimulation is due to negative regulation of TCR signals by PTEN. *J. Immunol.* 177, 4262–4266.

Cantley, L. C., and Neel, B. G. (1999). New insights into tumor suppression: PTEN suppresses tumor formation by restraining the phosphoinositide 3-kinase/AKT pathway. *Proc. Natl. Acad. Sci. U.S.A.* 96, 4240–4245.

Carpten, J. D., Faber, A. L., Horn, C., Donoho, G. P., Briggs, S. L., Robbins, C. M., Hostetter, G., Boguslawski, S., Moses, T. Y., Savage, S., Uhlik, M., Lin, A., Du, J., Qian, Y. W., Zeckner, D. J., Tucker-Kellogg, G., Touchman, J., Patel, K., Mousses, S., Bittner, M., Schevitz, R., Lai, M. H., Blanchard, K. L., and Thomas, J. E. (2007). A transforming mutation in the pleckstrin homology domain of AKT1 in cancer. *Nature* 448, 439–444.

Chen, M. L., Xu, P. Z., Peng, X. D., Chen, W. S., Guzman, G., Yang, X., Di Cristofano, A., Pandolfi, P. P., and Hay, N. (2006). The deficiency of Akt1 is sufficient to suppress tumor development in Pten+/− mice. *Genes Dev.* 20, 1569–1574.

Choi, J., Oh, S., Lee, D., Oh, H. J., Park, J. Y., Lee, S. B., and Lim, D. S. (2009). Mst1-FoxO signaling protects Naive T lymphocytes from cellular oxidative stress in mice. *PLoS ONE* 4, e8011. doi: 10.1371/journal.pone.0008011

Coffer, P. J. (2003). Transcriptional regulation of lymphocyte quiescence: as cunning as a FOX. *Trends Immunol.* 24, 470–471; author reply 471.

Deane, J. A., Kharas, M. G., Oak, J. S., Stiles, L. N., Luo, J., Moore, T. I., Ji, H., Rommel, C., Cantley, L. C., Lane, T. E., and Fruman, D. A. (2007). T-cell function is partially maintained in the absence of class IA phosphoinositide 3-kinase signaling. *Blood* 109, 2894–2902.

Dejean, A. S., Beisner, D. R., Ch'en, I. L., Kerdiles, Y. M., Babour, A., Arden, K. C., Castrillon, D. H., DePinho, R. A., and Hedrick, S. M. (2009). Transcription factor Foxo3 controls the magnitude of T cell immune responses by modulating the function of dendritic cells. *Nat. Immunol.* 10, 504–513.

Dejean, A. S., Hedrick, S. M., and Kerdiles, Y. M. (2011). Highly specialized role of Forkhead box O transcription factors in the immune system. *Antioxid. Redox Signal.* 14, 663–674.

Di Cristofano, A., Kotsi, P., Peng, Y. F., Cordon-Cardo, C., Elkon, K. B., and Pandolfi, P. P. (1999). Impaired Fas response and autoimmunity in Pten+/− mice. *Science* 285, 2122–2125.

Di Cristofano, A., Pesce, B., Cordon-Cardo, C., and Pandolfi, P. P. (1998). Pten is essential for embryonic development and tumour suppression. *Nat. Genet.* 19, 348–355.

Engelman, J. A., Luo, J., and Cantley, L. C. (2006). The evolution of phosphatidylinositol 3-kinases as regulators of growth and metabolism. *Nat. Rev. Genet.* 7, 606–619.

Fabre, S., Carrette, F., Chen, J., Lang, V., Semichon, M., Denoyelle, C., Lazar, V., Cagnard, N., Dubart-Kupperschmitt, A., Mangeney, M., Fruman, D. A., and Bismuth, G. (2008). FOXO1 regulates L-Selectin and a network of human T cell homing molecules downstream of phosphatidylinositol 3-kinase. *J. Immunol.* 181, 2980–2989.

Finlay, D., and Cantrell, D. (2010). Phosphoinositide 3-kinase and the mammalian target of rapamycin pathways control T cell migration. *Ann. N. Y. Acad. Sci.* 1183, 149–157.

Finlay, D. K., Sinclair, L. V., Feijoo, C., Waugh, C. M., Hagenbeek, T. J., Spits, H., and Cantrell, D. A. (2009). Phosphoinositide-dependent kinase 1 controls migration and malignant transformation but not cell growth and proliferation in PTEN-null lymphocytes. *J. Exp. Med.* 206, 2441–2454.

Francisco, L. M., Salinas, V. H., Brown, K. E., Vanguri, V. K., Freeman, G. J., Kuchroo, V. K., and Sharpe, A. H. (2009). PD-L1 regulates the development, maintenance, and function of induced regulatory T cells. *J. Exp. Med.* 206, 3015–3029.

Gao, B., Kong, Q., Kemp, K., Zhao, Y. S., and Fang, D. (2012). Analysis of sirtuin 1 expression reveals a molecular explanation of IL-2-mediated reversal of T-cell tolerance. *Proc. Natl. Acad. Sci. U.S.A.* 109, 899–904.

Guertin, D. A., Stevens, D. M., Saitoh, M., Kinkel, S., Crosby, K., Sheen, J. H., Mullholland, D. J., Magnuson, M. A., Wu, H., and Sabatini, D. M. (2009). mTOR complex 2 is required for the development of prostate cancer induced by Pten loss in mice. *Cancer Cell* 15, 148–159.

Guo, W., Lasky, J. L., Chang, C. J., Mosessian, S., Lewis, X., Xiao, Y., Yeh, J. E., Chen, J. Y., Iruela-Arispe, M. L., Varella-Garcia, M., and Wu, H. (2008). Multi-genetic events collaboratively contribute to Pten-null leukaemia stem-cell formation. *Nature* 453, 529–533.

Guo, W., Schubbert, S., Chen, J. Y., Valamehr, B., Mosessian, S., Shi, H., Dang, N. H., Garcia, C., Theodoro, M. F., Varella-Garcia, M., and Wu, H. (2011). Suppression of leukemia development caused by PTEN loss. *Proc. Natl. Acad. Sci. U.S.A.* 108, 1409–1414.

Gutierrez, A., Grebliunaite, R., Feng, H., Kozakewich, E., Zhu, S., Guo, F., Payne, E., Mansour, M., Dahlberg, S. E., Neuberg, D. S., den Hertog, J., Prochownik, E. V., Testa, J. R., Harris, M., Kanki, J. P., and Look, A. T. (2011). Pten mediates Myc oncogene dependence in a conditional zebrafish model of T cell acute lymphoblastic leukemia. *J. Exp. Med.* 208, 1595–1603.

Hagenbeek, T. J., Naspetti, M., Malergue, F., Garcon, F., Nunes, J. A., Cleutjens, K. B., Trapman, J., Krimpenfort, P., and Spits, H. (2004). The loss of PTEN allows TCR alphabeta lineage thymocytes to bypass IL-7 and Pre-TCR-mediated signaling. *J. Exp. Med.* 200, 883–894.

Hagenbeek, T. J., and Spits, H. (2008). T-cell lymphomas in T-cell-specific Pten-deficient mice originate in the thymus. *Leukemia* 22, 608–619.

Hand, T. W., Cui, W., Jung, Y. W., Sefik, E., Joshi, N. S., Chandele, A., Liu, Y., and Kaech, S. M. (2010). Differential effects of STAT5 and PI3K/AKT signaling on effector and memory CD8 T-cell survival. *Proc. Natl. Acad. Sci. U.S.A.* 107, 16601–16606.

Hedrick, S. M. (2009). The cunning little vixen: Foxo and the cycle of life and death. *Nat. Immunol.* 10, 1057–1063.

Hosaka, T., Biggs, W. H. III, Tieu, D., Boyer, A. D., Varki, N. M., Cavenee, W. K., and Arden, K. C. (2004). Disruption of forkhead transcription factor (FOXO) family members in mice reveals their functional diversification. *Proc. Natl. Acad. Sci. U.S.A.* 101, 2975–2980.

Hu, M. C., Lee, D. F., Xia, W., Golfman, L. S., Ou-Yang, F., Yang, J. Y., Zou, Y., Bao, S., Hanada, N., Saso, H., Kobayashi, R., and Hung, M. C. (2004). IkappaB kinase promotes tumorigenesis through inhibition of forkhead FOXO3a. *Cell* 117, 225–237.

Huang, Y. H., and Sauer, K. (2010). Lipid signaling in T-cell development and function. *Cold Spring Harb. Perspect. Biol.* 2, a002428.

Jaiswal, B. S., Janakiraman, V., Kljavin, N. M., Chaudhuri, S., Stern, H. M., Wang, W., Kan, Z., Dbouk, H. A., Peters, B. A., Waring, P., Dela Vega, T., Kenski, D. M., Bowman, K. K., Lorenzo, M., Li, H., Wu, J., Modrusan, Z., Stinson, J., Eby, M., Yue, P., Kaminker, J. S., de Sauvage, F. J., Backer, J. M., and Seshagiri, S. (2009). Somatic mutations in p85alpha promote tumorigenesis through class IA PI3K activation. *Cancer Cell* 16, 463–474.

Jensen, K. S., Binderup, T., Jensen, K. T., Therkelsen, I., Borup, R., Nilsson, E., Multhaupt, H., Bouchard, C., Quistorff, B., Kjaer, A., Landberg, G., and Staller, P. (2011). FoxO3A promotes metabolic adaptation to hypoxia by antagonizing Myc function. *EMBO J.* 30, 4554–4570.

Kerdiles, Y. M., Beisner, D. R., Tinoco, R., Dejean, A. S., Castrillon, D. H., DePinho, R. A., and Hedrick, S. M. (2009). Foxo1 links homing and survival of naive T cells by regulating L-selectin, CCR7 and interleukin 7 receptor. *Nat. Immunol.* 10, 176–184.

Kerdiles, Y. M., Stone, E. L., Beisner, D. R., McGargill, M. A., Ch'en, I. L., Stockmann, C., Katayama, C. D., and Hedrick, S. M. (2010). Foxo transcription factors control regulatory T cell development and function. *Immunity* 33, 890–904.

Kharas, M. G., Okabe, R., Ganis, J. J., Gozo, M., Khandan, T., Paktinat, M., Gilliland, D. G., and Gritsman, K. (2010). Constitutively active AKT depletes hematopoietic stem cells and induces leukemia in mice. *Blood* 115, 1406–1415.

Lee, J. W., Soung, Y. H., Kim, S. Y., Lee, H. W., Park, W. S., Nam, S. W., Kim, S. H., Lee, J. Y., Yoo, N. J., and Lee, S. H. (2005). PIK3CA gene is frequently mutated in breast carcinomas and hepatocellular carcinomas. *Oncogene* 24, 1477–1480.

Lee, J. Y., Nakada, D., Yilmaz, O. H., Tothova, Z., Joseph, N. M., Lim, M. S., Gilliland, D. G., and Morrison, S. J. (2010). mTOR activation induces tumor suppressors that inhibit leukemogenesis and deplete hematopoietic stem cells after Pten deletion. *Cell Stem Cell* 7, 593–605.

Li, A. G., Piluso, L. G., Cai, X., Wei, G., Sellers, W. R., and Liu, X. (2006). Mechanistic insights into maintenance of high p53 acetylation by PTEN. *Mol. Cell* 23, 575–587.

Lin, L., Hron, J. D., and Peng, S. L. (2004). Regulation of NF-kappaB, Th activation, and autoinflammation by the forkhead transcription factor Foxo3a. *Immunity* 21, 203–213.

Liu, X., Karnell, J. L., Yin, B., Zhang, R., Zhang, J., Li, P., Choi, Y., Maltzman, J. S., Pear, W. S., Bassing, C. H., and Turka, L. A. (2010). Distinct roles for PTEN in prevention of T cell lymphoma and autoimmunity in mice. *J. Clin. Invest.* 120, 2497–2507.

Locke, N. R., Patterson, S. J., Hamilton, M. J., Sly, L. M., Krystal, G., and Levings, M. K. (2009). SHIP regulates the reciprocal development of T regulatory and Th17 cells. *J. Immunol.* 183, 975–983.

Macintyre, A. N., Finlay, D., Preston, G., Sinclair, L. V., Waugh, C. M., Tamas, P., Feijoo, C., Okkenhaug, K., and Cantrell, D. A. (2011). Protein kinase B controls transcriptional programs that direct cytotoxic T cell fate but is dispensable for T cell metabolism. *Immunity* 34, 224–236.

Malstrom, S., Tili, E., Kappes, D., Ceci, J. D., and Tsichlis, P. N. (2001). Tumor induction by an Lck-MyrAkt transgene is delayed by mechanisms controlling the size of the thymus. *Proc. Natl. Acad. Sci. U.S.A.* 98, 14967–14972.

Medema, R. H., Kops, G. J., Bos, J. L., and Burgering, B. M. (2000). AFX-like Forkhead transcription factors mediate cell-cycle regulation by Ras and PKB through p27kip1. *Nature* 404, 782–787.

Miyamoto, K., Araki, K. Y., Naka, K., Arai, F., Takubo, K., Yamazaki, S., Matsuoka, S., Miyamoto, T., Ito, K., Ohmura, M., Chen, C., Hosokawa, K., Nakauchi, H., Nakayama, K., Nakayama, K. I., Harada, M., Motoyama, N., Suda, T., and Hirao, A. (2007). Foxo3a is essential for maintenance of the hematopoietic stem cell pool. *Cell Stem Cell* 1, 101–112.

Myers, M. P., Pass, I., Batty, I. H., Van der Kaay, J., Stolarov, J. P., Hemmings, B. A., Wigler, M. H., Downes, C. P., and Tonks, N. K. (1998). The lipid phosphatase activity of PTEN is critical for its tumor suppressor function. *Proc. Natl. Acad. Sci. U.S.A.* 95, 13513–13518.

Ouyang, W., Beckett, O., Ma, Q., Paik, J. H., DePinho, R. A., and Li, M. O. (2010). Foxo proteins cooperatively control the differentiation of Foxp3+ regulatory T cells. *Nat. Immunol.* 11, 618–627.

Paik, J. H., Kollipara, R., Chu, G., Ji, H., Xiao, Y., Ding, Z., Miao, L., Tothova, Z., Horner, J. W., Carrasco, D. R., Jiang, S., Gilliland, D. G., Chin, L., Wong, W. H., Castrillon, D. H., and DePinho, R. A. (2007). FoxOs are lineage-restricted redundant tumor suppressors and regulate endothelial cell homeostasis. *Cell* 128, 309–323.

Palomero, T., Sulis, M. L., Cortina, M., Real, P. J., Barnes, K., Ciofani, M., Caparros, E., Buteau, J., Brown, K., Perkins, S. L., Bhagat, G., Agarwal, A. M., Basso, G., Castillo, M., Nagase, S., Cordon-Cardo, C., Parsons, R., Zúñiga-Pflücker, J. C., Dominguez, M., and Ferrando, A. A. (2007). Mutational loss of PTEN induces resistance to NOTCH1 inhibition in T-cell leukemia. *Nat. Med.* 13, 1203–1210.

Podsypanina, K., Ellenson, L. H., Nemes, A., Gu, J., Tamura, M., Yamada, K. M., Cordon-Cardo, C., Catoretti, G., Fisher, P. E., and Parsons, R. (1999). Mutation of Pten/Mmac1 in mice causes neoplasia in multiple organ systems. *Proc. Natl. Acad. Sci. U.S.A.* 96, 1563–1568.

Puc, J., Keniry, M., Li, H. S., Pandita, T. K., Choudhury, A. D., Memeo, L., Mansukhani, M., Murty, V. V., Gaciong, Z., Meek, S. E., Piwnica-Worms, H., Hibshoosh, H., and Parsons, R. (2005). Lack of PTEN sequesters CHK1 and initiates genetic instability. *Cancer Cell* 7, 193–204.

Rao, R. R., Li, Q., Gubbels Bupp, M. R., and Shrikant, P. A. (2012). Transcription factor Foxo1 represses T-bet-mediated effector functions and promotes memory CD8(+) T cell differentiation. *Immunity* 36, 374–387.

Rathmell, J. C., Elstrom, R. L., Cinalli, R. M., and Thompson, C. B. (2003). Activated Akt promotes increased resting T cell size, CD28-independent T cell growth, and development of autoimmunity and lymphoma. *Eur. J. Immunol.* 33, 2223–2232.

Rolf, J., Bell, S. E., Kovesdi, D., Janas, M. L., Soond, D. R., Webb, L. M., Santinelli, S., Saunders, T., Hebeis, B., Killeen, N., Okkenhaug, K., and Turner, M. (2010). Phosphoinositide 3-kinase activity in T cells regulates the magnitude of the germinal center reaction. *J. Immunol.* 185, 4042–4052.

Salmena, L., Carracedo, A., and Pandolfi, P. P. (2008). Tenets of PTEN tumor suppression. *Cell* 133, 403–414.

Samuels, Y., Wang, Z., Bardelli, A., Silliman, N., Ptak, J., Szabo, S., Yan, H., Gazdar, A., Powell, S. M., Riggins, G. J., Willson, J. K., Markowitz, S., Kinzler, K. W., Vogelstein, B., and Velculescu, V. E. (2004). High frequency of mutations of the PIK3CA gene in human cancers. *Science* 304, 554.

Shen, W. H., Balajee, A. S., Wang, J., Wu, H., Eng, C., Pandolfi, P. P., and Yin, Y. (2007). Essential role for nuclear PTEN in maintaining chromosomal integrity. *Cell* 128, 157–170.

Sinclair, L. V., Finlay, D., Feijoo, C., Cornish, G. H., Gray, A., Ager, A., Okkenhaug, K., Hagenbeek, T. J., Spits, H., and Cantrell, D. A. (2008). Phosphatidylinositol-3-OH kinase and nutrient-sensing mTOR pathways control T lymphocyte trafficking. *Nat. Immunol.* 9, 513–521.

So, L., and Fruman, D. A. (2012). PI3K signalling in B- and T-lymphocytes: new developments and therapeutic advances. *Biochem. J.* 442, 465–481.

Song, M. S., Carracedo, A., Salmena, L., Song, S. J., Egia, A., Malumbres, M., and Pandolfi, P. P. (2011). Nuclear PTEN regulates the APC-CDH1 tumor-suppressive complex in a phosphatase-independent manner. *Cell* 144, 187–199.

Stambolic, V., Suzuki, A., de la Pompa, J. L., Brothers, G. M., Mirtsos, C., Sasaki, T., Ruland, J., Penninger, J. M., Siderovski, D. P., and Mak, T. W. (1998). Negative regulation of PKB/Akt-dependent cell survival by the tumor suppressor PTEN. *Cell* 95, 29–39.

Stiles, B., Gilman, V., Khanzenzon, N., Lesche, R., Li, A., Qiao, R., Liu, X., and Wu, H. (2002). Essential role of AKT-1/protein kinase B alpha in PTEN-controlled tumorigenesis. *Mol. Cell. Biol.* 22, 3842–3851.

Suzuki, A., Yamaguchi, M. T., Ohteki, T., Sasaki, T., Kaisho, T., Kimura, Y., Yoshida, R., Wakeham, A., Higuchi, T., Fukumoto, M., Tsubata, T., Ohashi, P. S., Koyasu, S., Penninger, J. M., Nakano, T., and Mak, T. W. (2001). T cell-specific loss of Pten leads to defects in central and peripheral tolerance. *Immunity* 14, 523–534.

Tandon, P., Gallo, C. A., Khatri, S., Barger, J. F., Yepiskoposyan, H., and Plas, D. R. (2011). Requirement for ribosomal protein S6 kinase 1 to mediate glycolysis and apoptosis resistance induced by Pten deficiency. *Proc. Natl. Acad. Sci. U.S.A.* 108, 2361–2365.

Tothova, Z., Kollipara, R., Huntly, B. J., Lee, B. H., Castrillon, D. H., Cullen, D. E., McDowell, E. P., Lazo-Kallanian, S., Williams, I. R., Sears, C., Armstrong, S. A., Passegué, E., DePinho, R. A., and Gilliland, D. G. (2007). FoxOs are critical mediators of hematopoietic stem cell resistance to physiologic oxidative stress. *Cell* 128, 325–339.

Tran, H., Brunet, A., Grenier, J. M., Datta, S. R., Fornace, A. J. Jr., DiStefano, P. S., Chiang, L. W., and Greenberg, M. E. (2002). DNA repair pathway stimulated by the forkhead transcription factor FOXO3a through the Gadd45 protein. *Science* 296, 530–534.

Trotman, L. C., Wang, X., Alimonti, A., Chen, Z., Teruya-Feldstein, J., Yang, H., Pavletich, N. P., Carver, B. S., Cordon-Cardo, C., Erdjument-Bromage, H., Tempst, P., Chi, S. G., Kim, H. J., Misteli, T., Jiang, X., and Pandolfi, P. P. (2007). Ubiquitination regulates PTEN nuclear import and tumor suppression. *Cell* 128, 141–156.

Van Parijs, L., and Abbas, A. K. (1996). Role of Fas-mediated cell death in the regulation of immune responses. *Curr. Opin. Immunol.* 8, 355–361.

Walsh, P. T., Buckler, J. L., Zhang, J., Gelman, A. E., Dalton, N. M., Taylor, D. K., Bensinger, S. J., Hancock, W. W., and Turka, L. A. (2006). PTEN inhibits IL-2 receptor-mediated expansion of CD4+ CD25+ Tregs. *J. Clin. Invest.* 116, 2521–2531.

Wang, R., Dillon, C. P., Shi, L. Z., Milasta, S., Carter, R., Finkelstein, D., McCormick, L. L., Fitzgerald, P., Chi, H., Munger, J., and Green, D. R. (2011). The transcription factor Myc controls metabolic reprogramming upon T lymphocyte activation. *Immunity* 35, 871–882.

Xue, L., Nolla, H., Suzuki, A., Mak, T. W., and Winoto, A. (2008). Normal development is an integral part of tumorigenesis in T cell-specific PTEN-deficient mice. *Proc. Natl. Acad. Sci. U.S.A.* 105, 2022–2027.

Yilmaz, O. H., Valdez, R., Theisen, B. K., Guo, W., Ferguson, D. O., Wu, H., and Morrison, S. J. (2006). Pten dependence distinguishes haematopoietic stem cells from leukaemia-initiating cells. *Nature* 441, 475–482.

You, H., Pellegrini, M., Tsuchihara, K., Yamamoto, K., Hacker, G., Erlacher, M., Villunger, A., and Mak, T. W. (2006). FOXO3a-dependent regulation of Puma in response to cytokine/growth factor withdrawal. *J. Exp. Med.* 203, 1657–1663.

Zhang, J., Xiao, Y., Guo, Y., Breslin, P., Zhang, S., Wei, W., and Zhang, Z. (2011). Differential requirements for c-Myc in chronic hematopoietic hyperplasia and acute hematopoietic malignancies in Pten-null mice. *Leukemia* 25, 1857–1868.

23

Regulation of glucose metabolism in T cells: new insight into the role of phosphoinositide 3-kinases

David K. Finlay[1,2]*

[1] School of Biochemistry and Immunology, Trinity Biomedical Sciences Institute, Trinity College Dublin, Dublin, Ireland
[2] School of Pharmacy and Pharmaceutical Sciences, Trinity Biomedical Sciences Institute, Trinity College Dublin, Dublin, Ireland

Edited by:
Klaus Okkenhaug, Babraham Institute, UK

Reviewed by:
Stephen Geoffrey Ward, University of Bath, UK
Lawrence Kane, University of Pittsburgh School of Medicine, USA

***Correspondence:**
David K. Finlay, School of Biochemistry and Immunology, Trinity Biomedical Sciences Institute, Trinity College, Dublin 2, Ireland.
e-mail: finlayd@tcd.ie

Naïve T cells are relatively quiescent cells that only require energy to prevent atrophy and for survival and migration. However, in response to developmental or extrinsic cues T cells can engage in rapid growth and robust proliferation, produce of a range of effector molecules and migrate through peripheral tissues. To meet the significantly increased metabolic demands of these activities, T cells switch from primarily metabolizing glucose to carbon dioxide through oxidative phosphorylation to utilizing glycolysis to convert glucose to lactate (termed aerobic glycolysis). This metabolic switch allows glucose to be used as a source of carbon to generate biosynthetic precursors for the production of protein, DNA, and phospholipids, and is crucial for T cells to meet metabolic demands. Phosphoinositide 3-kinases (PI3K) are a family of inositol lipid kinases linked with a broad range of cellular functions in T lymphocytes that include cell growth, proliferation, metabolism, differentiation, survival, and migration. Initial research described a critical role for PI3K signaling through Akt (also called protein kinase B) for the increased glucose uptake and glycolysis that accompanies T cell activation. This review article relates this original research with more recent data and discusses the evidence for and against a role for PI3K in regulating the metabolic switch to aerobic glycolysis in T cells.

Keywords: PI3K, Glucose metabolism, Akt, T lymphocyte, aerobic glycolysis, c-Myc, PDK1

PI3K IN T CELLS

Class 1 phosphoinositide 3-kinases (PI3K), lipid kinases that phosphorylate phosphatidylinositol-(4,5)-bisphosphate [PI(4,5)P_2] to generate the lipid signaling molecule phosphatidylinositol-(3,4,5)-trisphosphate [PI(3,4,5)P_3], play a crucial role in many aspects of T cell biology (Okkenhaug and Vanhaesebroeck, 2003). Class 1 PI3Ks consist of a catalytic subunit, responsible for the lipid kinase activity, and an adapter subunit which links the catalytic subunit to upstream activating signals. They are subdivided into Class 1A; p110α, β, or δ catalytic subunits coupled to p85 adapter subunits, and Class 1B; p110γ catalytic subunit coupled to the p101 adapter protein. The p85 subunit couples Class 1A PI3Ks to docking sites created by tyrosine-kinase signaling while the Class IB p101 links the p110γ kinase with G-protein-coupled receptors (Vanhaesebroeck et al., 2010). The levels of the lipid signaling molecule PI(3,4,5)P_3 are coordinately regulated by both class 1 PI3Ks and by the action of 3′ and 5′ phosphatases PTEN and SHIP1 that dephosphorylate PI(3,4,5)P_3 to generate PI(4,5)P_2 and PI(3,4)P_2 respectively (**Figure 1A**).

PI(3,4,5)P_3 is an important lipid signaling molecule in T cells, present at low levels in naïve T cells and elevated in response to signaling initiated by the T cell receptor (TCR) and various cytokine and chemokine receptors (Koyasu, 2003). Following TCR engagement by antigen presenting cells (APC) levels of PI(3,4,5)P_3 accumulate in the plasma membrane and are maintained for prolonged periods, requiring continual TCR engagement and activation of PI3K (Costello et al., 2002; Harriague and Bismuth, 2002; Huppa et al., 2003). Signals from co-stimulatory molecules such as CD28 are important for sustaining PI(3,4,5)P_3 levels following TCR engagement but are not in themselves sufficient to stimulate PI3K as PI(3,4,5)P_3 levels are only induced when the TCR engages APC presenting cognate peptide antigen (Costello et al., 2002; Garcon et al., 2007). Other physiological stimuli that can stimulate PI(3,4,5)P_3 levels in T cells include cytokines and chemokines (Koyasu, 2003). While PI(3,4,5)P_3 levels are induced by a number of cytokines it should be noted that the potency of these different cytokines can vary, e.g., IL2 maintains high levels of PI(3,4,5)P_3 while IL15 maintains comparatively low levels (Cornish et al., 2006 Sinclair et al., 2008).

In the thymus, PI3Kδ and PI3Kγ are the major isoforms required in developing thymocytes. While deletion of PI3Kδ or individually does not have a pronounced effect on thymopoiesis, deletion or inactivation of both isoforms in developing T cells results in a block early in thymocyte development at the CD4 CD8 double negative (DN) stage (Sasaki et al., 2000; Okkenhaug et al., 2002; Webb et al., 2005; Swat et al., 2006; Ji et al., 2007). Negative regulation of PI(3,4,5)P_3 signaling is also important in developing thymocytes. Thus, deletion of PTEN in early thymocyte progenitors results in constitutive PI(3,4,5)P_3 signaling that leads to the development of T cell leukemia or lymphoma (Suzuki et al., 2001 Hagenbeek and Spits, 2008; Finlay et al., 2009). In contrast to developing thymocytes, in mature T cells PI3Kδ appears to be the major PI3K isoform responsible for promoting PI(3,4,5)P_3 signaling in activated T cells. Thus, a point mutation that makes p110 catalytically inactive (D910A) abolishes PI(3,4,5)P_3 signaling in activated T cell subsets (Okkenhaug et al., 2002, 2006; Macintyre et al., 2011).

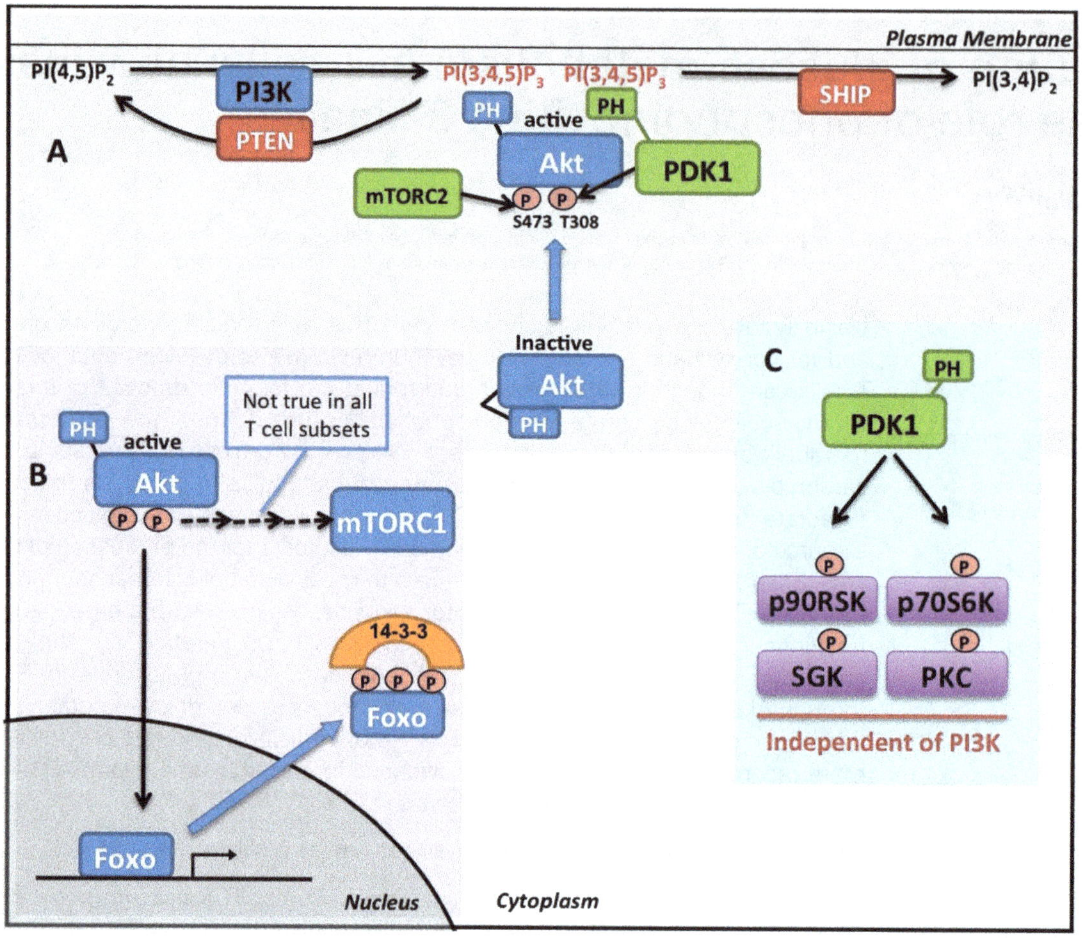

FIGURE 1 | PI3K and Akt signaling. (A) $PI(4,5)P_2$ is phosphorylated by Class 1 PI3K isoforms generating the second messenger molecule $PI(3,4,5)P_3$. Levels of $PI(3,4,5)P_3$ are negatively regulated by the lipid phosphatases PTEN and SHIP. Binding of the PH domain of Akt to $PI(3,4,5)P_3$ in the membrane results in a conformational change that allows for the phosphorylation of Akt on key residues(T308 and S473) by PDK1 and mTORC2. The recruitment of PDK1, via its PH domain, to the site of $PI(3,4,5)P_3$ is required for efficient Akt activation. **(B)** Active Akt phosphorylates Foxo transcription factors on multiple sites resulting in their translocation to the cytoplasm where they are retained in complex with 14-3-3 proteins. mTORC1 can be activated downstream of Akt, though this does not occur in all T cell types. **(C)** PDK1 also phosphorylates and activates a number of other members of the AGC kinase family in a PI3K independent manner.

PI3K SIGNALING

$PI(3,4,5)P_3$ acts as a signaling molecule through its interaction with the pleckstrin homology (PH) domains of a diverse array of signal transduction proteins. These proteins include Akt (also called PKB), Tec family kinases, and guanine-nucleotide-exchange proteins for Rho family GTPases. This interaction primarily controls the subcellular localization of PH domain containing proteins but can also control protein conformation and enzyme activity. Consider, for example, the activation of Akt, which is the best characterized $PI(3,4,5)P_3$ effector in T cells (for reviews Alessi and Cohen, 1998; Hanada et al., 2004; Cameron et al., 2007). The interaction of $PI(3,4,5)P_3$ with the PH domain of Akt stimulates its kinase activity by inducing a conformational change that allows Akt to be phosphorylated on threonine 308 and serine 473 by its upstream activating kinases phosphoinositide-dependent kinase 1 (PDK1) and mechanistic Target Of Rapamycin Complex 2 (mTORC2) respectively (**Figure 1A;** Calleja et al., 2007). PDK1 also contains a PH domain and co-localization of Akt and PDK1 to sites of $PI(3,4,5)P_3$ is required for efficient Akt activation (Bayascas et al., 2008; Waugh et al., 2009). Once activated, Akt phosphorylates a number of important signaling molecules including the Foxo transcription factors (Manning and Cantley, 2007). Foxo transcription factors localize to the nucleus where they promote the expression of target genes. Once phosphorylated by Akt, Foxos translocate into the cytoplasm where they are retained through their interaction with 14-3-3 proteins (**Figure 1B;** Coffer and Burgering, 2004; Burgering, 2008). PI3K/Akt signaling also activates the mTOR Complex 1 (mTORC1) in many cellular systems through multiple mechanisms (Laplante and Sabatini, 2009). mTORC1 is an important regulator of cellular metabolism that senses environmental cues such as nutrient availability and energy homeostasis (Delgoffe and Powell, 2009). However, it is now becoming apparent that mTORC1 activity is not universally dependent upon PI3K/Akt signaling in T cells. Thus, in activated

CD8 cells, mTORC1 activity is not blocked by the disruption of PI3K/Akt signaling by various pharmacological and genetic strategies (unpublished data; Macintyre et al., 2011).

MATCHING GLUCOSE METABOLISM TO METABOLIC DEMANDS

While naïve T cells only require energy to prevent atrophy and for survival and migration, activated T cell subsets have a greatly increased metabolic demand as they engage in rapid growth and proliferation, and the production of cytokines and other effector molecules. It is crucial that activated T cells increase their metabolism to meet the biosynthetic needs of the T cell as it responds either to developmental or pathogenic cues. To achieve this T cells respond to extrinsic signals from antigen receptors and cytokines to up-regulate the surface expression of key nutrient receptors: amino acid transporters, the transferrin receptor, and glucose transporters (Fox et al., 2005a; Kelly et al., 2007; Jacobs et al., 2008). Additionally, T cells switch their glucose metabolism from oxidative phosphorylation to aerobic glycolysis; i.e., glucose is metabolized to produce lactate even though oxygen is readily available (**Figure 2;** Greiner et al., 1994). Aerobic glycolysis is an inefficient route to generating ATP, producing two molecules ATP per molecule of glucose compared to >30 molecules ATP per glucose generated by oxidative phosphorylation. Therefore, cells must be able to sustain high levels of glucose uptake and an elevated glycolytic flux to generate sufficient ATP. This is achieved by increasing the expression of the GLUT1 glucose transporter and certain rate limiting enzymes within the glycolytic pathway (Vander Heiden et al., 2009; Marko et al., 2010). However, the real advantage of switching from oxidative phosphorylation to glycolysis is that it allows glucose to be used as a source of carbon to generate nucleic acid, amino acids and phospholipids (**Figure 2;** Vander Heiden et al., 2009). The generation of these biosynthetic precursors is critical for cells engaging in rapid growth, proliferation, and the synthesis of effector molecules. Therefore, to facilitate their differentiation and function, activated T cells up-regulate the expression of GLUT1, increase glucose uptake, and activate the switch to aerobic glycolysis

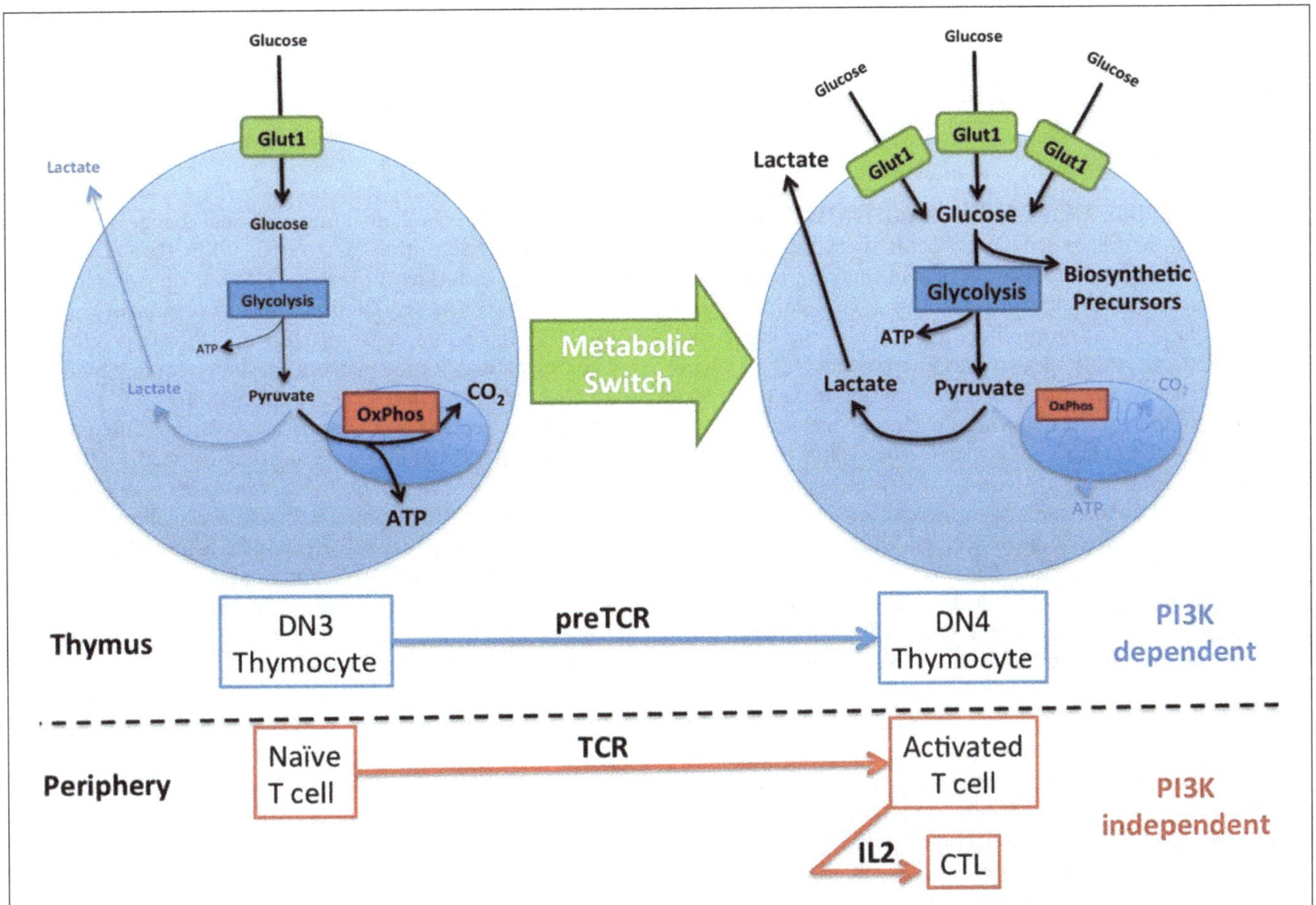

FIGURE 2 | PI3K controls the metabolic switch to aerobic glycolysis in thymocytes but not in mature T cells. Naïve T cells take up small amounts of glucose which is for the most part metabolized to CO_2 via mitochondrial oxidative phosphorylation (OxPhos) for the efficient generation of ATP. Activated T cells and certain thymocyte subsets increase the expression of the GLUT1 glucose transporter and thus glucose uptake, and increase glycolytic flux, primarily converting glucose to lactate. This metabolic switch increases the biosynthetic capacity of the T cells and is stimulated by antigen receptor signaling (PreTCR, TCR) and maintained by certain cytokines (IL2). PI3K signaling is required for this metabolic switch during thymopoiesis but not in peripheral activated T cells.

(Brand et al., 1984; Greiner et al., 1994; Frauwirth et al., 2002; Wofford et al., 2008).

PI3K AND GLUCOSE METABOLISM IN THE THYMUS

In the thymus discrete subpopulations, e.g., DN4 thymocytes, engage in rapid growth and robust proliferation. PI3K and Akt signaling is crucial in allowing these thymocyte subsets to match their metabolism with metabolic demands (Ciofani and Zuniga-Pflucker, 2005; Juntilla et al., 2007; Kelly et al., 2007; Finlay et al., 2010). Thus, mice lacking Akt or PDK1 or both PI3Kδ and γ isoforms during early thymopoiesis have a profound developmental block at the DN3/DN4 stage of T cell development(Hinton et al., 2004; Webb et al., 2005; Swat et al., 2006; Fayard et al., 2007; Juntilla et al., 2007; Mao et al., 2007). In the absence of PI3K/PDK1/Akt signaling DN4 thymocytes fail to up-regulate the expression of the glucose transporter, GLUT1, and also the expression of other key nutrient receptors for the uptake of amino acids (CD98, component of the L-amino acid transporter) and iron (transferrin receptor, CD71). Increased provision of these nutrients is a key requirement for these cells to meet the metabolic demands of rapid growth and proliferation and PI3K/PDK1/Akt deficient DN4 thymocytes that fail to do so atrophy and fail to develop (Juntilla et al., 2007; Kelly et al., 2007). Therefore, in T cells developing in the thymus, PI3K and Akt signaling is crucial to allow certain thymocyte subsets to match glucose metabolism with metabolic demands.

PI3K AND GLUCOSE METABOLISM IN ACTIVATED T CELLS

The metabolic switch to aerobic glycolysis is crucial during the activation and differentiation of T cells in the periphery. Thus, limiting glucose availability in activating T cells compromises TCR induced growth and proliferation and also the expression of certain effector molecules such as interferon γ (IFNγ; Cham et al., 2008; Jacobs et al., 2008). The transcription factor c-Myc is crucial for the metabolic switch in glucose metabolism that accompanies the activation of naïve T cells (Wang et al., 2011). Accordingly, deletion of c-Myc in naïve T cells prevents TCR induced glucose uptake and glycolysis, and activated c-Myc-null T cells completely fail to grow or proliferate (Trumpp et al., 2001; Iritani et al., 2002; Dose et al., 2006; Wang et al., 2011). Is PI3K and Akt signaling also required for the increase in glucose uptake and glycolysis in TCR activated T cells in the periphery? Certainly, antigen receptor induced c-Myc expression and glucose uptake have been attributed to PI3K signaling (Frauwirth et al., 2002; Grumont et al., 2002; Doughty et al., 2006; Jacobs et al., 2008; Wang et al., 2011). However, one criticism of these studies is that they rely on experiments involving the overexpression of Akt and the use of the PI3K inhibitor LY294002. Overexpression studies can be difficult to interrupt and while LY294002 was initially believed to be a highly specific PI3K inhibitor, and as such was used in good faith, it has since emerged that this inhibitor is rather non-specific. LY294002 potently inhibits a number kinases other than PI3K, including those with described roles in regulating T cell growth and proliferation, i.e., mTORC1 and Pim family kinases (Brunn et al., 1996; Davies et al., 2000; Fox et al., 2005b; Bain et al., 2007). The importance of these other LY204002 targets for T cell metabolism can be appreciated by a comparison of the cellular sizes of PI3K/Akt deficient CD8 cytotoxic T lymphocytes (CTL) and wild-type CTL cultured in the presence of LY294002. While PI3K/Akt deficient CTL are comparable in size to wild-type CTL, LY294002-treated CTL are substantially smaller (Cornish et al., 2006; Sinclair et al., 2008; Macintyre et al., 2011). Therefore, the question as to whether PI3K regulates TCR induced c-Myc expression has not been satisfactorily investigated to date. Nevertheless, a comparison of PI3K/Akt and c-Myc deficient T cells is extremely informative. In contrast to the failure of c-Myc-null T cells to engage in TCR stimulated growth and proliferation, PI3K deficient T cells show a relatively mild defect in growth and proliferation with activated T cells capable of completing numerous divisions, though at a reduced rate (Okkenhaug et al., 2002, 2006). Furthermore, T cells expressing a PDK1 K465E mutant which have defective TCR stimulated Akt activity, undergo normal TCR induced growth and proliferation (Waugh et al., 2009). These observations coupled to the fact that T cells activated in limiting concentrations of glucose do show a marked defect in proliferation argue that TCR induced c-Myc expression, glucose uptake and glycolysis is not compromised by disruption of PI3K and Akt signaling (Jacobs et al., 2008). More recently, PI3K/Akt independent glucose uptake and glycolysis in TCR activated T cells has been confirmed using pharmacological inhibitors of PI3Kδ (IC87114) and Akt (Akti1/2) with substantially greater selectivity than LY294002 (Macintyre et al., 2011). Akti1/2 is particularly selective toward Akt due to its unique allosteric mechanism of inhibition, binding to the PH domain of Akt and preventing the PH domain-PI(3,4,5)P_3 interaction and the resultant conformational change that is a prerequisite for Akt activation (Zhao et al., 2005; Bain et al., 2007). Both IC87114 and Akti1/2 prevent PI3K/Akt signaling in T cells while having no effect on TCR induced glucose uptake (Macintyre et al., 2011). Therefore, it seems clear that PI3K has differential roles in regulating glucose metabolism in developing thymocytes in the thymus and mature T cells in the periphery.

Once activated, T cells differentiate into various different effector T cell subsets depending on the local environment and cytokine availability. Many of these effector T cell subsets maintain an elevated glycolytic rate in response to cytokine signaling (Macintyre et al., 2011; Shi et al., 2011). For example, activated CD8 T cells undergo rapid growth and proliferation in response to interleukin 2 (IL2) as they differentiate into functional CTL. In response to IL2 signaling CTL maintain high levels of glucose uptake and lactate production indicative of elevated glycolysis (Macintyre et al., 2011). IL2 also promotes glucose uptake and glycolysis independently of PI3K and Akt but a key role has been revealed for PDK1. Thus, while IC87114 and Akti1/2 have no effect on CTL glucose uptake, a pronounced decrease is observed following the deletion of PDK1 using a Cre/loxP strategy (Macintyre et al., 2011). While PDK1 is responsible for the activation of Akt, it also activates a number of other members of the AGC kinase family including protein kinase C (PKC), 70-kDa ribosomal S6 kinase (p70S6K), 90-kDa ribosomal S6 kinase (p90RSK), and serum/glucocorticoid regulated kinase (SGK; Pearce et al., 2010). However, unlike the activation of Akt, PDK1 mediated activation of these other AGC family members are independent of PI3K signaling (**Figure 1C**). As members of this kinase family have overlapping substrate specificity it is likely that PDK1 dependent, Akt independent regulation of glucose metabolism reflects functional redundancy within the AGC family of protein kinases (Brunet et al., 2001; Zhang et al., 2006; Sapkota et al., 2007).

mTORC1 has described roles in regulating various aspects of cellular metabolism and given that its activity is independent of PI3K and Akt in some activated T cell subsets, it remains likely that mTORC1 is involved in maintaining glucose uptake and glycolysis (unpublished data; Duvel et al., 2010; Macintyre et al., 2011). Indeed, inhibition of mTORC1 decreases glycolysis in T cells activated under Th17 polarizing conditions (Shi et al., 2011). However, as mTORC1 inhibition also disrupts Th17 differentiation, it is difficult to interpret whether the effect of rapamycin on glycolysis is direct or as a result of the differentiation of different T cells. Therefore, a role for mTORC1 in controlling glycolysis in T cells has still to be formally demonstrated.

T CELL MIGRATION AND METABOLISM

The expression of adhesion molecules and chemokine receptors orchestrate the peripheral trafficking of activated T cells. The p110γ catalytic subunit is the major PI3K isoform in T cells that promotes $PI(3,4,5)P_3$ signaling in response to chemokines. Thus, migration to a range of chemokines is deficient in $p110\gamma^{-/-}$ T cells and these T cells fail to traffic normally to sites of inflammation (Reif et al., 2004; Smith et al., 2007; Martin et al., 2008; Thomas et al., 2008). T cell migration and motility are energy demanding processes and it is tempting to speculate that chemokine receptor signaling might promote T cell glucose metabolism to meet these energy demands. However, while there is some tentative data linking chemokine receptor signaling to cell growth and metabolism in transformed T cells and developing thymocytes the relationship between chemokine receptor signaling and T cell metabolism has not been directly studied (Janas et al., 2010; Lo et al., 2010). Nonetheless, it is worth mentioning that factors that influence T cell migration and/or homing, and thus the peripheral tissue destination of T cells, will affect T cell metabolism, albeit indirectly, by determining the cytokine environment to which they are exposed. A comparison of activated T cells responding to related cytokines IL2 and IL15 illustrates the differential regulation of T cell metabolism by distinct cytokine environments. IL2 promotes elevated glucose metabolism and glycolysis while IL15 does not maintain this metabolic state and T cells responding to IL15 are smaller with reduced nutrient uptake and glycolysis (Cornish et al., 2006; Macintyre et al., 2011; unpublished data). While PI3Kγ controls T cell migration in response to chemokines, PI3Kδ regulates the repertoire of adhesion and chemokine receptors expressed by activated T cells. PI3Kδ, signaling through Akt and the Foxo transcription factors, regulates the expression of key molecules required for T cell homing between the blood and the lymphoid organs; the adhesion molecule CD62L (also called L-selectin) and the chemokine receptors CC-chemokine receptor 7 (CCR7) and sphingosine-1-phosphate receptor 1 ($S1P_1$). Disruption of PI3Kδ/Akt signaling in activated CD8 T cells prevents the down-regulation of CD62L, CCR7, and $S1P_1$ and these T cells retain a lymph node trafficking pattern rather than migrating to non-lymphoid tissues and the sites of inflammation (Sinclair et al., 2008; Waugh et al., 2009; Finlay and Cantrell, 2010; Macintyre et al., 2011). Thus, PI3Kδ deficient T cells activated *in vivo* or wild-type T cells activated in mice treated with a PI3Kδ inhibitor fail to traffic into the periphery to antigenic sites (Jarmin et al., 2008). Therefore, both PI3Kγ and δ isoforms coordinately regulate T cell peripheral tissue homing thereby dictating the cytokine environments encountered and indirectly impacting upon T cell metabolism.

FINAL REMARK

It has recently become clear that the PI3K/Akt signaling axis is not the important regulator of glucose uptake and glycolysis in mature T cells, as initially described. However, disrupting PI3K may in fact impact upon T cell metabolism through indirect mechanisms, i.e., through altering their *in vivo* trafficking pattern, which will dictate the cytokines these T cells encounter.

REFERENCES

Alessi, D. R., and Cohen, P. (1998). Mechanism of activation and function of protein kinase B. *Curr. Opin. Genet. Dev.* 8, 55–62.

Bain, J., Plater, L., Elliott, M., Shpiro, N., Hastie, C. J., McLauchlan, H., Klevernic, I., Arthur, J. S., Alessi, D. R., and Cohen, P. (2007). The selectivity of protein kinase inhibitors: a further update. *Biochem. J.* 408, 297–315.

Bayascas, J. R., Wullschleger, S., Sakamoto, K., Garcia-Martinez, J. M., Clacher, C., Komander, D., van Aalten, D. M. F., Boini, K. M., Lang, F., Lipina, C., Logie, L., Sutherland, C., Chudek, J. A., van Diepen, J. A., Voshol, P. J., Lucocq, J. M., and Alessi, D. R. (2008). Mutation of the PDK1 PH domain inhibits protein kinase B/Akt, leading to small size and insulin resistance. *Mol. Cell. Biol.* 28, 3258–3272.

Brand, K., Williams, J. F., and Weidemann, M. J. (1984). Glucose and glutamine metabolism in rat thymocytes. *Biochem. J.* 221, 471–475.

Brunet, A., Park, J., Tran, H., Hu, L. S., Hemmings, B. A., and Greenberg, M. E. (2001). Protein kinase SGK mediates survival signals by phosphorylating the forkhead transcription factor FKHRL1 (FOXO3a). *Mol. Cell. Biol.* 21, 952–965.

Brunn, G. J., Williams, J., Sabers, C., Wiederrecht, G., Lawrence, J. C., and Abraham, R. T. (1996). Direct inhibition of the signaling functions of the mammalian target of rapamycin by the phosphoinositide 3-kinase inhibitors, wortmannin and LY294002. *EMBO J.* 15, 5256—5267.

Burgering, B. M. T. (2008). A brief introduction to FOXOlogy. *Oncogene* 27, 2258–2262.

Calleja, V., Alcor, D., Laguerre, M., Park, J., Vojnovic, B., Hemmings, B. A., Downward, J., Parker, P. J., and Larijani, B. (2007). Intramolecular and intermolecular interactions of protein kinase B define its activation in vivo. *PLoS Biol.* 5, e95. doi: 10.1371/journal.pbio.0050095

Cameron, A. J., De Rycker, M., Calleja, V., Alcor, D., Kjaer, S., Kostelecky, B., Saurin, A., Faisal, A., Laguerre, M., Hemmings, B. A., McDonald, N., Larijani, B., and Parker, P. J. (2007). Protein kinases, from B to C. *Biochem. Soc. Trans.* 35, 1013–1017.

Cham, C. M., Driessens, G., O'Keefe, J. P., and Gajewski, T. F. (2008). Glucose deprivation inhibits multiple key gene expression events and effector functions in CD8 + T cells. *Eur. J. Immunol.* 38, 2438–2450.

Ciofani, M., and Zuniga-Pflucker, J. C. (2005). Notch promotes survival of pre-T cells at the beta-selection checkpoint by regulating cellular metabolism. *Nat. Immunol.* 6, 881–888.

Coffer, P. J., and Burgering, B. M. (2004). Forkhead-box transcription factors and their role in the immune system. *Nat. Rev. Immunol.* 4, 889–899.

Cornish, G. H., Sinclair, L. V., and Cantrell, D. A. (2006). Differential regulation of T-cell growth by IL-2 and IL-15. *Blood* 108, 600–608.

Costello, P. S., Gallagher, M., and Cantrell, D. A. (2002). Sustained and dynamic inositol lipid metabolism inside and outside the immunological synapse. *Nat. Immunol.* 3, 1082–1089.

Davies, S. P., Reddy, H., Caivano, M., and Cohen, P. (2000). Specificity and mechanism of action of some commonly used protein kinase inhibitors. *Biochem. J.* 351, 95–105.

Delgoffe, G. M., and Powell, J. D. (2009). mTOR: taking cues from the immune microenvironment. *Immunology* 127, 459–465.

Dose, M., Khan, I., Guo, Z., Kovalovsky, D., Krueger, A., von Boehmer, H., Khazaie, K., and Gounari, F. (2006). c-Myc mediates pre-TCR-induced proliferation but not developmental progression. *Blood* 108, 2669–2677.

Doughty, C. A., Bleiman, B. F., Wagner, D. J., Dufort, F. J., Mataraza, J. M., Roberts, M. F., and Chiles, T. C. (2006). Antigen receptor-mediated changes in glucose metabolism in B lymphocytes: role of phosphatidylinositol 3-kinase signaling in the glycolytic control of growth. *Blood* 107, 4458–4465.

Duvel, K., Yecies, J. L., Menon, S., Raman, P., Lipovsky, A. I., Souza, A. L., Triantafellow, E., Ma, Q., Gorski, R., Cleaver, S., Vander Heiden, M. G., MacKeigan, J. P., Finan, P. M., Clish, C. B., Murphy, L. O., and Manning, B. D. (2010). Activation of a metabolic gene regulatory network downstream of mTOR complex 1. *Mol. Cell* 39, 171–183.

Fayard, E., Gill, J., Paolino, M., Hynx, D., Hollander, G. A., and Hemmings, B. A. (2007). Deletion of PKBalpha/Akt1 affects thymic development. *PLoS ONE* 2, e992. doi: 10.1371/journal.pone.0000992

Finlay, D., and Cantrell, D. (2010). Phosphoinositide 3-kinase and the mammalian target of rapamycin pathways control T cell migration. *Ann. N. Y. Acad. Sci.* 1183, 149–157.

Finlay, D. K., Kelly, A. P., Clarke, R., Sinclair, L. V., Deak, M., Alessi, D. R., and Cantrell, D. A. (2010). Temporal differences in the dependency on phosphoinositide-dependent kinase 1 distinguish the development of invariant Valpha14 NKT cells and conventional T cells. *J. Immunol.* 185, 5973–5982.

Finlay, D. K., Sinclair, L. V., Feijoo, C., Waugh, C. M., Hagenbeek, T. J., Spits, H., and Cantrell, D. A. (2009). Phosphoinositide-dependent kinase 1 controls migration and malignant transformation but not cell growth and proliferation in PTEN-null lymphocytes. *J. Exp. Med.* 206, 2441–2454.

Fox, C. J., Hammerman, P. S., and Thompson, C. B. (2005a). Fuel feeds function: energy metabolism and the T-cell response. *Nat. Rev. Immunol.* 5, 844–852.

Fox, C. J., Hammerman, P. S., and Thompson, C. B. (2005b). The Pim kinases control rapamycin-resistant T cell survival and activation. *J. Exp. Med.* 201, 259–266.

Frauwirth, K. A., Riley, J. L., Harris, M. H., Parry, R. V., Rathmell, J. C., Plas, D. R., Elstrom, R. L., June, C. H., and Thompson, C. B. (2002). The CD28 signaling pathway regulates glucose metabolism. *Immunity* 16, 769–777.

Garcon, F., Patton, D. T., Emery, J. L., Hirsch, E., Rottapel, R., Sasaki, T., and Okkenhaug, K. (2007). CD28 provides T-cell costimulation and enhances PI3K activity at the immune synapse independently of its capacity to interact with the p85/p110 heterodimer. *Blood* 111, 1464–1471.

Greiner, E. F., Guppy, M., and Brand, K. (1994). Glucose is essential for proliferation and the glycolytic enzyme induction that provokes a transition to glycolytic energy production. *J. Biol. Chem.* 269, 31484–31490.

Grumont, R. J., Strasser, A., and Gerondakis, S. (2002). B cell growth is controlled by phosphatidylinosotol 3-kinase-dependent induction of Rel/NF-kappaB regulated c-myc transcription. *Mol. Cell* 10, 1283–1294.

Hagenbeek, T. J., and Spits, H. (2008). T-cell lymphomas in T-cell-specific Pten-deficient mice originate in the thymus. *Leukemia* 22, 608–619.

Hanada, M., Feng, J., and Hemmings, B. A. (2004). Structure, regulation and function of PKB/AKT – a major therapeutic target. *Biochim. Biophys. Acta* 1697, 3–16.

Harriague, J., and Bismuth, G. (2002). Imaging antigen-induced PI3K activation in T cells. *Nat. Immunol.* 3, 1090–1096.

Hinton, H. J., Alessi, D. R., and Cantrell, D. A. (2004). The serine kinase phosphoinositide-dependent kinase 1 (PDK1) regulates T cell development. *Nat. Immunol.* 5, 539–545.

Huppa, J. B., Gleimer, M., Sumen, C., and Davis, M. M. (2003). Continuous T cell receptor signaling required for synapse maintenance and full effector potential. *Nat. Immunol.* 4, 749–755.

Iritani, B. M., Delrow, J., Grandori, C., Gomez, I., Klacking, M., Carlos, L. S., and Eisenman, R. N. (2002). Modulation of T-lymphocyte development, growth and cell size by the Myc antagonist and transcriptional repressor Mad1. *EMBO J.* 21, 4820–4830.

Jacobs, S. R., Herman, C. E., Maciver, N. J., Wofford, J. A., Wieman, H. L., Hammen, J. J., and Rathmell, J. C. (2008). Glucose uptake is limiting in T cell activation and requires CD28-mediated Akt-dependent and independent pathways. *J. Immunol.* 180, 4476–4486.

Janas, M. L., Varano, G., Gudmundsson, K., Noda, M., Nagasawa, T., and Turner, M. (2010). Thymic development beyond beta-selection requires phosphatidylinositol 3-kinase activation by CXCR4. *J. Exp. Med.* 207, 247–261.

Jarmin, S. J., David, R., Ma, L., Chai, J. G., Dewchand, H., Takesono, A., Ridley, A. J., Okkenhaug, K., and Marelli-Berg, F. M. (2008). T cell receptor-induced phosphoinositide-3-kinase p110delta activity is required for T cell localization to antigenic tissue in mice. *J. Clin. Invest.* 118, 1154–1164.

Ji, H., Rintelen, F., Waltzinger, C., Bertschy Meier, D., Bilancio, A., Pearce, W., Hirsch, E., Wymann, M. P., Ruckle, T., Camps, M., Vanhaesebroeck, B., Okkenhaug, K., and Rommel, C. (2007). Inactivation of PI3Kgamma and PI3Kdelta distorts T-cell development and causes multiple organ inflammation. *Blood* 110, 2940–2947.

Juntilla, M. M., Wofford, J. A., Birnbaum, M. J., Rathmell, J. C., and Koretzky, G. A. (2007). Akt1 and Akt2 are required for alphabeta thymocyte survival and differentiation. *Proc. Natl. Acad. Sci. U.S.A.* 104, 12105–12110.

Kelly, A. P., Finlay, D. K., Hinton, H. J., Clarke, R. G., Fiorini, E., Radtke, F., and Cantrell, D. A. (2007). Notch-induced T cell development requires phosphoinositide-dependent kinase 1. *EMBO J.* 26, 3441–3450.

Koyasu, S. (2003). The role of PI3K in immune cells. *Nat. Immunol.* 4, 313–319.

Laplante, M., and Sabatini, D. M. (2009). mTOR signaling at a glance. *J. Cell. Sci.* 122, 3589–3594.

Lo, B. K., Yu, M., Zloty, D., Cowan, B., Shapiro, J., and McElwee, K. J. (2010). CXCR3/ligands are significantly involved in the tumorigenesis of basal cell carcinomas. *Am. J. Pathol.* 176, 2435–2446.

Macintyre, A. N., Finlay, D., Preston, G., Sinclair, L. V., Waugh, C. M., Tamas, P., Feijoo, C., Okkenhaug, K., and Cantrell, D. A. (2011). Protein kinase B controls transcriptional programs that direct cytotoxic T cell fate but is dispensable for T cell metabolism. *Immunity* 34, 224–236.

Manning, B. D., and Cantley, L. C. (2007). AKT/PKB signaling: navigating downstream. *Cell* 129, 1261–1274.

Mao, C., Tili, E. G., Dose, M., Haks, M. C., Bear, S. E., Maroulakou, I., Horie, K., Gaitanaris, G. A., Fidanza, V., Ludwig, T., Wiest, D. L., Gounari, F., and Tsichlis, P. N. (2007). Unequal contribution of Akt isoforms in the double-negative to double-positive thymocyte transition. *J. Immunol.* 178, 5443–5453.

Marko, A. J., Miller, R. A., Kelman, A., and Frauwirth, K. A. (2010). Induction of glucose metabolism in stimulated T lymphocytes is regulated by mitogen-activated protein kinase signaling. *PLoS ONE* 5, e15425. doi: 10.1371/journal.pone.0015425

Martin, A. L., Schwartz, M. D., Jameson, S. C., and Shimizu, Y. (2008). Selective regulation of CD8 effector T cell migration by the p110 gamma isoform of phosphatidylinositol 3-kinase. *J. Immunol.* 180, 2081–2088.

Okkenhaug, K., Bilancio, A., Farjot, G., Priddle, H., Sancho, S., Peskett, E., Pearce, W., Meek, S. E., Salpekar, A., Waterfield, M. D., Smith, A. J., and Vanhaesebroeck, B. (2002). Impaired B and T cell antigen receptor signaling in p110delta PI 3-kinase mutant mice. *Science* 297, 1031–1034.

Okkenhaug, K., Patton, D. T., Bilancio, A., Garcon, F., Rowan, W. C., and Vanhaesebroeck, B. (2006). The p110delta isoform of phosphoinositide 3-kinase controls clonal expansion and differentiation of Th cells. *J. Immunol.* 177, 5122–5128.

Okkenhaug, K., and Vanhaesebroeck, B. (2003). PI3K in lymphocyte development, differentiation and activation. *Nat. Rev. Immunol.* 3, 317–330.

Pearce, L. R., Komander, D., and Alessi, D. R. (2010). The nuts and bolts of AGC protein kinases. *Nat. Rev. Mol. Cell Biol.* 11, 9–22.

Reif, K., Okkenhaug, K., Sasaki, T., Penninger, J. M., Vanhaesebroeck, B., and Cyster, J. G. (2004). Cutting edge: differential roles for phosphoinositide 3-kinases, p110gamma and p110delta, in lymphocyte chemotaxis and homing. *J. Immunol.* 173, 2236–2240.

Sapkota, G. P., Cummings, L., Newell, F. S., Armstrong, C., Bain, J., Frodin, M., Grauert, M., Hoffmann, M., Schnapp, G., Steegmaier, M., Cohen, P., and Alessi, D. R. (2007). BI-D1870 is a specific inhibitor of the p90 RSK (ribosomal S6 kinase) isoforms in vitro and in vivo. *Biochem. J.* 401, 29–38.

Sasaki, T., Irie-Sasaki, J., Jones, R. G., Oliveira-dos-Santos, A. J., Stanford, W. L., Bolon, B., Wakeham, A., Itie, A., Bouchard, D., Kozieradzki, I., Joza, N., Mak, T. W., Ohashi, P. S., Suzuki, A., and Penninger, J. M. (2000). Function of PI3Kgamma in thymocyte development, T cell activation, and neutrophil migration. *Science* 287, 1040–1046.

Shi, L. Z., Wang, R., Huang, G., Vogel, P., Neale, G., Green, D. R., and Chi, H. (2011). HIF1alpha-dependent glycolytic pathway orchestrates a metabolic checkpoint for the differentiation of TH17 and Treg cells. *J. Exp. Med.* 208, 1367–1376.

Sinclair, L. V., Finlay, D., Feijoo, C., Cornish, G. H., Gray, A., Ager, A., Okkenhaug, K., Hagenbeek, T. J., Spits, H., and Cantrell, D. A. (2008). Phosphatidylinositol-3-OH kinase and nutrient-sensing mTOR pathways control T lymphocyte trafficking. *Nat. Immunol.* 9, 513–521.

Smith, L. D., Hickman, E. S., Parry, R. V., Westwick, J., and Ward, S. G. (2007). PI3Kgamma is the dominant isoform involved in migratory responses of human T lymphocytes: effects of ex vivo maintenance and limitations of non-viral delivery of siRNA. *Cell. Signal.* 19, 2528–2539.

Suzuki, A., Yamaguchi, M. T., Ohteki, T., Sasaki, T., Kaisho, T., Kimura, Y., Yoshida, R., Wakeham, A., Higuchi, T., Fukumoto, M., Tsubata, T., Ohashi, P. S., Koyasu, S., Penninger, J. M., Nakano, T., and Mak, T. W. (2001). T cell-specific loss of Pten leads to defects in central and peripheral tolerance. *Immunity* 14, 523–534.

Swat, W., Montgrain, V., Doggett, T. A., Douangpanya, J., Puri, K., Vermi, W., and Diacovo, T. G. (2006). Essential role of PI3Kdelta and PI3Kgamma in thymocyte survival. *Blood* 107, 2415–2422.

Thomas, M. S., Mitchell, J. S., DeNucci, C. C., Martin, A. L., and Shimizu, Y. (2008). The p110gamma isoform of phosphatidylinositol 3-kinase regulates migration of effector CD4 T lymphocytes into peripheral inflammatory sites. *J. Leukoc. Biol.* 84, 814–823.

Trumpp, A., Refaeli, Y., Oskarsson, T., Gasser, S., Murphy, M., Martin, G. R., and Bishop, J. M. (2001). c-Myc regulates mammalian body size by controlling cell number but not cell size. *Nature* 414, 768–773.

Vander Heiden, M. G., Cantley, L. C., and Thompson, C. B. (2009). Understanding the Warburg effect: the metabolic requirements of cell proliferation. *Science* 324, 1029–1033.

Vanhaesebroeck, B., Guillermet-Guibert, J., Graupera, M., and Bilanges, B. (2010). The emerging mechanisms of isoform-specific PI3K signalling. *Nat. Rev. Mol. Cell Biol.* 11, 329–341.

Wang, R., Dillon, C. P., Shi, L. Z., Milasta, S., Carter, R., Finkelstein, D., McCormick, L. L., Fitzgerald, P., Chi, H., Munger, J., and Green, D. R. (2011). The transcription factor Myc controls metabolic reprogramming upon T lymphocyte activation. *Immunity* 35, 871–882.

Waugh, C., Sinclair, L., Finlay, D., Bayascas, J. R., and Cantrell, D. (2009). Phosphoinositide (3,4,5)-triphosphate binding to phosphoinositide-dependent kinase 1 regulates a protein kinase B/Akt signaling threshold that dictates T-cell migration, not proliferation. *Mol. Cell. Biol.* 29, 5952–5962.

Webb, L. M., Vigorito, E., Wymann, M. P., Hirsch, E., and Turner, M. (2005). Cutting edge: T cell development requires the combined activities of the p110gamma and p110delta catalytic isoforms of phosphatidylinositol 3-kinase. *J. Immunol.* 175, 2783–2787.

Wofford, J. A., Wieman, H. L., Jacobs, S. R., Zhao, Y., and Rathmell, J. C. (2008). IL-7 promotes Glut1 trafficking and glucose uptake via STAT5-mediated activation of Akt to support T-cell survival. *Blood* 111, 2101–2111.

Zhang, H. H., Lipovsky, A. I., Dibble, C. C., Sahin, M., and Manning, B. D. (2006). S6K1 regulates GSK3 under conditions of mTOR-dependent feedback inhibition of Akt. *Mol. Cell* 24, 185–197.

Zhao, Z., Leister, W. H., Robinson, R. G., Barnett, S. F., Defeo-Jones, D., Jones, R. E., Hartman, G. D., Huff, J. R., Huber, H. E., Duggan, M. E., and Lindsley, C. W. (2005). Discovery of 2,3,5-trisubstituted pyridine derivatives as potent Akt1 and Akt2 dual inhibitors. *Bioorg. Med. Chem. Lett.* 15, 905–909.

Permissions

All chapters in this book were first published in IHTCFEIRTL, by Frontiers; hereby published with permission under the Creative Commons Attribution License or equivalent. Every chapter published in this book has been scrutinized by our experts. Their significance has been extensively debated. The topics covered herein carry significant findings which will fuel the growth of the discipline. They may even be implemented as practical applications or may be referred to as a beginning point for another development.

The contributors of this book come from diverse backgrounds, making this book a truly international effort. This book will bring forth new frontiers with its revolutionizing research information and detailed analysis of the nascent developments around the world.

We would like to thank all the contributing authors for lending their expertise to make the book truly unique. They have played a crucial role in the development of this book. Without their invaluable contributions this book wouldn't have been possible. They have made vital efforts to compile up to date information on the varied aspects of this subject to make this book a valuable addition to the collection of many professionals and students.

This book was conceptualized with the vision of imparting up-to-date information and advanced data in this field. To ensure the same, a matchless editorial board was set up. Every individual on the board went through rigorous rounds of assessment to prove their worth. After which they invested a large part of their time researching and compiling the most relevant data for our readers.

The editorial board has been involved in producing this book since its inception. They have spent rigorous hours researching and exploring the diverse topics which have resulted in the successful publishing of this book. They have passed on their knowledge of decades through this book. To expedite this challenging task, the publisher supported the team at every step. A small team of assistant editors was also appointed to further simplify the editing procedure and attain best results for the readers.

Apart from the editorial board, the designing team has also invested a significant amount of their time in understanding the subject and creating the most relevant covers. They scrutinized every image to scout for the most suitable representation of the subject and create an appropriate cover for the book.

The publishing team has been an ardent support to the editorial, designing and production team. Their endless efforts to recruit the best for this project, has resulted in the accomplishment of this book. They are a veteran in the field of academics and their pool of knowledge is as vast as their experience in printing. Their expertise and guidance has proved useful at every step. Their uncompromising quality standards have made this book an exceptional effort. Their encouragement from time to time has been an inspiration for everyone.

The publisher and the editorial board hope that this book will prove to be a valuable piece of knowledge for researchers, students, practitioners and scholars across the globe.

List of Contributors

Hugo A. van den Berg
University of Warwick, Coventry, UK

Kristin Ladell, Kelly Miners, Bruno Laugel, Sian Llewellyn-Lacey, Mathew Clement, David K. Cole, Emma Gostick, Linda Wooldridge, Andrew K. Sewell and John S. Bridgeman
Institute of Infection and Immunity, Cardiff University, Cardiff, UK

David A. Price
Institute of Infection and Immunity, Cardiff University, Cardiff, UK
Vaccine Research Center, National Institute of Allergy and Infectious Diseases, National Institutes of Health, Bethesda, MD, USA

Johanne M. Pentier and Andrew K. Sewell
Institute of Infection and Immunity, Cardiff University School of Medicine, Heath Park, Cardiff, Wales, UK

John J. Miles
Institute of Infection and Immunity, Cardiff University School of Medicine, Heath Park, Cardiff, Wales, UK
Human Immunity Laboratory, Queensland Institute of Medical Research, Brisbane, QLD, Australia
School of Medicine, The University of Queensland, Brisbane, QLD, Australia

Barbara Szomolay and Hugo Antonius van den Berg
University of Warwick, Coventry, UK

Tamsin Williams
Institute of Infection and Immunity, Cardiff University School of Medicine, Cardiff, UK

Linda Wooldridge
Faculty of Medical and Veterinary Sciences, University of Bristol, Bristol, UK

Yili Li and Roy A. Mariuzza
W. M. Keck Laboratory for Structural Biology, Institute for Bioscience and Biotechnology Research, University of Maryland, Rockville, MD, USA
Department of Cell Biology and Molecular Genetics, University of Maryland, College Park, MD, USA

Scott R. Burrows
Human Immunity Laboratory and Cellular Immunology Laboratory, Queensland Institute of Medical Research, Brisbane, QLD, Australia
School of Medicine, The University of Queensland, Brisbane, QLD, Australia

YiyuanYin
Department of Antibody Engineering, Genentech, South San Francisco, CA, USA

John J. Miles
Human Immunity Laboratory and Cellular Immunology Laboratory, Queensland Institute of Medical Research, Brisbane, QLD, Australia
School of Medicine, The University of Queensland, Brisbane, QLD, Australia
Institute of Infection and Immunity, Cardiff University School of Medicine, Cardiff, Wales, UK

Linda Wooldridge
Institute of Infection and Immunity, Cardiff University School of Medicine, Heath Park, Cardiff, UK

Julien Schmidt and and Immanuel Luescher
Ludwig Center, University of Lausanne, Epalinges, Switzerland

Danijel Dojcinovic and Philippe Guillaume
TCMetrix Sàrl, Epalinges, Switzerland

Niels Schaft, Miriam Coccoris, Joost Drexhage, Christiaan Knoop and Reno Debets
Laboratory of Experimental Tumor Immunology, Department Medical Oncology, Erasmus MC Cancer Institute, Rotterdam, Netherlands

I. Jolanda M. de Vries and Gosse J. Adema
Department Tumor Immunology, Nijmegen Center for Molecular Life Sciences, Radboud University Nijmegen Medical Center, Nijmegen, Netherlands

Christopher J. Holland and David K. Cole
Institute of Infection and Immunity, Cardiff University School of Medicine, Cardiff, UK

Andrew Godkin
Institute of Infection and Immunity, Cardiff University School of Medicine, Cardiff, UK
Department of Integrated Medicine, University Hospital of Wales, Cardiff, UK

David K. Cole, Pierre J. Rizkallah and Jonathan M. Boulter
Cardiff University School of Medicine, Heath Park, Cardiff, UK

Malkit Sami, Penio T. Todorov and Bent K. Jakobsen
Immunocore Limited, Oxon, UK

Daniel R. Scott, Oleg Y. Borbulevych and Brian M. Baker
Department of Chemistry and Biochemistry, University of Notre Dame, Notre Dame, IN, USA

Ruth K. Moysey
Immunocore Limited, Oxon, UK
Oxford Nanopore Technologies Ltd., Oxford, UK

Yi Li
Immunocore Limited, Oxon, UK
Center for Infection and Immunity, Guangzhou Institutes of Biomedicine and Health, Chinese Academy of Sciences, Guangzhou, China

Sid P. Kerkar
Laboratory of Pathology, Center for Cancer Research, National Cancer Institute, National Institutes of Health, Bethesda, MD, USA

Andre Kunert, Trudy Straetemans, Coen Govers, Cor Lamers and Reno Debets
Laboratory of Experimental Tumor Immunology, Erasmus MC Cancer Institute, Rotterdam, Netherlands
Department of Medical Oncology, Erasmus MC Cancer Institute, Rotterdam, Netherlands

Ron Mathijssen and Stefan Sleijfer
Department of Medical Oncology, Erasmus MC Cancer Institute, Rotterdam, Netherlands

Verena Brucklacher-Waldert, Edward J. Carr, Michelle A. Linterman and MarcVeldhoen
Laboratory for Lymphocyte Signalling and Development, The Babraham Institute, Cambridge, UK

Jennifer D. Stone and David M. Kranz
Department of Biochemistry, University of Illinois, Urbana, IL, USA

Andreas A. Hombach and Hinrich Abken
Center for Molecular Medicine Cologne, University of Cologne, Cologne, Germany
Department I Internal Medicine, University Hospital Cologne, Cologne, Germany

V. Zoete and M. Ferber
Molecular Modeling Group, Swiss Institute of Bioinformatics, Lausanne, Switzerland

M. Irving
Molecular Modeling Group, Swiss Institute of Bioinformatics, Lausanne, Switzerland
Lausanne Cancer Center, Lausanne, Switzerland

M. A. Cuendet
Molecular Modeling Group, Swiss Institute of Bioinformatics, Lausanne, Switzerland
Department of Chemistry, NewYork University, NewYork, USA

O. Michielin
Molecular Modeling Group, Swiss Institute of Bioinformatics, Lausanne, Switzerland
Lausanne Cancer Center, Lausanne, Switzerland
Department of Research, University Hospital Center and University of Lausanne, Lausanne, Switzerland
Ludwig Center for Cancer Research of the University of Lausanne, Lausanne, Switzerland

J. Lori Blanchfield, Shayla K. Shorter and Brian D. Evavold
Department of Microbiology and Immunology, Emory University, Atlanta, GA, USA

Angharad Lloyd, Owen N. Vickery and Bruno Laugel
Institute of Infection and Immunity, Cardiff University School of Medicine, Cardiff, Wales, UK

Michael Hebeisen and Danilo Presotto
Department of Oncology, Lausanne University Hospital Center (CHUV), University of Lausanne, Lausanne, Switzerland

Susanne G. Oberle
Swiss Vaccine Research Institute, Epalinges, Switzerland
Division of Immunology and Allergy, Department of Medicine, Lausanne University Hospital (CHUV), Lausanne, Switzerland

Daniel E. Speiser and Nathalie Rufer
Department of Oncology, Lausanne University Hospital Center (CHUV), University of Lausanne, Lausanne, Switzerland
Ludwig Center for Cancer Research, University of Lausanne, Lausanne, Switzerland

Dietmar Zehn
Swiss Vaccine Research Institute, Epalinges, Switzerland
Division of Immunology and Allergy, Department of Medicine, Lausanne University Hospital (CHUV), Lausanne, Switzerland

Nicolas Kluger and Annamari Ranki
Department of Dermatology, Allergology and Venereology, Institute of Clinical Medicine, Skin and Allergy Hospital, Helsinki University Central Hospital, University of Helsinki, Helsinki, Finland

Kai Krohn
Clinical Research Institute HUCH Ltd, Helsinki, Finland

Anita Schuch
Department of Medicine II, University Hospital of Freiburg, Freiburg, Germany
Faculty of Biology, University of Freiburg, Freiburg, Germany

Alexander Hoh
Department of Medicine II, University Hospital of Freiburg, Freiburg, Germany
Faculty of Biology, University of Freiburg, Freiburg, Germany
Spemann Graduate School of Biology and Medicine, University of Freiburg, Freiburg, Germany

Robert Thimme
Department of Medicine II, University Hospital of Freiburg, Freiburg, Germany

Christopher J. Gamper and Jonathan D. Powell
Department of Oncology, Johns Hopkins University, Baltimore, MD, USA

Ryan H. Newton and Laurence A. Turka
Department of Medicine, Beth Israel Deaconess Medical Center, Harvard Medical School, Boston, MA, USA

David K. Finlay
School of Biochemistry and Immunology,Trinity Biomedical Sciences Institute,Trinity College Dublin, Dublin, Ireland
School of Pharmacy and Pharmaceutical Sciences, Trinity Biomedical Sciences Institute, Trinity College Dublin, Dublin, Ireland

Index

www.ingramcontent.com/pod-product-compliance
Lightning Source LLC
LaVergne TN
LVHW060525210926
848485LV00005B/1143